DECISION MAKING
ONCOLOGY
EVIDENCE-BASED MANAGEMENT

With a special contribution by
GEETHA JOSEPH, M.D.

Associate Professor
Division of Medical Oncology/Hematology
Department of Medicine
University of Louisville School of Medicine
James Graham Brown Cancer Center
Lousiville, Kentucky

DECISION MAKING IN
ONCOLOGY
EVIDENCE-BASED MANAGEMENT

Edited by

BENJAMIN DJULBEGOVIĆ, M.D., PH.D.

Associate Professor
Division of Medical Oncology/Hematology
Department of Medicine
University of Louisville School of Medicine
James Graham Brown Cancer Center
Lousiville, Kentucky

DANIEL M. SULLIVAN, M.D.

Associate Professor
Division of Bone Marrow Transplantation
Department of Internal Medicine
Associate Professor
Department of Biochemistry and Molecular Biology
H. Lee Moffitt Cancer Center and Research Institute
University of South Florida College of Medicine
Tampa, Florida

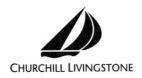

CHURCHILL LIVINGSTONE

New York, Edinburgh, London, Madrid, Melbourne, San Francisco, Tokyo

Library of Congress Cataloging-in-Publication Data

Decision making in oncology : evidence–based management / Benjamin
   Djulbegović, Daniel M. Sullivan ; with a special contribution by
   Geetha Joseph
       p.   cm.
     Includes bibliographical references and index.
     ISBN 0–443–08989–2 (alk. paper)
       1. Oncology—Decision making.   2. Cancer—Decision making.
   3. Medical protocols.   I. Djulbegović, Benjamin.
       [DNLM: 1. Neoplasms—diagnosis.   2. Neoplasms—therapy.
   3. Evidence–Based Medicine.   QZ 241 D2944 1997]
   RC262.D446   1997
   616.99′4—dc21
   DNLM/DLC
   for Library of Congress   97–3873
                                                                        CIP

Distributed in the United Kingdom by Churchill Livingstone, Robert Steven-
son House, 1–3 Baxter's Place, Leith Walk, Edinburgh EH1 3AF, and by associated companies, branches, and representatives throughout the world.

Medical knowledge is constantly changing. As new information becomes
available, changes in treatment, procedures, equipment and the use of drugs
become necessary. The editors/authors/contributors and the publishers have,
as far as it is possible, taken care to ensure that the information given in this
text is accurate and up to date. However, readers are strongly advised to confirm that the information, especially with regard to drug usage, complies with
the latest legislation and standards of practice.

The Publishers have made every effort to trace the copyright holders for bor-
rowed material. If they have inadvertently overlooked any, they will be
pleased to make the necessary arrangements at the first opportunity.

Acquisitions Editor: *Michael Houston*
Production Supervisor: *Laura Mosberg Cohen*
Desktop Coordinators: *Jo-Ann Demas and Alice Terry*

Printed in the United States of America

First published in 1997   7   6   5   4   3   2   1

This book is dedicated to my daughter, Mia and my son, Mak, who have made every aspect of life worthwhile and who have brought a joy and new meaning to the lives of Mira and me.

B.Dj.

For their love and support, this book is dedicated to Kim, Kelly, and Alex.

D.M.S.

Life is short
And the art long
The occasion instant
Experiment perilous
Decision difficult

Hippocrates, circa 350 B.C.

Nature is probabilistic
And information incomplete
Outcomes are valued
Resources limited
Decision unavoidable

Milton C. Weinstein and Harvey V. Fineberg,
Clinical Decision Analysis (1980)

It has often been said that a person does not really understand something until he teaches it to someone else. Actually, a person does not really understand something until he/she ... can express it as an algorithm.

D. E. Knuth,
coinventor of BASIC computer language (~1965)

Contributors

Biljana Baškot, M.D.

Attending Physician, InPhyNet Medical Management, Fort Lauderdale, Florida

Sead Beganović, M.D., Ph.D.

Research Fellow, Division of Medical Oncology/Hematology, Department of Medicine, University of Louisville School of Medicine, James Graham Brown Cancer Center, Louisville, Kentucky

Leela Bhupalam, M.D.

Fellow, Division of Medical Oncology/Hematology, Department of Medicine, University of Louisville School of Medicine, James Graham Brown Cancer Center, Louisville, Kentucky

James R. Bosscher, M.D.

Assistant Professor, Division of Gynecologic Oncology, Department of Obstetrics and Gynecology, University of Louisville School of Medicine, James Graham Brown Cancer Center, Louisville, Kentucky

Maribeth Brune, Pharm.D.

Oncology Pharmacist, Pharmacy Department, H. Lee Moffitt Cancer Center and Research Institute, Tampa, Florida

Jeffrey M. Bumpous, M.D.

Assistant Professor, Department of Surgery, University of Louisville School of Medicine, James Graham Brown Cancer Center, Louisville, Kentucky

Alfonso Cervera, M.D.

Fellow, Division of Medical Oncology/Hematology, Department of Medicine, University of Louisville School of Medicine, James Graham Brown Cancer Center, Louisville, Kentucky

Robert A. Clark, M.D.

Professor and Chairman, Department of Radiology, University of South Florida College of Medicine; Chief of Diagnostic Imaging, Department of Radiology, H. Lee Moffitt Cancer Center and Research Institute, Tampa, Florida

C. Edgar Davila, D.D.S.

Assistant Clinical Professor, Division of Otolaryngology, Department of Surgery, University of South Florida College of Medicine; Attending Physician, Section of Maxillofacial Prosthedontics and Dental Oncology, H. Lee Moffitt Cancer Center and Research Institute; Prosthedontist, Medical Arts Center, Tampa, Florida

Srdjan Denić, M.D.

Medical Oncologist-Hematologist, Division of Oncology and Hematology, Department of Medicine, Lewistown Hospital, Lewistown, Pennsylvania

William R. Dinwoodie, M.D.

Associate Professor, Division of Oncology and Hematology, Department of Internal Medicine, University of South Florida College of Medicine; Associate Director, Pain Management Program, H. Lee Moffitt Cancer Center and Research Institute, Tampa, Florida

Benjamin Djulbegović, M.D., Ph.D.

Associate Professor, Division of Medical Oncology/Hematology, Department of Medicine, University of Louisville School of Medicine, James Graham Brown Cancer Center, Lousiville, Kentucky

David L. Doering, M.D.

Assistant Professor, Division of Gynecologic Oncology, Department of Obstetrics and Gynecology, University of Louisville School of Medicine, James Graham Brown Cancer Center, Louisville, Kentucky

Michael Edwards, M.D.

Associate Professor, Department of Surgery, University of Louisville School of Medicine, James Graham Brown Cancer Center, Louisville, Kentucky

Karen K. Fields, M.D.

Associate Professor, Department of Internal Medicine, University of South Florida College of Medicine; Leader, Bone Marrow Transplant Program, Division of Bone Marrow Transplantation, Department of Internal Medicine, H. Lee Moffitt Cancer Center and Research Institute, Tampa, Florida

Donald R. Fleming, M.D.

Assistant Professor, Division of Medical Hematology/Oncology, Department of Medicine, University of Louisville School of Medicine, James Graham Brown Cancer Center, Louisville, Kentucky

Michael B. Flynn, M.D.

Professor, Division of Oncology, Department of Surgery, University of Louisville School of Medicine; Associate Director, Cancer Control and Community Relations, James Graham Brown Cancer Center; Consultant, Department of Surgical Oncology, Veterans Affairs Medical Center, Louisville, Kentucky

Linda Garland, M.D.

Assistant Professor, Division of Oncology and Hematology, Department of Internal Medicine, H. Lee Moffitt Cancer Center and Research Institute, Tampa, Florida

Ellen Gesser, R.D., C.N.

Nutritional Consultant, Caritas Home Health, Bardstown, Kentucky

Randall Gibb, M.D.

Fellow, Division of Gynecologic Oncology, Department of Medicine and Obstetrics and Gynecology, University of Louisville School of Medicine, James Graham Brown Cancer Center, Louisville, Kentucky

Shawn D. Glisson, M.D.

Fellow, Division of Medical Oncology/Hematology, Department of Medicine, University of Louisville School of Medicine, James Graham Brown Cancer Center, Louisville, Kentucky

Steven C. Goldstein, M.D.

Assistant Professor, Department of Internal Medicine, University of South Florida College of Medicine; Attending Physician, Division of Bone Marrow Transplantation, Department of Internal Medicine, H. Lee Moffitt Cancer Center and Research Institute, Tampa, Florida

Michael S. Gordon, M.D.

Associate Professor, Department of Medicine, Indiana University School of Medicine; Director, Clinical Hematology and Cytokine Program, Section of Hematology/Oncology, Department of Medicine, University Medical Center, Indianapolis, Indiana

Terence Hadley, M.D.

Associate Professor, Division of Medical Oncology/Hematology, Department of Medicine, University of Louisville School of Medicine, James Graham Brown Cancer Center, Louisville, Kentucky

James I. Harty, M.D.

Associate Professor, Department of Medicine, and Professor, Division of Urology, Department of Surgery, University of Louisville School of Medicine, James Graham Brown Cancer Center, Louisville, Kentucky

A. K. Huang, M.D.

Assistant Professor, Division of Infectious Diseases, Department of Medicine, University of Louisville School of Medicine, James Graham Brown Cancer Center, Louisville, Kentucky

Baby O. Jose, M.D.

Professor, Department of Radiation Oncology, University of Louisville School of Medicine, James Graham Brown Cancer Center, Louisville, Kentucky

Geetha Joseph, M.D.

Associate Professor, Division of Medical Oncology/Hematology, Department of Medicine, University of Louisville School of Medicine, James Graham Brown Cancer Center, Lousiville, Kentucky

Ward Katsanis, M.D.

Fellow, Department of Obstetrics and Oncology, University of Louisville School of Medicine; Lecturer, Division of Gynecologic Oncology, Department of Obstetrics-Gynecology, James Graham Brown Cancer Center, Louisville, Kentucky

Jacqueline A. LaPerriere, R.Ph.

Clinical Assistant Professor, Department of Neurology, University of South Florida College of Medicine, Tampa, Florida; Clinical Assistant Professor, Department of Pharmacy Practice, University of Florida College of Pharmacy, Gainesville, Florida; Coordinator, Interdisciplinary Pain Program, H. Lee Moffitt Cancer Center and Research Center, Tampa, Florida

Renato V. La Rocca, M.D., F.A.C.P.

Associate Clinical Professor, Division of Medical Oncology/Hematology, Department of Medicine, University of Louisville School of Medicine, James Graham Brown Cancer Center; Associate Clinical Professor, Department of Medicine, University of Kentucky College of Medicine, Lexington, Kentucky

Paul Mangino, Pharm.D.

Clinical Pharmacist, Department of Pharmacy, University of Louisville Hospital, Louisville, Kentucky

Koji Nakagawa, M.D., Ph.D.

Assistant Professor, Hepatobiliary Unit, First Department of Surgery, Chiba University School of Medicine, Chiba, Japan

M. Jane Nolte, Pharm.D.

Pharmacy Specialist, Drug Information Center, Division of Pharmacy Services, Memorial Sloan-Kettering Cancer Center, New York, New York

Nermina Obralić, M.D.

Attending Physician, Department of Radiation Oncology, Institute of Oncology, Sarajevo, Bosnia-Herzegovina

Ivana Pavlić-Renar, M.D.

Head, Department of Diabetology, University of Zagreb Medical School, Vuk Vrhovac Institute for Diabetes, Endocrinology and Metabolic Diseases, Zagreb, Croatia

Hiram C. Polk, M.D.

Ben A. Reid, Sr., Professor and Chairman, Department of Surgery, University of Louisville School of Medicine, James Graham Brown Cancer Center, Louisville, Kentucky

Zoran Potparić, M.D.

Fellow, Division of Plastic Surgery, Department of Surgery, Eastern Virginia Medical School, Norfolk, Virginia

Carol Rodriguez, A.R.N.P.

Clinical Assistant Professor, Department of Neurology, University of South Florida College of Medicine; Nurse Practictioner, Interdisciplinary Pain Program, H. Lee Moffitt Cancer Center and Research Institute, Tampa, Florida

Nolan Sakow, M.D.

Assistant Professor, Division of Nuclear Medicine, Department of Diagnostic Radiology, University of Louisville School of Medicine, James Graham Brown Cancer Center, Louisville, Kentucky

Gerry Sheehan, R.D., M.Ed.

Nutritional Consultant, Chicago, Illinois

Daniel M. Sullivan, M.D.

Associate Professor, Division of Bone Marrow Transplantation, Department of Internal Medicine, and Associate Professor, Department of Biochemistry and Molecular Biology, H. Lee Moffitt Cancer Center and Research Institute, University of South Florida College of Medicine, Tampa, Florida

Beverly Taft, R.N., O.C.N.

Oncology Nurse Clinician, Division of Medical Oncology, Department of Medicine, University of Louisville School of Medicine, James Graham Brown Cancer Center, Louisville, Kentucky

Wayne Tuckson, M.D.

Assistant Professor, Department of Surgery, University of Louisville School of Medicine, James Graham Brown Cancer Center, Louisville, Kentucky

Rambabu Tummala, M.D.

Attending Physician, Lake County Oncology and Hematology, Tavares, Florida

Aaron I. Vinik, M.D., Ph.D., F.C.P., F.A.C.P.

Professor, Division of Endocrinology and Metabolism, Departments of Medicine, Anatomy, and Neurobiology, Eastern Virginia Medical School; Director, Diabetes Research Institute, and Vice-Chairman for Research, The Diabetes Institutes, Norfolk, Virginia

Jane M. Weaver, M.D.

Surgical Resident, Department of Surgery, University of Louisville School of Medicine, Louisville, Kentucky

Sheron R. Williams, M.D.

Attending Physician, Cancer Care Center, Louisville, Kentucky

Lung T. Yam, M.D.

Professor, Department of Medicine, University of Louisville School of Medicine, James Graham Brown Cancer Center; Chief of Hematology, Division of Hematology/Oncology, Department of Medicine, Veterans Affairs Medical Center, Louisville, Kentucky

Preface

The primary aim of this book is to outline diagnostic and treatment strategies for medical oncology based on the supporting evidence that exists in the literature. This aim was realized by (1) considering the key reasoning strategies for the management of a particular cancer; (2) establishing the goal of the treatment as a leading reasoning principle; (3) grading the quality of supporting evidence for the recommended strategies; (4) assessing the risk/benefit ratio of available treatment options; and (5) providing practical physicians' orders in the appendices.

We have elected to use algorithms as the major teaching tool. The text that accompanies the algorithms explains the principles behind their construction, lists the quality of data used to support the recommendations, and provides additional key clinical information. To construct these algorithms, an enormous amount of clinical literature has been reviewed. We have cited key references at the end of each chapter, and apologize if we have inadvertently overlooked any important references.

This book is intended for everyone who deals with the patient suffering from cancer: students, residents, fellows, general internists, surgeons, and radiation and medical oncologists. Students and residents can learn essential principles behind many practical decisions, while practicing physicians may find useful explicit recommendations on how to deal with a particular oncologic problem. As medical oncology is a dynamic field, we would be grateful for any advice, comments or criticism so that any potential future edition of this text can live up to the expectations of its readers.

No human endeavor, including the writing of a book, is an isolated experience. We would like to thank our contributors, who have made their best effort to comply with our often excessive requests concerning the contents and format of their chapters. Ms. Katrina Morris deserves special thanks for providing us with the necessary resources when we needed them most. Many other people helped in the creation of the manuscripts in indirect ways, and we take this opportunity to thank them.

For further details on the aim and scope of the book, the reader is referred to the Introduction and Chapter 1.

Benjamin Djulbegović, M.D., Ph.D.
Daniel M. Sullivan, M.D.

Introduction

Several years ago we took an explicit approach[1] (as opposed to an implicit approach, which relies on the problem-solving expertise of individuals instead of on the evidence existing in the literature) to identify reasoning and decision making strategies that lie behind diagnostic and therapeutic problem solving during the care of patients with blood diseases. That effort culminated in the book *Reasoning and Decision Making in Hematology*. The book was well received both in the United States and abroad, creating the necessary impetus to extend this evidence-based approach to another area in which we are actively participating as practicing physicians: oncology. As defined by the Evidence-Based Medicine Working Group at McMaster's University, evidence-based medicine is an approach to the practice of medicine in which clinicians are aware of the evidence in support of their practice and of the strength of that evidence.[2] Our aim this time was again to (1) identify the reasoning strategies in the management of the most common cancers; (2) define clinical practice guidelines in oncology for the practicing physician; and (3) identify the core information in oncology.

This aim was accomplished by stressing the following aspects of the management of patients with malignant diseases:

1. Identification of the key reasoning strategies during the management of a particular cancer. These strategies are derived from an understanding of the underlying principles of the biology and clinical behavior of a given cancer.

2. Establishing the goal of the treatment as a leading reasoning principle in the management of the patient with a malignant disorder (see Ch. 1).

We have explicitly defined the goal of the treatment at every decision point during the "natural history" of treatment of a specific disease.

3. Enumerating and grading the quality of supporting evidence for recommended management stategies (see Table 1-7). For each disease in particular, and for the field of oncology in general, this step enables the reader to estimate how much of the practice of oncology is evidence-based.

4. Formulation of a principle of administration of treatment according to the best benefit/risk ratio (see Ch. 1). In many cases, supporting evidence for recommendations are accompanied by tables of benefits/risks of the available treatment alternatives.

5. Translation of these guidelines into practical steps through detailed therapeutic physicians' orders, shown in the appendices.

In a word, this book should help transform knowledge in the field of oncology into practical steps.

We again elected to use algorithms as the major tool in teaching and diagnostic/therapeutic problem solving in oncology. Information is presented in condensed algorithmic form, with each algorithm summarizing tens of pages of written text. We have sacrificed simplicity for thoroughness. The text that accompanies the algorithms explains the principles behind the construction of each algorithm, lists the quality of data used to support the recommendations, and provides additional key clinical information. The reader is strongly encouraged to study these algorithms carefully. We believe that the core information in oncology provided through these algorithms is probably equal to a textbook of several thousand pages in length. To construct these algorithms, a thorough search of the literature was performed. Because of space limitations, we could not cite all references reviewed, and it is possible that some important references were inadvertently overlooked and have not been listed among the suggested readings. If this is the case, we apologize for such omissions.

Our recommendations or guidelines convert "all accumulated research, development, and experience" into practical steps since "it is unrealistic to think that individuals can synthesize in their heads scores of pieces of evidence and accurately estimate the outcomes of different options."[1] As evidence is collected to formulate specific management recommendations, it becomes clear that the quality of medical evidence varies considerably and that there is inherent variability and uncertainty about diagnostic or treatment decisions and patient outcomes.

This is the key reason that most of our recommendations are just that—recommendations or guidelines that allow deviations from original proposals "up to 40% percent of the time."[1] For example, there is high-quality evidence from a large randomized trial that a doxorubicin-containing regimen (ABVD) is superior to MOPP chemotherapy in the treatment of advanced Hodgkin's disease (see Ch. 8). However, this evidence was obtained from a population of patients that had no patients older than 72 years or with cardiopulmonary diseases. It is conceivable, therefore, that many patients could be treated with non-ABVD chemotherapeutic regimens that would fit such patients' needs better as judged by the physician in charge. Our recommendations, therefore, should be interpreted as an effort to achieve balance between "benefits of standardization and the prerogatives of physicians to make decisions tailored to individual patients."[3]

Rarely, our proposals should be considered as standards that should be followed in almost every case (with expected deviations of less than 5%).[1] For example, high-level evidence has demonstrated the efficacy of annual screening mammography in every woman older than 50 years.

Often, however, outcomes are not known and our proposals are in the form of "options"[1] with decisions about treatment being left to the physician in charge and to the patient. For example, chronic lymphocytic leukemia cannot be cured at this time with any known modality of treatment. However, high-dose chemotherapy followed by bone marrow transplantation can eradicate disease. Whether this will lead to cures or improved survival compared with other forms of therapy currently available is not known at this time (in the algorithms, this uncertainty is indicated by a question mark following the statement of the intended treatment goals).

Sometimes outcomes may be known but patient preferences may not be known. In such cases our proposals would also be "options,"[1] and selection of intervention would be based on individual patients' preferences. For example, the survival outcome for the treatment of early-stage prostate cancer with surgery versus radiation therapy versus watchful waiting is almost identical. However, complications and the actual course of disease may be different with each of these treatment options. In such cases, the treatment would be strongly influenced by individual patients' preferences regarding each of these therapeutic options (such as impotence as a complication after surgery versus rectal bleeding after radiation therapy) (see Ch. 45).

Of even more importance to us is that an evidence-based approach lays ground for new ethics in the practice of medicine. Evidence-based medicine dispels the older ethics of practice based on infallible authorities[4] and brings increasing democratization to the practice of medicine.[5] Decisions should be based on the evidence rather than authority. "'Authoritarian medicine' has been gradually replaced by 'authoritative medicine'."[4,5] The approach taken in this book signifies a contemporary shift from consensus-based medicine to evidence-based medicine.

Benjamin Djulbegović, M.D., Ph.D.
Daniel M. Sullivan, M.D.

REFERENCES

1. Eddy DM: A Manual for Assessing Health Practices and Designing Practice Polices: The Explicit Approach. American College of Physicians, Philadelphia, 1992
2. Howard R, Haynes B, Jadad A et al: Evidence-based medicine: a new approach to teaching the practice of medicine. http://hiru.mcmaster.ca/ebm/overview/htm
3. Pearson SD, Polak JL, Cartwright S et al: A critical pathway to evaluate suspected deep vein thrombosis. Arch Intern Med 155:1773
4. McIntyre N, Popper K: The critical attitude in medicine: the need for a new ethics. Br Med J 287:1919–1923, 1983
5. Davidoff F, Case K, Fried P: Evidence-based medicine: why all the fuss? Ann Intern Med 122:727, 1995

Abbreviations

@, at
bid., two times a day
BSA, body surface area
Ca, calcium
CBC c diff., complete blood count with differential count
CBC, complete blood count
ccu, cubic
chemoRx, chemotherapy
CR, complete response
CT, computed tomography
D, day
D5 or D5W, 5% dextrose in water
Dx, diagnosis
FF, free flowing
HT, height
IV, intravenous
IVPB, intravenous piggy back
Mg, magnesium
ml, milliliter
mo, month
MRI, magnetic resonance imaging
MS, median survival
N/V, nausea and vomiting
NS, normal saline
p, post
PPD, purified protein derivative (tuberculin)

PR, partial response
prn, as needed
q, every
qam, every morning
qhs, prior to bedtime
qid, four times a day
Rx, treatment
sc or sq, subcutaneous
SMA-18, sequential multiple analyzer (which provides a result on 18 analytes from one blood sample; i.e., GOT [glutamate oxalacetate transaminase]; GPT [glutamate pyruvate transaminase]; LDH [lactate dehydrogenase]; GGT [γ-glutamyltranspeptidase]; AP [alkaline phosphatase]; phosphorus; calcium; TP [total proteins]; ALB [albumin]; CO_2 [carbon dioxide]; BUN [blood urea nitrogen]; uric acid; creatinine; sodium; potassium; chloride; glucose; bilirubin; cholesterol)
SMA-7, sequential multiple analyzer (which provides a result on 7 analytes from one blood sample; i.e., BUN; creatinine; sodium; potassium; chloride; glucose; CO_2)
STAT, urgently
tid, three times a day
wk, week
WT, weight
yr, year

Contents

Principles of Reasoning and Decision Making in Oncology

Benjamin Djulbegović

Medical information is doubled every decade. To keep up with the 10 leading journals in internal medicine, clinicians must read 200 articles and 70 editorials per month. Today, there are more than 20,000 biomedical journals. Medical students are expected to read 11,161 pages per year and practicing physicians need to recall more than 2 million information. We know more than 30,000 diseases, which can present with an infinite number of combinations. More than 15,000 drugs are currenty available with an average annual increase of 250. Considering the abundance of information and the brain's limited capacity for storage and processing of information, it is clear that clinical problem solving and decision making have become severely compromised. An obvious question would be: Is it possible to identify some reasoning strategies that can help us deal with information overload and improve problem solving and decision making in medicine? We believe the answer is a resounding "yes." Below are outlined some of the principles of clinical reasoning and decision making that may be helpful in oncologic practice.

BASIC ELEMENTS OF THE CLINICAL PROCESS

The clinical process bears remarkable similarity to the process of scientific discovery, in that it is an inferential process during which a clinician quickly generates a hypothesis (diagnostic triggering). Hypotheses are continually being excluded or confirmed as new data are gathered. Studies estimate that a first hypothesis is generated 28 seconds after hearing the patient's chief complaint. An average of 5.5 hypotheses are generated for each case and no more than 7 hypotheses are active at any one time. The hypothesis forms a context (model) within which further information gathering takes place. Verifying a diagnostic hypothesis is the next step in

the diagnostic process. Competing hypotheses are eliminated and a hypothesis that will serve as the basis for a patient's management is formed. Figure 1-1 shows the basic elements of this hypotheticodeductive method.

DIAGNOSIS

Studies on cognitive aspects of reasoning processes in clinical medicine show that overall a diagnosis is made using three reasoning techniques: (1) probabilistic, (2) causal, and (3) deterministic. The first two processes constitute what is known as knowledge-based reasoning, while deterministic reasoning is also known as rule-based functioning.

PROBABILISTIC REASONING

The probabilistic reasoning strategy is based on an estimate of the likelihood that the patient has a specified disease. This strategy is rarely used initially in oncology, since the usual diagnostic standard is based on surgical biopsy or excision as the single most important procedure in establishing a diagnosis of a tumor. This, in turn, implies that tolerance for uncertainty in diagnosis in oncology is small. Oncologists usually believe that histologic diagnosis provides 100% diagnostic certainty and that further management is largely dependent on this information. (Some theoretical work suggests that 100% diagnostic certainty is not achievable and therefore should not be attempted. Likewise, histopathologic diagnosis may be associated with false-positive and false-negative results as any other diagnostic tests. Despite theoretical postulates, most oncologists consider histopathologic diagnosis as a gold standard test where cancer management begins.)

Once the initial diagnosis of cancer has been established on histologic grounds, the next step is

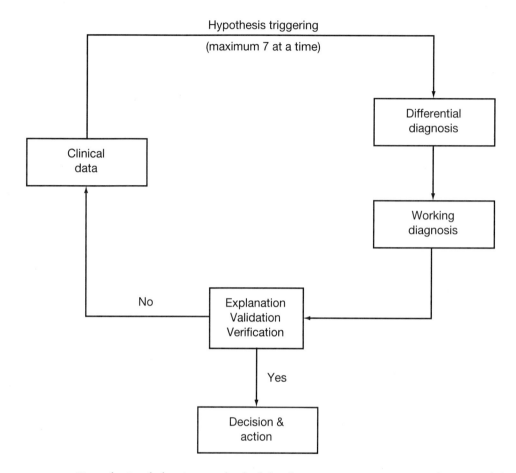

FIGURE 1-1 *Hypotheticodeductive method of the diagnostic process. It can be argued that the clinical process is only a special case of the scientific method. In general, application of the probabilistic and production-rule reasoning is effective in hypothesis triggering, while causal reasoning is powerful in validating and verifying hypotheses (see text for details).*

to try to establish the extent of a disease by using the diagnostic staging process. The staging information can be obtained by noninvasive methods, such as physical examination, laboratory findings, and imaging studies (*clinical staging*), or by surgical procedures and histopathologic analysis of tissue specimens (*surgical pathologic staging*). It is during staging workup that probabilistic reasoning strategy is widely used.

Examples of typical questions requiring probabilistic estimates include the following:

In a patient who has Hodgkin's disease with cervical and hilar adenopathy, and palpable spleen, what is the likelihood of stage III?

What is the probability of metastatic cancer in a patient with breast cancer whose primary tumor is 2.5 cm and there is no axillary node involvement?

Are these probabilities increased after imaging studies?

These estimates are not calculated precisely, usually because data are not available. Nevertheless, the role of new information as gathered by ordering diagnostic tests is to *increase the level of (diagnostic) certainty*.

How certain we are that a particular malignant process has spread beyond a specific stage will depend on the validity of the diagnostic methods used. Since our clinical tools are not perfect, it is important to understand their limitations while measuring the information they provide as precisely as possible. This is done by determining the *diagnostic test operating characteristics* (i.e., the set of characteristics that reflect the information about patients with and without disease), which are sensitivity, specificity, false-positive (α-error) rate and a false-negative rate (β-error) (see Table 1-1 for definitions of terms). Information collected from diagnostic tests is best represented by plots drawn in terms of receiver operating characteristics (ROC).

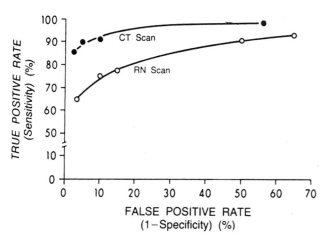

FIGURE 1-2 *Receiver operating characteristics (ROC) plot is the best way to express information content of diagnostic tests. The ROC curve is a plot of sensitivity vs false-positive rate, each point on the curve being associated with a different threshold-decision level. The graph shows ROC data for computed tomography (CT) and radionuclide (RN) scan for detection of brain tumor. Area under curve of an ideal test is equal to 1 (S = 1, Sp = 1). ROC for a completely uninformative test corresponds to a 45° line. The performance of most tests is between these two extremes. Note inverse relationship between sensitivity and specificity—as one increases, the other decreases. (Data from Swets et al. Science 205:753–9, 1979.)*

The ROC curve is a plot of sensitivity against a false-positive rate (Fig. 1-2). When these test characteristics are mathematically manipulated with the pretest estimate of disease (Bayes theorem), the post-test probability of disease (the true estimate of the certainty level) can be calculated (see Fig. 1-3 and Table 1-1 for formula). For most diagnostic tests, Bayes theorem is most useful when the prior probability of disease is between 30% and 70%. The calculation for post-test probability is rarely done, usually because quantitative data on sensitivity and specificity of many clinical tests are lacking. However, when ROC data are known, the following strategy can be formulated during clinical workup: the use of highly sensitive tests when we want to exclude disease (e.g., an advanced stage of cancer) and highly specific tests when we want to confirm a diagnostic possibility (e.g., cancer being in an advanced stage) (Fig. 1-4).

Most of the time, the information content of our diagnostic armamentarium is assessed qualitatively rather than quantitatively. In general, the validity of diagnostic methods in oncology can be qualitatively expressed by comparing their certainty or C factor. The definitions for C factor are shown in Table 1-2 and can be used to gauge the level of certainty in a diagnosis of cancer and the probability of its extent.

CAUSAL REASONING

When the pathophysiology of the process is known, the application of causal reasoning (cause-and-effect relationship) is a powerful method. The causal model is particularly powerful in validating and verifying the strength of generated hypotheses. When applicable, causal reasoning is an irreplaceable type of clinical reasoning. In oncology, causal reasoning is dependent on an understanding of the biology of disease and the natural spread of tumors. For example, the knowledge that tumors can produce various factors that cause an increase in calcium levels would help the clinician to recognize changes in the mental status of patients in whom cancer has been diagnosed. Similarly, it is justified to order imaging studies such as magnetic resonance imaging (MRI) in a patient presenting with severe low back pain and known history of breast cancer based on an understanding of metastatic cancer as a cause of spinal cord compression. Probabilistic and causal reasoning processes are part of what is known as *knowledge-based reasoning*, or *synthetic thinking*, which is

TABLE 1-1 GLOSSARY OF TERMS AND USEFUL "DECISION FORMULAS"

Operating test characteristic
> A set of characteristics that reflect the information a diagnostic test conveys about a patient with and without disease (sensitivity, specificity, false-negative, false positive rate)

Sensitivity (S) (true positives, TP), $P(T+ \mid D+)$
> Probability that a test will be positive when a disease is present.

Specificity (true negatives, TN) (Sp), $P(T- \mid D-)$
> Probability that a test result will be negative when a disease is not present.

False-negative rate (FN = 1-S), $P(T- \mid D+)$
> Probability that a test result will be negative when a disease is present.

False-positive rate (FP = 1-Sp), $P(T+ \mid D-)$
> Probability that a test result will be positive when a disease is not present.

Pretest probability, $P(D+)$
> Probability that a condition exists before a test is performed (It often means prevalence of a specific disorder, but it can be related to the clinician's estimate of the probability of a disease before a test is performed).

Post-test probability of disease, $P(D+ \mid T+)$ or $P(D+ \mid T-)$
> Probability of a disease, given positive or a negative test result.

Odds (O)
> The ratio of number of patients with a disease to the number of patients without a disease. It can be converted to probability (P) and vice versa according to the following relationships:

$$O = P/(1\text{-}P) \quad P = O/(1 + O).$$

Likelihood ratio (LR)

$$LR = \frac{\text{frequency of clinical finding in disease}}{\text{frequency of clinical finding in no-disease}}$$

$$LR+ = \frac{\text{frequency of clinical finding is present in disease}}{\text{frequency of clinical finding is present in no-disease}} = S/FP$$

$$LR- = \frac{\text{frequency of clinical finding is absent in disease}}{\text{frequency of clinical finding is absent in no-disease}} = FN/Sp$$

Bayes' theorem for calculating the post-test probability of disease:

$$\text{Posttest Odds} = \text{Pretest Odds} * LR+ \quad \text{(a positive result)}$$

$$\text{Posttest Odds} = \text{Pretest Odds} * LR- \quad \text{(a negative result)}$$

A general formula for calculation of decision thresholds[a,b]

$$p_t = \frac{1}{LR \cdot \dfrac{B}{R} + 1}$$

---

[a]*From Djulbegović B, Desoky A: Equation and Nomogram for Calculation of Testing and Treatment Probability Thresholds. Med Decis Making 16:198, 1996. This formula is valid only if risks of diagnostic tests is negligible. If risks of the testing is substantial then the threshold level should be calculated according to Pauker SG, Kassirer JP: The threshold approach to clinical decision making. N Engl J Med 302:1109–1117, 1980.*

[b]*This equation can be used for easy calculation of the threshold probability of interest. LR is the likelihood ratio, B is the benefit experienced by treated patients with the disease, and R is the risk experienced by treated patients without the disease. To calculate a testing decision threshold (p_{tt}), use LR+ (LR > 1); to calculate a treatment threshold (p_{rx}) use LR– (LR < 1). When no further tests are available, assume LR = 1 and calculate the treatement threshold (p_{rx}). (See also Fig. 1-6.)*

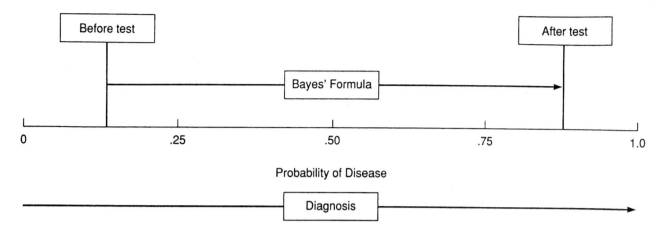

FIGURE 1-3 *The role of Bayes theorem. Note how diagnostic certainty is increased after application of diagnostic test. (For Bayes formula, see Table-1.) (From Sox HC et al: Medical Decision Making, 1988:68, with permission.)*

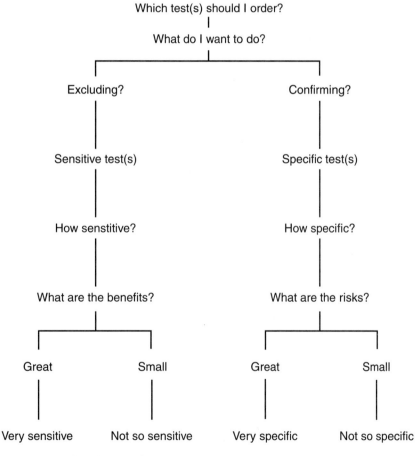

FIGURE 1-4 *Strategy for choice of diagnostic tests. Note that this strategy is valid for tests with very high sensitivities and specificities. For tests with lower sensitivities and specificities, one should use likelihood ratios (LR) to rule in or rule out disease. (From Burke DM: Test strategies in selected clinical problems. Clin Labor Med 1982;2:789–802, with permission.)*

TABLE 1-2   CERTAINTY (C) FACTOR

C Factor	Definition
C factor	Reflects the validity of classification according to diagnostic methods used
C1	Evidence from standard diagnostic means (e.g., inspection, palpation, and standard radiography; intraluminal endoscopy for tumors of certain organs)
C2	Evidence obtained by special diagnostic means (e.g., radiographic imaging in special projections, tomography, CT, ultrasonography, lymphography, angiography, scintigraphy, MRI, endoscopy, biopsy, and cytology)
C3	Evidence from surgical exploration, including biopsy and cytology
C4	Evidence of the extent of disease following definitive surgery and pathologic examination of the resected specimen
C5	Evidence from an autopsy

(From Rubin P: Clinical Oncology: A Multidisciplinary Approach. p. 11. 7th Ed. WB Saunders, Philadelphia, 1993, with permission.)

used for novel situations requiring conscious analytic processing and stored knowledge.

DETERMINISTIC REASONING

From probabilistic or causal association between clinical findings, one may derive clinical rules that can be applied in various settings. These rules are based on compilation of knowledge in a certain medical field. Ideally, one would like to develop a catalog of all these rules for the particular field. These rules are examples of deterministic or categorical reasoning, which is often used in clinical medicine. They are also called production rules (if-then rules). *Rule-based reasoning* is widely used in oncology, both for diagnostic and treatment purposes. Classical examples would be, *"If* the patient with histologic diagnosis of Hodgkin's disease has mesenteric lymph node involvement, then challenge a diagnosis," that is, review the histopathology because it is likely that non-Hodgkin's lymphoma is mistaken for Hodgkin's lymphoma. "If the female patient presents with axillar adenopathy due to adenocarcinoma, then suspect a breast cancer as a primary origin of the tumor even if the mammogram was normal," because breast cancer is the most probable source of adenocancarcinoma cells in axillar lymph nodes in a female.

When these production rules are organized in an ordered set of instructions that analyze the problem in stepwise fashion, the whole strategy is being presented in the form of *algorithms*. The major advantage of presenting the clinical strategies in algorithmic form is that explicit definitions of the clinical problem preclude ambiguity. Algorithms seem to be a more effective teaching method than prose, particularly in preventing information overload, which is the primary reason for using them in this book. Information is presented in a condensed algorithmic form, each algorithm summarizing tens and sometimes hundreds of pages of written text.

However, there are problems with algorithms. They are usually unsuitable for patients with multiple problems since the usual starting point is identification of one particular problem (patient's complaints, abnormal diagnostic finding). They often do not allow the clinician to bypass essential steps in the clinical workup, and they usually become so complicated, it is difficult to present them as a ready-print figure. Nevertheless, we believe that construction of the algorithms based on categorical and probabilistic reasoning represents the optimal way to teach oncology as we approach the end of the twentieth century.

SKILL-BASED REASONING

Besides knowledge-based and rule-based reasoning, physicians often use skill-based reasoning, which relates to patterns of thought and actions that are governed by stored models of preprogrammed instructions, largely unconscious. Skill-based reasoning is usually performed using *heuristics*, that is, ad hoc rules of thumb, clinical shortcuts. They are particularly important in hypothesis triggering. The following two heuristics are often used:

Availability heuristic—a diagnostic event is invoked because it is easily remembered.

Representative heuristic—a diagnostic event is invoked because a set of findings resembles a well-defined clinical entity.

Humans prefer pattern recognition to calculation, so they are strongly biased to search for a prepackaged solution, that is a "rule," before resorting to more tedious knowledge-based cognition. The difference between the novice and the experienced clinician lies in the capability of the latter to move from knowledge-based to skill-based reasoning. Experts have a much larger reportoire of skill-based schemata and problem-solving rules than novices. However, exclusive use of heuristics may lead to diagnostic or treatment failure (see below). Any departure from a routine, that is, a new problem, requires a rule-based or knowledge-based solution.

In general, all the reasoning processes identified here serve to answer the following three questions:

(1) Does my patient have malignancy?

(2) What type of malignancy does my patient have?

(3) What is the extent of the disease?

TREATMENT

The treatment of patients with malignant disorders is characterized by the following reasoning principles:

(1) What is a goal of the treatment?

(2) Do benefits outweigh risks in achieving these goals?

(3) Is difference between potential benefit and harm worth the cost?*

A goal-oriented management in oncology typically starts with the question: Can I cure the disease in this patient? If the answer is yes, the questions that follow are

What is the price of this cure?

Do the benefits of treatment exceed the risks?

For example, we can cure chronic myelogenous leukemia (CML) in a 70-year-old patient by using a bone marrow transplantation (BMT) procedure with a very high risk of short-term mortality. In this situation, we usually opt for a conservative, less risky treatment that cannot cure the disease, but would consistently result in several additional years of life.

If we cannot cure the disease, the next question we must ask is can we prolong survival in our patient? Again, if the answer is yes, the question is, Does the benefit of treatment justify its risk? For example, survival in patients with acute myelogenous

nous leukemia (AML) can be prolonged with autologous BMT, but not in a 67-year-old man because of the high risk of treatment mortality.

If we cannot prolong survival, the following question is usually asked: Can we improve the quality of life in our patient? The decision to administer palliative treatment will again depend on the treatment's risk/benefit ratio. For example, we would not administer chemotherapy to a patient with metastatic colon cancer and advanced liver failure because chemotherapy would just add to the misery of our patient. Our treatment would focus on supportive care.

Figure 1-5 illustrates the basics of reasoning processes in oncology.

THRESHOLD APPROACH TO DECISION MAKING

Clinical medicine can be defined as a discipline of decision making under circumstances of uncertainties. As discussed earlier, physicians poorly tolerate any level of uncertainty. A very low level of diagnostic suspicion would regularly trigger a battery of tests available in today's enormous diagnostic armamenatarium. Treatment would be administered only at the maximum level of diagnostic certainty. It is believed that nonoptimal and unnecessary use of medical technology and treatments is a consequence of large variation in physicians' practice patterns. In turn, this variation was thought to result from physicians' uncertainty about the most optimal diagnostic and treatment actions. The threshold model can help define acceptable levels of diagnostic uncertainty at which diagnostic or treatment actions should be made.

According to the threshold model (Fig. 1-6; Table 1-1 [equation]), the level of diagnostic certainty for clinical decisions is a function of the characteristics of available therapies and the diagnostic test characteristics. A clinical strategy—observation vs testing vs treatment—is dictated by the probability of a disease (P_D) exceeding two relevant threshold probabilities. If the probability of disease is smaller than the testing threshold (P_{tt}) the testing should be withheld. If the probability of a disease is greater than the treatment threshold (P_{rx}) then treatment should be given. The test should be done only if the probability of a disease is between the two thresholds (Fig. 1-6). Table 1-1 gives a simple equation showing how to calculate threshold levels. When a specific therapy result in high benefit and low risk, one can tolerate substantial diagnostic uncertainty not only because the treatment is effective, but also because it will cause little harm

---

*This aspect of the clinical process is usually adressed by cost-effectiveness analysis (CEA) which measures additional benefit of one strategy over another and additional costs of that strategy in dollars. CEA then combines these two assessments to give dollars per clinical outcome (say $ per year of life saved). The most controversial aspect of CEA is estimate of upper limit for cost-effectiveness ratio, but values of more than $100,000 per year of life saved are generally considered high.

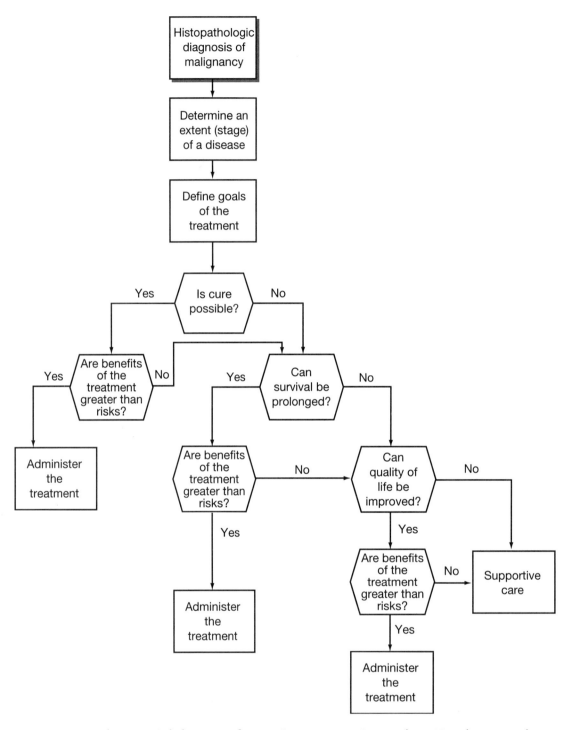

FIGURE 1-5 *The essential elements of reasoning processes in oncology. Note how a goal-oriented reasoning intertwined with estimates of benefits and risks of available treatment options dominate the approach to the management of the patients with malignant disorders. This can occur at any point of cancer presentation (newly diagnosed malignancy, first relapse, second relapse, etc.).*

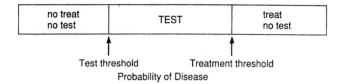

FIGURE 1-6 *Threshold concept of decision making. Note two thresholds: (1) test threshold-probability at which choice between testing or not testing is equal, (2) treatment threshold-probability at which choice between treating or not treating is equal. Action (to test or to treat) is made when the probability of disease exceeds these decision threshold levels. Threshold probabilities are functions of operating characteristics of the test, risk of the test and efficacy and risk of the treatment. These thresholds can be calculated according to formula depicted in Table 1-1 or with the nomogram shown in Fig. 1-7. (Adapted from Pauker SG, Kassirer DP: The threshold approach to eliminate decision making. N Engl J Med 302:1109–1117, 1980, with permission.)*

FIGURE 1-7 *Nomogram to calculate threshold probabilities. To use the nomogram determine benefit/risk (B/R) ratio on the right-hand scale and positive and negative likelihood ratios on the center axis, and then connect these lines with the left-hand scale. For example, you are seeing 45-year-old women in your office with a palpable, movable mass with round borders. Should you obtain a mammogram, perform surgery, or do nothing? The literature data suggest that the chance this woman has a breast cancer is about 10% (see Panzer et al.). LR+ of mammogram for detection of breast cancer is about 8, and LR– is .2 (see Sox et al.). Benefit/risk ratio of treatment for early breast cancer is at least 13 (JAMA 273:142, 1995). Connecting B/R point (13) with straight lines through LR+ = 8 and LR–=.2 and extending them to intercept the left-hand scale, we obtain that the test–no test threshold is 0.95% and the test–treatment threshold is 27%. This means that we should do nothing only if our assessment of the probability of cancer is less than 0.95% and that the surgery would be justified if estimated probability of disease is above 27%. In our case the estimated probability of disease is 10%. Therefore, our decision should be to obtain biopsy, and depending on a result proceed with the surgery or the follow-up strategy. (From Djulbegovic B and Desoky A: Equation and Nomogram for Calculation of Testing and Treatment Probability Thresholds. Med Decis Making 16:198 1996, with permission.)*

to patients who do not have the disease. Similarly, if the test has a high positive likelihood ratio (LR+), the testing threshold is reached at very low level of diagnostic suspicion. By contrast, any therapy that is not highly effective or carries considerable risk must be given only when the level of diagnostic uncertainty is minimal. If a particular therapy combines low efficacy with high risk, one would want to give it to as few patients as possible who do not have the disease. To do this, a substantial diagnostic certainty is required, for the attainment of which more testing may be justified. Tests with low negative likelihood ratios (LR–) have a small number of false-positive results; the equation in Table 1-1 also predicts that higher diagnostic certainty would be required for tests with lower LR–, as well as smaller benefit/risk (B/R) ratio.

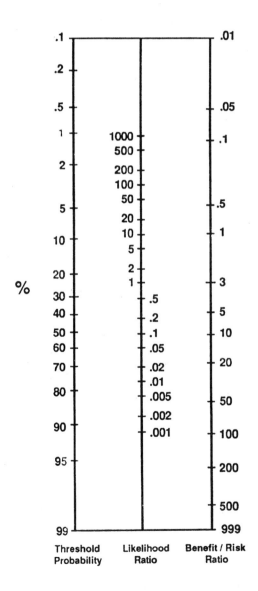

A nomogram has been devised to enable easy determination of diagnostic and treatment thresholds, combining operating characteristics of diagnostic tests as likelihood ratios (LRs) and estimates of therapeutic benefit/risk ratios (Fig 1-7). One has to be careful not to take calculated decision threshold results at face value without trying to understand the accuracy of their assessment. One method that takes into account the measurement of the uncertainty in the calculated threshold values is shown in Figure 1-8, which demonstrates that *practicing physicians should aim for diagnostic certainty only when the benefit of treatment is equal to its associated risk*, which is a familiar situation to all oncologists who would, for example, never expose a patient with AML to BMT procedures if they are not absolutely certain of their diagnosis. Treatment benefit almost equals risk under these clinical settings. In all other cases, decisions about treatment do not have to rely on maximum diagnostic certainty. When benefit greatly exceeds risk, such as in the settings of adjuvant chemotherapy for breast cancer, we may administer therapy even when our certainty of disease recurrence is quite low (Fig. 1-8).

Overall, decisions involving treatment thresholds are predominant in oncology (Fig. 1-8), rather than decisions concerning diagnostic thresholds, since risks of most diagnostic tests are negligible. Evidently knowledge of the benefits and risks of available therapies is the most important aspect of the clinical management of patients with oncologic diseases. This conclusion implies that medical personnel should be careful to catalog these important data. Ironically, data on the benefits and risks of various treatment for malignant diseases are usually lacking. As it has been pointed out by some authors, if the data on the testing and treatment are not available, then "you have to wonder what practitioners are basing decisions on." Therefore, an important goal for clinical medicine in the next 10 years is to develop a catalog of benefits risk ratios for the "1,000 most important clinical decisions." Table 1-3 shows current best estimates of various treatment results with contemporary therapy. Data regarding treatments of specific malignancies are amply provided in this book.

It is important to note that treatment benefits and risks can be expressed in different ways. In oncology the outcomes of interest are usually overall survival, disease-free survival, response rates, mortality, grade of toxicity and the measurements of the quality of life (Tables 1-4 to 1-7).

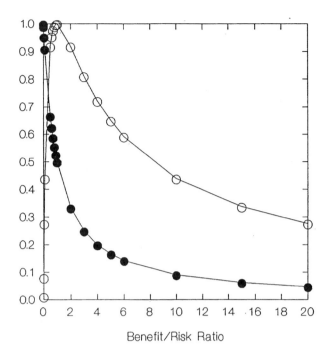

Benefit/Risk Ratio

FIGURE 1-8 *The relation between benefits (B) and risks (R) of a treatment and the threshold probability and the threshold entropy. In contrast to the method shown in Figure 1.6, this graph also illustrates the importance of the error or uncertainty in the measurements of the decision thresholds. Entropy (empty circles) represents the measure of uncertainty in the threshold probability (solid circles.) For a given B/R ratio, treatment is preferred when an estimate of the probability of a disease, p(D), in a patient is greater than the corresponding threshold entropy value. Note that when benefit equals risk, the theoretical probability of a disease at which we can start treatment is slightly higher than 50% (see also Table 1–1). However, under these circumstances the acceptable level of diagnostic certainty is not 50%, but rather 100% because the entropy around the threshold level is maximum. On the other hand, when benefit greatly exceeds risk, the treatment can be given even when the probability of disease is quite low (e.g., adjuvant chemotherapy in breast cancer). (Modified from Djulbegović B et al: Med Hypoth 45:503–509, 1995, with permission.)*

MINIMIZATION OF ERRORS

As discussed above, it seems that our reasoning skills are directly proportional to the knowledge in the field with more rule-based and skill-based functioning being acquired as we develop our expertise. However, all reasoning processes are prone to error. It is estimated that clinical medicine usually func-

TABLE 1-3   VARIOUS TREATMENT RESULTS WITH CURRENT THERAPIES

	No. Patients	(%)
Outcome of Treatment in Patients with Localized Disease Using Current Therapies	985,000	
Total New – 1988	985,000	
Total with localized disease	630,000	
Cured with surgery	275,000	(43.7)
Cured with radiation therapy	113,000	(18.0)
Cured (?) with adjuvant chemotherapy	25,000	(3.9)
Cured with chemotherapy	15,000	(2.4)
Will relapse after initial treatment	202,000	(32.0)
Local recurrence	133,000	(21.0)
Distant metastases	68,000	(11.0)
Estimated Treatment Results of Radiation Therapy in Incurable Patients		
Treated by Radiation with Curative Intent	226,000	
Will be Cured of Cancer	113,000	(50.0)
Will Recur Locally	76,000	(33.4)
Will Relapse with Distant Metastases	34,000	(16.6)
Estimated Benefits from Chemotherapy in Cancer Patients with Metastatic Spread		
Distant metastases	582,000	
Estimated cures with chemotherapy	18,000	(3.1)
Significant remissions (~ 2 yr)	34,000	(5.7)
Satisfactory remissions (~ 1 yr)	87,000	(14.9)
Minimal or no prolongation of life	443,000	(76.3)

(Adapted from Devita VT, Hellman S, Rosenberg SA: Cancer: Principles and Practice of Oncology. 4th Ed. Lippincott-Raven, Philadelphia, 1993, with permission.)

TABLE 1-4 NEOPLASTIC DISEASES AND THEIR RESPONSE TO CHEMOTHERAPY

Type of cancer	% Therapeutic Response (PR + CR)	Survival of Responders
Prolonged survival or cure		
Gestational trophoblastic tumors	70–95	60% cured with high tumor burden
		90% cured with moderate tumor burden
Burkitt's tumor	>50–60	50% cured
Seminoma	95	90% cured
Nonseminomatous testicular	90	90% cured
Wilms' tumor	60–80	65% cured with adjuvant CT
Osteogenic sarcoma	60–80	65% cured with adjuvant CT
Neuroblastoma	50–80	>20% cured
Acute lymphocytic leukemia (adults)	50–60	30% cured
Acute lymphoblastic leukemia (children)	90	70% cured
Non-Hodgkin's lymphoma (children)	90	60% cured
Non-Hodgkin's (DLC) lymphoma (adults)	75	50% cured
Rhabdomyosarcoma	90	70% cured with adjuvant CT
Hodgkin's disease	90	80% cured
Acute myelogenous leukemia	50–80	15% cured
Palliation and prolongation of survival		
Prostate cancer	70	Increased
Breast cancer	60	Increased with adjuvant CT
Chronic lymphocytic leukemia	50	Slightly increased
Non-Hodgkin's indolent lymphoma (adults)	60	Increased
Multiple myeloma	60	Slightly increased

(Continues)

TABLE 1-4 *(Continued)*

Type of cancer	% Therapeutic Response (PR + CR)	Survival of Responders
Small-cell carcinoma of the lung	60	2–5% cured
Chronic myelocytic leukemia	90	Increased
Palliation with uncertain prolongation of life		
Ovarian cancer	30–50	Probably increased
Endometrial cancer	25	Probably increased
Soft tissue sarcoma	30–50	Probably increased with adjuvant CT
Gastric cancer	30	Probably increased
Colorectal cancer	30–40	Increased with adjuvant CT
Anal cancer (CT + RT)	70	Probably increased
Bladder cancer	30–40	Probably increased
Uncertain palliation		
Pancreatic cancer	10–15	Brief
Liver cancer	10–15	Brief
Cervical cancer	20	Brief
Melanoma (cutaneous)	20	Brief
Adrenal cortical cancer	20	Brief
Kidney cancer	10–20	Brief

Abbreviations: CT, chemotherapy; RT, radiation therapy; PR, partial response; CR, complete response; DLC, diffuse large cell.

(From Fischer DS: Follow-Up of Cancer: A Handbook for Physcians. 4th Ed. Lippincott-Raven, Philadelphia, 1996, with permission.)

TABLE 1-5 HOW TO MEASURE EFFECTIVENESS OF THE TREATMENT?

To measure effectiveness of our interventions, we must be able to identify outcomes clearly, which we want to modify with the treatments. Each treatment is associated with benefits (good outcomes) and risks (bad outcomes). In oncology, benefits are usually measured in terms of overall survival, disease-free survival, complete and partial remissions, tumor mortality; risks are usually measured as mortality and the grade of toxicity; [a]finally, effect of intervention on the quality of life can be used to express both benefits and the risks of a particular treatment.

Statistically, effects of the treatment can be expressed in numerous ways. In oncology, calculation of reduction in mortality in relative risk or odds ratio is often used as a measurement of the effectiveness of the treatment. While this is statistically correct, these calculations frequently do not convey meaning of real clinical significance (as opposed to statistical significance) of the effectiveness of a particular treatment. The number of patients needed to be treated (NNT) to produce a therapeutic difference for one person has been proposed as a useful summary measurement for the description of medical treatment.[b] NNT is equal to the reciprocal of difference in probability of outcomes between two treatment alternatives according to $1/(p_{rx1} - p_{rx2})$.[c] To calculate NNT for an intervention to produce, on average, one additional benefit use the following formula:

$$NNT = \frac{1}{(B1 - B2)},$$

where $B1$ = probability of benefit under treatment alternative 1, and $B2$ = probability of benefit under treatment alternative 2. To calculate NNT for an intervention to produce, on average, one additional harm use the following formula:

$$NNT = \frac{1}{(H1 - H2)},$$

where $H1$ = probability of harm under treatment alternative 1, and $H2$ = probability of harm under treatment alternative 2. To combine both benefits and risk, use the following formula:

$$NNT = \frac{1}{(B1 - B2) + (H1 - H2)}.$$

For example, tamoxifen given to node-positive breast cancer patients[d] resulted in ten year survival of 50.4% in comparison with a control group that had 42.2% ten year survival. This benefit for tamoxifen as expressed in relative risk reduction in mortality is equal to 16.2% [(50.4–42.2)/50.4) = 16.2%]. When a reciprocal of absolute reduction in mortality is calculated (1/(0.504–0.422) = 1/.082 = 12.1), one may calculate that we need to treat 12 women with node positive breast cancer in order for one to have benefit. In node negative patients, this absolute reduction in mortality is 3.5% indicating that we need to treat 28 (NNT = 1/.035) females with a node negative tumor in order for one to experience benefit.

Tamoxifen is, however, not associated only with benefits. Prolonged use of tamoxifen has been associated with increased risk of endometrial cancer. Number of endometrial cancer after four years on tamoxifen is 9/1000 in comparison to .7/1000 in female not receiving tamoxifen. Some studies show that an average death rate in tamoxifen-associated endometrial cancer is about 33% comparing with 2.6% in patients not treated with tamoxifen.[e] Thus, absolute risk of dying due to endometrial cancer after four years of tamoxifen therapy is about [(.7/1000*.026)–(9/1000*.33)] =–.0029518.[f] Number of patients needed to be treated (NNT) with tamoxifen for one female to experience one fatal complication is 1/–.0029518 = 338.7. When benefits and risks of tamoxifen are calculated together NNT for node-positive women = 1/(.082–.0029518) = 12.6 and for node-negative women NNT = 1/(.035–.0029518) = 31.2.

[a]*Uniform toxicity grading criteria are defined by many institutions such as NCI, WHO, SWOG, etc. (Appendix 1 shows one of these grading scales.)*

[b]*See N Engl J Med 1988;318:1728; Med Decision Making 1993;13:247; Am J Med 1992;92:117.*

[c]*It is important to note that absolute differences rather than relative differences in probabilities are entered in the formulas (see the example).*

[d]*Lancet 1992;339:1.*

[e]*Oncology 1995;9:129.*

[f]*A positive NNT index indicates desirable outcome, and negative NNT unfavorable outcome.*

TABLE 1-6. OUTCOMES OF CANCER TREATMENT (SEE ALSO FIG. 1-5)

Survival is the most important outcome of cancer treatment.

An improvement in at least disease-free survival is a prerequisite for recommending adjuvant therapy.

Treatment can be recommended even without an improvement in survival (e.g., in case of metastatic cancer) if it improves quality of life.

Complete responses is an important outcome when it predicts survival.

(The value of outcomes like tumor responses and change in bio-markers depends on their ability to predict patient outcomes, i.e., survival and quality of life.)

Progression is an important outcome because it signals the need to change or stop treatment.

Cost-effectiveness is outcome that should be particularly considered when the benefits of treatments are modest and costs high.

Patient outcomes (e.g., survival and quality of life) are more important than cancer outcomes (i.e., response rate).

There is no minimum benefit above which treatment is justified; rather, benefits should be balanced against risks and costs.

(From the Outcome Working Group, Health Services Research Committee, American Society of Clinical Oncology. J Clin Oncol 14:671–679, 1996, with permission.)

TABLE 1-7. LEVELS OF EVIDENCE AND GRADING OF EVIDENCE FOR RECOMMENDATIONS

	Type of Evidence
Level	
I	Evidence obtained from meta-analysis of multiple, well-designed, controlled studies or from high-power randomized, controlled clinical trial
II	Evidence obtained from at least one well-designed experimental study or low-power randomized, controlled clinical trial
III	Evidence obtained from well-designed, quasi-experimental studies such as nonrandomized, controlled single-group, pre-post, cohort, time, or matched case-control series
IV	Evidence from well-designed, nonexperimental studies, such as comparative and correlational descriptive and case studies
V	Evidence from case reports and clinical examples
Grade	
A	There is evidence of type I or consistent findings from multiple studies of types II, III, or IV
B	There is evidence of types II, III, or IV and findings are generally consistent
C	There is evidence of types II, III, or IV but findings are inconsistent
D	There is little or no systematic empirical evidence

(From the Canadian Medical Association: The Canadian Task Force on the periodic health examination. Can Med Assoc J 121:1193, 1979, with permission.)

tions at a 1% failure rate, which is substantially higher than in any other industry.* Skill-based errors are called *slips*, and rule-based and knowledge-based errors are called *mistakes*. Particular attention should be paid to commonly used heuristics, which are often dysfunctional—for example, extrapolation of the results from the small samples, "treat patient, not numbers," correcting abnormality slowly, achieving diagnostic certainty (see above), and operate now to avoid "greater" risk in the future—although widely disseminated in practice are found to be inaccurate in many cases. These and other rules must be first identified for each field, and then scrutinized. Studies in prevention of errors have shown that standardization of processes wherever possible is one of the best ways to reduce and avoid errors. Algorithms are particularly useful for this purpose. However, to enable standardization in clinical medicine, rules upon which recommended strategy is based have to be of highest quality possible. Understanding quality of evidence, upon which the physician bases diagnos-

tic or treatment decisions is, therefore, very important. Table 1-7 list types of evidence that are generally used to summarize the strength of therapeutic recommendations. This book provides data on type of evidence of recommended strategies in the management of malignant diseases.

SUGGESTED READINGS

Diamond GA, Forrester JS: Metadiagnosis: an epistemologic model of clinical judgement. Am J Med 75:129–137, 1983

Djulbegović B: Decision making, algorithms and clinical reasoning. In: Reasoning and Decision Making in Hematology. Churchill Livingstone, New York, 1992

Djulbegović B, Hozo I, Abdomerovic A, Hozo S: Diagnostic entropy as a function of therapeutic benefit/risk ratio. Med Hypoth 45:503–509, 1995

Eddy DM. Comparing benefits and harms: the balance sheet. JAMA 263:2493–2505, 1990

Eddy DM: Cost-effectiveness analysis: is it up to the task? JAMA 267:3342–3348, 1992

Kassirer JP: Diagnostic reasoning. Ann Intern Med 110:893–900, 1989

Kassirer JP, Kopelman RI: Learning Clinical Reasoning. Williams & Wilkins, Baltimore, 1991

Leape LL: Error in medicine. JAMA 272:1851–1857, 1994

McDonald CJ: Medical heuristics: the silent adjudicators of clinical practice. Ann Intern Med 124:56–62, 1995

If we had to live with 99.9% accuracy, we would have 2 unsafe plane landings per day at O'Hare Airport, 16,000 pieces of lost mail every hour, and 32,000 bank checks deducted from the wrong bank account every hour.

Moskowitz AJ, Kuipers BJ, Kassirer JP: Dealing with uncertainty, risks and tradeoffs in clinical decisions: a cognitive science approach. Ann Intern Med 108:435–449, 1988

Panzer JR, Black ER, Griner PF: Diagnostic Strategies for Common Medical Problems. ACP, Philadelphia, 1991

Pauker SG, Kassirer JP: Therapeutic decision making: a cost-benefit analysis. N Engl J Med 293:229–234, 1975

Pauker SG, Kassirer JP. The threshold approach to clinical decision making. N Engl J Med 302:1109–1117, 1980

Sacket DL, Haynes RB, Guyatt GH, Tugwell P: Clinical Epidemiology: A Basic Science for Clinical Medicine. 2nd Ed. Little, Brown, Boston, 1991

Sox HC, Blatt MA, Higgins M, Marton KI: Medical Decision Making. Butterworth, Boston, 1988

2 | Myelodysplastic Syndromes

Michael S. Gordon

Prevalence: 3–5/100,000 population (most patients are men over 60 years)

Key reasoning principle: Identification of those patients who can be managed with supportive treatment versus those patients who will require aggressive treatment.

Goal of treatment: Supportive except for the minority of (young) patients who may be treated aggressively in the curative manner.

Prognosis: Median survival

Refractory anemia, (RA) and refractory anemia with ringed sideroblasts (RARS), 60 months

Refractory anemia with excess blasts (RAEB), 10–12 months

RAEB in transformation (RAEB-t), 5–8 months

Chronic myelomonocytic leukemia (CMML), 10–18 months

The myelodysplastic syndromes (MDS) are a family of heterogeneous hematologic disorders characterized by ineffective hematopoiesis and cytopenias. The diagnosis of an MDS is usually suspected when a patient presents with anemia, leukopenia, or thrombocytopenia. Many patients will present with complex cytopenias.

Anemia is present in about 90% of patients at the time of diagnosis; pancytopenia in about 50%; the combination of anemia and thrombocytopenia in 20 to 25%; anemia and neutropenia in 5% to 10%; and cytopenia or monocytosis in the absence of anemia in less than 5% of patients. The peripheral blood (PB) smear can be very helpful in supporting this diagnosis. Often, patients have a macrocytic anemia with reticulocytopenia. As stated, patients with MDS are often leukopenic with a concomitant neutropenia and may have evidence for dysmyelopoiesis with hypogranular or pseudo-Pelger-Huet neutrophils. A mild peripheral monocytosis is often associated with the neutropenia.

MDS usually occurs in elderly patients with a median age of about 65 years. Less than 10% of patients are younger than 50 years, and about 1% of patients are younger than 40 years.

DIAGNOSIS

A bone marrow (BM) aspiration with cytogenetics and review of the PB smear are the most useful tools for confirming the diagnosis. In the bone marrow, dysplastic features in all three hematologic lineages, the erythroid (megaloblastoid changes, multinucleation, nuclear chromatin abnormalities), myeloid (hypogranularity, pseudo-Pelger-Huet cells), and megakaryocytic (micromegakaryocytes, monolobed forms), are often seen. These marrows are often hyperplastic although a small percentage of patients

15

may have a hypoplastic appearance that can be confused with aplastic anemia. The PB may show evidence of isolated or multiple cytopenia. In addition, common findings include macrocytosis, monocytosis, myeloid abnormalities (hypogranularity and pseudo-Pelger-Huet cells).

Physical examination is not particularly helpful in the diagnosis of MDS. Lymphadenopathy is usually not seen, and the spleen and liver are palpable in 20% and 10% of patients, respectively.

The percentage of bone marrow blasts, the presence or absence of ringed sideroblasts, and the PB absolute monocyte count are critical for determining the correct MDS classification. The French-American-British (FAB) group has defined diagnostic criteria for the five subsets for MDS. They include RA (BM blasts <5%); RARS (BM blasts <5% with >15% ringed sideroblasts); RAEB (BM blasts 5%–20%); RAEB-t (BM blasts 20%–30%); and CMML (BM blasts <20% and absolute PB monocyte count >1,000 cells/µl). BM blast percentages greater than 30% are consistent with the diagnosis of acute myeloid leukemia. A recent update of the diagnostic criteria for CMML suggests that patients with a leukocytosis greater than 13,000 cells/µl behave more like a myeloproliferative disorder than an MDS and should be considered as such for the purposes of clinical intervention.

PROGNOSIS

The prognosis of patients with MDS is intimately linked to their FAB classification and cytogenetics. Table 2-1 shows data on survival and the natural history of a disease (risk to transformation to AML). In general, the greater the percentage of BM blasts, the poorer the prognosis. Patients with RA or RARS often have median survivals greater than 60 months. This compares favorably to those

patients with CMML (median survival of 10–18 months) and RAEB/RAEB-t median survivals of 5–10 months. For patients with more advanced disease, morbidity and mortality are often associated with transformation to AML. For patients with RA/RARS, this occurs in 10–15%, compared with rates of 30% for CMML and 40 to 60% for patients with RAEB/RAEB-t. The rate of transformation, and hence the survival of the MDS patient, appears to be linked to the presence of abnormal cytogenetics at the time of diagnosis. Patients with abnormal karyotypes do worse than those with normal cytogenetics. In addition, complex karyotypic abnormalities perform worst and often are associated with the highest rates of leukemic transformation. In contrast, several syndromes, such as that associated with the 5q- abnormality, may be associated with a more indolent course. Those patients who do not suffer from leukemic transformation often develop progressive pancytopenia with resultant complications of infectious or hemorrhagic deaths.

TREATMENT

While the standard therapy, based upon randomized phase III trials, continues to be expectant observation and supportive care with transfusions, new options are opening for increasing numbers of MDS patients. Therapy with hormones (either corticosteroids or androgens) is generally ineffective and associated with various side effects. Low-dose

TABLE 2-1. MYELODYSPLASTIC SYNDROMES: NATURAL HISTORY AND PROGNOSIS

Syndrome	AML Risk	Median Survival[a]
RA/RARS	10%–15%	60 months
RAEB	40%–50%	10–12 months
RAEB-t	50%–75%	5–8 months
CMML	~30%	10–18 months

[a]Leading cause of death: infections, 65%.

Abbreviations: CMML, chronic myelomonocytic leukemia; RAEB, refractory anemia with excess blasts; RAEB-t, refractory anemia with excess blasts in transformation; RA/RARS, refractory anemia/refractory anemia with ringed sideroblasts.

———————————————————→

FIGURE 2-1. *Management of myelodysplastic syndromes (MDS). The key reasoning principle relates to the identification of those patients who can be managed with supportive treatment versus those patients who will require aggressive treatment. Using FAB (French-American-British) classifications and various prognostic factors may aid with this decision. Understanding the benefits/risks of the available treatments further helps decide which patients should be treated aggressively and which should be managed with supportive care only. The goal of the treatment in the management of MDS is largely supportive, except for the minority of (young) patients who may be treated aggressively in the curative manner. Recommended strategy is mainly based on indirect evidence (level IV data) but also on level I and II evidence for the use of growth factors and observation in a stable disease, respectively. (Modified from Djulbegović B: Reasoning and Decision Making in Hematology. Churchill Livingstone, New York, 1992, with permission.)*

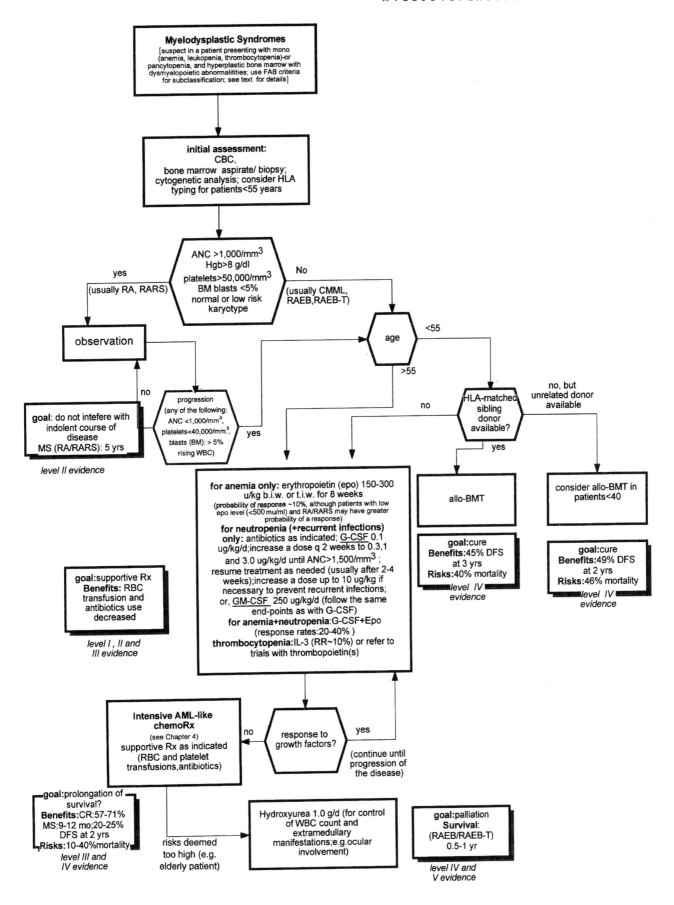

Myelodysplastic Syndromes
[suspect in a patient presenting with mono (anemia, leukopenia, thrombocytopenia)-or pancytopenia, and hyperplastic bone marrow with dysmyelopoietic abnormalitities; use FAB criteria for subclassification; see text for details]

initial assessment:
CBC,
bone marrow aspirate/ biopsy;
cytogenetic analysis; consider HLA typing for patients<55 years

ANC >1,000/mm^3
Hgb>8 g/dl
platelets>50,000/mm^3
BM blasts <5%
normal or low risk karyotype

yes
(usually RA, RARS)

No
(usually CMML, RAEB,RAEB-T)

observation

age

<55

>55

HLA-matched sibling donor available?

no, but unrelated donor available

no

yes

no

progression
(any of the following:
ANC <1,000/mm^3,
platelets<40,000/mm.^{3},
blasts (BM): > 5%
rising WBC)

yes

goal: do not intefere with indolent course of disease
MS (RA/RARS): 5 yrs

level II evidence

for anemia only: erythropoietin (epo) 150-300 u/kg b.i.w. or t.i.w. for 8 weeks
(probability of response ~10%, although patients with low epo level (<500 mu/ml) and RA/RARS may have greater probability of a response)
for neutropenia (+recurrent infections) only: antibiotics as indicated; G-CSF 0.1 ug/kg/d;increase a dose q 2 weeks to 0.3,1 and 3.0 ug/kg/d until ANC>1,500/mm^3; resume treatment as needed (usually after 2-4 weeks);increase a dose up to 10 ug/kg if necessary to prevent recurrent infections; or, GM-CSF 250 ug/kg/d (follow the same end-points as with G-CSF)
for anemia+neutropenia:G-CSF+Epo (response rates:20-40%)
thrombocytopenia:IL-3 (RR~10%) or refer to trials with thrombopoietin(s)

allo-BMT

goal:cure
Benefits:45% DFS at 3 yrs
Risks:40% mortality
level IV evidence

consider allo-BMT in patients<40

goal:cure
Benefits:49% DFS at 2 yrs
Risks:46% mortality
level IV evidence

goal:supportive Rx
Benefits: RBC transfusion and antibiotics use decreased

level I, II and III evidence

Intensive AML-like chemoRx
(see Chapter 4)
supportive Rx as indicated (RBC and platelet transfusions,antibiotics)

no

response to growth factors?

yes

(continue until progression of the disease)

goal:prolongation of survival?
Benefits:CR:57-71%
MS:9-12 mo;20-25% DFS at 2 yrs
Risks:10-40%mortality
level III and IV evidence

risks deemed too high (e.g. elderly patient)

Hydroxyurea 1.0 g/d (for control of WBC count and extramedullary manifestations;e.g.ocular involvement)

goal:palliation
Survival:
(RAEB/RAEB-T)
0.5-1 yr

level IV and V evidence

chemotherapy yields poor response rates with clinically significant toxicity and, compared in a randomized trial with observation, was inferior in quality of life and survival.

Various hematopoietic growth factors have been studied in patients with MDS. At present, the three that are most widely used include the myeloid factors, granulocyte colony stimulating factor (G-CSF) and granulocyte-macrophage colony stimulating factor (GM-CSF), and erythropoietin. While they have been aggressively studied in controlled trials, a survival advantage has not been associated with their use in randomized trials. In general, G-CSF and GM-CSF have the ability to induce increases in the number and function of circulating neutrophils in the PB. This effect is seen in nearly all patients treated and has not, in randomized trials, been associated with an increased rate of leukemic transformation. In contrast, the use of erythropoietin remains controversial. A recent meta-analysis of all erythropoietin clinical trials in MDS suggests that early use (before the need for red blood cell [RBC] transfusions) in patients with low risk MDS (e.g., RA/RARS) with low erythropoietin levels may yield optimal results. In general though, the use of erythropoietin in patients with MDS is associated with a 10% to 15% response rate characterized by decreased RBC transfusion requirement. The combination of G-CSF and erythropoietin has been studied by the group at Stanford and subsequently in a multicenter trial. The concomitant use of these two agents appears to promote an enhanced erythroid response, although the exact magnitude of this effect is unclear. It is likely in the range of 20% to 30% improvement.

The use of aggressive therapy for MDS is limited to patients with good performance status and includes allogeneic BM transplant (BMT) or induction chemotherapy. In the former, the use of a sib-matched donor may be associated with as many as 50% of patients obtaining long-term disease-free survival (DFS). The cure rates for this disease appear to be related to the timing of BMT with regard to MDS classification. Patients transplanted at the Fred Hutchinson Cancer Research Center in Seattle demonstrated a 0% relapse rate for those with fewer than 5% BM blasts at the time of BMT. This compares to higher rates of relapse, approaching 50% to 60% for patients with more advanced disease. Transplant-related morbidity and mortality are the most problematic issues for this approach. In addition, the availability of a sib-matched donor for these patients remains a rate-limiting step. The use of matched unrelated donors for allogeneic

BMT in MDS patients has demonstrated an actuarial 2-year DFS of 49%. Unfortunately, this procedure is associated with a high risk of severe graft-versus-host disease, and a 2-year actuarial mortality of 46%. Finally, the use of intensive induction chemotherapy, while associated with a significant risk of death, may be associated with as much as a 20% to 25% 2-year DFS.

The critical aspect of decision making in the management of MDS relates to the use of *aggressive treatment versus supportive care*. As discussed above, several randomized trials (level II evidence) have compared low-dose chemotherapy and hormonal therapy with supportive care only in patients with a stable disease. Increased toxicity (poor benefit/risk ratio) with no survival benefit in the treatment arm indirectly confirmed superiority of supportive care in this patient group. Our algorithm recommends active interventions in the patient with progressive disease and poor prognostic factors (increased blasts, multiple chromosomal abnormalities, low platelets, low absolute neutrophil counts). These factors were found to be able to predict the course of MDS in several prognostic systems. However, none of several prognostic systems described in the literature was prospectively validated with respect to the tailoring of the treatment toward a specific risk category. A new international risk analysis system designed to take into account specific cytogenetic and morphologic risk factors will likely aid in determining optimal timing for initiation of various potentially toxic therapies.

TREATMENT GOALS

What should be our goals in the management of MDS? As discussed above, retrospective data (level IV evidence) suggest that MDS can be cured with BMT at the cost of high mortality associated with this procedure. Unfortunately, this goal of cure can be pursued for relatively rare young patients with MDS. For most other patients, the goal of the management is largely supportive, with the aim of correction of anemia, prevention of bleeding associated with thrombocytopenia, and prophylaxis against recurrent infections. Figure 2-1 shows a recommended strategy for the management of MDS. It is mainly based on indirect data (level III and IV evidence). Note, however, that high quality evidence (level I and II) demonstrated no efficacy of low-dose ara-C (cytosine-arabinoside), retinoic acid, vitamin D3, and hormonal therapy with androgens and steroids. Consequently, these management options are not listed in our algorithm.

SUGGESTED READINGS

Anderson JE, Appelbaum FR, Fisher LD et al: Allogeneic bone marrow transplantation for 93 patients with myelodysplastic syndrome. Blood 82:677–681, 1993

Anderson JE, Appelbaum FR, Storib R: An update on allogeneic marrow transplantation for myelodysplastic syndrome. Leukemia Lymphoma 17:95–99, 1995

Beris P: Primary clonal myelodysplastic syndrome. Semin Hematol 26:216, 1989

Boultwood J, Lewis S, Wainscoat JS: The 5q- syndrome. Blood 84:3253–3260, 1994

Deiss A: Acquired disorders associated with hematologic malignancies. Myelodysplastic syndromes. pp. 1949–1968. In Lee GR, Bithell TC, Foerster J, Athens JW, Lukens JN (eds): Wintrobe's Clinical Hematology. 9th Ed. Lea & Febiger, Philadelphia, 1993

Estey E, Pierce S, Kantarjian H et al: Treatment of myelodysplastic syndromes with AML-type chemotherapy. Leukemia Lymphoma 11 (suppl. 2):59–63, 1993

Greenberg P, Fenaux P, Morel P et al: International workshop consensus risk analysis system for myelodysplastic syndromes (MDS). Blood 86:270a, 1995

Hellstrom-Lindberg E: Efficacy of erythropoietin in the myelodysplastic syndromes: a meta-analysis of 205 patients from 17 studies. Br J Haematol 89:67–71, 1995

Koeffler HP: Myelodysplastic Syndromes (Preleukemia). Semin Hematol 23:284–299, 1986

Keoffler HP, Heitjan D, Mertelsmann J, et al: Randomized study of 13-cis retinoic acid v placebo in the myelodysplastic disorders. Blood 71:703–708, 1988

Miller KB, Kyungmann K, Morrison FS et al: The evaluation of low-dose cytarabine in the treatment of myelodysplastic syndromes: a phase III intergroup study. Ann Hematol 65:162–168, 1992

Negrin RS, Stein R, Vardiman J, et al: Treatment of the anemia of myelodysplastic syndromes using recombinant human granulocyte colony-stimulating factor in combination with erythropoietin. Blood 82:737–743, 1993

3 Acute Lymphoblastic Leukemia

Alfonso Cervera

Incidence: 1/100,000/year (20% of all acute leukemias)

Goal of the treatment: Cure

Main modality of the treatment: Chemotherapy

Prognosis (overall): 30%–40% of patients are long-term survivors

Acute lymphoblastic leukemia (ALL) is a malignant disease characterized by the proliferation and accumulation of cells of the lymphoid series that have suffered arrest at some point in the maturation process. ALL is the most common malignant disease in childhood; however, in adults it constitutes less than 5% of all the leukemias and only 20% of the acute leukemias. The age-adjusted incidence rate goes from 5.3 per 100,000 before the age of 5 years to less than 1 per 100,000 in people between 20 and 65 years of age, after which it increases to reach 2.3 per 100,000 in people older than 80. It is interesting to note that the incidence of ALL in the black population is approximately half that of the white population. There is a small predominance of male patients.

The survival of children and adults with ALL differs. In children, remission can be obtained in more than 90% of the patients and long-term survival can be expected in at least 75% of them, as opposed to adults in whom most series report achieving a remission in 65% to 85% of the patients, and only 30% to 40% are long-term survivors. While the better tolerance of children to intense chemotherapy plays an important role in this, differences in biologic characteristics of the childhood and adult forms of the disease also participate. The chromosomal abnormalities that are common in the childhood form, and that are believed to confer good prognosis, are uncommon in adults; on the other hand, the Philadelphia chromosome, a particularly unfavorable translocation, is present in 5% of children and, in contrast, in about 30% of cases among adults.

Those patients with ALL who receive only supportive care have a median survival of 1 to 2 months, as opposed to those who receive therapy, in whom the median survival is about 24 months. Survival in excess of 5 years can be achieved in at least a third of all patients. Therefore, all patients should be offered treatment. Because life-taking complications can develop rapidly, ALL constitutes a hematologic emergency.

DIAGNOSIS AND CLASSIFICATION

ALL, unlike acute myelogenous leukemia (AML), is seldom preceded by a myelodysplastic phase. The clinical presentation is thus acute, and the patient usually has symptoms of only a few weeks' duration. The clinical picture is nonspecific, and while fever (not secondary to infection), weight loss, and bone or joint pain can occur, most symptoms are attributable to varying degrees of anemia, thrombocytopenia, and neutropenia that are almost universal. Lymphoblasts can be found in the peripheral

21

blood in more than 90% of patients, regardless of the total white blood cell count. The diagnosis of ALL, therefore, should be considered in the differential diagnosis of the patient with bone marrow (BM) dysfunction or circulating blasts.

The BM aspirate shows hypercellular particles with paucity or even absence of normal hematopoietic elements and abundant lymphoblasts. Cytochemistry is extremely important for the differential diagnosis between AML and ALL. To diagnose ALL, less than 3% of the blasts should be positive for Sudan black, myeloperoxidase, or nonspecific esterase; on the other hand, most cases are positive for periodic acid-Schiff, and at least 20% are positive for acid phosphatase. Flow cytometry can be very helpful in those patients in whom the light microscopic findings alone are not enough to reach an adequate diagnosis.

ALL is a heterogeneous disorder, and characterization and classification of the patient's disease has both therapeutic and prognostic implications. The first *classification* that correlated with prognosis used morphologic criteria and was published by the French-American-British cooperative group in 1976 (Table 3-1). Later, the use of monoclonal antibodies allowed the realization of two important facts: first, the series of events involved in the differentiation and maturation of normal lymphoid-committed precursors is associated with changes in the expression of cell surface markers and, second, malignant lymphoblasts have surface markers that mimic the immunophenotypes of some normal lymphocyte precursors. A classification of ALL based upon the immunophenotype of the lymphoblasts (Table 3-2) has allowed, to some extent, the successful use of species-specific therapy (Fig. 3-1). Finally, the identification of some nonrandom chromosomal abnor-

malities can aid in the classification of some patients, but most important, it provides useful prognostic information (Tables 3-3 and 3-4).

At the time of initial evaluation, investigation of cardiac (echocardiogram and ejection fraction), hepatic, and renal function as well as metabolic status, including serum electrolytes, uric acid, and lactic dehydrogenase are mandatory, so that abnormalities can be corrected (Appendix 3-1) and drug doses can be modified accordingly. Disseminated intravascular coagulation is rare in ALL; however, coagulation should be assessed in every patient to exclude incidental clotting abnormalities that, in conjunction with thrombocytopenia, could lead to significant bleeding. Aggressive search for microbial pathogens is indicated in the neutropenic and febrile patient and empiric as well as prophylactic antibiotics, in the neutropenic afebrile patient, should be initiated immediately (Appendix 3).

Involvement of the central nervous system (CNS) at presentation is found in 5% to 10% of adult patients and, while it can produce signs of increased intracranial pressure and even palsy of cranial nerves, it is frequently asymptomatic; therefore, examination of the cerebrospinal fluid (CSF) is very important. The timing of this examination is controversial. One approach is to delay it until the malignant cells have been cleared from the peripheral blood because of the theoretical concern of seeding the CSF with circulating blasts; however, this has not been shown to occur, and we recommend that it be done at diagnosis, given the high mortality of the condition when left untreated.

TREATMENT

The chemotherapeutic treatment of ALL has traditionally been divided into three phases: (1)

TABLE 3-1 MORPHOLOGIC CLASSIFICATION OF ACUTE LYMPHOBLASTIC LEUKEMIA[a]

	L1	L2	L3
Cell Size	Small cells predominate	Large cells, heterogeneous in size	Large and homogeneous
Nuclear chromatin	Homogeneous in any one case	Variable-heterogeneous in any one case	Finely stippled and homogeneous
Nuclear shape	Regular occasional clefting or indentation	Irregular; clefting and indentation common	Regular—oval to round
Nucleoli	Not visible, or small and inconspicuous	One or more present, often large	Prominent; one or more vesicular
Amount of cytoplasm	Scanty	Variable; often moderately abundant	Moderately abundant
Basophilia of cytoplasm	Slight or moderate, rarely intense	Variable; deep in some	Very deep
Cytoplasmic vacuolation	Variable	Variable	Often prominent

[a]*In 1976 the French-American-British Cooperative group, using morphology alone, divided ALL into three subtypes. This classification gained acceptance, and some modifications have been introduced.*

TABLE 3-2 IMMUNOLOGIC CLASSIFICATION OF ACUTE LYMPHOBLASTIC LEUKEMIA

Subtype	%	Usual Morphology	Immunophenotype[a]
B Lineage			
Early pre-B	11	L1 or L2	CD19+,CyD22+,CD24+,HLADR+,TdT+,CyIgM–
Pre-B	9	L1	CD10±,CD19+,CyCD22+,CD24+,CyIgM+,HLADR+,TdT+
C ALL	52	L1 or L2	CD10+,CD19+,CyCD22+,CD24+,CyIgM–,HLADR+TdT+
B ALL	4	L3	CD10±,CD19+,CyCD22+,CD24+,CyIgM–,SIgM+,HLADR+ TdT–
T Lineage			
Pre-T	6	L1 or L2	CD7+,CD3+,CD2–,HLADR±,TdT+
Pre-T	18	L1 or L2	CD7+,CD3+,CD2+,HLADR–.TdT±

[a]*The immunologic classification of ALL is based on the expression of surface (S) and cytoplasmic (Cy) markers. The morphologic subtypes were added to show the fact that the microscopic characteristics of the lymphoblasts are not completely specific.*

induction (reduction of the tumor burden to the point at which blasts are not detectable by light microscopy), (2) consolidation (reduction of the residual leukemic cells to minimal level), and (3) maintenance. Clearly children with ALL benefit from the use of all three phases. However, in adult patients, randomized trials show no clear advantage to consolidation or maintenance; despite this, the consensus is that therapy has to be continued once remission has been achieved with induction because recent large prospective nonrandomized multicenter trials suggest that leukemia-free survival (LFS) is improved by including the latter two phases, without adding major toxicity.

The exception to the previous statement are those patients with mature B-cell ALL, which is the least common subtype in all age groups and for which the use of conventional ALL regimens invariably yields poor results. The outlook for children

with this variant improve remarkably with short but intense protocols that include fractionated cyclophosphamide or ifosfamide in moderate doses, high-dose methotrexate and cytarabine. Application of similar protocols in adults has also made a positive difference. The German experience, recently published (Fig. 3-1A and Appendix 3) supports this concept and provides evidence for the use of low-dose cyclophosphamide and prednisone as pretreatment for those patients with large tumor burden. It is likely that cranial irradiation, for CNS prophylaxis, will be deleted from the protocol in the future. However, at this point there is not enough information to recommend its routine omission.

For patients with other B-cell ALL subtypes and T-cell ALL, induction with the combination of vincristine, an anthracycline, and steroids has consistently produced remission rates of about 80%. The addition of cyclophosphamide and asparaginase, in randomized trials, has not increased the remission rate. However, some recent prospective nonran-

TABLE 3-3 COMMON CYTOGENETIC ABNORMALITIES IN ACUTE LYMPHOBLASTIC LEUKEMIA

Lineage	Karyotype
Early pre-B	t(4;11)(q21;q23)
	t(9;22)(q34;q11)
Pre-B	t(1;14)(p32;q11)
	t(1;19)(q23;p13)
	t(9;22)(q34;q11)
C ALL	t(9;22)(q34;q11)
B ALL	t(8;14)(q24;q32)
	t(2;8)(p12;q24)
	t(8;22)(q24;q12)
T ALL	t(8;14)(q24;q11)
	t(10;14)(q24;q11)
	t(11;14)(p13;q11)

It is useful to determine the cytogenetic characteristics of ALL, both because it aids in establishing prognostic factors and because it can have relevance in the treatment of some patients.

TABLE 3-4 FACTORS THAT CORRELATE WITH REMISSION DURATION IN ALL[a]

Factor	Good Prognosis	Bad Prognosis
Time to complete remission	<4 weeks	>4 weeks
Age	<35 years	>35 years
Leukocyte count	<30,000/μl	>30,000/μl
Immunophenotype	c-ALL T-ALL	
Cytogenetic abnormalities		t(4;11) t(9;22)

[a]*Prognostic factors in ALL. T-ALL was considered a bad prognostic subtype until recently, when with modern chemotherapy it has become a favorable subtype. The prognosis of t(9;22)-positive and t(4;11)-positive ALL is dismal with standard chemotherapy.*

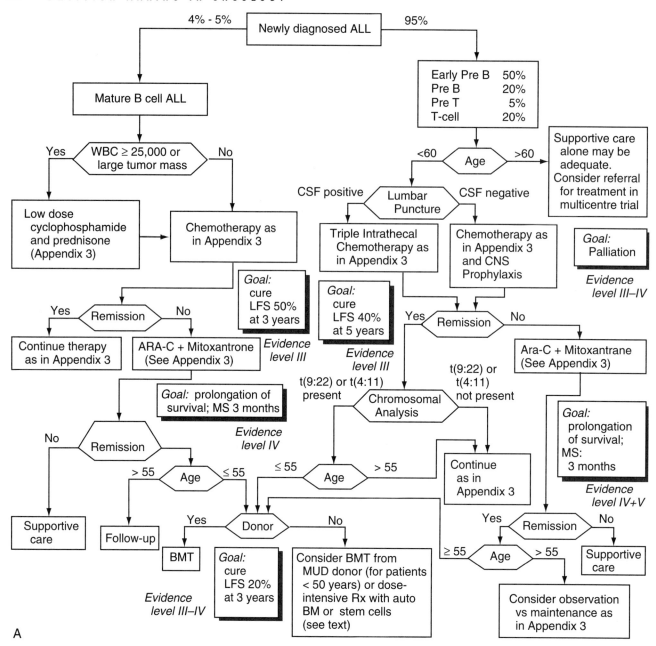

FIGURE 3-1 *(A & B) Acute lymphoblastic leukemia (ALL) is a hematologic emergency because of the high incidence of metabolic and hematologic complications associated with untreated disease. The most important distinction in the initial approach to all patients is whether mature B-cell ALL is present because specific treatment yields better results. The goal in the young patient is cure, and although results have been improving, this is achievable in only 40% of patients. In elderly patients treatment with intense chemotherapy does not improve survival, and some patients benefit more from supportive care alone. Bone marrow transplantation (BMT) should be reserved for patients with Philadelphia-chromosome-positive ALL, for those with t(4;11), and for those who relapse and achieve a second remission. Justification exists for BMT for those patients who do not respond to chemotherapy; for patients with mature B-cell ALL, BMT should be considered only if remission is not obtained after 2 cycles of the proposed chemotherapy. Relapse after BMT can be treated with some experimental measures, but specific recommendations at this point are hard to make. (Figure continues.)*

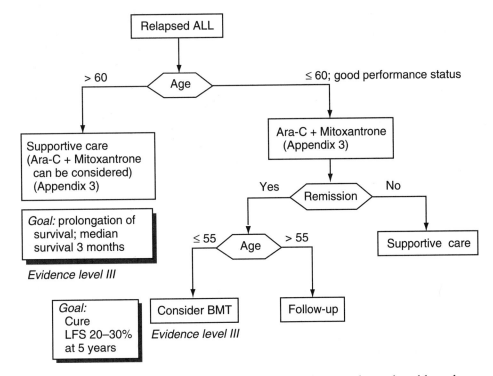

FIGURE 3-1 (Continued) *Second transplants or the infusion of peripheral lymphocytes from the donor with or without interleukin-2 activation are available. See Tables 3-5 to 3-9 for details on benefits and risks of various treatment alternatives. The quality of evidence for the proposed initial treatment is of II–III levels and IV–V levels for relapsed disease. LFS, leukemia-free survival; MUD, matched unrelated donor; MS, median survival; CNS, central nervous system.*

domized multicenter trials suggest that the duration of overall survival and LFS are improved, without a major change in toxicity, by intensifying the induction regimen.

In the latest trial of the Cancer and Leukemia Group B, study 8811, a complete remission rate of 85% and a median survival longer than 45 months were found. These results are better than what has

been previously published. However, in this study lumbar puncture was not done at diagnosis, and only one patient had symptomatic CNS disease at presentation, yet 10 patients (6%) either developed overt symptoms of CNS involvement during consolidation or were found to have blasts in their CSF three months after diagnosis. While all 10 responded initially to treatment, none was a long-term survivor.

TABLE 3-5 COMPARISON OF RISK/BENEFIT BETWEEN BONE MARROW TRANSPLANT AND CHEMOTHERAPY FOR ALL IN FIRST REMISSION[a]

	Leukemia-Free Survival at 5 Years ($P=0.2$)	Probability of Relapse at 5 Years ($P=0.0001$)	Treatment-Related Death ($P=0.0001$)	Level of Evidence	References
Chemotherapy	32%	66%	5%		Ann Intern Med 115:13–18, 1991
BMT	34%	30%	53%	III	Ann Intern Med 123:428–431, 1993

[a]*Bone marrow transplantation (BMT) does not offer an advantage for most patients in first remission. Evidence from small single-institution series suggests that patients who are Philadelphia chromosome positive or t(9;22) and with t(4;11) may benefit from BMT in first remission. The quality of evidence supporting this inference is of levels III, IV, and V. P, statistical significance.*

TABLE 3-6 COMPARISON OF RISK/BENEFIT BETWEEN BONE MARROW TRANSPLANT AND CHEMOTHERAPY IN T(4;11) AND T(9;22) POSITIVE ALL

	Leukemia-Free Survival, 3 Years (%)	Overall Survival 3 Years (%)	Level of Evidence	References
Chemotherapy	11	19		Blood 78: 1923–1927, 1991
			IV–V	Blood 85: 2025–2037, 1995
Bone marrow transplant	46	65		Bone Marrow Transpl 16:663–667, 1995

Bone marrow transplant does not offer an advantage in most patients in first remission. Evidence from small single-institution series suggests that patients with Philadelphia-chromosome-positive or t(9;22) and with t(4;11) may benefit from BMT in first remission. The quality of evidence supporting this inference is of levels IV and V.

Thus while this protocol offers the highest complete remission rate and longest median survival in adults so far, it leaves unanswered the issue of the treatment of CNS involvement at diagnosis. Furthermore, relapse in the CNS either concomitantly or preceding relapse in the BM occurred in a significant number of their patients. This suggests that the prophylactic treatment employed was not optimal.

The German Cooperative Multicentre ALL Trials Group (GMALL) has published consistently good results with the protocol outlined in Appendix 3-3 (see Fig. 3-1). The role of early treatment and prophylaxis of the CNS is underscored by their results and those of the M.D. Anderson Cancer Center recently published. With this approach, complete remission can be expected in more than 80% of patients, long-term LFS in 60% of low-risk patients, and 35% of high-risk patients.

Allogeneic BM transplantation (BMT) in first remission should be reserved for patients less than 55 years old with Philadelphia-chromosome-positive ALL and for those with t(4;11), as their prognosis with standard chemotherapy is extremely poor. Those patients in this category but younger than 50 years of age, without an HLA-identical sibling, should be considered for a BMT from a matched unrelated donor (MUD). Currently BMT is not indicated in first remission in patients with other bad prognostic indicators, such as high WBC count at presentation or slow response to induction chemotherapy, because these seem to affect the outcome of BMT as well. The role of dose-intensive chemotherapy with autologous BM or peripheral stem-cell support is still unknown. For this reason, those patients who are not eligible for BMT should be referred for inclusion in prospective trials testing this modality.

Those patients who fail to achieve a remission constitute a major challenge because they tend to be older and, even if remission is obtained after a different chemotherapeutic combination, the chances of long-term survival are extremely low. Little information exists in the literature regarding these patients. However, it is reasonable to try to induce a remission with high-dose cytarabine and mitoxantrone (Appendix 3), after which some patients could undergo BMT when feasible. If a HLA-identical sibling is not available, a transplant from a MUD can be considered. However, it must be kept in mind that obtaining a donor from the registries may take several months. In any event, the outlook for there patients is dismal, and 3-year LFS with BMT is only around 20%.

Age as a prognostic factor should be viewed as a continuous variable in that disease-free survival

TABLE 3-7 RISK/BENEFIT BETWEEN STANDARD CHEMOTHERAPY AND METHOTREXATE–CYCLOPHOSPHAMIDE-BASED CHEMOTHERAPY IN MATURE B-CELL ALL

	Complete Remission (%)	Leukemia-Free Survival (%)	Overall Survival (%)	Level of Evidence	References
Standard	44	0	0		Blood 87:495–508, 1996
				III	
Specific (see Appendix 3)	74	71	51		

Mature B-cell acute lymphoblastic leukemia is the only variant of the disease for which specific chemotherapy is available. The long-term survival of patients with this subtype and treated with the conventional protocols is close to 0% as opposed to that of patients treated with moderate-dose cyclophosphamide- and methotrexate-containing regimens, which is around 70%, especially for young patients. The quality of evidence to support this inference is of level III.

TABLE 3-8 RISK/BENEFIT SUPPORTIVE CARE AND CHEMOTHERAPY IN PATIENTS OVER 60 YEARS OF AGE

	Complete Remission (%)	Survival at 5 Years (%)	Mean Survival	Level of Evidence	References
Supportive care	0	0	1 month	III	Blood 80:1813–1817, 1992
Chemotherapy	20	4	3 months	III	Blood 87:495–508, 1996

The decision of whether to treat an elderly patient with chemotherapy or with supportive care alone has to be made on an individual basis. The series that report the results of intense chemotherapy in patients within this age group show no clear advantage when compared with those patients who receive only supportive care. The quality of evidence supporting this inference is of level III, IV.

suffers progressive decrements with increasing age. The reason for this is not completely understood but, very likely, several factors participate. ALL in elderly patients is not very common. However, some authors have found that individuals older than 60 years constitute almost a third of their adult cases. Long-term LFS can be achieved in probably less than 10% of these patients, and there is usually no significant difference in the mean survival of those patients treated with supportive care alone and those treated with aggressive chemotherapy. For this reason we believe that chemotherapeutic treatment in these patients is adequate, mainly in the context of prospective trials.

Despite treatment, approximately 50% to 60% of patients will eventually relapse. The outlook after this is dismal, specially if the first remission is shorter than 24 months; the median survival with standard dose chemotherapy ranges from 2 to 7 months, and less than 5% of the patients are long-term survivors. In these patients, allogeneic BMT if a second remission is achieved, can produce 20% to 30% long-term survival, especially in young patients. The pediatric literature reveals that those patients who relapse more than 36 months after the initial remission may fare as well with conventional chemotherapy as with BMT but there is not enough information in the adult literature to make a specific recommendation. Adult patients should be

evaluated on an individual basis to decide which treatment modality has the highest chance of inducing a prolonged remission. Again, the role of dose-intensive chemotherapy with autologous BM or peripheral stem-cell rescue is uncertain, but some studies have produced promising reports, and thus those patients who can be considered good candidates for this type of treatment should be included in multicenter trials.

Those patients who relapse after BMT are extremely difficult to treat, both because of the resistance of their disease to treatment and because of the amount of chemotherapy to which they have been exposed. There are still some options available for these patients, and frequently a new remission can be achieved with further chemotherapy although, as to be expected, this is extremely short lived. Another possibility is the transfusion of peripheral blood lymphocytes from the original donor (when this is applicable and feasible), which has shown promising results, especially in cytogenetic relapses of chronic myelogenous leukemia. A recent report from Israel describes the successful treatment using this modality 4 of 6 patients with ALL who had relapsed after BMT. Activation of the transfused lymphocytes with interleukin-2 seems to have been beneficial in two of these patients.

The use of granulocyte colony-stimulating factor (G-CSF) during the induction phase of treat-

TABLE 3-9 COMPARISON OF RISK/BENEFIT OF BMT AND CHEMOTHERAPY OF ALL IN SECOND REMISSION

	Disease-Free Survival 3 Years	Probability of Relapse	Treatment-Related Mortality	Level of Evidence	References
Chemotherapy	5–11%	65–70%	15%	III and IV	Bone Marrow Transplant 7 (suppl 2):38, 1991
BMT	20–30%	25%	50%	III and IV	Blood 80(suppl1):80, 1992

Bone marrow transplantation (BMT) in those patients that relapse and achieve a second remission seems to be superior to treatment with conventional chemotherapy; however, no definite conclusion can be made, since a prospective comparative trial is still lacking. The quality of evidence at this time is of level III and IV.

ment has shown benefit in a prospective randomized trial reported by GMALL. Other nonrandomized trials support this concept, and thus the use of G-CSF (Appendix 3) seems to be justified.

Several strategies currently being developed are very likely going to improve the long-term outlook for patients with ALL. One is the measurement and quantification of minimal residual disease and the adjustment of the treatment to this. Another is the individualization of dosages of antileukemic drugs to achieve a target level of systemic exposure whereby the therapeutic effect is increased and toxicity reduced. Finally, the circumvention of drug resistance will very likely prove to be the most useful strategy.

SUGGESTED READINGS

Bennett JM, Catovsky D, Daniel MT et al: Proposals for the classification of the acute leukemias. Br J Haematol 33:451–458, 1976

Billet AL: High-dose therapy in acute lymphoblastic leukemia. In Armitage JO, Antman KH (eds): High Dose Cancer Therapy. Williams & Wilkins, Baltimore, 1995

Boucheix C, David B, Sebban C et al: Immunophenotype of adult acute lymphoblastic leukemia, clinical parameters and outcome: an analysis of a prospective trial including 562 tested patients (LALA 87). Blood 84:1603–1612, 1994

Copelan EA, McGuire EA: The biology and treatment of acute lymphoblastic leukemia in adults. Blood 85:1151–1168, 1995

Cortes J, O'Brien SM, Pierce S et al: The value of high-dose systemic chemotherapy and intrathecal therapy for central nervous system prophylaxis in different risk groups of adult acute lymphoblastic leukemia. Blood 86:2091–2097, 1995

Djulbegović B, Herzig R: Adult acute lymphoblastic leukemia pp. 107–111. In Djulbegović B (ed): Reasoning and Decision Making in Hematology. Churchill Livingstone, New York, 1992

Evans WE, Rodman J, Relling MV et al: Individualized dosages of chemotherapy as a strategy to improve response for acute lymphoblastic leukemia. Semin Hematol 28:15–21, 1991

Fiere D, Lepage E, Sebban C et al: Adult acute lymphoblastic leukemia: a multicentric randomized trial testing bone marrow transplantation as postremission therapy. J Clin Oncol 11:1990–2001, 1993

Hernandez JA, Land KJ, McKenna RW: Leukemias, myeloma and other lymphoreticular neoplasms. Cancer 1(supp. 1):381–394, 1995

Hoelzer D: Prognostic factors in acute lymphoblastic leukemia Leukemia 6 (suppl. 6): 49–51, 1992

Hoelzer D, Ludwig WD, Thiel E et al: Improved outcome in adult B-cell acute lymphoblastic leukemia. Blood 87:495–508, 1996

Hoelzer D, Thiel E, Ludwig WD et al: The German multicentre trials for treatment of acute lymphoblastic leukemia in adults. Leukemia 6(suppl 2):175–177, 1992

Hoelzer E, Thiel E, Loffler H et al: Prognostic factors in a multicentre study for treatment of acute lymphoblastic leukemia in adults. Blood 71:123–131, 1988

Hoelzer E, Thiel H, Loffler H et al: Intensified therapy in acute lymphoblastic and acute undifferentiated leukemia in adults. Blood 64:38–47, 1984

Horowitz MM, Messerer D, Hoelzer D et al: Chemotherapy compared with bone marrow transplantation for adults with acute lymphoblastic leukemia in first remission. Ann Intern Med 115:13–18, 1991

Kantarjian HM: Adult acute lymphocytic leukemia: critical review of current knowledge. Am J Med 97:176–184, 1994

Larson RA, Dodge RK, Burns P et al: A five-drug remission induction regimen with intensive consolidation for adults with acute lymphoblastic leukemia: cancer and leukemia group B study 8811. Blood 85:2025–2037, 1995

Lejune C, Tubiana N, Gastaut JA: High dose cytosine arabinoside and mitoxantrone in previously treated acute leukemia patients. Eur J Haematol 44:240–246, 1990

Ottman OG, Hoelzer D, Gracien D et al: Concomitant granulocyte colony-stimulating factor and induction chemotherapy in adult acute lymphoblastic leukemia: a randomized phase III trial. Blood 86:444–450, 1995

Preti A, Kantarjian HM: Management of adult acute lymphocytic leukemia: present issues and key challenges. J Clin Oncol 12:1312–1322, 1994

Slavin S, Naparstek E, Nagler A et al: Allogeneic cell therapy with donor peripheral blood cells and recombinant human interleukin-2 to treat leukemia relapse after allogeneic bone marrow transplantation. Blood 87:2195–2204, 1996

Stockschlader M, Hegewisch-Becker S, Kruger W et al: Bone marrow transplantation for Philadelphia-chromosome-positive acute lymphoblastic leukemia. Bone Marrow Transpl 16:663–667, 1995

Traweek T: Immunophenotypic analysis of acute leukemia. Am J Clin Pathol 99:504–512, 1993

Zhang MJ, Hoelzer D, Horowitz MM et al: Long-term follow-up of adults with acute lymphoblastic leukemia in first remission treated with chemotherapy or bone marrow transplantation. Ann Intern Med 123:428–431, 1995

4 Acute Myelogenous Leukemia

Alfonso Cervera
Benjamin Djulbegović

Incidence: Age dependent

<20 years old, 0.5/100,000

21–69 years old, 0.6–6/100,000

>70 years old, 10–17/100,000

Goal of Treatment: Cure is achievable in young patients

In elderly patients, palliation and prolongation of survival

Main modality of treatment: Chemotherapy

Prognosis: 20% overall 5-year survival

Acute myelogenous leukemia (AML) is a malignant disease characterized by the accumulation of clonal neoplastic cells of the myeloid series. AML accounts for approximately one fourth of all the leukemias diagnosed in the United States each year and affects all age groups, although it is more common in the elderly. Its age-adjusted incidence is less than 1 per 100,000 in people younger than 20 years and increases to slightly more than 10 per 100,000 in those older than 70.

AML should be included in the differential diagnosis of the patient with evidence of bone marrow (BM) dysfunction or circulating blasts. The diagnosis is based on the findings of the BM biopsy/aspirate, which is usually hypercellular, with decreased or absent megakaryocytes; by convention, to differentiate AML from other conditions, the blasts should constitute at least 30% of all the nucleated cells in the aspirate. The disease is classified into different subtypes according to the French-American-British (FAB) criteria (Table 4-1).

AML is universally and rapidly fatal when left untreated. However, modern chemotherapeutic protocols can achieve a remission in most affected individuals, and disease-free survival in excess of 5 years can be expected in up to 40% of patients. Therefore, all patients should be offered treatment.

Upon diagnosis the morphologic subtype, immunophenotype, and chromosomal abnormalities should be determined, and supportive treatment instituted (see Appendix 4). Life-taking complications can develop rapidly, and thus treatment should be considered as an emergency.

The probability of long-term survival depends, on one hand, on the biologic characteristics of the disease and some demographic qualities of the host and, on the other, on the type and intensity of the treatment. In certain patient populations, more intense regimens may mean a higher likelihood of sustained remission. In other groups, the positive effects of such therapy can be offset by a higher morbidity and mortality. Thus, the reasoning process in treatment selection is based on the knowledge of clinical and biologic markers that correlate with treatment outcome (Table 4-2). Some of these markers are believed to be useful to predict

TABLE 4-1 CLASSIFICATION OF ACUTE MYELOGENOUS LEUKEMIA

	Subtype	Frequency (%)	Characteristic Features
M0	Undifferentiated myeloblasts	2–3	Large agranular blasts. Immunophenotype usually CD34+, HLADR–
M1	Myeloblastic leukemia without differentation	20	Frequently associated with t(9;22) cytogenetic abnormality. Immunophenotype CD34+,HLADR+
M2	Myeloblastic leukemia with differentiation	30	Large granular blasts
M3	Promyelocytic leukemia	10	Heavily granulated promyelocytes with bilobed nuclei and Auer rods. Demonstration of translocation of t(15;17) is required for diagnosis. Immunophenotype CD14–, CD34– HLADR.
	M3V		Contains small granules that are evident only on electron microscopy
M4	Myelomonocytic leukemia	25–30	Monocytic cells compose 20% to 80% of nonerythroid nucleated marrow cells. Immunophenotype: CD14+, CD34–, HLADR+
	M4EO		More than 5% abnormal eosinophilic precursors in bone marrow. Associated with Inv(16) cytogenetic abnormality
M5	Monocytic leukemia	10	More than 80% of nonerythroid bone marrow nucleated cells are monocytic. Immunophenotype CD14+, CD34–, HLADR+
M6	Erythroleukemia	4–5	More than 50% of all nucleated bone marrow cells are erythroblasts. Immunophenotype: CD13–, CD41–
M7	Megakaryoblastic leukemia	1–3	Bone marrow biopsy may show fibrosis. Large granular blasts. Immunophenotype: CD13–, CD41+, CD42b+

early mortality, and the others correlate with intrinsic resistance to chemotherapy (manifested by failure to achieve a remission or by rapid relapse). While some of the nonrandom chromosomal abnormalities found in the blast cells of AML seem to confer sensitivity to cytarabine and idarubicin and thus are associated with a better prognosis, others identify a group of patients with extremely poor prognosis (Table 4-2).

TREATMENT

The cornerstone of the treatment of AML is the combination of *cytarabine with an anthracyclic antibiotic*. Evidence from prospective trials suggests that idarubicin is superior to daunorubicin and doxorubicin and is, currently, the agent of choice. The dose and schedule of administration of cytarabine has been debated for many years. While some groups advocate the use of high-dose cytarabine (HDAC) for induction, two prospective trials have shown that in the newly diagnosed patient, the "7+3" schedule yields equivalent results with less toxicity; in this regimen, cytarabine is given at 100 or 200 mg/m^2/day as a continuous infusion during 7 days and idarubicin 12 mg/m^2/day is given on three consecutive days during the cytarabine infusion. There is some evidence to support the use of the higher cytarabine dosage in patients younger than 60 years. A BM aspirate should be performed 14 to 21 days after the start of treatment to determine whether the marrow has become profoundly hypocellular and the percentage of blasts has been reduced to less than 5%. Remission should be documented later according to standard criteria (Table 4-3). (See Appendix 4.)

In the patient with previous exposure to antineoplastic chemotherapy or with a history of a preced-

TABLE 4-2 FACTOR THAT AFFECT PROGNOSIS IN ACUTE MYELOGENOUS LEUKEMIA

Risk Factors Associated With Early Mortality	Risk Factors Associated With Resistance to Chemotherapy	Factors Associated With Favorable Outcome
Poor performance status	Preceding myelodysplasia	Cytogenetics: t(15;17), t(8;21); inv 16
Age over 60	Secondary acute myelogenous leukemia	
Low pretreatment serum albumin level	Cytogenetics: –5, 5q–, –7, 7q–, +8, 11q–	
Abnormal renal or hepatic function before treatment	Slow cytoreduction	
	White blood cell count >10,000/mm^3	

TABLE 4-3 CRITERIA FOR REMISSION IN ACUTE MYELOGENOUS LEUKEMIA

Less than 5% myeloblasts in the bone marrow
Restoration of normal hematopoieis
Resolution of cytogenetic abnormalities
Resolution of any evidence of extramedullary leukemia (granulocytic sarcomas)

TABLE 4-4 RISK/BENEFIT OF STANDARD DOSE CYTARABINE VS HDAC

Regimen	In Induction for AML		
	Complete Remission (%)	Mortality (%)	Evidence Type
Standard dose (1)	59–74	7	I
HDAC(2)	55–70	17	I

Regimen	For Consolidation in AML			
	Overall Survival (%)	Disease-Free Survival (%)	Mortality (%)	Evidence Type
Standard dose (3)	31	21	1	I
HDAC (3)	46	39	5	I

References: (1) Proc Am Soc Clin Oncol 11:849, 1992; (2) Proc Am Soc Clin Oncol 11:856, 1992; (3) N Engl J Med 331:896, 1994

Abbreviations: AML, acute myelogenous leukemia; HDAC, high-dose cytarabine.

ing myelodysplastic syndrome, the approach for remission induction should be different, given the poor results obtained with the conventional treatment. Some small series suggest that HDAC can induce a remission in more patients than the same drug in the conventional doses. However, most of these remissions are short lived. Allogeneic BM transplantation (BMT) can achieve disease-free long-term survival in some of the patients in whom a remission is obtained and should be considered in this particular subgroup. If a sibling donor is not available, a BMT from a matched unrelated donor (MUD) should be evaluated.

Promyelocytic blasts are extremely sensitive to the usual chemotherapeutic agents, and patients with acute promyelocytic leukemia (APL) have, with the standard therapy, a better long-term outcome than the patients with other morphologic variants,

even considering that the disseminated intravascular coagulation (DIC) associated with it produces a significant mortality during the induction phase. Recently all-trans retinoic acid (ATRA) has been shown to induce a remission in more than two-thirds of APL patients, but more important is the observation that the coagulopathy is quickly con-

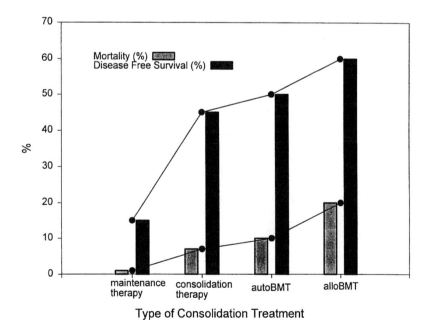

FIGURE 4-1 *Benefit/risk ratio of different types of postremission therapies. Note that as outcomes improve with intensive regimens, so do the risks. The careful balancing of benefits and risks in individual patients represents a key reasoning principle in the management of acute myelogenous leukemia (for details, see text and also Figs. 4-2 and 4-3 and Tables 4-4 to 4-7).*

TABLE 4-5 RISK/BENEFIT OF ATRA FOLLOWED BY HDAC VS 7+3 FOLLOWED BY HDAC FOR THE TREATMENT OF APL[a]

Regimen	Complete Remission (%) (P=0.25)	One-year Disease-Free Survival (%) (P=0.0001)	One-Year Overall Survival (%) (P=0.01)	Mortality (%) (P=NS)	Type of Evidence	References
7+3 followed by HDAC	81	50	74	5		Blood 82: 3241, 1993
					II	Lancet 343: 1033, 1994
ATRA followed by HDAC	91	83	91	5		

[a]The major criticism of this study is that some patients on the ATRA arm received standard chemotherapy concomitantly with ATRA. ATRA, all-trans retinoic acid; HDAC, high dose cytarabine; P, statistical significance.

trolled and few fatal hemorrhagic events occur with its use. Some evidence suggests that disease-free long-term survival is superior in patients who receive ATRA for induction followed by intense chemotherapy compared with patients who receive chemotherapy only.

It is very important to stress that this approach is not free of toxicity and that high mortality from the so-called retinoic acid syndrome has been reported. This consists of leukocytosis, which appears as soon as 2 days after the start of treatment, associated with fever, respiratory distress, pleural effusions, and pulmonary infiltrates in the absence of demonstrable infection. Peripheral edema, pericardial effusions, renal and hepatic failure, and episodic hypotension have also been described. It is particularly common in patients who present with elevated white blood cell (WBC) count. Given the high mortality of the syndrome, two approaches have been developed. One is to give dexamethasone 10 mg twice a day for 3 days, should any symptoms of respiratory distress appear. The other is to start standard chemotherapy if the WBC increases above 6,000/mm³ by day 5, above 10,000/mm³ by day 10, or more than 15,000/mm³ by day 15, without discontinuing ATRA. To avoid the complications of neutropenia associated with chemotherapy, we prefer the use of steroids and reserve the use of concomitant chemotherapy for patients who present with hyperleucocytosis.

POSTREMISSION THERAPY

Two comparative trials have shown that, in patients younger than 60 years, postremission therapy with HDAC increases the duration of remission. Unfortunately, how high the doses should be and how many courses are necessary to obtain the maximal benefit is not known. Our recommendation is that cytarabine 3 g/m² every 12 hours for six days and idarubicin 12 mg/m² on three consecutive days be given once after the patient has recovered from induction therapy. Maintenance therapy in AML has not shown any benefit. Allogeneic marrow transplants done in first remission have consistently yielded lower relapse rates than both standard dose chemotherapy and HDAC (Tables 4-4 to 4-7); however, this does not translate into longer survival, because of the high mortality associated with it. For this reason, its use in first remission is still very controversial and probably indicated only in special circumstances (see Fig. 4-1, which shows the benefit/risk ratio for the different postremission treatments).

The long-term results of chemotherapy in patients with one or more bad prognostic indica-

TABLE 4-6 RISK/BENEFIT OF BMT VS HDAC IN FIRST REMISSION OF AML

Regimen	4-year Actuarial Relapse Rate (%) (P=0.05)	4-year Disease Free Survival (%) (P=NS)	4-Year Overall Survival (%) (P=NS)	Mortality (P=0.002)	Type of Evidence	Reference
HDAC	60	38	53	6	II	Clin Oncol 10:41, 1992
BMT	32	48	45	32		

Abbreviations: AML, acute myelogenous leukemia; BMT, bone marrow transplantation; HDAC, high-dose cytarabine; P, statistical significance; NS, not significant.

TABLE 4-7 RISK/BENEFIT OF INTENSIVE CHEMOTHERAPY VS. ALLOGENEIC BMT OR MYELOABLATIVE CHEMOTHERAPY WITH AUTOLOGOUS BM SUPPORT FOR AML IN FIRST REMISSION[a]

Treatment Modality	4-Year Estimate of Disease-Free Survival (%)	4-Year Estimate of Overall Survival (%) (P=NS)	Mortality (%)	Relapse Rate (%)	Evidence Type	References
Intensive chemotherapy	30	46	5.8	57		N Engl J Med 332:217–223
Myeloablative chemotherapy with autologous BM	48	56	10.4	40	I	
Allogenic BMT	35	59	20	24		

[a]One potential problem in the interpretation of this study is that the dose of cytarabine in the intensive chemotherapy was only 2 g/m² × 8 doses, which may have been insufficient.

Abbreviations: AML, acute myelogenous leulkemia; BM, bone marrow; BMT, bone marrow transplantations; NS, not significant.

tors are extremely poor, even if remission is achieved initially; for this reason this is a population that may benefit from BMT in first remission after standard chemotherapy. Those patients who lack a suitable related donor and who are younger than 40 years may be candidates for a BMT from a MUD. Myeloablative doses of chemotherapy with autologous BM or peripheral stem cell (PSC) support is an option for patients who, because of age constraints or lack of a suitable donor, would not be considered for BMT. Some studies have suggested that the results with this approach are the same as with BMT, and for this reason autologous stem cell

TABLE 4-8 FOLLOW-UP OF PATIENT WITH ACUTE MYELOGENOUS LEUKEMIA

After discharge from the hospital following initial chemotherapy, the frequency with which patients treated for acute leukemia need follow-up depends on the efficacy of the induction regimen. Those patients in complete remission need frequent observation until the peripheral blood is reconstituted: this usually requires a twice-weekly measurement of counts and administration of blood component therapy as needed (packed red blood cells at hematocrit less than 22%–25%; platelets for counts less than 20,000). In the setting of leukopenia, vigilant attention to any signs or symptoms of infection is essential, with rehospitalization for any fever higher than 100.6°F.

Once the peripheral blood is reconstituted, the frequency of blood checks can be lengthened to monthly intervals. Since consolidation or intensive therapy is subsequently administered, a return to the pancytopenia state requires a repetition of the initial frequent laboratory measurements and examinations. At the completion of chemotherapy, patients should be seen monthly for the first 3 years. The intervals between appointments for patients in complete bone marrow remission may then be lengthened to 3 months. Repeat marrows are done at the times indicated by the managing hematologist/oncologist.

Failure to enter a remission calls for rehospitalization.

(From Wiernik PH: Acute myeloid leukemia. In Fischer DS (ed): Follow-up Cancer: A Handbook for Physicians. Lippincott-Raven, Philadelphia, 1996, with permission.)

procurement should be a priority in this group of patients once remission has been achieved.

Failure to induce profound BM aplasia or the presence of more than 5% blasts in the BM aspirate 21 days after the start of therapy has been considered an independent predictor of short duration of remission if this is finally achieved. For this reason in the young patient (younger than 50 years) with a suitable sibling donor, BMT is indicated at this point. The patient who is not a candidate for BMT may benefit from HDAC. An important exception to this are the APL patients, in whom, regardless of the agents used, it takes longer to obtain complete remission (CR); patients on ATRA achieve remission at a mean of 5 to 6 weeks, but periods of treatment as long as 78 days may be required.

With this approach between 50% and 70% of the patients, depending on the risk category, can be expected to relapse. With aggressive therapy, some of them can still be long-term survivors. However, most will die of progressive disease or complications of the treatment. The factors that can predict prognosis in the newly diagnosed patient are still applicable, so that a patient with bad prognosis at diagnosis is less likely to have a durable second remission than a patient that at diagnosis was found to have fewer poor prognosis indicators. At this point the duration of the first remission becomes crucial. The patients who relapse more than 6 months after standard therapy can usually achieve a remission with the same drugs. However, in the patient younger than 50 years with a suitable donor, a BMT is probably preferable; if a sibling donor is not available, BMT from a MUD should be considered for the patient younger than 40 years. If autologous BM or PSC were collected more than 6 months before the relapse, myeloablative therapy with reinfusion of the autologous cells can be tried, provided a second remission has been achieved.

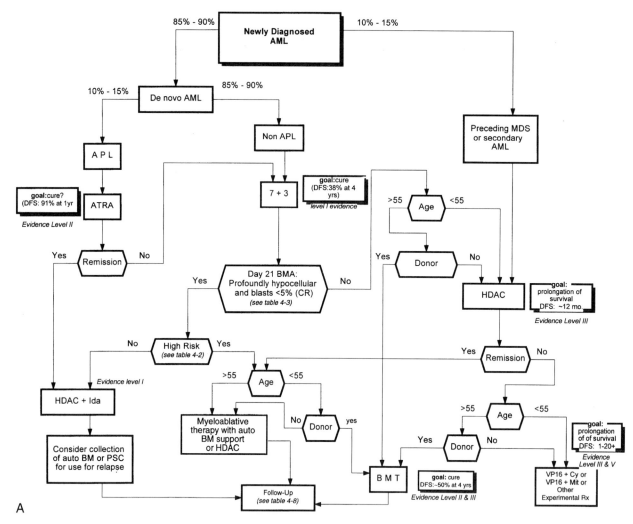

A

FIGURE 4-2 *(A & B) Treatment of acute myelogenous leukemia (AML). Understanding the natural history of AML coupled with benefit/risk estimates of various treatments available dominates the clinical approach to the management of AML. If left untreated, median survival of patients with AML is about 6 weeks, and only 3% of patient will survive 1 year. Therefore, AML should be considered a medical emergency. At the same time, treatment is not innocuous and careful estimates of benefits and risks are of crucial importance (see Fig. 4-1 and Tables 4-4, 4-7). The goal of the treatment should be cure in young patients and prolongation survival in older patients. Recommended strategy for induction treatment and consolidation is largely based on level I and II evidence; treatment of relapsed patients is mainly based on level IV and some level III evidence. (For dosages and practical details of the management, see Appendix 4.) ATRA, all-trans retinoic acid; APL, acute promyelocytic leukemia; HDAC, high dose cytarabine; BM, bone marrow; PSC, peripheral stem cell; BMA, bone marrow aspirate; IDA, idarubicin; MDS, myelodysplastic syndrome; VP16, etoposide; CY, cyclophosphamide; MIT, mitoxantrone; DFS, disease-free survival.*

Relapse less than 6 months after the initial remission identifies a group of patients in whom an inherently resistant subpopulation of blasts was selected by the therapy; these patients should be considered for a different induction plan. Resistance to standard dose cytarabine can be overcome by HDAC. Again, BMT is indicated in the young patient with an available sibling or unrelated donor.

Between 10% and 40% of the patients who undergo BMT in first remission will eventually

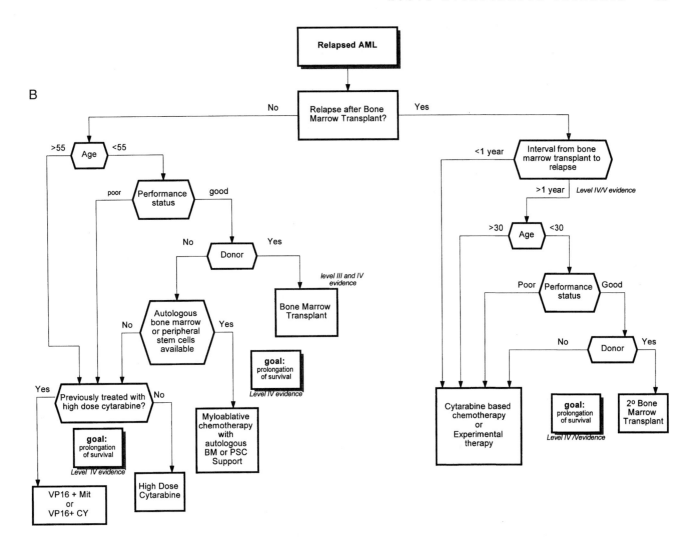

relapse. The interval between transplant and relapse is again important. A second transplant should be considered for young patients who relapse more than a year after the initial transplant and have a good performance status and no major sequelae from prior treatment. IL-2 has been given after BMT in an attempt to prevent relapse, and this is probably adequate. However, no clear evidence to support its use in this context is yet available. Those patients who relapse less than a year from the transplant constitute a more serious problem, because they are frequently debilitated from the previous treatment. Withdrawal of cyclosporine or donor buffy coat transfusions with or without IL-2 could be tried, especially if the graft has not been entirely replaced by the leukemic process. It must be stressed that while this therapy has shown benefit in some patients with chronic myelogenous leukemia (see Ch. 5), in AML most attempts have had disappointing results.

Those patients who will not be considered for a second BMT can be treated with cytarabine-based combination chemotherapy or other experimental approaches. Clearly, the goal in these patients should be palliation and prolongation of survival.

Treatment of AML in patients over 60 years of age is difficult, both because older people tolerate chemotherapy poorly and because their leukemias are often resistant to chemotherapy. Intensive therapy is of no benefit in this group. Comparative trials of standard chemotherapy versus supportive care alone have shown longer survival in the chemotherapy arm, and thus it seems reasonable to propose standard chemotherapy for remission induction. In this age group the decision to give postremission therapy should be individualized and based not only upon age but also upon performance status.

The use of growth factors in AML is still controversial. The randomized trials reported so far yield conflicting results. If anything, the use of granulocyte colony-stimulating factor (G-CSF) or granulocyte macrophage colony-stimulating factor (GM-CSF) shortens the duration of neutropenia without modifying survival. The use of these drugs has no adverse effects in the treatment of AML (see Ch. 60).

The therapy of AML continues to evolve. A few years ago long-term survivors were a medical curiosity and now it is an achievable goal for some individuals afflicted with it. The use of newer methods to detect minimal residual disease and molecular techniques to identify resistance to chemotherapy and its mechanisms, along with newer therapeutic agents will surely improve the cure rate.

Figure 4-2 shows the recommended strategy for the management of AML and Tables 4-4 to 4-8 show benefits and risks of treatment options at various decision points, which are depicted in Figure 4-2.

SUGGESTED READINGS

Anasetti C, Etzioni R, Petersdorf EW, et al: Marrow transplantation from unrelated donors. Ann Rev Med 46:169–180, 1995

Estey EH: Treatment of acute myelogenous leukemia and myelodysplastic syndromes. Semin Hematol 32:132–151. 1995

Fenaux P, Le Deley MC, Castaigne S et al: Effect of all-trans retinoic acid in newly diagnosed acute promyelocytic leukemia. Results of a multicenter randomized trial. Blood 82:3241–3249, 1993

Giralt SA, Champlin RE: Leukemia relapse after allogeneic bone marrow transplantation. A review. Blood 84:3603–3612, 1994

Mayer RJ, Davis RB, Schiffer CA et al: Intensive postremission chemotherapy in adults with acute myeloid leukemia. N Engl J Med 331:896–903, 1994

Schiller GJ, Nimer SD Territo MC et al: Bone marrow transplantation versus high dose cytarabine-based chemotherapy for acute myelogenous leukemia in first remission. J Clin Oncol 10:41–46, 1992

Stone RM, Berg DT, George SL et al: Granulocyte-macrophage colony-stimulating factor after initial chemotherapy for elderly patients with primary acute myelogenous leukemia. N Engl J Med 332:1671–1677, 1995

Wiley JS, Firkin FC: Reduction of pulmonary toxicity by prednisolone prophylaxis during all-trans retinoic acid treatment of acute promyelocytic leukemia. Leukemia 9:774–778, 1995

Willezme R, Suciu S, Mandelli F, et al: Treatment of patients with acute promyelocytic leukemia. The EORTC-LCG experience. Leukemia 8(suppl 2):48–55, 1994

Zittoun RA, Mandelli F, Willezme R et al: Autologous or allogeneic bone marrow transplantation compared with intensive chemotherapy in acute myelogenous leukemia. N Engl J Med 332:217–223, 1995

5 Chronic Myelogenous Leukemia

Benjamin Djulbegović

Incidence: 1.5 per 100,000 population

Goal of treatment: Cure if a patient is a bone marrow transplant BMT candidate; prolongation of survival with α-interferon; palliation with chemotherapy

Prognosis: BMT: survival 40–70% at 7– 10 years if transplanted in chronic phase; α-interferon: 61–89 months (median survival); busulfan/hydroxyurea: 45–56 months (median survival)

Chronic myelogenous leukemia (CML) accounts for about 20% of all leukemia cases with a death rate of about 1.5/100,000 population. The disease is rather rare among the young population with only 10% of cases occurring between ages 5 and 20. The median age of diagnosis reported from individual centers is about 43 years but is close to 60 for patients not selected by referral.

DIAGNOSIS

Diagnosis of CML does not present major clinical difficulty. It is usually suspected in a patient with increased white blood cell (WBC) count on account of increased neutrophils, basophils, or eosinophils. Typical clinical features include splenomegaly, neutrophilia, basophilia (sensitivity ~ 100%), and thrombocytosis with hypercellular bone marrow (Fig. 5-1) Specific laboratory findings include a low level of leukocyte alkaline phosphatase (LAP). Philadelphia chromosome (Ph) was found in 90% to 95% of cases CML and *bcr-abl* gene rearrangement. (Low LAP is found rarely in other diseases; it can, however, also be low in PNH, and sometimes in MDS, ITP, infectious mononucleosis, pernicious anemia, and congenital hypophosphatasia.) Philadelphia chromosome is a hallmark of the disease: it is the result of breaks on chromosome 9 and 22, with a reciprocal translocation of the distal genetic material, t(9;22)(q34;q11), and transposition of *c-abl* proto-oncogene in proximity to the breakpoint cluster region (BCR). This new hybrid *bcr-abl* oncogene encodes proteins (p210 or p190), which have a causal relationship to CML development. Only a minority of patients (3%–5%) are both Ph-negative and do not show BCR rearrangement. Ph-negative, BCR-positive CML have a similar clinical picture, response to therapy, and outcome as Ph-positive CML. True Ph[1]-negative, BCR-negative CML has an intermediate prognosis between chronic myelomonocytic leukemia (CMML) (with which it is often confused) and Ph-positive CML.

NATURAL HISTORY

The natural history of CML is characterized by an evolution of the disease from a chronic phase through an accelerated to a terminal phase of acute leukemia, the so-called blast crisis or blast transformation. However, some patients may go directly into the blast phase without a previously documented "accelerated phase," or may even present in the blast phase of the disease (Table 5-1). Patients with CML may live from a few months to 14 years with a median survival rate between 2 and 4 years. Prognostic systems have been developed to help predict the course of the disease in individual patients (Table 5-2).

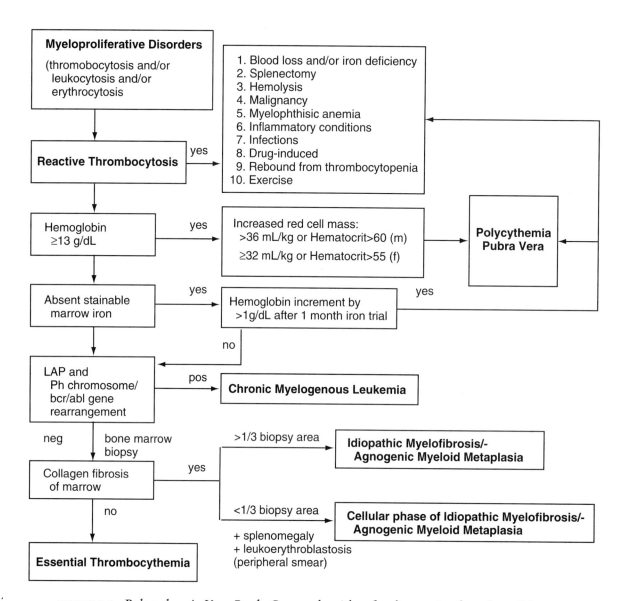

FIGURE 5-1. *Polycythemia Vera Study Group algorithm for diagnosis of myeloprolifera-tive disorders. CML, chronic myeloid leukemia; P. Vera, polycythemia vera; IMF/AMM, idiopathic myelofibrosis; LAP, leukocyte alkaline phosphatase. (From Murphy S: Primary thrombocytopenia. p. 234. In Williams JD et al (eds): Hematology, 4th Ed. McGraw-Hill, New York, 1990, with permission.)*

TABLE 5-1 DEFINITIONS OF ACCELERATED AND BLASTIC PHASES OF CML

A. Blastic phase CML
   30% or more blasts in the marrow or peripheral blood
   Extramedullary disease with localized immature blasts
B. Accelerated phase CML
   1. Multivariate analysis-derived criteria
      Peripheral blasts 15% or more
      Peripheral blasts plus promyelocytes 30% or more
      Peripheral basophils 20% or more
      Thrombocytopenia $<100 \times 10^3/\mu l$ unrelated to therapy
      Cytogenetic clonal evolution
   2. Other criteria used in common practice
      Increasing drug dosage requirement
      Splenomegaly unresponsive to therapy
      Marrow reticulin or collagen fibrosis
      Marrow or peripheral blasts $\geq 10\%$
      Marrow or peripheral basophils $\pm$ eosinophils 10% or
         greater
      Triad of WBC $> 50 \times 10^3/\mu l$, hematocrit <25% and
         platelets $<100 \times 10^3/\mu l$ not controlled with therapy
      Persistent unexplained fever or bone pains

(From Kantarjian HM, Deisseroth A, Kurzrock R, Estrov Z, Talpaz M: Chronic myelogenous leukemia: a concise update. Blood 82:691–703, 1993, with permission.)

TABLE 5-2 SYNTHESIS PROGNOSTIC STAGING SYSTEM FOR CML

Stage	No. of Poor-Prognosis Characteristics	Prognostic Determinants
1	0 or 1	Poor-Prognosis Characteristics
2	2	Age ≥ 60
		Spleen ≥ 10 cm below costal margin
		Blasts $\geq 3\%$ in blood or $\geq 3\%$ in marrow
3	≥ 3	Basophils $\geq 7\%$ in blood or $\geq 3\%$ in marrow
		Platelets $\geq 700 \times 10^3/\mu l$
4	Any accelerated phase characteristic	Accelerated-Phase Characteristics
		Cytogenetic clonal evolution
		Blasts $\geq 15\%$ in blood
		Blasts + promyelocytes $\geq 30\%$ in blood
		Basophils $\geq 20\%$ in blood
		Platelets $<100 \times 10^3/\mu l$

(From Kantarjian HM, Deisseroth A, Kurzrock R et al: Chronic myelogenous leukemia: a concise update. Blood 82:691–703, 1993, with permission)

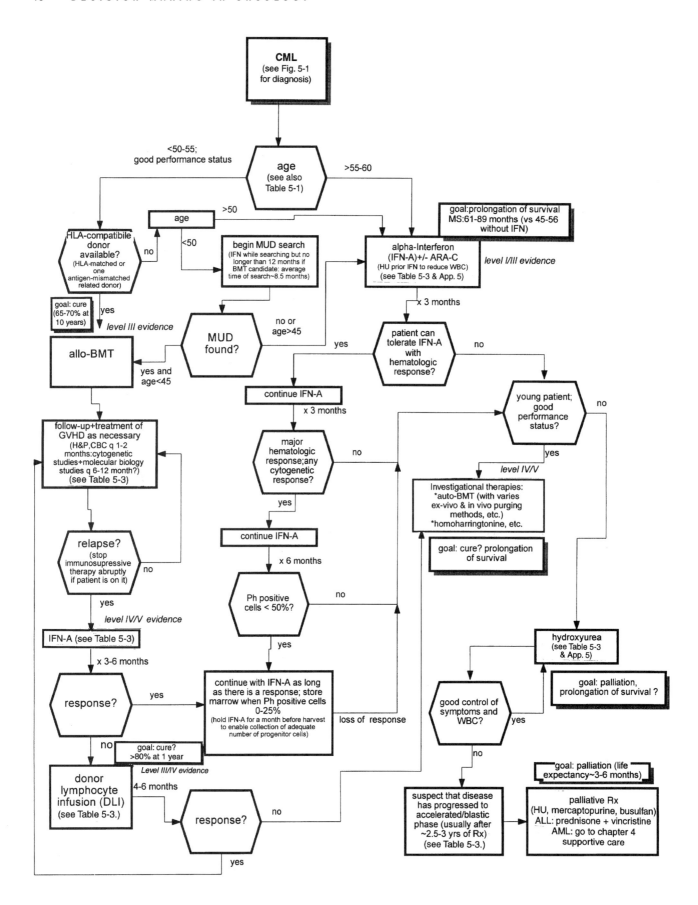

FIGURE 5-2 *Treatment of chronic myelogenous leukemia (CML). The goal of treatment is cure or prolongation of survival. Which goal will be pursued depends on the estimates of the risk/benefit of available treatment options. The major decision revolves around whether and when to perform the only known curative, but high-risk, procedure: bone marrow transplantation (BMT). The new element appears in the management of CML: determination of the optimal timing for BMT. Note that age cutoff when to offer BMT vs interferon therapy should not be taken as an absolute, and may vary depending on biological age of the patient (see also Table 5-3). Recommendations for BMT and interferon are based on solid evidence (level I and II); recommendations for other treatment options listed are based on less solid evidences (mainly level III and IV). WBC, white blood cell count; HLA, human leukocyte antigen; GVHD, graft vs host disease.*

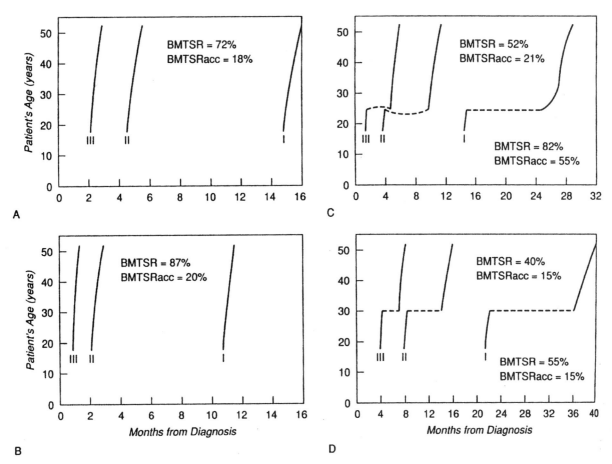

FIGURE 5-3 *(A–D) Time-threshold for BMT as a function of the survival in prognostic groups of CML (I, II, III), BMT success rates in the chronic (BMTSR) and accelerated/blastic (BMTSRacc) phases of a disease and patient's age. To determine optimal timing of BMT in the individual patient, first inquire about results of BMT at the particular center to which you are referring your patient (some results reported in the literature are shown in the figure). Second, determine prognostic group of CML for your patient. Third, draw the line from your patient's age on the ordinate to the corresponding prognostic group and then from this intersection draw a vertical line to the abscissa. Read this value as the optimal timing of BMT after CML is diagnosed. (From Denić S et al: Period Biol 91:394, 1989, with permission.) Prognostic groups are determined according to Sokal et al: Blood 63:789, 1984. A = exp.116 · (age—43.4), B = .0345 · (spleen size [cm]–7.51); C =.188 · (platelets/700)²–.563; D = 8.86·10⁻²· (% blast–2.1); G = A + B + C + D. If G <.78 then patient is in group I. If G> =.78 < = 1.3 then patient is in group II. If G > 1.3 then patient is in group III. Table 5-2 can also be used to determine prognostic group. Note that this method applies only if the estimated risk for leukemia relapse is negligible.*

TABLE 5-3 BENEFITS/RISKS OF PREFERRED MANAGEMENT ALTERNATIVES FOR CML

Type of Treatment	Complete Remission (CR) (%)	Disease-Free Survival (DFS) (%)	Outcomes Overall Survival (OS) (%)	Mortality (%)	Type of Evidence	References	Comment
			Decision point # 1: Who should be transplanted (how old) and when BMT should be performed?				

Numerous type III evidences (study on natural history of disease) have demonstrated that BMT is currently only curative treatment for CML. However, BMT is not risk-free procedure and appears that success is highly age-dependent. Most authors believe that BMT with HLA-matched or one-antigen mismatched related donor (MRD) should be offered to patients up to 55 years old (up to 65 according to Seattle group) and BMT with MUD (matched unrelated donor) should be considered in patients younger than 40–45 (younger than 56 according to Seattle group). Evidences for this recommendations are not solid (type IV and V). (Contemp Oncol 1994; Oct:46; Blood 1993;82:691; Blood 1993;82:2235; Semin Hematol 1993;30:1). Type III and IV evidences suggest that BMT should be performed preferably within 1 year of diagnosis (90% and 81% surviving 1 and 5 years after BMT, respectively): decision analysis suggest that optimal timing of BMT is function of patient's age, success of BMT procedure and prognostic stage of the disease (see Fig 5-2). Patients who are BMT candidates should not be treated with busulfan at all or with α-interferon longer than 12 months (see below).

Type of Treatment	CR (%)	DFS (%)	OS (%)	Mortality (%)	Type of Evidence	References	Comment
BMT (best preparative regimen not known: similar results reported with BU/CY and CY/TBI and VP-16/TBI)	85–99% (graft failure between 1% for MRD and16% for MUDs)	MRD By phase (at 5–10 years) Chronic phase: 40–70% Accelerated phase: 15–40% Blastic phase: 10% By age (chronic phase): <20 years 60–70% 20–29 years: 40–50% >30 years: 40% MUD 45 ± 21% (within 1 year of diagnosis) 36% ± 11% (after 1 year of diagnosis)	By phase Chronic phase: 65% 70% (10 years) Accelerated phase: 30–40% (7 years) Blastic phase: 10%–15% (5 years)	MRD Early 10–25% Late 10–25% Leukemia relapse Chronic phase: 5–30% Accelerated 50–60% Blastic: 60–80% MUD: 63%	Most evidences are level III and IV; data on preparative regimens are of level I; data on MUD of level IV	Contemp Oncol 1994;Oct:46, Blood 1993,82: 691, Blood 1993, 82:2235, Blood 1993;81:543, Blood 1994;84: 2036 Blood 1994, 84: 4368 J Clin Oncol 1992;10: 779 Ann Intern Med 1989,73:861 Blood 1995;85: 2263, Blood 1993, 83:2723	Data from single institutions studies are somewhat superior than ones listed; some data suggest that data might be poorer for centers performing less than 5 BMT/ year (Blood 1992;79:2771; level IV evidence)

Decision point # 2: α-interferon (IFN) vs. hydroxyurea (HU) (vs. busulfan) (BU)?

At least 4 randomized trials (level I evidence) and several single-arm studies (level III evidence) have demonstrated that α-interferon changes the natural history of CML leading to prolongation of survival (N Engl J Med 1994;330:820, Lancet 1995;345:1392, Blood 1994;84:4064, Blood 1995;86:906, Ann Intern Med 1995;122;124, Blood 1993;82:2975). Interferon was superior to busulfan in two randomized trials (Blood 1994;84:4064; Blood 1995;86: 906) and to hydroxyurea in at least one randomized trial (N Engl J Med 1994;330:820). However, in German randomized trial IFN was as effective as HU; survival was better both for IFN and HU if WBC where tightly controlled (Blood 1994;84:4064). HU was superior to BU in another randomized trial (Blood 1993;82:2235). Several level III evidences suggest that use of busulfan was associated with poorer outcome if BU was used prior BMT (Blood 1993;82:2235). BU, therefore, should not be used as a first line chemotherapy. One level I evidence (Leukemia Lymphoma 1992;11:181) and one level III evidence (J Clin Oncol 1992;10:772) suggest that treatment with IFN in combination with ARA-C result in better survival than IFN alone. Prolonged administration of IFN (> 12 months) has been associated with adverse BMT outcomes (level IV evidence: Blood 1995;10:2981).

| α-Interferon | Hematologic response: 60–80% Cytogenetic response: major [(Ph) suppression %]: 30–40% Complete: 7–24% | Median karyotypic response duration for nonrelapsing patients (months): 30–46 Relapse-free karyotypic response: 35–82% | Median survival: 61–89 months (45 months for BU; 56.4 months for HU) | Mortality: 0.45%, flu-like side effects: ~90% (10–25% will discontinue because of adverse effects); other grade III/IV toxicity occur in ~5% immune-mediated (hypothyroidsm, hemolytic anemia; SLE): 5% | Level I and level III | N Engl J Med 1994; 330:820 Lancet 1995;345:1392 Blood 1994;84: 4064 Blood 1995; 86:906 Ann Intern Med 1995;122:124, Blood 1993;82: 2975 Lancet 1995; 346:984 Lancet 1996;347:57 J Clin Oncol 1995;13: 2401 | Which is optimal dose of IFN is currently unresolved. Most data suggest that 5 million U/m^2 daily is associated with better responses than lower doses (Blood 1993;82:691). However, one type III evidence suggest that 2 million U/m^2 for 28 days and then 3 times a week is as effective as higher doses (and yet less toxic and less costly). (Ann Intern Med 1994; 121:736) |
| Donor lymphocyte infusion (optimal dose not known, but can be as little as 10^7/kg) | 60–70% | 85–100% (at 1–2 years of follow-up) | 85–100% (at 1–2 years of follow-up) | Overall mortality: 22% pancytopenia GVHD: 80–90% | Level III and IV | Blood 1993;82:3211, Blood 1994;83: 3377, Blood 1993; 82:2310, N Engl J Med 1994;330: 100, J Clin Oncol 1993;11:513 | Should we commence treatment after molecular relapse is detected or wait until patient is in hematologic and cytogenetic relapse? Some data suggest that better response is obtained if treatment starts in molecular relapse (level V evidence; Blood 1994;83:3377 |

Decision Point #3: What is the best salvage treatment after BMT failed?
(Donor Lymphocyte Infusion vs. Interferon vs. Second BMT)

All evidences indirect (level III or IV). Second BMT is feasible but associated with high mortality (~65%). Donor lymphocyte infusion (DLI) appears to be very effective but are also associated with severe adverse effects (see below). IFN induced complete cytogenetic response in 31% patients with 25% remaining in CR after 4–6.5 years of follow-up (Blood 1992;80:1437 Contemp Oncol 1994;oct 4). However, in another retrospective study IFN improved survival only at 2 years with no difference in 6 years survival from conservatively treated group (Blood 1993;82:3211). Most authors recommend stopping cyclosporine if patient is taking it (Bone Marrow Transplant 1992;10:391) followed by trial with IFN and DLI in those patients who failed IFN.

Decision Point #4: How to follow the patient?

Patient should be clinically seen every 2–3 months if he/she is stable (level V evidence). Serial cytogenetic and polymerase chain reaction (PCR) studies to detect 1 abnormal cell out of 1 million cells is performed every 6 months. Results of positive bcr/abl transcripts have been associated with conflicting results. Positive PCR reaction at 3 months was of no value in predicting CML relapse. At 6 and 12 months PCR positivity indicates likelihood of 38% and 30% relapse, respectively, but is not predictive for any particular patient (Blood 1995;85:2632). Other studies showed lack of prediction for CML relapse (Blood 1993;81:1089). Also, bcr/abl transcripts are frequently at low levels detected in healthy adults (~ 30%; Blood 1995;86:3118). Therefore, we believe that positive Southern blot analysis (equivalevent to cytogenetic studies) can be used to diagnose relapse but that PCR studies for bcr/abl should be pursued only within the context of investigational studies.

TREATMENT

Goals of treatments in managements of CML vary from cure to prolongation of survival to maintaining good quality of life by effective palliative treatment. Traditional treatment of CML includes chemotherapy agents such as *busulfan* or *hydroxyurea*. This treatment, however, does not lead to cytogenetic remission (Ph[1] does not disappear) and thus does not change the natural history of the disease. The role of these agents is mainly palliative. In several trials, patients treated with *α-interferon* have prolonged survival in comparison with conservative treatment. Currently, *bone marrow transplantation (BMT)* is considered the only possible curative treatment for CML. This is not a risk-free procedure, however, and carries a mortality rate between 5% and 30% (and up to 46% in some series). *Given the high risk associated with BMT, and the chronic nature of the disease, determination of benefit/risks of available treatment options and the optimal timing of BMT represent the key reasoning element in the management of patients with CML.* Figure 5-2 shows a method for determination of this time-threshold for BMT in *an individual patient* (for a group of CML patients as a whole, some data indicate that optimal timing would be within first year of diagnosis; see also Table 5-3.). Figure 5-3. outline details of clinical management of CML.

SUGGESTED READINGS

Clift RA, Appelbaum FR, Thomas ED: Treatment of chronic myeloid leukemia by marrow transplantation. Blood 82:1954–1956, 1993

Denic S, Djulbegovic B, Ridzanovic Z: Optimal timing of bone marrow transplantation in chronic myelogenous leukemia. Period Biol 91:391–396, 1989

Kantarjian HM, Deisseroth A, Kurzrock R et al: Chronic myelogenous leukemia: a concise update. Blood 82:691–703, 1993

Kumar L, Gulati SC: Alpha-interferon in chronic myelogenous leukaemia. Lancet 346:984–985, 1995

Kurzrock R, Kantarjian HM, Shtalrid M et al: Philadelphia chromosome-negative chronic myelogenous leukemia without breakpoint cluster region rearrangement: a chronic myeloid leukemia with a distinct clinical course. Blood 75:445–452, 1990

Shtalrid M, Talpaz M, Blick M et al: Philadelphia chromosome-negative chronic myelogenous leukemia with breakpoint cluster region rearrangement:molecular analysis, clinical characteristics and response to therapy. J Clin Oncol 6:1569–1575, 1988

6 Chronic Lymphocytic Leukemia

Benjamin Djulbegović

Incidence: 6/100,000 population

Main modality of treatment: Observation; chemotherapy

Goal of treatment: Prolongation of survival and palliation

Prognosis (median survival):

Stage A: 14 years

Stage B: 5 years

Stage C: 2.5 years

Chronic lymphocytic leukemia (CLL) is a disease characterized by the clonal proliferation and accumulation of neoplastic lymphocytes. The etiology of CLL is not known, but it is the only type of leukemia that is not associated with exposure to irradiation. CLL is the most common type of leukemia, with an age-adjusted incidence of 5.2 per 100,000 in the 55 to 59 age range and 30.4 per 100,000 in the 80 to 84 age range; the incidence in men is about twice that in women. This is a disease predominantly of the older population with a median age of an onset in the seventh decade. It is seen in less than 10% to 15% of people younger than 50.

DIAGNOSIS

Diagnosis of CLL is easy. It is usually suspected and diagnosed after the blood count test discloses an increased number of lymphocytes (see Table 6-1 for diagnostic criteria). Phenotypically, CLL is a B-cell disease in more than 95% of all cases. Monoclonality is proven by the presence of either κ or λ light chains on the cell surface. A unique feature of CLL is the presence of CD5 antigen. Some investigators feel that if CD5 is not found on cells, a diagnosis of CLL should be questioned (the sensitivity of this test is close to 100%).

TABLE 6-1 CHRONIC LYMPHOCYTIC LEUKEMIA: DIAGNOSTIC CRITERIA[a]

1.	Absolute lymphocytosis in peripheral blood > 5 × 10⁹/L (NCI/Working Group) > 10 × 10⁹/L (IWCLL)
2.	The majority of lymphocytes should be small and mature in appearance Morphologic subtypes:
2.1	Typical or classic CLL: <10% atypical lymphocytes
2.2	CLL/PLL: prolymphocytes in blood between 11% and 54%
2.3	Atypical or mixed: variable proportion of atypical lymphocytes; < 10% prolymphocytes
3.	Characteristic immunophenotype SmIg +/–, CD5+, CD19+, CD20+, CD21+, CD23+, FM7–/+, CD22 +/–
4.	Bone marrow infiltration > 30% lymphocytes in bone marrow aspirate, or consistent pattern in bone marrow biopsy

Abbreviations: IWCLL, international workshop on CLL; PLL, prolymphocytic leukemia; SmIg, surface membrane immunoglobulin.

[a]CD5 and CD19 antigens are present in 98% to 100% of cases; CD21 in about 90% of cases, other antigens are expressed less frequently; flow-cytometry is the best test to make a distinction between CLL and other differential diagnostic possibilities (such as reactive lymphocytosis, PLL, lymphoplasmacytoid lymphoma, hairy cell leukemia, splenic lymphoma with villous lymphocytes, marginal zone B-cell lymphoma, mantle-cell lymphoma, or follicular lymphoma).

(From Montserrat E, Rozman C: Chronic lymphocytic leukemia: present status. Ann Oncol 6:223, 1995, with permission.)

TABLE 6-2 **STAGING SYSTEM USED FOR CLL**

Staging System	Stage	Clinical Features	Median Survival (yr)
Rai			
Low risk	0	Lymphocytosis alone	14.5
Intermediate risk	I	Lymphocytosis, lymphadenopathy	(9)
	II	Lymphocytosis, spleen or liver enlargement (or both)	7.5 (5)
High risk	III	Lymphocytosis, anemia (hemoglobin < 11 g/dl)	
	IV	Lymphocytosis, thrombocytopenia (<100,000/mm³)	2.5
Binet[a]	A	No anemia, no thrombocytopenia <3 lymph-enlarged lymphoid areas	14
	B	No anemia, no thrombocytopenia >3 lymph-enlarged lymphoid areas	5
	C	Anemia (hemoglobin < 10 g/dl), thrombocytopenia (<100,000/mm³), or both	2.5

[a]The Binet staging system evaluates enlargement of the following: lymph nodes (unilateral or bilateral) in the head and neck, axillae, and groin; spleen; and liver.

(From Rozman C, Montserat E: Chronic lymphocytic leukemia. N Engl J Med 333: 1055, 1995, with permission.)

TABLE 6-3 **CHRONIC LYMPHOCYTIC LEUKEMIA: PROGNOSTIC FACTORS[a]**

Parameter	Median Survival (yr)
Bone marrow histopathologic pattern	
Nondiffuse	14
Diffuse	3–5
Number of lymphocytes in blood	
< 50,000/mm³	12
>50,000/mm³	4
Doubling time	
> 12 months	15
≤ 12 months	6
Lymphocyte morphology in peripheral blood	
< 5% prolymphocytes	5–6
> 5% prolymphocytes	3–4
Cytogenetic abnormalities	
Normal karyotype	>10
Multiple and complex abnormalities	5–6

[a]Number of lymphocytes and prolymphocytes in blood as well as doubling time behave as continuous variables: the higher the number of cells or the shorter the doubling time, the poorer the prognosis. In most instances, these poor-risk factors are not found alone but accompanying advanced disease.

(From Rozman C, Montserat E: Chronic lymphocytic leukemia. N Engl J Med 333: 1055, 1995, with permission.)

The diagnosis of CLL does not imply the need for therapy. CLL is a heterogeneous disease with a natural history that can vary from an indolent course and normal life expectancy to progressive, ultimately fatal, disease and short life expectancy. *The key reasoning process in the management of patients with CLL relates to identification of those patients with an indolent course of disease (and thus no need for therapy) and those with progressive disease (where therapeutic intervention may lead to prolongation of survival).* The use of two staging systems and prognostic factors are widely used to help differentiate patients who require therapy from those for whom follow-up is sufficient. The survival correlates very well with the tumor burden, which is measured by determination of the stage (Table 6-2). However, determination of the stage does not provide information on a likelihood of the progression of the disease in a given patient. In this regard, identification of other variables may help provide additional prognostic information (Tables 6-3, 6-4, and 6-5). Combining the staging systems with prognostic variables serve to define the disease at low risk, intermediate risk, or high risk for rapid progression. This categorization helps to formulate the treatment strategy regarding whether and when a patient with CLL should be treated. As shown in Figure 6-1, this management can vary from watchful waiting to aggressive therapy.

TREATMENT GOALS

At the present time, CLL is not a curative disease. Goals of the treatment are, therefore, prolongation

FIGURE 6-1 *Treatment of chronic lymphocytic leukemia (CLL). Note that the diagnosis of CLL does not imply the need for therapy. The strategy shown is according to a current literature consensus based on some type I, but mainly type III, evidence (see also Table 6-6). (For doses and treatment protocols, see Appendix 6.) XRT, radiation therapy; BMT, bone marrow transplant; TBI, total body irradiation.*

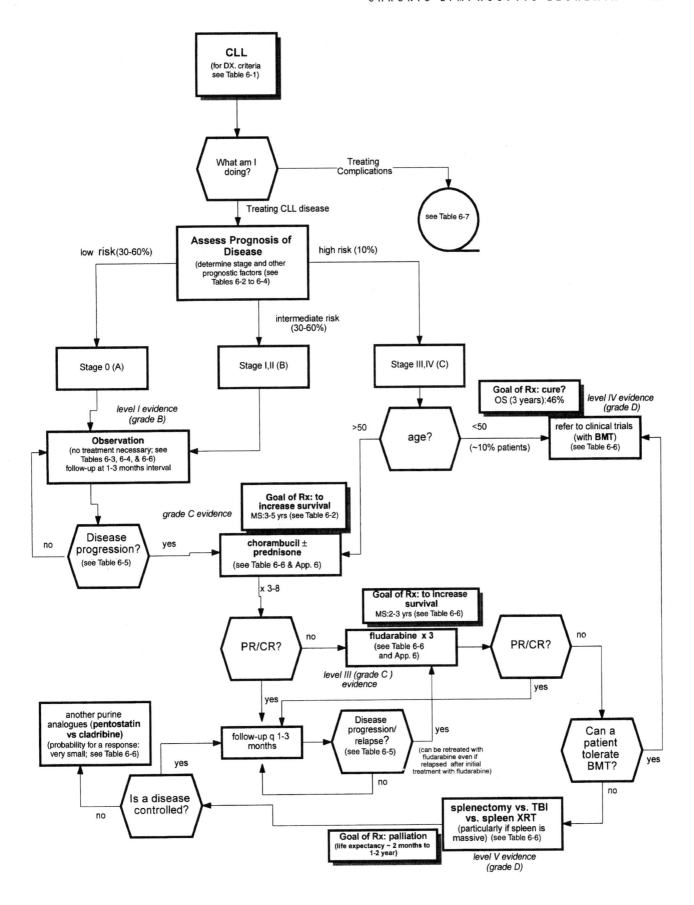

TABLE 6-4 SMOLDERING CLL[a]

Montserrat and Rozman criteria (1988)
Stage A
  Nondiffuse bone marrow histopathology
  Hemoglobin ≥13 g dl
  Blood lymphocytes ≤ 30 × 10⁹/L
  Lymphocyte doubling time > 12 months
French Cooperative Group on CLL criteria
A-1
  Stage A
  Hemoglobin >12 g/dl
  Blood lymphocytes <30,000/mm³
A-2
  Stage A
  Hemoglobin <12 g dl
    Blood lymphocytes ≥ 30,000/mm³
    Lymphocytes in bone marrow aspirate <80%
    Number of lymphoid areas[b] enlarged <2

[a]The patients with "smoldering" CLL have a life expectancy that is not different from the sex and age-matched population. After 3 years, only about 5% of these patients show disease progression.

[b]Lymphoid areas considered are cervical, axillary, and inguinal lymphadenopathy (whether unilateral or bilateral), spleen, and liver.

(From Montserrat E, Rozman C: Chronic lymphocytic leukaemia: prognostic factors and natural history. Baillières Clin Haematol 6:860, 1993, with permission.)

TABLE 6-5 INDICATIONS FOR INSTITUTION OF THERAPY IN CLL

1. Progressive disease-related symptoms.
2. Evidence of progressive marrow failure (i.e., worsening anemia, thrombocytopenia, recurrent sepsis associated with hypogammaglobulinemia).
3. Autoimmune hemolytic anemia or immune thrombocytopenia.
4. Massive splenomegaly with or without evidence of hypersplenism.
5. Bulky disease as evidenced by large lymphoid masses.
6. Progressive hyperlymphocytosis.

    The rate of increase of blood lymphocyte count is usually a more reliable indicator than the absolute number. Therapy is generally not withheld when the count is higher than 150,000/mm³. Leukostasis, which is associated with a high leukocyte count in other leukemias, is seldom encountered in CLL, but complications from hyperviscosity syndrome of hyperleukocytosis have been reported in CLL Leukopheresis should be the first step when the starting blood count is in excess of 350,000/mm³ followed by chemotherapy (after 3–4 treatments on a cell separator machine). In these cases, allopurinol should always be added to prevent tumor lysis syndrome (see also Appendix 6.)

(Adapted from Rai KR, Kalra J: Chronic lymphocytic leukemia. p. 251. In Brain MC, Carbone PP (eds): Current Therapy in Hematology/Oncology. CV Mosby, St. Louis, 1995, with permission.)

of survival and maintaining good quality of life. To achieve these goals, the optimal answer to decisions listed in Table 6-6 must be found. Figure 6-1 and Table 6-6 provide current answers to these questions.

COMPLICATIONS

Beside treatment of the disease, treating complications of the disease is very important, such as infections, hemolytic anemia, and thrombocytopenia. The most common cause of death in CLL is related to infections secondary to disease-induced or treatment-induced neutropenia or immunodeficiency. The second common cause of death is related to bleeding complications, hepatic failure, and wasting and inanition. Finally, death may result from progression to large-cell lymphoma, acute leukemia, or prolymphocytoid leukemia. Table 6-7 shows the most common complications

associated with CLL along with their optimal management.

SUGGESTED READINGS

Cheson BD: Chronic Lymphocytic Leukemia. Marcel Dekker, New York, 1993

Dighiero G, Travedo P, Chevret S et al. B-cell chronic lymphocytic leukemia present status and future directions. Blood 78:1901–1914, 1991

Faguet GB: Chronic lymphocytic leukemia: an updated review. J Clin Oncol 12:1974–1990, 1994

Foon KA, Rai KR, Gale PR. Chronic lymphocytic leukemia: new insights into biology and therapy. Ann Intern Med 113:525–539, 1990

International Workshop on Chronic Lymphocytic Leukemia: Chronic Lymphocytic leukemia: recommendations for diagnosis, staging and response criteria. Ann Intern Med 110:236–238, 1989

Molica S: Progression and survival in early chronic lymphocytic leukemia. Blood 78:895–899, 1991

O'Brien S, del Giglio A, Keating M: Advances in the biology and treatment of B-cell chronic lymphocytic leukemia. Blood 85:307–318, 1995

Rozman C, Montserat E: Chronic lymphocytic leukemia. N Engl J Med 333:1052–1057, 1995

TABLE 6-6 BENEFITS/RISKS OF PREFERRED MANAGEMENT ALTERNATIVES FOR CLL (AS SHOWN IN FIG. 6-1)

Type of Treatment	Complete Remission (CR) (%)	Disease-Free Survival (DFS)(%)	Overall Survival (OS) (%)	Outcomes Mortality (%)	Type of Evidence	References	Comment

Decision Point #1: What is the best treatment for early stages CLL?
(observation with deferred treatment vs chemoRx)

Type I evidence and numerous type III evidences (study on natural history of disease; e.g., Blood 1991;78:1545, Blood 1991;78:1545) favors no treatment until progression of a disease (see also Table 6-4).

Observation (deferred treatment)	1%(CR)+2% (PR)	Stable disease 74%	85% (at 8 years)	0%	Level I	Blood 1990;75:1414	Survival appears to be worse in treated group secondary to increase incidence of epithelial cancers

Decision Point #2: What is the best first line treatment for progressive and advanced disease?
(Chlorambucil vs. CVP vs. CHOP vs. Fludarabine)

Chlorambucil is still recommended because inconsistent results from randomized trials. CHOP was superior to CVP in stage C in French trial (Nouv Rev Fr Hematol 1988;30:449) but not to chlorambucil in Danish trial (Nouv Rev Fr Hematol 1988;30:433); finally fludarabine demonstrated a higher response rate to CHOP, CAP or chlorambucil, but longer follow-up is needed to determine if this higher CR will result in improvement in survival (Blood 1995;86:607a; Blood 1994;84:461a; Blood 1993;82:199a). In recent European randomized trial of patients with Binet stage B or C, fludarabine showed higher CR than CAP (60 vs 44%); in previously untreated group median duration of CR was 179 days for CAP and was not reached for fludarabine; this may translate into survival advantage for fludarabine which was 4.3 years for CAP and still has not been reached for fludarabine (p = 0.087) (at 4.3 years 67% of patients treated with fludarabine are alive) (Lancet 1996;347:1422–38)

| Chlorambucil | 1%–10% | 38–87% | 45% (5 years, B stage) 25%–36% (C stage) | 0 (?) (usually well tolerated drug, but can aggravate pancytopenia if given in pancytopenic phase without steroids) | Grade C (inconsistency in results from level II evidences) | JOCO 1994;12:1974, NEJM1995;333: 1052, Blood 1995; 85:307 | In recent U.S. randomized trial CR for fludarabine was 33% vs. 8% for chlorambucil (Blood 1995); in European trial (Lancet 1996; 347:1432) fludarabine also induced more CRs (60 vs 44%) than CAP; these CRs were more durable and may translate into survival advantage for previously untreated patients. However, 5% mortality was noted in fludarabine group (which was not different from CAP toxicity) but it is almost certainly higher than for chlorambucil. |

(Continues)

TABLE 6-6 (Continued)

Type of Treatment	Complete Remission (CR) (%)	Disease-Free Survival (DFS)(%)	Overall Survival (OS) (%)	Mortality (%)	Type of Evidence	References	Comment
			Outcomes				

Decision Point #3: What is the best salvage treatment after chlorambucil failed?

(Which purine analogue?)

Type III evidence favors use of purine analogue after first line treatment failed. Most data exist regarding the use of fludarabine, but no direct comparison exists between fludarabine vs. cladribine vs. pentostatin. Fludarabine seems to have higher response rate than other two purine analogues (type III and IV evidences)

Type of Treatment	Complete Remission (CR) (%)	Disease-Free Survival (DFS)(%)	Overall Survival (OS) (%)	Mortality (%)	Type of Evidence	References	Comment
Fludarabine	28–57%	10–36%	29 months ~20% (5 years for responding patients; 9 weeks for non-responding patients)	1.5% (sepsis:3%–13%); long-term immuno-suppressive effects with prolonged lymphocytopenia (CD4) exists for about 1 year; antibiotic prophylaxis is, therefore, recommended (JOCO 1995; 13:2431)	Level III	Blood 1993;81: 2878, Blood 1993;82:1695	Median time to progression: 21 months; response rates higher in previously untreated patients (CR ~ 35% + PR ~ 45%)
Cladribine	0–37%	28–31%	8–28 months (median survival) for responding patients; 3.5 months for non-responding patients)	18% (mostly due to fungal infections); thrombocytopenia is usual dose-limiting toxicity	Level III	JOCO 1993;11: 679, JOCO 1995; 13:983	Median time to progression: 16 months; response rates higher in previously untreated patients (CR ~ 25% + PR ~ 60%)

Decision Point #4: Is there effective salvage therapy after fludarabine failed?

Conflicting type III evidence points to the existence of non-cross resistance between fludarabine and other purine analogues (cladribine). Most data, however, suggest that use of cladribine will likely not benefit patient after fludarabine failure.

Type of Treatment	Complete Remission (CR) (%)	Disease-Free Survival (DFS)(%)	Overall Survival (OS) (%)	Mortality (%)	Type of Evidence	References	Comment
Cladribine	0–25%	7–75%	~10% at 18 months 3 months (median survival)	35% (within 2 months) (mostly due to infection)	Level III and IV	NEJM1992;327: 1056, NEJM 1994; 330:319	One small study (NEJM 1992; 327:1056) with 4 patients suggested non-cross resistance; larger study (28 patients) suggested opposite

Decision Point #5: Who and when should be transplanted with CLL?

Type III evidence favors use of purine analogue after first line treatment failed. Type III and IV evidence suggest high long-term disease-free survival but follow-up is still short. Type V evidence suggest that patients younger than 55 with HLA identical donor should be eligible for allo-transplant, and patients younger than 65 should be eligible for auto-BMT. No conclusive evidence suggest that allo-BMT is superior to auto-BMT. Very few data exist for BMT with MUD (matched-unrelated donor). Optimal timing of BMT is not known, but most authors believe it should be attempted with minimal residual disease being present (after CR or solid PR is achieved) or shortly after disease progressed after treatment with purine analogues.

(Molecular remissions have been achieved with **BMT**. It is not known whether this will translate into the cure. Type III and **IV** evidence suggest high long-term disease-free survival but follow-up is still short. Type **V** evidence suggest that patients younger than 55 with **HLA** identical donor should be eligible for allo-transplant, and patients younger than 65 should be eligible for auto-BMT. No conclusive evidence suggest that allo-BMT is superior to auto-BMT. Very few data exist for **BMT** with **MUD** (matched-unrelated donor). Optimal timing of **BMT** is not known, but most authors believe it should be attempted with minimal residual disease being present (after **CR** or solid **PR** is achieved) or shortly after disease progressed after treatment with purine analogues.

Auto-BMT	80–90%	10–15% 3 years	40–45% at 5 years	7–18%	Level III and IV	JOCO 1994;12:748; Blood 1995;86:1813a	The studies cited included 40 patients only; mixed patients characteristics; some had marrow purged
Allo-BMT	70–80%	10–15%	48–90% at 3 years (68% in stage I, 57% in stage II, 34% in stage IV)	10–50% (47% in largest series reported for matched HLA-identical siblings)	Level IV/V	JOCO 1994;12: 748, Blood 1995; 86:1813a, Ann Intern Med 1996; 124:311	Patients with mixed clinical characteristics; some patients received T-cell depleted marrow; usual conditioning regimen;TBI + cyclophosphamide

Decision Point # 6: Splenectomy vs. Splenic Irradiation (XRT) for palliation?

(Type IV/V evidence suggest that splenectomy or splenic XRT can prolong survival in patients with advanced stages but role of these treatment modalities is usually reserved for palliation. No comparative studies exist, but most authors would operate on patients with refractory cytopenias and symptomatic splenomegaly and reserve splenic XRT for patients who are poor surgical candidates. However, one randomized trial (chlorambucil vs. penta COP vs. Splenic XRT) showed increased survival for irradiated patients (59 months vs 36 months)(Nouv Re Fr Hematol 1988;30:423)

Spenectomy	hemoglobin increased >11 g/dll in 77%; platelets increased > 100,000 mm^3 in 70%; both hemoglobin and platelets increased in 64% cases	41 months (median survival); ~ 20% at 8 years; 14 months (median survival) in non-responders (none alive at 5 years)	Operative mortality 4% (morbidity 26%)	Level IV	Am J Med 1992;93: 435	Response to splenic XRT is about 25%

TABLE 6-7 MANAGEMENT OF COMPLICATIONS ASSOCIATED WITH CLL

Complication/Management	% Patients Affected
Direct antiglobulin test (positive results)	8–35
Hemolytic anemia	
Prednisone at .8 mg/kg BW per day by mouth for two weeks. If anemia has started to improve, the prednisone dose is reduced by 50% at each two-week interval for an overall continous therapy of 6 weeks. Thereafter, prednisone may be given for 1 week every month at 0.5 mg/kg BW for an additional 4–6 months.[a]	
Immune thrombocytopenia	2
See above	
Anemia (nonhemolytic)[b]	
Recombinant erythropoietin (epo) 150 U/kg three times a week subcutaneous with an escalation of 50 U/kg up to a maximum of 300 U/kg three times a week.Response rate:55% independent of epo levels.	
Neutropenia	0.5
G-CSF or GM-CSF may overcome neutropenia related to treatment[c].	
Pure red-cell aplasia	0.5
Cyclosporine at 7–12 mg/kg[d] by mouth daily in single dose with breakfast. Titrate the dose to maintain the whole blood through level at 200–700 ng/ml or plasma level of 40–200 ng/ml. Administer prednisone at 40–60 mg/day along with cyclosporine. Monitor liver and renal functions regularly.	
Expected time to response: 14 ± 3 days. If response is noted, discontinue steroids and cyclosporine slowly over several months. If side effects or infection occur, stop treatment.[e]	
Hypogammaglobulinemia	20–60
Infections	
Most frequent causes—*Streptococcus pneumoniae, Staphylococcus, Haemophilus influenzae, Candida, Aspergillus,* varicella-zoster virus.	
Other causes—*Legionella, Pneumocystis carinii, Listeria, Toxoplasma gondii,* cytomegalvirus.[f]	
High-dose immunoglobulin (400 mg/kg body weight) every three weeks. (Number of infections are decreased, but survival is not affected. This therapy results in gain of 0.8 quality-adjusted day per patient per year at a cost of $6,000,000 per quality-adjusted year of life gained.)[g]	
Disease transformation	
Prolymphocytoid leukemia	10
Disease not responsive to alkylating agents or prednisone: fludarabine may be effective (?)	
Large-cell lymphoma (Richter syndrome)	3–5
Combined chemotherapy. (CHOP-Bleo, VAD, MACOP-B); response rate: 42%; median survival: 5 months. (Patients who responded: median survival: ~1 year)[h]	
Acute leukemia (see Ch. 3)	<1
Multiple myeloma (see Ch. 11)	<1
Second cancers	5–15
Most frequent sites: skin, lung, gastrointestinal tract.	

[a]*Data from Rai KR and Kalra J. Chronic lymphocytic leukemia. p. 251. In Brain MC, Carbone PP (eds): Current Therapy in Hematology/Oncology. Mosby, St. Louis, 1995.*

[b]*Type III evidence. Br J Haematol 89:627, 1995.*

[c]*Ann Hematol 62:32–34, 1991.*

[d]*In the USA, cyclosporine (Sandimmune) is manufactured as capsules of 25 and 100 mg.*

[e] *Type IV evidence (Am J Hematol 41:5, 1992); if there is contraindication to cyclosporine, try conventional therapy with alkylating agents (response time: 154 ± 97 days).*

[f] *These infections are especially common in patients treated with both purine analogues and prednisone.*

[g] *Type I evidence: N Engl J Med 319:902, 1988; cost-effectiveness analysis: N Engl J Med 325:81, 1991.*

However, lower doses (250 mg/kg) every four weeks may be as effective as higher doses (Br J Haematol 88:2309, 1994); cost-effectiveness analysis of lower doses is not, however, known.

[h] *JOCO 11:1985, 1993.*

(Modified from Rozman C and Montserat E: N Engl J Med 333:1055, 1995, with permission; treatment of infections related to hypogamma-globulinemia is based on level I evidence, the treatment of most other complications are based on levels III, IV, and V evidence.)

7 Hairy Cell Leukemia

Lung T. Yam

Incidence: 0.2 per 100,000/year (2% of all adult leukemias in the United States

Goal of treatment: Cure (?)

Main modality of treatment: Chemotherapy

Prognosis (median survival): Normal life expectancy for patients in complete remission (?) (82% disease-free survival at 3 years)

PRESENTING SIGNS

Hairy cell leukemia (HCL) is a rare disease characterized by splenomegaly, cytopenias, and neoplastic "hairy cells" in blood, marrow, and other hematopoietic organs. It composes 2% of all adult leukemias and occurs four times as often in males. Splenomegaly is found in 85%–95% of patients with massively enlarged spleens in 25%. The hairy cells possess distinct morphologic features and can be identified either by light or phase contrast microscopy. Since there may be few hairy cells in blood, and because bone marrow aspirate is not obtainable in 50% of cases, a bone marrow biopsy is recommended to confirm the diagnosis. Hairy cells are also identified by demonstration of tartrate-resistant acid phosphatase (in 95% or more of patients), and the expression of monoclonal surface immunoglobulin CD11c, CD19, CD20, CD22, and CD25.

MANAGEMENT

The natural course of HCL varies widely. About 10% of patients are asymptomatic and live a relatively normal, productive life for as long as 25 years with little or no medical intervention. Others may die within 1 year after diagnosis. The median survival of patients with HCL is 4 to 5 years. The primary cause of death is hematopoietic failure, particularly severe granulocytopenia, and fatal infections.

Treatment of HCL should be given according to the severity of the disease (Fig. 7-1). It may not be necessary for patients who are asymptomatic and have a hemoglobin of more than 10 g/dL, neutrophils equal to or more than 1,000/mm³, and platelets of 100,000/mm³ or more. However, such patients should be monitored by close observation. Patients who are symptomatic will need specific treatment. *Splenectomy* is indicated for those with massive splenomegaly, painful or ruptured spleen, and with infections or severe thrombocytopenia that precludes chemotherapy. The procedure is palliative and not curative. Those who respond to splenectomy may be monitored by close observation and may receive supportive care if needed. All other symptomatic patients should be treated with *systemic therapy*. These include patients with progressive disease, severe cytopenias, frequent infections, moderate splenomegaly, and those who either did not respond to or relapsed after splenectomy.

Systemic treatment for HCL is aimed at achieving durable, long-term remission and possible cure. Systemic chemotherapy is highly effective for HCL. A single course of 2-chloro-deoxyadenosine (2-

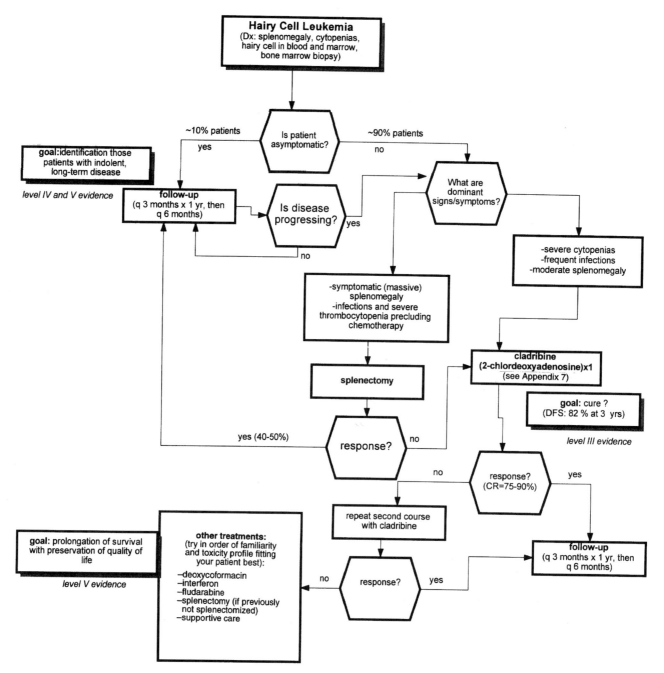

FIGURE 7-1 *Management of hairy cell leukemia (HCL). Assessment of a requirement for the treatment represents a key reasoning principle in the management of HCL. The goal of treatment is to achieve long-term remission and possible cure. Note need for awareness of the increased risk for secondary malignancies in the long-term follow-up of patients with HCL. Recommended strategy for the first-line treatment is based on level III evidence, and for the treatment of a relapse, on level V evidence. (Note that three randomized trials were performed to evaluate the effectiveness of pentostatin versus interferon [J Clin Oncol 13:974, 1995], splenectomy versus interferon [Am J Hematol 41:13, 1992], and low-versus high-dose of interferon [Blood 78:3133, 1991]. Based on single-arm studies, cladribine appears to be the most effective treatment with the most favorable toxicity profile and is considered the treatment of choice despite the lack of randomized trials, comparing its efficacy with other known active modalities in HCL.)*

CdA), 0.1 mg/kg/day for seven days is recommended. The response rate may be as high as 90%, and long-term complete remissions may reach 75% to 82%. Patients who do not respond or relapse on this form of treatment may be given a second course. Alternatively, they may be treated with deoxycoformycin or interferon-α. The treatment results of deoxycoformycin are very encouraging, although this drug is more toxic, more expensive, and less effective than 2-CdA. Treatment with interferon-α will result in complete remission in 5% of patients, normalization of the complete blood count in an additional 75%, and minor or no response in the remaining patients. The rare patient who fails on these treatments may be treated with fludarabine, splenectomy, and supportive measures.

SUGGESTED READINGS

Annino L, Ferrari A, Giona F et al: Deoxycoformycin induces long-lasting remissions in hairy cell leukemia: Clinical and biological results of two different regimens. Leukemia Lymphoma 14 (suppl 11):115, 1994

Beutler E: New chemotherapeutic agent: 2-chlorodeoxyadenosine. Semin Hematol 30:40, 1994

Bouroncle BA: The history of hairy cell leukemia: Characteristics of long-term survivors. Semin Oncol 11 (suppl 2):479, 1987

Cassileth PA, Cheuvart B, Spiers AS et al: Pentostatin induces durable remissions in hairy cell leukemia. J Clin Oncol 9:243, 1991

Golomb HM, Catovsky D, Golde DW: Hairy cell leukemia: a clinical review based on 71 cases. Ann Intern Med 89:677, 1978

Jaiyesimi IA, Kantarjian HM, Estey EH: Advances in therapy for hairy cell leukemia. Cancer 72:5, 1993

Kampmeier P, Spielberger R, Dickshin T et al: Increased incidence of second neoplasms in patients treated with interferon alpha 2b for hairy cell leukemia: a clinopathologic correlation. Blood 83:2931, 1991

Kantarjian HM, Schachner J, Keating MJ: Fludarabine therapy in hairy cell leukemia. Cancer 67:1291, 1991

Piro LD, Carrera CJ, Carson DA, Beutler E: Lasting remissions in hairy cell leukemia induced by a single infusion of 2-chlorodeoxyadenosine. N Engl J Med 322:1117, 1990

Quesada JR, Reuben J, Manning JT et al: Alpha interferon for induction of remission in hairy cell leukemia. N Engl J Med 310:15, 1984

Ratain MJ, Vardiman JW, Barker CM et al: Prognostic variables in hairy cell leukemia after splenectomy as initial therapy. Cancer 62:2420, 1988

Schwarting R, Stein H, Wang CY: The monoclonal antibodies as HCL I (α Leu 14) and aS HCL₃ (α Leu M5) allow the diagnosis of hairy cell leukemia. Blood 65:974, 1985

Yam LT, Janckila AJ, Lam KWK, Li CY: Cytochemistry of tartrate-resistant acid phosphatase: 15 years experience. Leukemia 1:285, 1987

8 Hodgkin's Lymphoma

Lung T. Yam
Benjamin Djulbegović

Prevalence: 1% of all malignancies

Incidence: ~7,400 new cases per year in the United States (2.8/100,000)

Goal of treatment: Cure in all stages

Main modality of treatment: Chemotherapy in advanced stages; radiation therapy (XRT) in early stages; combined modality (CMT) (chemo+XRT) for disease with unfavorable characteristics

Prognosis:

Stages IA and IIB:	OS (overall survival): ~80–85% at 10 years DFS (disease-free survival): ~70–75% at 10 years
Stage IIIA and IIIB:	OS: ~65–70% at 10 years DFS: ~30–45% at 10 years
Stage IVA + B:	OS: ~42 at 10 years DFS: ~18% at 10 years

Hodgkin's disease (HD) is a neoplastic disorder of the lymphoid tissues characterized by the presence of Reed-Sternberg giant cells in the appropirate cellular background of the involved tissues. It is an uncommon disorder comprising less than 1% of all malignancies. HD has a bimodal age distribution with peaks of incidence in the first and fifth decades. Overall, it affects males more often than females. However, the nodular subtype with mediastinal involvement predominates in females. The etiology of the disorder is uncertain, but viral infection has been implicated. Patients with this disease often present with painless lymphadenopathy. Table 8-1 show the prevalence of lymph node involvement in different areas of the lymph node system. Other findings include weight loss, fever, and excessive night sweats, especially in patients with advanced disease. Laboratory studies may help to assess activity or extent of disease, but are not diagnostic.

DIAGNOSIS

The diagnosis of HD rests primarily on histopathologic examination of involved tissues. The detection of Reed-Sternberg cells *and* the appreciation of the appropriate cellular background is essential to establish the diagnosis and to subclassify HD (Table 8-2). Immunophenotypic and molecular genetic techniques are not diagnostic, but may help to identify non-Hodgkin's lymphomas (NHL) in some cases of HD of the follicular lymphocyte predomi-

TABLE 8-1 APPARENT SITE OF ONSET OF HODGKIN'S DISEASE AS JUDGED BY THE LARGEST AREA OF INVOLVEMENT AT THE TIME OF DIAGNOSIS (348 PATIENTS)

Site	Percent
High cervical nodes	29
Supraclavicular nodes	41
Mediastinal structures	11
Axillary nodes	4
Abdominal nodes	13
Spleen	1

(Adapted from Teillet F et al: A reappraisal of clinical and biological signs in staging Hodgkin's disease. Cancer Res 31:1723, 1971, with permission.)

nance or lymphocyte depletion subtypes. Extent of disease is estimated by assessment of clinical findings and histopathologic examination of the involved tissues (Tables 8-3 and 8-4). The disease can be classified into limited (I and II) or extended (III and IV) stages and A or B subcategories. In contrast to NHL (see Chapter 9), which are usually disseminated at the time of diagnosis, HD appears to "spread" by sequential involvement of contagious nodes. Therefore, accurate staging is much more important in management of HD than in NHL, largely because treatment of early stages (e.g., I and II) may be radiation therapy (XRT) alone without systemic chemotherapy (see below).

TREATMENT

The treatment goal in HD is a cure with minimum morbidity and long-range toxicity. Many different effective therapeutic options are available. Selection of therapy with the least morbidity is equally important. Therefore, choosing the treatment with the best benefit/risk ratio dominates clinical reasoning in the management of patients with HD.

TABLE 8-2   HISTOPATHOLOGY OF HODGKIN'S DISEASE

Histologic Types	% Cases	Clinical Features
Lymphocyte predominance[a] (LP)	10	Limited disease; may progress to MC or LD if not cured
Nodular sclerosis (NS)	60	Mediastinal involvement common, often in young women
Mixed cellularity (MC)	20	B symptoms frequent
Lymphocyte depletion (LD)	10	Usually advanced (stage IV), often anergic

[a] Including the follicular and diffuse subtypes.

TABLE 8-3 ASSESSMENT OF HODGKIN'S DISEASE

History and physical examination
Complete blood counts
Erythrocyte sedimentation rate
Biochemical studies of blood (SMA-18)
Radiographic studies of chest (posteroanterior and lateral views)
Computed tomography of neck, chest, abdomen, and pelvis
Bipedal lymphangiography
Bilateral iliac crest marrow aspiration and biopsy
Studies used in special circumstances
    Radionuclide scanning (bone, gallium, liver, & spleen)
    Ultrasonography
    Magnetic resonance imaging
    Laparotomy

Abbreviation: SMA, sequential multichannel autoanalyzer.

The exact definition of stage of disease forms a basis for the choice of treatment(s). An optimal management include minimizing both the extent of treatment and extent of staging. (See Tables 8-3 and 8-4 and Figure 9-1 and Table 9-4 for the optimal

TABLE 8-4 STAGING AND CLASSIFICATION OF HODGKIN'S DISEASE[a]

Stage I	Involvement of a single lymph node region (I) or single extralymphatic site (I_E)
Stage II	Involvement of two or more lymph node, regions on the same side of the diaphragm (II) or localized involvement of an extralymphatic site and one or more lymph node regions on the same side of the diaphragm (II_E)
Stage III_1	Involvement of lymph nodes on both side of diaphragm; abdominal disease is limited to the upper abdomen (i.e., spleen, splenic hilar nodes, celiac nodes, porta hepatis node)
Stage III_2	Involvement of lymph nodes on both sides of diaphragm; abdominal disease includes para-aortic, mesenteric, and iliac involvement with or without disease in the upper abdomen
Stage IV	Disseminated involvement of one or more extralymphatic organs or tissues with or without associated lymph node disease
A	No symptoms
B	Fever, night sweats, or weight loss of more than 10% of body weight in the previous 6 months
X	Bulky disease (greater than 10 cm in maximum dimension; greater than one-third of the internal transverse diameter of the thorax at the level T5–T6)
E	Limited involvement of a single extranodal site
CS	Clinical stage: when based solely on physical examination and imaging techniques
PS	Pathologic stage: when based on biopsies

[a] The Ann Arbor staging classification, Cotswolds modification.
(From Lister et al: J Clin Oncol 7:1630, 1989, with permission.)

approach to staging in HD). It is important to note that there is an *inverse relationship between tumor burden and curability and between staging and the extent of treatment*. Overall the choice of treatment will depend on whether the patient is in an *early stage* (stage IA–IIB), *intermediate stage* (IIIA₁), or *advanced stage* (IIIA₂–IVB). The majority of authors consider presence of B symptoms beyond stage II of very important significance; accordingly advanced stages comprise all stages from IIB to IVB; we also accept this approach to HD, but consider patients with IIB with one or two symptoms only and ESR <30 mm to have a more favorable clinical course (see Figure 8-1 and Table 8-6).

Sometimes, however, patients present with the disease contiguous to nodal involvement (E disease; see Table 8-4) or with disseminated or diffuse organ involvement. An additional separate category will comprise patients with *bulky disease*, such as large mediastinal lymphadenopathy. Some modification of the general plan of the treatment may be necessary for those patients with less typical presentations.

In the management of HD several critical decisions can be identified. A major decision in the treatment of HD is *when to use XRT alone and when to use chemotherapy (CRx) or a combined modality (CMT) approach* (i.e., XRT+CRx). Intertwined with the decision about the use of XRT is the problem of *whether to perform staging laparotomy* to make sure that the disease is truly in the early stage before XRT is administered. Two solutions to this problem are as follows:

1. Always avoid laparotomy. Most authors believe that treatment should be based on the consideration of prognostic factors (Table 8-5): Use XRT in patients with favorable and CMT in patients with unfavorable prognostic factors.

2. Perform laparotomy if the laparotomy will alter determination of the stage, and this information will alter the treatment plan. XRT can be used when the estimated probability of early stages is greater than 90% to 95% (see Table 8-5). Conversely, if the estimated probability of an advanced stage is greater than 90% to 95%, the patient should be treated with systemic therapy, and laparotomy should be avoided. Laparotomy should be considered only in those patients with the probability of HD being in advanced stage greater than 10% and less than 90%.

The second decision-making problem is the *selection of a specific chemotherapy regimen* from among the more than 40 regimens described in the

TABLE 8-5 ESTIMATION OF THE PROBABILITY OF HODGKIN'S DISEASE BEING IN EARLY VS ADVANCED STAGE

Finding	PS(I+II) (%)	PSIII (%)	PSIV (%)
MC B male	19	46	35
MC B female	35	46	19
NS B male	37	50	13
NS B female	56	38	6
Age			
<16	61	35	4
>15<31	61	36	3
>30<46	54	40	4
>45	41	44	15
Left neck+	54	44	2
Left neck–	63	38	1
Right neck+	54	45	1
Mediastinum+	59	39	2
Mediastinum	55	42	3
Mediastinum			
Bulky disease		>50[a]	
CSIA female	91–93[a]		
CSIIA females			
<26 years old	91–93[a]		
CSIA LP males	91–93[a]		
CSIA above thyroid notch,			
LP or NS, ESR <10 mm	~95[a]		
CSI or CSII₂, no bulky			
disease, with ESR <30 mm			
if B symptoms present or			
ESR <50 mm if B symptoms			
absent	>81[a]		
PI >7.5[b]		>37	

CS, clinical stage; PS, pathological stage; LP Lymphocyte predominant; NS, nodular sclerosis; MC, mixed celllularity; ESR, erythrocyte sedimentation rate.

[a]Estimated from relapse risk.

[b]Prognostic Index (PI)=0.05* (age in years) + 1.0* (mediastinal involvement [1=no; 2=yes])+2.0* (pathologic grade [1=LP and NS1; 2=NS2 and MC])+1.0* (ESR [1=0–9; 2=10–39; 3=40+])–1.2* (sex [1=M; 2=F]). Note that survival for patients with clinical stage IA and IIA but with PI>7.5 is only about 60% at 10 years in comparison for patients with <5 that is about 95%.

(Data from Br J Heamatol 44: 347, 1980; J Clin Oncol 11:2258, 1993; J Clin Oncol 12:288, 1994; Blood 83:318, 1994; Lancet 1:967, 1985.)

literature. Cancer and leukemia group B (CALGB) randomized trial showed that a doxorubicin-containing regimen (ABVD) has a better benefit/risk ratio than two other popular regimens (MOPP and MOPP/ABVD) (see Table 8-6 and Appendix 8). Therefore, in patients in whom administration of doxorubicin is not contraindicated (e.g., older patients with cardiopulmonary disease) ABVD has emerged as preferred treatment for patients with advanced stage of HD.

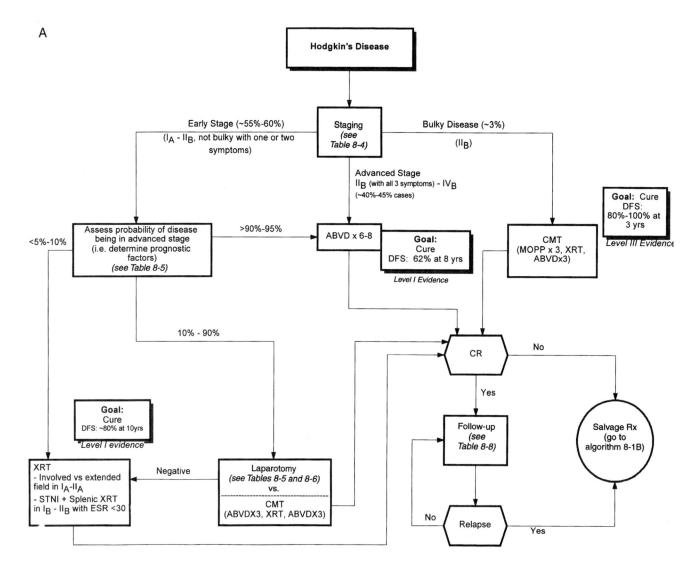

FIGURE 8-1 *(A & B) Management of Hodgkin's disease (HD). Accurate determination of the stage represents a key principle in the management of HD. This serves as a basis to enable formulation of **risk/benefit estimates** to tailor risk of the treatment without compromising the curative potential of the selected therapy to the individual patient. The goal of the treatment is cure in all stages. Data used for construction of the algorithm for primary treatment are of high-quality (mainly level I evidence). Data used to construct management of the patient with resistant/recurrent or residual disease are mainly indirect (level IV or are based on decision analyses). See Table 8-6 for supporting data for the constructions of the algorithms. Note: Patients themselves will play an increasing role in the decision management, since the treatment risk/benefit ratio could be highly individualized (e.g., wish for fertility or hair preservation; choice between alkylating agents and doxorubicin-containing regimens in patients over 50). See Table 8-7 for details on short- and long-term toxicities of commonly employed treatment modalities. See Appendix for details on administration of MOPP and ABVD regimens, which are the basis for all other chemotherapy regimens described in the literature; broken arrow indicates alternative strategy (see Table 8-6). XRT, radiation therapy; STNI, subtotal lymph node irradiation; CMT, combination modality treatment (i.e., XRT and chemotherapy); DFS, disease-free survival; Rx, treatment; LT, long term; BMT, bone marrow transplant; PBSC, peripheral blood system cells.*

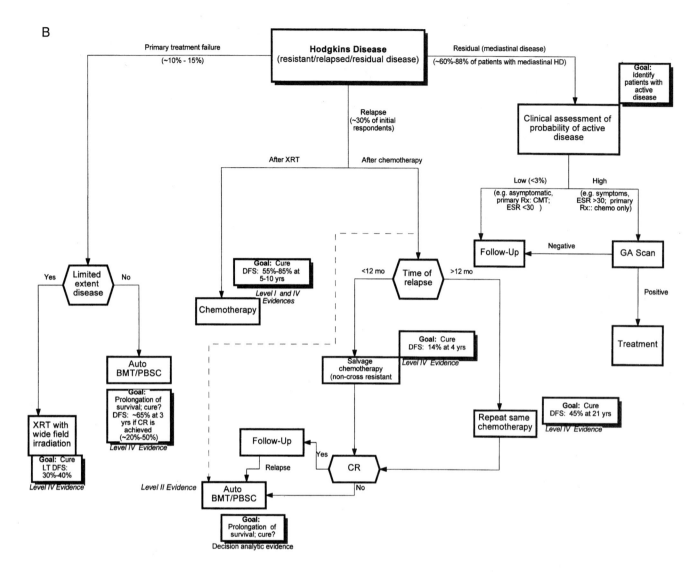

B

Controversy still exists about the optimal treatment for stages IIB to IIIA₁. Recommendations range from XRT to chemotherapy to CMT. However, most authors recommend full-course chemotherapy for these patients and we adopted this regimen (see Figure 8-1A and Table 8-6). However, patients in stage IIB with only one or two symptoms and ESR <30 mm can be successfully treated with XRT only (Fig. 8-1A).

Two further decision-making problems as to treatment are a *choice of salvage treatment and management of a residual mass after completion of initial treatment*. Figure 8-1B shows recommendation for the management of residual and refractory/relapsed disease, and Table 8-6 specifies supporting data for these recommendations.

Figures 8-1 and 8-2 are constructed on high-quality data (most are of level I, and good level III evidence). However, equally good evidence exists for some alternative treatments that are not incorporated in our algorithms (see Table 8-6). All these data indicate that in the management of HD we have not the treatment of choice but rather the choice of treatments. The reasoning principle, therefore, must rely on the individual estimate of the risk of treatment without compromising the curative potential of the selected therapy.

The high success in the management of HD has not come without cost. Table 8-7. show short- and long-term toxicities of the MOPP and ABVD regimens, which are the basis for all other chemotherapy regimens described in the literature. Figure 8-2 shows the cumulative risk of death from HD and treatment-related complications during the follow-up of patients with HD. Quality of life is also significantly impaired. Table 8-8. show recommendations for the follow-up.

With contemporary management, 70% to 80% of patients may expect to be cured. An additional

TABLE 8-6 BENEFITS/RISKS OF PREFERRED MANAGEMENT ALTERNATIVES FOR HODGKIN'S DISEASE (HD) AS SHOWN IN FIG. 8-1

Type of Treatment	Outcomes				Type of Evidence	References	Comment
	Complete Remission (CR) (%)	Disease-Free Survival (DFS) (%)	Overall Survival (OS) (%)	Mortality/Toxicity (%)			

Decision point # 1: What is the best first line treatment for early stages? Is staging laparotomy necessary?

XRT vs. ChemoRx vs. "gentle: chemoRx + XRT.

It appears that all these modalities have equal efficacy but that their toxicity profiles differ (see Table 8–7). XRT appears to be the treatment of choice for true early stage disease (PS IA–IIB) or for early clinical stages with favorable prognostic factors (see Table 8–5). In patients with unfavorable characteristics, the disease will be found intraabdominally in 24–36% of cases. These patients can be treated with combined XRT + chemoRx or undergo staging laparotomy. Decision analysis (Br J Haematol 1980;44:347) showed that XRT should be reserved for patients with probability of a disease being in early stages >90–95%; chemoRx should be given to the patients who have a probability of advanced HD > 90%; and laparotomy should be considered for all other patients. However, European randomized H6 trial demonstrated that XRT can be safely given to patients with favorable characteristics without resorting to laparotomy; the patients with unfavorable prognostic features should be given CMT (combined XRT + chemoRx), again without performing laparotomy (J Clin Oncol 1993;11:2258). At this point using "gentle" chemoRx + XRT cannot be considered a standard of care because of conflicting data on its toxicity despite its apparent efficacy (J Clin Oncol 1988;6:1822; J Clin Oncol 1994;12:288).

Type of Treatment	CR (%)	DFS (%)	OS (%)	Mortality/Toxicity (%)	Type of Evidence	References	Comment
XRT (STNI + splenic XRT)	98%	78 (at 6 years)	>93% (at 6 years)	0% (immediate treatment related deaths) (see Table 8-7 for long-term complications)	Level I	J Clin Oncol 1993; 11; 2258 Blood 1994; 83:318	Staging laparotomy can be avoided in the favorable prognostic group; no difference in outcome was found between the patients who were clinically and surgically staged. In general OS and FFP for stage PS IA–IIA is about 80% at 15 yrs; for PS IB–IIB OS and FFP is about 78% and 76% at 15 yrs, respectively.
ABVDx3 followed by XRT followed by ABVDx3	98%	88% (at 6 years)	91% (at 6 years)	1.3%; Decreased vital capacity in 12% of patients; 1-2% of secondary cancer	Level I	J Clin Oncol 1993; 11;2258	No staging laparotomy necessary in the unfavorable prognostic group; ABVD + XRT superior to MOPP + XRT in terms longer DFS and less toxicity

Decision point #2: What is the best first line treatment for IIB with all systemic symptoms and IIB bulky disease?

Five years freedom from relapse (FFR) in patients with all systemic symptoms (fever, night sweats weight loss) treated with XRT only is about 40%. Similarly, patients with IIB bulky disease treated with XRT only have 54% FFR at 12 years. Consequently, these patients should be treated with CMT (combined XRT + chemoRx programs).

| CMT (XRT + ChemoRx) | 85-100% | 91% (FFR at 12 years) 88-100% at 3 years | 90% at 12 years 85-100% at 3 years | Toxic death: 1.8% (due to XRT pneumonitis + *Pneumocystis carinii*) XRT pneumonitis: 18%; pericarditis: 3% (see also Table 8–7) | Level IV Level III | J Clin Oncol 1989; 7:1059 J Clin Oncol 1991: 9:227 Haematologica 1987;72:237 | Longer follow-up exists for MOPP +XRT; however, MOPP followed by XRT followed by ABVD is currently considered the treatment of choice for IIB bulky disease (data shown for IIB bulky disease only) |

Decision Point # 3: What is the best therapy for advanced stages? What is the best regimen?

For stages IIIA2-IVB most authors believe that chemoRx is the standard treatment of choice. Numerous regimens have been described in the literature (for dosages of the most common ones, see Appendix 8). Most physicians believe that overall ABVD regimen has the best benefit/risk ratio. In direct comparison with MOPP and MOPP/ABVD, ABVD therapy was superior to MOPP and was less toxic than MOPP/ABVD (level I evidence). Treatment of IIIA1 is less standardized. XRT alone appears to be inferior to chemoRx or CMT (J Clin Oncol 1985:3:1166) except for minimal stage IIIA1 disease (Int Radiat Oncol Bio Phys 1987: 13:1437). XRT also may play a role in a subgroup patients with bulky disease or nodular sclerosis where it did improve remission duration when used in adjuvant setting (Ann Intern Med 1994; 120:903). However, CMT does not appear to be superior to chemoRx alone (J Clin Oncol 1994::2:894) leading to recommendation that all patients with stage IIIA should be treated with chemoRx (N Engl J Med 1992;326:678). However, some single arm studies (level III evidence) show excellent benefit/risk ratio with short-term chemoRx (MOPPx2) followed by XRT (see below).

| ABVD | 82% | 61% (FFR at 5-8 years) | 73% at 5-7 years | Fatal: 3.2% (due to pulmonary and cardiac toxicity) (see also Table 8-7.) | Level I | N Engl J Med 1992 327:1478 | Data shown for stages IIIA2-IVB; while ABVD appears to be the regimen of choice, the choice of the treatment should be individualized according to the patient's other comorbid conditions (e.g., avoid ABVD in patients with cardiac/pulmonary disease) |

(Continues)

TABLE 8-6 *(Continued)*

Type of Treatment	Outcomes				Type of Evidence	References	Comment
	Complete Remission (CR) (%)	Disease-Free Survival (DFS) (%)	Overall Survival (OS) (%)	Mortality/toxicity (%)			
MOPPx2 followed by XRT		86% (FFP at 10 years)	84% at 10 years	1% of AML at 15 years; fertility preserved	Level III	J Clin Oncol 1988; 6:1293	Overall prognosis according to stage: OS and FFP at 11 yrs:IIIA: 70% and 30%; IIIB: 65% and 45%; IVA + B: 42% and 18% (from review of British National Lymphoma randomized studies) (Lancet 1985;1:1967)
ABVDx3, XRT, ABVDx3		80.8% at 7 years	87.7 at 7 years	radiation fibrosis (59%) no leukomogenesis no irreversible gonadal dysfunction; no cardiac toxicity	Level I	J Clin Oncol 1987; 5:27	Data shown for stages IIB-III; ABVD-XRT superior to MOPP-XRT

Decision Point #4: What is the best treatment of relapse/resistant disease (salvage therapy)?

About 10–5% patients with HD will experience primary treatment failure and about 30% of initial responders will relapse. Half of relapses occur within 1 year of CR and the rest within 3 years. Only 4% of patients will relapse after five years of CR (J Clin Oncol 1992;10:210). The approach to the patient with relapse (see Fig 8-1B) largely depends on the timing of relapse (< 1 yr vs. > 1 yr) and the type of primary therapy that preceded relapse (XRT vs. chemoRx). The overall outcome depends on three risk factors: time of relapse, stage at relapse (poor prognosis for stage IV) and presence of B symptoms. The key question in the management relates to the optimal timing of high-dose Rx with autoBMT or PBSC rescue. All data to support various recommendations in the literature are indirect. Results of decision analysis (J Clin Oncol 1992; 10:200) indicate that the best timing might be second relapse but some authorities recommend transplant at first relapse from any front-line chemoRx, regardless of the length of remission (based on level IV and V evidences) (Blood 1994:83:1161); one small randomized study showed FFP advantage of high-dose chemoRx (BEAM + autoBMT) over conventional chemoRx doses (mini-BEAM) (Lancet 1993:341:1051; Oncology 1996:10:233).

| ChemoRx (salvage after XRT failure) | 72–94% | 54–84% | 45–81% (at 7 years) | See above and Table 8-7 | Level I Level IV | Contemp Oncology 1992; Oct:16 J Clin Oncol 1986;4:838 Oncology 1996; 10:233 | Retrospective data to suggest that doxorubicin containing regimens are superior to other chemo Rx; one randomized trial showed no advantage of doxorubicin-containing regimens over other chemo Rx regimens |

Conventional salvage chemoRx (after chemoRx failure)	32–59%	14 % at 4 years (relapse < 1 year) 45% at 21 years (relapse > 1 year)	11% at 22 years (relapse < 1 year) 24% at 22 years (relapse > 1 years)	0–8%	Level IV and V	J Clin Oncol 1992; 10:210 J Clin Oncol 1992;10:200	Note that prognosis in patients not entering CR is poor (median survival ~1.3 years with 0–12% surviving 5 years) (Proc Am Soc Clin Oncol 1993; 12:364)
Salvage with auto BMT (various regimens described; most commonly used are CBV and BEAM)	46–79% (mean: 60%)	40–90% at 3 years (mean: 65%)	52–85% at 3 years	0–24% (mean 11%)	Level IV and V	Contemp Oncology 1992; Oct: 16 Blood 1995; 86: 451 Blood 1994;83: 1193	Note that alloBMT has a limited role in the treatment of HD (J Clin Oncol 1996; 14:572)

Decision Point #5: What is optimal approach to the management of residual (usually mediastinal) mass after treatment is completed?
Residual mediastinal disease occurs in 60–80% with mediastinal HD. Overall probability that a residual mass represents an active disease is about 19% (16–24%) This probability increases in symptomatic patients, those with increased ESR (erythrocyte sedimentation rate), those patients presenting with mass after treatment with chemotherapy only and those patients with positive gallium scan (sensitivity and specificity for detection of active disease about 90%) (Data supporting the algorithm in Fig. 8-2 are based on two retrospective studies, results of a decision analysis and one prospective study on gallium scan) (J Clin Oncol 1988;6:940; J Clin Oncol 1985;3:637; Med hypotheses 1992;38:166; Eur J Haematol 1989;42:344). FFP, freedom from progression; PBSC, peripheral blood stem cells.

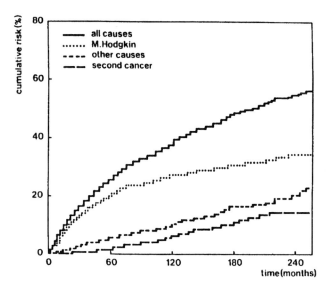

FIGURE 8-2 *Cumulative risk of death from specific causes in patients with Hodgkin's disease. (From van Leeuwen FE, Klokman WJ, Hagenbeek A et al: Second cancer risk follow Hodgkin's disease: a 20-year follow-up study. J Clin Oncol 12:312, 1994, with permission.)*

TABLE 8-7 ACUTE AND LONG-RANGE TOXICITIES ASSOCIATED WITH CURRENT TREATMENT MODALITIES FOR HODGKIN'S DISEASE (SEE ALSO FIG 8-2)

Short-term toxicities
    Mortality (~2–3%)
    Vomiting (almost 100%)
    Leukopenia
    (MOPP: 20–25% ABVD: 40%)
    Thrombocytopenia (MOPP: 15–20%; ABVD: 25%)
    Peripheral neuropathy (more with vincristine than with vinblastine)
    Alopecia (doxorubicin: 56 %; MOPP: 30%)
    Skin hyperpigmentation (bleomycin): 19%

Long-term toxicities
    Male sterility (MOPP: 90–100%, with 10–20% of recovery)
    Amenorrhea & premature ovarian failure (MOPP: 75–85% in women >30; 20% in women < 30)
    Pericarditis (XRT: 15–30%)
    Hypothyroidism (52% at 20 yr; 67% at 26 yr) (XRT-related)
    Graves' disease (~4%) (XRT-related)
    Thyroid cancer (1.7%) (XRT-related)
    Pneumonitis+chronic restrictive fibrositis (XRT: ~20%)
    Cardiomyopathy (doxorubicin: when dose > 400–450 mg/m²)
    Lung fibrosis (bleomycin: when dose >150 mg/m²)
    Acute leukemia (1–4% 10 yr after MOPP; 0.7% 10 yr after ABVD; 10–15% 10 yr after XRT+MOPP)
    Non-Hodgkin's lymphoma (2–4% at 10 yr after chemotherapy)
    Solid tumors (13% at 15 years after XRT; continue to rise)

Abbreviations: XRT, radiation therapy.

TABLE 8-8 FOLLOW-UP SCHEDULE FOR PATIENTS WITH HODGKIN'S DISEASE

Every 3 months for 1–2 years after treatment
Every 6 months after 3 years of treatment
To perform:
    History and physical examination
    Complete blood counts
    Erythrocyte sedimentation rate
    Blood chemistries
    Radiographic studies of chest (posteroanterior and lateral views (annually after 5 years)
    Computed scanning per year or as indicated
For patients with mantle or total nodal XRT, check
    TSH, T$_3$, T$_4$ semiannually for 5 years, then annually thereafter
        Screening mammography (in young women start 8–10 years after treatment); annual gynecological exam for women

Abbreviations: TSH, thyroid-stimulating hormone; XRT, radiation therapy. (Long-term follow-up after Blood 87:3625, 1996)

15% to 20% who fail initial therapy will achieve a durable complete response to secondary treatment, and the rest of patients will succumb either to disease or to effects of continuous therapy.

SUGGESTED READING

Behar RA, Horning SJ, Hoppe RT: Hodgkin's disease with bulky mediastinal involvement: effective management with combined modality therapy. Int J Radiat Oncol Biol Phys 25:771, 1993

Canellos GP, Anderson JR, Propert KJ et al: Chemotherapy of advanced Hodgkin's disease with MOPP, ABVD, or MOPP alternating with ABVD. N Engl J Med 327:1478, 1992

Chopra R, McMillan AK, Linch DC et al: The place of high-dose BEAM therapy and autologous bone marrow transplantation in poor-risk Hodgkin's disease: a single-center eight year study of 155 patients. Blood 81:1137, 1993

DeVita VT, Hubbard SM: Hodgkin's disease. N Engl J Med 328:560–565, 1993

Haybittle JL, Easterling MJ, Bennett MH et al: Review of British National Lymphoma Investigation Studies of Hodgkin's disease and development of prognostic index. Lancet 1:967, 1985

Henkelmann GC, Hagemeister FB, Fuller LM: Two cycles of MOPP and radiotherapy for stage III$_1$B and stage III$_1$B Hodgkin's disease. J Clin Oncol 6:1293, 1988

Leopold FA, Canellos GP, Rosenthal D et al: Stage IA-IIB-Hodgkin's disease: staging and treatment of patients with large mediastinal adenopathy. J Clin Oncol 6:1822, 1988

Longo, Young RC, Wesley M et al: Twenty years of MOPP therapy for Hodgkin's disease. J Clin Oncol 4:1295, 1986

Longo DL, Glatstein E, Duffey FL et al: Radiation therapy versus combination chemotherapy in the treatment of early stage Hodgkin's disease: seven year results of a prospective randomized trial. J Clin Oncol 9:906, 1991

Mauch, Goffman T, Rosenthal DS et al: Stage III Hodgkin's disease: Improved survival with combined modality therapy as compared with radiation therapy alone. J Clin Oncol 3:1166, 1985

Rosenberg SA, Kaplan HS: The evolution and summary results of the Stanford randomized clinical trials for the management of Hodgkin's disease 1963–1984. Int J Radiat Oncol Biol Phys 11:5–22, 1985

Santoro A, Bonadonna G, Valagussa P et al: Long-term results of combined chemotherapy-radiotherapy approach in Hodgkin's disease: superiority of ABVD plus radiotherapy versus MOPP plus radiotherapy. J Clin Oncol 5:27, 1987

Tucker MA, Coleman CN, Cox RL et al: Risk of second cancers after treatment for Hodgkin's disease. N Engl J Med 318:76, 1988

Urba WJ, Longo DL: Hodgkin's disease. N Engl J Med 326:678–686, 1992

Wheeler C, Antin JH, Churchill WH et al: Cyclophosphamide, carmustine, and eloposide with autologous bone marrow transplantation in refractory Hodgkin's disease and non-Hodgkin's lymphoma: a dose-finding study. J Clin Oncol 8:648, 1990

Yellen SB, Cella DF, Bonomi A: Quality of life in people with Hodgkin's disease. Oncology 7:41, 1993

9 Non-Hodgkin's Lymphoma

Benjamin Djulbegović

Incidence: 16/100,000 population

Main modality of treatment: Chemotherapy

Goal of treatment: Cure in aggressive and rapidly progressive cases

Prolongation of survival in low-grade cases

Prognosis (overall):

Low-grade: 6–7 years (median survival)

Aggressive: 3–4 years (median survival)

Rapidly progressive: 60% (5-year survival)

Non-Hodgkin's lymphoma (NHL) includes about 3% of all cancers in the United States, with an estimated annual incidence of about 16 per 100,000 population. NHL represents an extremely heterogeneous group of neoplasms of the immune system, each of which is characterized by its own particular histology, immunophenotype, and in some cases genotype. The clinical course of NHL most closely correlates with histologic type. Enlargement of peripheral lymph nodes is the most common presenting clinical feature in lymphomas (60%–70%), but involvement of extranodal sites also occurs, sometimes being the only site of disease. This fact can be translated into a clinical production rule: *Malignant lymphomas should always be considered in a differential diagnosis of enlarged lymph nodes and splenomegaly but also in any patient presenting with unexplained fever, weight loss, pruritus, or superior vena cava syndrome* (Table 9-1).

DIAGNOSIS

The diagnosis of NHL rests entirely on a biopsy of a lymph node or an affected extranodal site. The key decision is when to perform a lymph node biopsy (Table 9-2). An adequate surgical biopsy is of utmost importance. Inguinal nodes should not be biopsied if equally suspicious peripheral nodes are present elsewhere. Fine needle aspirates do not suffice. Although not a substitute for morphologic examination, use of immunohistochemistry or determination of phenotype by flow cytometry and molecular biology techniques is a very useful supplement to an accurate diagnosis. Interobserver concordance of diagnoses rises substantially when these techniques are combined with hematoxylin and eosin morphologic examination. Determination of a histologic subtype, a stage of disease (a prognostic subgroup), human immunodeficiency virus (HIV) status and anatomic location define basic elements of the clinical approach to the management of non-Hodgkin's lymphoma. The reasoning process is goal-oriented (cure, prolongation of survival, palliation) and depends on these five variables.

Once the histologic diagnosis of NHL is made, the translation of a histologic subtype into clinical action follows. This is done with assistance of one of many pathologic classification systems that essen-

TABLE 9-1 WORKING FORMULATION CLASSIFICATION SYSTEM FOR NON-HODGKIN'S LYMPHOMA AND DISEASE CHARACTERISTICS

Malignant Lymphoma	Median Age	Male: Female	Lymph Node Involvement (%)		Bone Marrow Involved (%)	Median Survival (Years)[a]
			Local	Generalized		
Working Formulation						
Low grade (33.8%)						
Small lymphocytic	60	1:1	—	100	75	6+
Follicular, small cleaved cell (22.5%)	55	1:1	20	80	50–75	6+
Follicular, mixed small cleaved and large cell	55	1:1	30–40	60–70	30	5
Intermediate grade (aggressive) (37.1%)						
Follicular, large cell	55	2:1	50+	(1)[b]	33	3
Diffuse, small cleaved cell (6.9%)	55	2:1	25	(2)[b]	Common	3
Diffuse, mixed small and large cell (6.7%)	60	1:1	50	ND	15	3
Diffuse, large cell (19.7%)	55	1:1	50	(3)[b]	10	1.5
High grade (rapidly progressive) (17.1%)						
Large cell, immunoblastic (7.9%)[c]	50	1.5:1	50+	ND	10	1
Lymphoblastic (4.2%)	17	2:1	25	75	100	2
Small, noncleaved cell (5%)	30	3:1	33	ND	15	NS
Miscellaneous (12%)						

[a] See also Tables 9-11 through 9-13. [c] Treat as aggressive non-Hodgkin's lymphoma (see Fig. 9-4 and Table 9-12).

[b] Extranodal Involvement: (1), 50%; (2), 67%; (3), frequent.

Abbreviations: NS, not specified but 25% disease-free at 5 years; ND, not determined.

tially try to relate a histologic subtype with natural history and potential curability of NHL. Tables 9-1 and 9-3 show new Revised European American Lymphoma (REAL) classification along with the still widely popular Working Formulation system for classification of NHL. (Table 9-1 also shows important clinical information on NHL.)

STAGING

The next step in the evaluation of patients with NHL is determination of the stage of disease (i.e., the tumor burden). Staging is important because of the relatively good correlation between the stage of disease and prognosis for a given histologic type of NHL. None of the other clinical, pathologic, immunologic, and (molecular) biologic characteristics of NHL correlates with the natural history of disease and response to treatment better than histologic subtype. (An impressive amount of information on the significance of T and B subtyping, various chromosome aberrations, presence of specific oncogenes, and numerous other prognostic variables have not as yet had a bearing on clinical management.) Likewise,

TABLE 9-2 RULES REGARDING WHEN TO PERFORM LYMPH NODE BIOPSY

Any peripheral lymph node 1 cm or greater that does not show signs of regression after 6 weeks of observation should be biopsied.

In patients with nondiagnostic biopsy or with atypical hyperplasia of lymph nodes, there should be little hesitation to repeat the biopsy since 25% to 30% of such patients will subsequently develop a disease (usually a lymphoma).

The probability of malignancy in enlarged peripheral lymph nodes increases steadily with age: 10% of neck masses in children are malignant, compared with 80% of neck masses in adults older than 40 years.

A firm nontender mass in the neck of a patient over 40 is probably metastatic cancer, while soft nodes are more likely to be either benign or are lymphomas. The probability of lymphoma is much larger in the young population than metastatic carcinoma. Enlarged supraclavicular nodes should be considered malignant until proven otherwise.

Note that fine needle aspiration of a suspicious lymph node in the head and neck area should precede excisional lymph node biopsy (because of the possibility of compromise of the field of neck dissection should carcinoma cells be detected). When biopsy is performed, it is important to provide adequate material for information on clonality and CD phenotype.

(Modified from Djulbegović B: Reasoning and Decision Making in Hematology. Churchill Livingstone, New York, 1992.)

TABLE 9-3 RELATION BETWEEN REAL (REVISED EUROPEAN AMERICAN LYMPHOMA) AND WORKING FORMULATION LYMPHOMA CLASSIFICATION SYSTEMS

Low-grade lymphomas of B-cell origin
  A. Small B-lymphocytic lymphoma/leukemia
    B lymphocytic, CLL or CLL type
    B lymphocytic with plasmacytoid differentiation
    B lymphocytic, mantle cell (e.g., lymphomatous polyposis)
  B. Follicular center lymphomas
    Predominantly small cleaved cell (follicular or follicular/diffuse)
    Mixed small and large cell (follicular or follicular/diffuse)
    Diffuse, small cleaved cell of follicular center origin
  C. Parafollicular small B-cell lymphoma
    Marginal-zone B-cell lymphoma of spleen (with or without villous lymphocytes)
    Low-grade B-cell lymphoma of MALT type (with or without plasma cells)
    Monocytoid B-cell lymphoma (with or without plasma cells)
  D. Other
    Hairy cell leukemia
    Extramedullary plasmacytoma
    Medullary plasmacytoma

Intermediate-grade lymphomas of B-cell origin
  E. Mantle cell lymphoma (usual or blastic type, mantle, or diffuse pattern)
  F. Follicular center large-cell lymphoma (follicular or follicular/diffuse)
  G. Diffuse large-cell lymphomas
    Predominantly large noncleaved and/or cleaved (including multilobated)
    Immunoblastic (with or without plasmablastic differentiation)
    Paraimmunoblastic (prolymphocytic leukemia)
    Primary mediastinal large B-cell (with or without sclerosis)
    Anaplastic large-cell of B-cell origin
    Lymphoproliferative disease (usually Epstein-Barr, virus-associated)
  H. Diffuse mixed small- and large-cell lymphoma
    Of B-cell origin
    T-cell-rich B-cell lymphoma

High-grade lymphomas of B-cell origin
  I. Small noncleaved cell lymphoma
    Burkitt's lymphoma (usually Epstein Barr, virus associated)
    non Burkitt lymphoma
  J. Lymphoblastic lymphoma/leukemia of B-cell origin
    Precursor B lymphoblastic (CALL type)
    Pre-B lymphoblastic
    B lymphoblastic

Low-grade lymphomas of T (or NK)-cell origin
  K. Small lymphocytic lymphoma/leukemia
    T-cell chronic lymphocytic leukemia
    Large granular lymphocyte leukemia (T or NK type)
    Sézary syndrome
  L. Mycosis fungoides

(Continues)

TABLE 9-3 *(Continued)*

Intermediate-grade lymphomas of T/NK-cell origin
  M. Peripheral T-cell lymphomas (with or without angiocentric growth)
    Medium-sized cell pleomorphic (with or without clear cells)
    Mixed small- and large-cell (with or without clear cells)
    Large cell (including immunoblastic and multilobated)
  N. Adult T-cell lymphoma/leukemia (HTLV1-associated)
  O. ALCL (T or O-cell)
  P. Other (provisional) T-cell entities
    Lennert's lymphoma (T-lymphocytic with epithelioid histiocytes)
    Angioimmunoblastic T-cell lymphoma (AILD like)
    Intestinal T-cell lymphoma (with or without enteropathy)
    Nasal NK cell lymphoma (angiocentric growth, usually Epstein-Barr-virus associated)
    Lymphomatoid granulomatosis (angiocentric growth)
    Subcutaneous panniculitic T-cell lymphoma
    Hepatosplenic $\gamma\delta$ T-cell lymphoma

High-grade lymphomas of T-cell origin
  Q. T-lymphoblastic lymphoma/leukemia

Hodgkin's disease (HD)
  IA. Lymphocyte predominance (NLPHD and diffuse variant)
  IB. Lymphocyte-rich classical HD
  II. Nodular sclerosis
  III. Mixed cellularity
  IVA. Lymphocyte depletion HD
  IVB. Anaplastic large-cell lymphoma-like HD

Abbreviations: CLL, chronic lymphocytic leukemia; CALL, common acute lymphoblastic leukemia; HTLV1, human T-cell lymphotropic virus type 1; ALCL, anaplastic large cell lymphoma.

(From Poppema C: Lymphoma classification proposal, comment. Blood 87:412–413, 1996, with permission.)

selection of the treatment is stage dependent. Table 9-4 shows the Ann Arbor staging classification of NHL (Cotswold modification along with staging system for gastric NHL). Table 9-5 shows the NCI staging system for small noncleaved lymphoma. Figure 9-1 and Table 9-6 show diagnostic strategies in the evaluation of patients with NHL. One, however, has to recognize that a staging system is limited and cannot be the sole variable that determines the course of disease. Table 9-7 shows the international prognostic index (IPI), which can predict a prognosis for patients much better than the Ann Arbor staging system alone (Tables 9-8 and 9-9). The IPI, however, has not yet been used to tailor treatment toward an individual patient. Clinical trials using this approach are in progress (Figs. 9-2, 9-4, and Table 9-10).

TABLE 9-4 ANN ARBOR STAGING CLASSIFICATION COTSWOLDS MODIFICATIONS OF HODGKIN'S DISEASE

Stage I	Involvement of a single lymph node region (I) or single extralymphatic site (I_E)
Stage II	Involvement of 2 or more lymph node regions on the same side of the diaphragm (II) or localized involvement of an extralymphatic site and one or more lymph node regions on the same side of the diaphragm (II_E)
	The number of anatomic sites involved is indicated by a suffix (e.g., II_3)
Stage III_1	Involvement of lymph nodes on both sides of diaphragm. Abdominal disease is limited to the upper abdomen (i.e., spleen, splenic hilar nodes, celiac nodes, porta hepatitis node)
Stage III_2	Involvement of lymph nodes on both sides of diaphragm. Abdominal disease includes para-aortic, mesenteric, and iliac involvement with or without disease in the upper abdomen
Stage IV	Disseminated involvement of one or more extralymphatic organs or tissues with or without associated lymph node disease
A	No symptoms
B	Fever, night sweats, or weight loss of more than 10% of body weight in the previous 6 months
X	Bulky disease (greater than 10 cm in maximum dimension; greater than 1/3 of the internal transverse diameter of the thorax at the level T5/T6)
E	Limited involvement of a single extranodal site
U	Unconfirmed/uncertain complete remission (as in the persistent radiologic abnormalities of uncertain significance)
CS	Clinical stage: when based solely on physical examination and imaging techniques
PS	Pathologic stage: when based on biopsies

The Ann Arbor staging classification modified according to recommendation published in J Clin Oncol 7:1630–1636, 1989. Note that subdivision of stage III is more applicable in the staging of Hodgkin's disease.

Stage III is not applicable to gastrointestinal (GI) lymphoma. GI lymphoma are staged as follows: stage I, tumor confined to GI tract; stage II, tumor extending into abdomen from primary GI site (II_1, local; II_2, distant, IIE, penetration of serosa to involve adjacent organs or tissues); IV, disseminated extranodal involvement or a GI tract lesion with supradiaphragmatic nodal involvement (Ann Oncol 5:397–400, 1994).

TABLE 9-5 NCI STAGING SYSTEM FOR SMALL NON-CLEAVED LYMPHOMA

Stage I	Single extra-abdominal tumor
Stage IR	Resected (< 90~) intra-abdominal tumor
Stage II	Multiple extra-abdominal sites excluding bone marrow and CNS
Stage IIIA	Unresected intra-abdominal tumor
Stage IIIB	Intra- and extra-abdominal tumor except bone marrow
Stage IVA	Bone marrow involvement without abdominal or CNS tumor
Stage IVB	Bone marrow and abdominal tumor or CNS disease

TABLE 9-6 CLINICAL FEATURES OF LYMPHOMA THAT ARE IMPORTANT IN MEDICAL DECISION MAKING

	Hodgkin's Disease	*Non-Hodgkin's Lymphoma*	*Comment*
Histologic subtype	Not so important as in NHL	Crucial	Treatment strategies in low-grade, intermediate-grade, and high-grade NHL are quite different
Ann Arbor staging system	Essential for planning appropriate management	Much less important in NHL than in HD	Radiation has very limited role in the primary treatment of NHL, and chemotherapy is initial treatment of choice in most NHL, even in early stages
Bilateral bone marrow biopsy	Bone marrow biopsies are required in patients with advanced disease, splenic involvement, and elevated serum alkaline phosphatase	Standard work-up; essential in all patients with high-grade lymphomas	Bone marrow involvement occurs in 5%–20% of patients with HD and in 60%–80% of patients with low-grade NHL
Bilateral lymphogram of lower extremities	Required in all patients with nodes <1.5 cm by CT (but only if radiation therapy is considered)	Not required as a routine procedure	Overall S and Sp, 90%, comparable to CT, better than CT for para-aortic nodes (S, 82%; Sp, 100% vs S, 76% and Sp, 90%, respectively); CT better for high para-aortic nodes and mesenteric nodes
Osseous involvement	Rare (from 0.6% in CS IA to 17.7% in CS IVB) (J Clin Oncol 13:403, 1995)	5% to 15% of all patients as initial presentation	Bone scan required more often in NHL than in HD; prognosis does not seem to be affected by marrow involvement
Liver involvement	Rare (5% of patients at diagnosis) without splenic involvement	40% to 60% in small lymphocytic and small cleaved-cell lymphomas	Liver biopsy is rarely required (more often in NHL than in HD); diagnostic criteria by imaging technique: multiple focal defects that are neither cystic nor vascular noted with at least two techniques; spleen involvement: clearly palpable spleen or equivocal palpable spleen confirmed by radiologic technique (radiologic enlargement alone is not adequate)
CNS disease	Quite rare	25% of patients with diffuse histology and bone marrow disease	Lumbar puncture is recommended in NHL patients with high-grade histology, aggressive histology with bone marrow, testicular, or epidural tumor involvement; and HIV + NHL

Abbreviation: CS, clinical stage; CT, computed tomography; HIV, human immunodeficiency viruses; HD, Hodgkin's disease; NHL, non-Hodgkin's lymphoma; S, sensitivity; Sp, specificity.

(From Djulbegović B: Reasoning and Decision Making in Hematology. Churchill Livingstone, New York, 1992, with permission.)

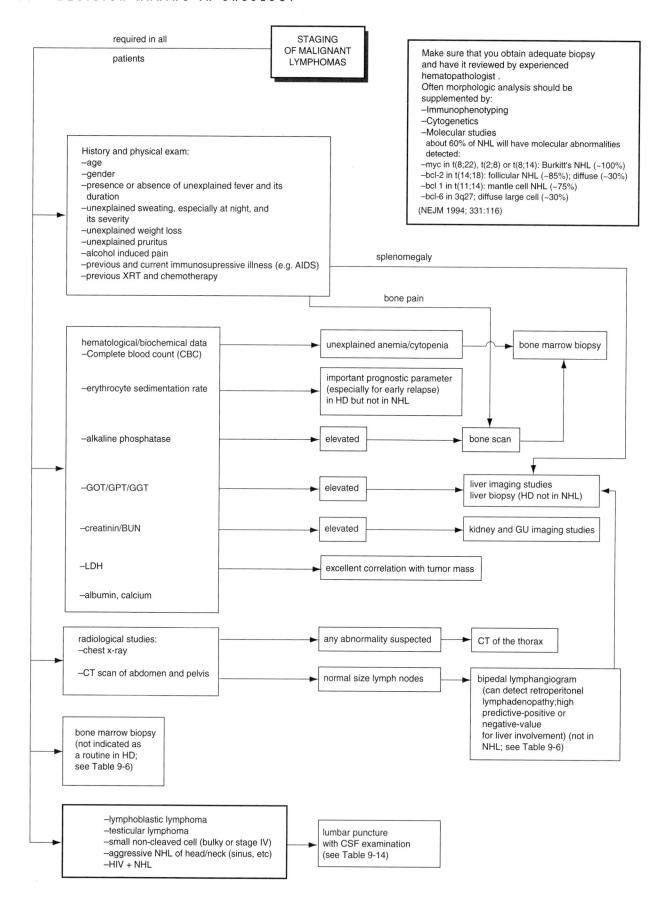

required in all
patients

STAGING
OF MALIGNANT
LYMPHOMAS

Make sure that you obtain adequate biopsy
and have it reviewed by experienced
hematopathologist .
Often morphologic analysis should be
supplemented by:
–Immunophenotyping
–Cytogenetics
–Molecular studies
 about 60% of NHL will have molecular abnormalities
 detected:
–myc in t(8;22), t(2;8) or t(8;14): Burkitt's NHL (~100%)
–bcl-2 in t(14;18): follicular NHL (~85%); diffuse (~30%)
–bcl 1 in t(11;14): mantle cell NHL (~75%)
–bcl-6 in 3q27; diffuse large cell (~30%)
(NEJM 1994; 331:116)

History and physical exam:
–age
–gender
–presence or absence of unexplained fever and its
 duration
–unexplained sweating, especially at night, and
 its severity
–unexplained weight loss
–unexplained pruritus
–alcohol induced pain
–previous and current immunosupressive illness (e.g. AIDS)
–previous XRT and chemotherapy

splenomegaly

bone pain

hematological/biochemical data
–Complete blood count (CBC)

unexplained anemia/cytopenia

bone marrow biopsy

–erythrocyte sedimentation rate

important prognostic parameter
(especially for early relapse)
in HD but not in NHL

–alkaline phosphatase

elevated

bone scan

–GOT/GPT/GGT

elevated

liver imaging studies
liver biopsy (HD not in NHL)

–creatinin/BUN

elevated

kidney and GU imaging studies

–LDH

excellent correlation with tumor mass

–albumin, calcium

radiological studies:
–chest x-ray

any abnormality suspected

CT of the thorax

–CT scan of abdomen and pelvis

normal size lymph nodes

bipedal lymphangiogram
(can detect retroperitonel
lymphadenopathy;high
predictive-positive or
negative-value
for liver involvement) (not in
NHL; see Table 9-6)

bone marrow biopsy
(not indicated as
a routine in HD;
see Table 9-6)

–lymphoblastic lymphoma
–testicular lymphoma
–small non-cleaved cell (bulky or stage IV)
–aggressive NHL of head/neck (sinus, etc)
–HIV + NHL

lumbar puncture
with CSF examination
(see Table 9-14)

TABLE 9-7 INTERNATIONAL PROGNOSTIC INDEX [a]

Patients older than 60 years
  Age (≤ 60 vs. > 60)
  Serum LDH (≤ 1 × normal vs. > 1 × normal)
  Performance status (0 or 1 vs. 2–4) (See Appendix 1)
  Stage (I or II vs. III or IV)
  Extranodal involvement (≤ 1 site vs. > 1 site)

Patients younger than 60 years
  Stage (I or II vs. III or IV)
  Serum LDH (≤ 1 × normal vs. > 1 × normal)
  Performance status (0 or 1 vs. 2–4) (See Appendix 1)

[a] *To arrive at the score sum number of risk factors present at diagnosis, assign 1 to each prognostic factor present.*

(Modified from N Engl J Med 329: 987; 1993, with permission.)

TABLE 9-8 OUTCOME ACCORDING TO RISK GROUP DEFINED BY THE INTERNATIONAL INDEX AND THE AGE-ADJUSTED INTERNATIONAL INDEX IN AGGRESSIVE NON-HODGKIN'S LYMPHOMA

Risk Group	No of Risk Factors	Complete Response (%)	Relapse-Free Survival 2-Year Rate (%)	Relapse-Free Survival 5-Year Rate (%)	Survival 2-Year Rate (%)	Survival 5-Year Rate (%)
International Index (all patients)						
Low	0 or 1	87	79	70	84	73
Low intermediate	2	67	66	50	66	51
High intermediate	3	55	59	49	54	43
High	4 or 5	44	58	40	34	26
Age-Adjusted Index (patients ≤ 60 years)						
Low	0	92	88	86	90	83
Low intermediate	1	78	74	66	79	69
High intermediate	2	57	62	53	59	46
High	3	46	61	58	37	32
Age-Adjusted Index, (patients > 60 years)						
Low	0	91	75	46	80	56
Low intermediate	1	71	64	45	68	44
High intermediate	2	56	60	41	48	37
High	3	36	47	37	31	21

(Modified from N Engl J Med 329:987; 1993, with permission.)

FIGURE 9-1 *Guidelines for staging malignant lymphomas (see also Table 9-6). The goal of staging is to describe accurately the extension of disease. These guidelines are based on the Ann Arbor staging classification and its Cotswalds modification for staging of lymphomas (see Table 9-4).*

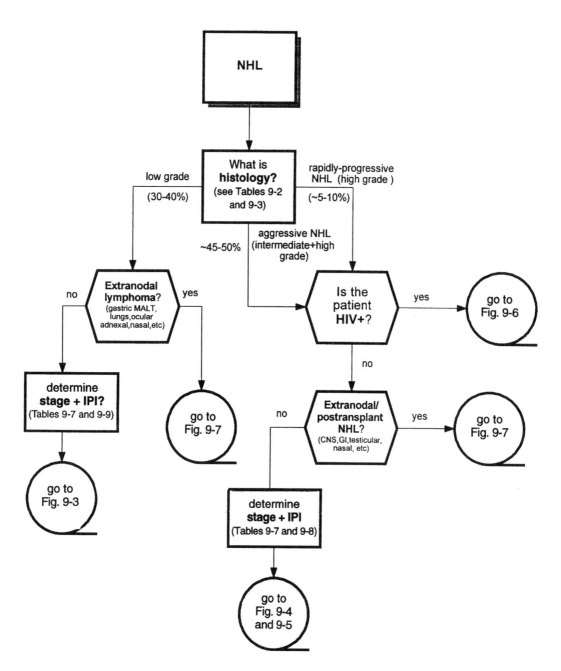

FIGURE 9-2 *An approach to the management of non-Hodgkin's lymphoma. A strategy is formulated based on determination of a histologic subtype, a stage of disease (a prognostic subgroup), human immunodeficiency virus status and anatomic location. The goal of treatment depends on the knowledge of these essential five variables.*

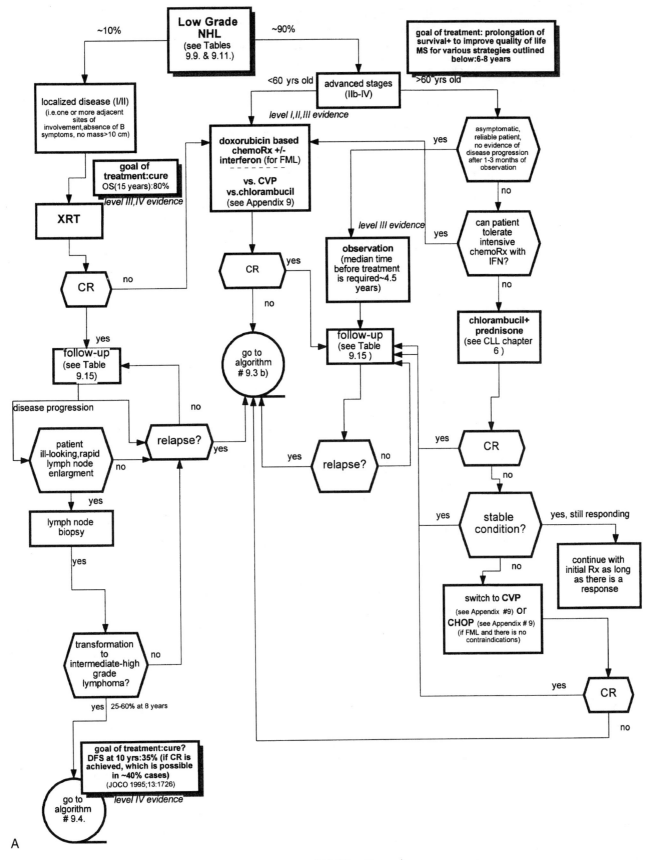

A

FIGURE 9-3 *(A)* (Continues).

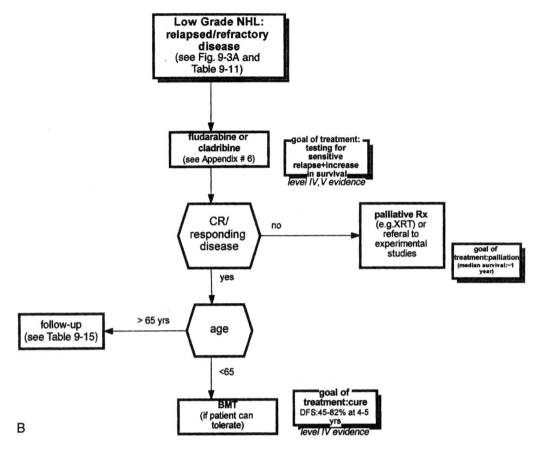

B

FIGURE 9-3 *(A & B) Management of patient with low grade non-Hodgkin's lymphoma (NHL) (use this algorithm with Table 9-11). Reasoning principles are based on understanding the natural history of disease, the tumor burden upon presentation (stage of disease) and probabilities of response, outcomes (disease-free and overall survival), and risk of specific types of treatment. Note that the course of disease is manifested with many remissions and relapses, each remission having shorter duration. To a certain extent survival correlates with response to therapy, although the main goal of treatment is still palliation. Presented is the current literature consensus regarding treatment approach to NHL. As seen in Table 9-11, the evidences gathered for initial treatment with any treatment alternatives are of high-quality (level I, II, or long-term single-arm studies); evidences for recommended strategy in relapse are mainly indirect. (For doses and treatment protocols see Appendices 6 and 9.)*

FIGURE 9-4 *Management of patient with aggressive non-Hodgkin's lymphoma (NHL) (use this algorithm with Table 9-12). Reasoning principles are based on understanding the natural history of disease, the tumor burden upon presentation (stage of disease) and probabilities of response, outcomes (cure, disease-free and overall survival), and risk of specific types of treatment. The main goal of treatment remains cure, which is not always possible. Presented is the current literature consensus regarding the treatment approach to NHL. As seen in Table 9-11, the evidences gathered for this recommended strategy are quite solid. Note that mantle-cell lymphoma can occasionally have an indolent course and should be treated according to principles outlined in Figure 9-3 and Table 9-11. Similarly, localized Ki-1 + ALCL (anaplastic large cell lymphoma) should be treated less aggressively (usually radiation therapy). (For doses and treatment protocols, see Appendix 9.)*

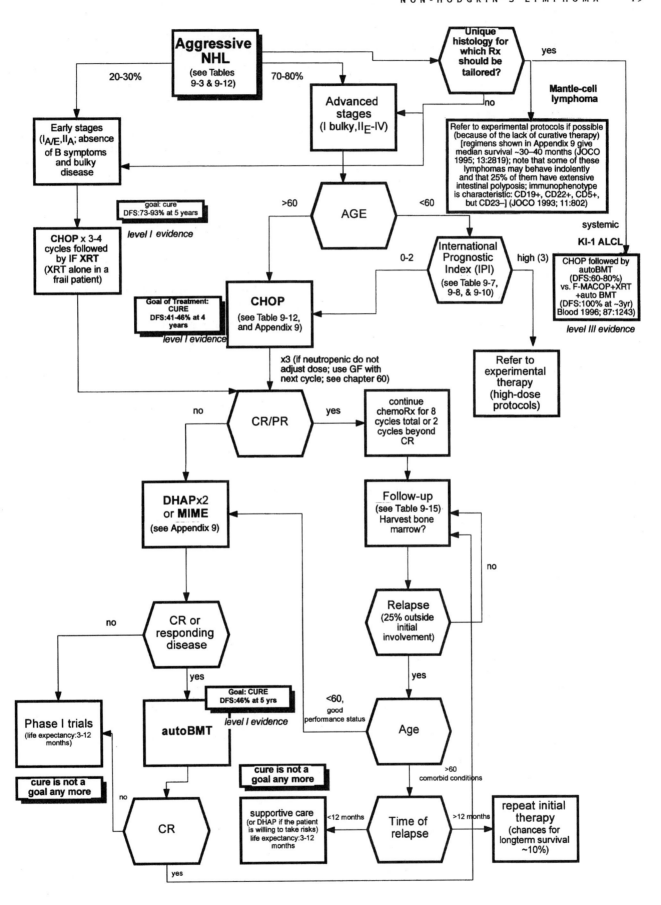

TABLE 9-9 RESPONSE TO THERAPY AND SURVIVAL OF 125 PATIENTS ACCORDING TO THE INTERNATIONAL INDEX IN LOW-GRADE NON-HODGKIN'S LYMPHOMA

Risk Group	All Low-Grade NHL Patients (N = 125)		Follicular Lymphoma Patients (N = 107)	
	Complete Response (%)	10-Year Survival (%)	Complete Response (%)	Complete Survival (%)
Low	60	73.6	61.5	75
Low intermediate	35	45.2	41.2	47
High intermediate	23	53.5	25	55
High	21	0	21.4	0

(From Lopez-Guillelmo A et al: Applicability of the International Index for aggressive lymphomas to patients with low-grade lymphoma. J Clin Oncol 12:1343–1348, 1994, with permission.)

Finally, the approach to the patient with NHL will depend on HIV status and anatomic presentation of NHL (Fig. 9-2).

The principles outlined above are then coupled with an estimate of probabilities of response and cure and risk of specific types of treatment to help define the goals of treatment as the major reasoning principle employed in the management of patients with NHL (see also Ch. 1, Fig. 1-5).

LOW-GRADE LYMPHOMA

Low-grade lymphomas, although indolent in their course, are rarely cured. Before the advent of chemotherapy, half of patients diagnosed with low-grade lymphoma died within 5 years. The goal of treatment in the management of these lymphomas should be prolongation of survival. Since early institution of treatment does not seem to alter prognosis versus deferred treatment, timing of the treatment is usually guided by the need to improve patients' quality of life by controlling their symptoms, with minimal induced treatment-related toxicity (Fig. 9-3 and Table 9-11).

HIGH-GRADE LYMPHOMA

In contrast to low-grade lymphoma, aggressive and high-grade lymphomas can be cured, despite a rapid clinical course if left untreated (overall median survival in untreated patients is about 1 year). Therefore, the goal of treatment should be cure, which unfortunately is not always possible (Figs. 9-4 and 9-5; Tables 9-12 to 9-13).

The goal of treatment of *HIV-associated lymphoma* is also to achieve prolongation of life although treatment usually focuses on palliation and control of symptoms (Fig. 9-6).

The course of disease in *extranodal lymphoma* (called *special sites NHL*) depends largely on anatomic involvement (e.g., central nervous or gastrointestinal systems, testicular), and the goals of treatment will differ in each case (e.g., prolongation of survival in central nervous system lymphoma, potential curability in gastrointestinal lymphoma) (Fig. 9-7).

TABLE 9-10 OTHER RELEVANT DECISIONS IN TREATMENT OF NON-HODGKIN'S LYMPHOMA [a]

Initial decision dilemma: tailoring therapy according to age, International Prognostic Index (IPI), and new (REAL) lymphoma classification

    All evidences are indirect (type IV and V) and the use IPI, REAL classification or age to tailor management cannot be standard at this time.

Decision dilemma: timing of salvage therapy

    AutoBMT for younger patients (< 60 years) preferred; for older patients, time of relapse (< 12 months vs > 12 months) is probably important; however, this issue has never been studied in NHL, and practice is based on physicians' experience and analogy to the management of Hodgkin's disease (level V evidence)

Decision dilemma: follow-up tests and timing (see Table 9-15)

    Levels IV and V evidence

Decision dilemma: indications for prophylactic intrathecal therapy (see Table 9-14)

    Levels IV and V evidence

---

[a] *As shown in Figures 9-2, 9-4*

Abbreviation: NHL, non-Hodgkin's lymphoma.

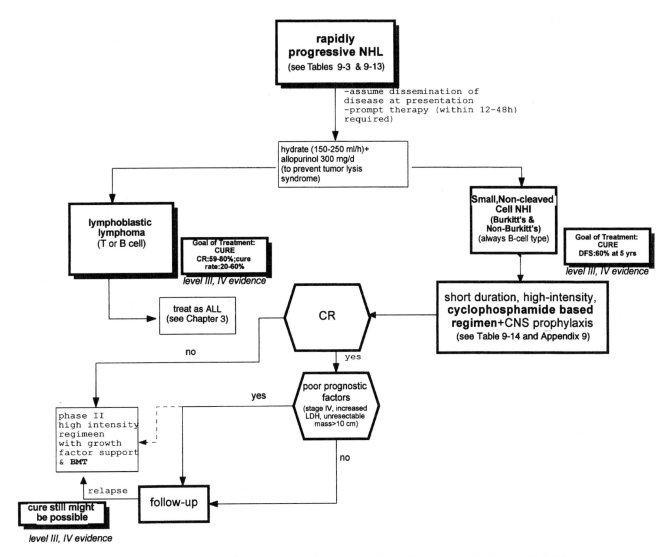

FIGURE 9-5 *Management of patient with high-grade (rapidly progressive) non-Hodgkin's lymphoma (see also Table 9-13). Reasoning principles are based on understanding the natural history of disease, the tumor burden upon presentation (stage of disease), and probabilities of response, outcomes (cure, disease-free and overall survival), and risk of specific types of treatment. Treatment of high-grade lymphomas is a medical emergency, and rapid institution of management is essential. The goal of treatment is a cure. The evidences for recommended strategy are largely indirect (see Table 9-13). (For doses and treatment protocols, see Appendix 9.)*

TABLE 9-11 BENEFITS/RISKS OF PREFERRED MANAGEMENT ALTERNATIVES FOR LOW-GRADE NON-HODGKIN'S LYMPHOMA[a]

Decision Point 1: What is the best first-line treatment for advanced stages of low-grade non-Hodgkin's lymphoma

(observation with deferred treatment vs single agent chemotherapy vs combined chemotherapy with and without doxorubicin or interferon)

Evidences for recommended strategy are direct (level I) and indirect (type III, IV and V); no trial demonstrated superiority of any management available; one randomized trial between deferred treatment and aggressive chemotherapy showed no difference in DFS (55% at 4 yrs) and OS (84% at 4 years) (Semin Hematol 1988;25:11), multiple randomized trials between single agent and combined chemotherapy containing no doxorubicin with or without radiation therapy showed no difference in CR, DFS or OS (Semin Oncol 1990;17:51); whether doxorubicin-containing regimens offer any advantage is not clear at this time; adding interferon to doxorubicin-based chemotherapy lead, however, to prolongation of DFS and OS; most authors believe that follicular mixed (FM) lymphoma should be treated with doxorubicin-based chemotherapy because of the more aggressive course of this disease and potential curability with more aggressive regimens (Ann Intern Med 1984;100:651; Proc Am Soc Clin Oncol 1990;9:259; JOCO 1993;11:644). However, long-term follow-up at NCI showed no positive impact of doxorubicin-containing regimens on survival of FML or other subtypes of low-grade NHL (level IV evidence) (J Clin Oncol 1993;11:644).

Type of Treatment		Outcomes				References	Comment
	Complete Remission (CR) (%)	Disease-Free Survival (DFS) (%)	Overall Survival (OS) (%)	Mortality (%)	Type of Evidence		
Observation (deferred treatment)	23 (overall) 14 (SL) 30 (FSC) 17 (FM) (spontaneous regressions)	Freedom from requiring therapy: 3 years (all subtypes) SL: 72 months FSC: 48 months FM: 16.5 months	50 (11 years) (all subtypes) SL: 92 (5 years) FSC: 92 (5 years) FM: 66 (5 years)	NA	Level III	NEJM 1984;311: 1471	Neither incidence nor time to histologic transformation (HT), as a primary determinant of length of survival, was influenced by starting time of therapy
Chlorambucil	65	50 (median)	60 + months	0 (?)	Level I, II, and III	Semin Oncol 1990;17:51	Note that CR and survival decreases with every new relapse; median survival drops from 9.2 years at presentation to 2 years at third relapse (JOCO 1995;13:140)
CVP	83	50 (median)	60 + months	0 (?)	Level I, II, III	Semin Oncol 1990;17:51	Addition of interferon to chemotherapy seems to be superior to chemotherapy alone in one trial (at the expense of increase toxicity)
TBI	77	48 (median)	60 months	1–2 (?)	Level I,II, III	Semin Oncol 1990;17:51	
Interferon+ doxorubicin based chemotherapy	20 (CR+PR=76) 32 (CR+PR=86)	50 (34 months) 71 (2 years)	86 (3 years) 87 (2 years) (No difference in survival with respect to chemotherapy after 5 years of follow-up)	0 (Severe adverse reactions in 11%–34%)	Level I Level I	NEJM 1993;329: 1608 NEJM 1992;327: 1336 NEJM 1993;329: 1821	

Decision Point 2: What is the best treatment of a relapse (salvage therapy)?

(Recommendations for use of purine analogues are based on indirect evidences, levels III, IV, and V, that response rates seems to be higher with these agents than with standard chemotherapy; however, direct comparative trials between these drugs and standard therapy are lacking.)

Treatment	Response			Toxicity	Level	Reference	Comments
Cladribine	13 + 43 (CR+PR)	33 (durable response) (follow-up: 2–29 months)	Not reported	29	Level III	JOCO 1994;12:788	Less toxicity and higher response rates are seen in previously untreated patients (Blood 1995; 86:1710). Infections are major complications with use of purine analogues (JOCO 1995;13:2431)
Fludarabine	60 (CR+PR)	Durable responses noted	Not reported	62 (neutropenia) 19 (life-threatening infections)	Level III	Semin Hematol 1994;31:28	See also above; another purine analogue with activity in low grade NHL is pentostatin; however, the author has not had personal experience with its use

Decision Point 3: What is the best first-line treatment for early stages of disease?

Treatment	Response			Toxicity	Level	Reference	Comments
Radiation therapy>90 (?)	69–100	80 (15 years)		0	Level III	Semin Oncol 1990;17:51	A plateau after 5 years suggest curability (particularly in young patients of 40–60 years old)

Decision Point 4: What is optimal timing of bone marrow transplantation (BMT)?

All evidences are indirect, level IV and V; most authors recommend a second remission as optimal timing for autoBMT for patients younger than 65 (or who can tolerate treatment); most authors favor autoBMT over alloBMT because considerably less mortality and morbidity. However, some authors recommend alloBMT.

Treatment	Response			Toxicity	Level	Reference	Comments
AlloBMT	80 (8 out 10)	82 (5 years)		20	Level III	JOCO 1995;13:1096	Small study (10 patients) with young patients (23–45 years)
AutoBMT		45(4 years)		5	Level III	JOCO 1994;12:1177	

Decision Point 5: Is achievement of molecular remission necessary? Should follow-up include routine measurement of molecular markers for minimal residual disease?

All evidences indirect, level IV and V. No conclusive recommendation possible. Reciprocal chromosomal translocation t(14;18) is a characteristic molecular marker of follicular NHL found in about 85% of cases. Early studies report significant decrease in DFS in patients with positive t(14:18) translocation (NEJM 1991;325:1525). However, subsequent studies found positive cells in up to 38% patients who were in apparent long-term remission (JOCO 1993;11:1668; JOCO 1994;12:1532). Also, in 6 of 9 healthy persons tested, this translocation was detected, with frequency of 1 in 100,000 B cells. Blood 1995;85:2528.

[a] as shown in Figure 9-3.

TABLE 9-12 BENEFITS/RISKS OF PREFERRED MANAGEMENT ALTERNATIVES FOR AGGRESSIVE NON-HODGKIN'S LYMPHOMA[a]

Type of Treatment	Outcomes					References	Comment
	Complete Remission (CR) (%)	Disease-Free Survival (DFS) (%)	Overall Survival (OS) (%)	Mortality (%)	Type of Evidence		

Decision Point 1: What is the best first-line treatment for advanced stages of non-Hodgkin's lymphoma?

Third generation regimen vs second generation regimen vs first-generation regimen? The third generation regimen did not demonstrate any advantage in randomized prospective trials over first generation regimens. (Level I evidence.)

Type of Treatment	CR (%)	DFS (%)	OS (%)	Mortality (%)	Type of Evidence	References	Comment
CHOP	44–59	41 (3 years) 32 (4 years)	54 (3 years) 51 (4 years)	1–4	Level I	NEJM 1992;327: 1342; NEJM 1993;328:1002 JOCO 1994;12: 709	No difference demonstrated in any of randomized trials; selection is usually clinician and institution dependent. Most clinicians favor CHOP (least costly in dollar terms)
MACOP-B	51	46 (3 years) 44 (4 years)	50 (3 years) 56 (4 years)	4–6	Level I	NEJM 1993; 328: 1002, JOCO 1994; 12:709	
m-BACOD	48–56	46	52 (3 years) 49 (5 years)	5–6	Level I	NEJM 1992;327: 1342; NEJM 1993;328:1002	
ProMACE -CytaBOM	56	41 (3 years)	50 (3 years)	3	Level I	NEJM 1993;328: 1002	

Decision Point 2: What is the best therapy for slow (partial responders?

Some studies suggested (level IV evidence) that slow-responders have poor prognosis and should be treated aggressively with bone marrow transplantation (BMT) early in therapy to change the course of disease. However, a prospective randomized trial did not demonstrate superiority of BMT over first-generation chemotherapy (level I evidence)

Type of Treatment	CR (%)	DFS (%)	OS (%)	Mortality (%)	Type of Evidence	References	Comment
CHOP	74	72 (4 years)	85 (4 years)	0	Level I	NEJM 1995;332: 1045	CHOP equally effective to autoBMT

Decision Point 3: What is the best treatment of relapse (salvage therapy)?

The patients with relapsed disease have poor prognosis.

(A randomized trial demonstrated advantage of treating these patients with aggressive therapy if disease responds to conventional therapy. No advantage was found for primary refractory disease.)

Type of Treatment	CR (%)	DFS (%)	OS (%)	Mortality (%)	Type of Evidence	References	Comment
autoBMT (BEAC with radiation therapy to bulky disease)	84	46 (5 years)	53 (5 years)	5.5	Level I Level IV	NEJM 1995;333: 1540 JOCO1994; 12:2524	Superior to conventional chemotherapy (DHAP) (only patients < 60 years studied, with no central nervous system or bone marrow involvement); alloBMT= aBMT purging = nonpurging (mortality with DHAP or MIME were reported to be between 0%–8%)

Decision Point 4: What is the best first-line treatment for early stages?

Most patients with early stages can be cured. Randomized prospective trials demonstrated superiority of doxorubicin-containing regimens. A recent randomized trial showed that CHOP × 3 followed by XRT was superior to CHOP × 8 (level I evidence) (ASCO, 1996).

Type of Treatment	CR (%)	DFS (%)	OS (%)	Mortality (%)	Type of Evidence	References	Comment
CHOP + IF radiation therapy	95–100	77 (at 4 years)	90–95 (stage I) (at 4 years) 75 (stage II) (at 4 years)	1 (?)	Level IV	ASCO 1996;15:411 Ann Intern Med 1987;107:25 Oncology 1991; 5:127	CHOP × 3 followed by XRT was better than CHOP × 8 for stage I and asymptomatic patients. For stage II and symptomatic patients results were not so good (OS less than 75% and 65% respectively)

[a] as shown in Figure 9-4. Abbreviations: NEJM, N Engl J Med; JOCO, J Clin Oncol; ASCO, American Society of Clinical Oncology; (annual meeting).

TABLE 9-13 BENEFITS/RISKS OF PREFERRED MANAGEMENT ALTERNATIVES FOR RAPIDLY PROGRESSIVE NHL[a]

Type of Treatment	Outcomes						Comment
	Complete Remission (CR) (%)	Disease-Free Survival (DFS) (%)	Overall Survival (OS) (%)	Mortality (%)	Type of Evidence	References	
Decision Point 1: What is the best first-line treatment for small, non-cleaved cell NHL?							
(Best regimen not identified; no randomized trial available; most authors believe that the best therapy is a short-duration, high-intensity cyclophosphamide-based regimen). (Level III evidence)							
Cyclophosphamide, etoposide, vincristine, bleomycin, doxorubicin, methotrexate, prednisone	85	60 (5 years)	60 (5 years)	10	Level III	JOCO 1991;9:941	Better results for early-stage disease
Variable	80	60 (5 years)	30–90 (5 years) (depending on stage)	0 (20% septic episodes)	Level III	JOCO 1990;8:615	
ProMACE-CytaBOM or PROM-ACE-MOPP	63–100	71–100 (15 years)	51–88 (15 years)	3–6	Level III	JOCO 1994;12:215	
Decision Point 2: What is the best treatment of relapse (salvage therapy) for small, non-cleaved cell non-Hodgkin's lymphoma?							
Most authors believe that second-line chemotherapy will produce short CR, and that only hope for cure might be BMT; alloBMT might be preferable to autoBMT (level IV and V evidence)							
autoBMT		30 (5 years)	30 (5 years)	14%	Level IV	JOCO 1994;12:1358	These are data for lymphoblastic NHL; few data exists for small, non-cleaved cell NHL
			72% (transplanted in CR vs 37% transplanted in chemosensitive relapse vs 7% for chemoresistant disease) (at 3 years)	8.5%	Level IV	JOCO 1996;14:2465	Second cited study included adults with Burkitt's and Burkitt's like NHL: it appears that autoBMT with peripheral stem cell rescue is superior salvage treatment to conventional therapy. The results for patient stransplanted in first CR require, however, comparison with modern dose-intensive regimens.
Decision Point 3: Should consolidation with BMT be used in patient with poor prognostic factors for small, non-cleaved cell NHL?							
(A chance for relapse in patients with poor prognosis is high; outcome with second-line therapy is poor; however, consolidation with BMT carries significant morbidity/mortality)							
Auto vs alloBMT		The presence of CNS disease at the transplant adversely affects prognosis (27% DFS); however, if CNS disease is cleared, the results with BMT were as good as in those without CNS disease (DFS at 5 years, 42%)			Level IV	JOCO 1994;12:2415	Results refer to all histologies not only to those with small, non-cleaved NHL
Decision Point # 4: Indications for prophylactic intrathecal therapy of small, non-cleaved cell NHL (see Table 9-14)							
Most authors administer CNS prophylaxis to high-risk patients; however, some use it routinely, believing that it is an essential component of therapy (type IV and V evidence)						Level IV Level V	
Methotrexate i.t. (12 mg twice weekly × 5)		Spread in CNS occurs in 28% of patients who receive no i.t. prophylaxis vs 8% who have i.t prophylaxis				JOCO 1991;9:1973	

[a]As shown in Figure 9-5. Abbreviations: BMT, bone marrow transplantation; CNS, central nervous system; NHL, non-Hodgkin's lymphoma.

TABLE 9-14 INDICATIONS FOR CNS PROPHYLAXIS

Lymphoblastic lymphoma

Testicular lymphoma

Small non-cleaved cell (all patients?)

Aggressive NHL of head/neck (sinus, etc.)

HIV + lymphoma (if marrow is involved or histology is
  small, non-cleaved cell NHL)

Aggressive lymphoma with bone marrow involvement

*Based on indirect data (types IV and V evidence); see also Figure
9-1.*

**TABLE 9-15 FOLLOW-UP TIMING AND OPERATING CHARAC-
TERISTICS OF DIAGNOSTIC TESTS IN DETECTION OF
RELAPSE IN AGGRESSIVE NON-HODGKIN'S LYMPHOMA**[a]

Timing[b]: every 3 months for 2 years, then every 6 months for
another year, then annually (65%–70% of relapses are detected
at initially involved sites, 25%–35% at new sites)

Diagnostic Test	Sensitivity (%)[c]	Specificity(%)
Physical examination	80	99
Complete blood count	21	98
LDH	65	85
Chest X-ray	21	95
Chest CT scan	45	83
Abdominal/pelvic CT[d]/US	55	94
Gallium scan	90	90
Bone marrow biopsy	26	100

[a] *Adapted from Weeks JC et al: JOCO 9:1196–1203, 1991, with permission. Probability of relapse (after m BACOD therapy) is 2.1% per
year for early stages; in advanced stages this increases to 13.3%/year
for the first 2 years, 7.7% per year for years 2 through 5, and 1.6%
per year of relapse thereafter; these probabilities may be used as
pretest estimates that can be combined with the values below to
obtain post-test probability of relapse (see also Ch. 1) (type IV evidence)*

[b] *Indirect evidences for recommended strategy (mainly type V)*

[c] *At the time of relapse, sensitivity as a screening test (performed
within 3 months before clinical relapse) is notoriously low, ranging from 0 for chest CT to 42% for elevated LDH.*

[d] *About 60% of patients who presented with an abdominal mass
larger than 10 cm had residual mass detectable by CT after therapy.
In these cases, surgical evaluation is unlikely to show residual lymphoma. These patients are no more likely to relapse than those without mass. Consequently, additional therapy is not indicated in these
patients. (JOCO 6:1832–1837, 1988 (type IV evidence).*

Abbreviations: CT, computed tomography; LDH, US, ultrasound.

FIGURE 9-6 *Management of human immunodeficiency virus (HIV) associated lymphoma. Reasoning
principles are based on understanding the natural
history of disease, the tumor burden upon presentation (stage of a disease) and probabilities of response,
outcomes (disease-free and overall survival), and risk
of specific types of treatment and concurrent therapy
for HIV disease and pneumocystis carinii pneumonia. These factors determine the goal of treatment
that mostly focuses on slight prolongation of survival
and palliation. Evidences for recommended strategy
are mainly of type III and IV. A recent randomized
trial showed that median survival (MS) does not differ between treatment with chemotherapy at 60%
dose reduction and full dose chemotherapy with
growth factor supports. (Mayo Clin Proc
1995;70:665; Cancer Control 1995; March/April:97.)
Note that staging for an immunocompetent patient
presenting with a central nervous system mass is
essentially the same, except for bypassing the empirical treatment for toxoplasmosis (Ann Intern Med
1993;119:1093).*

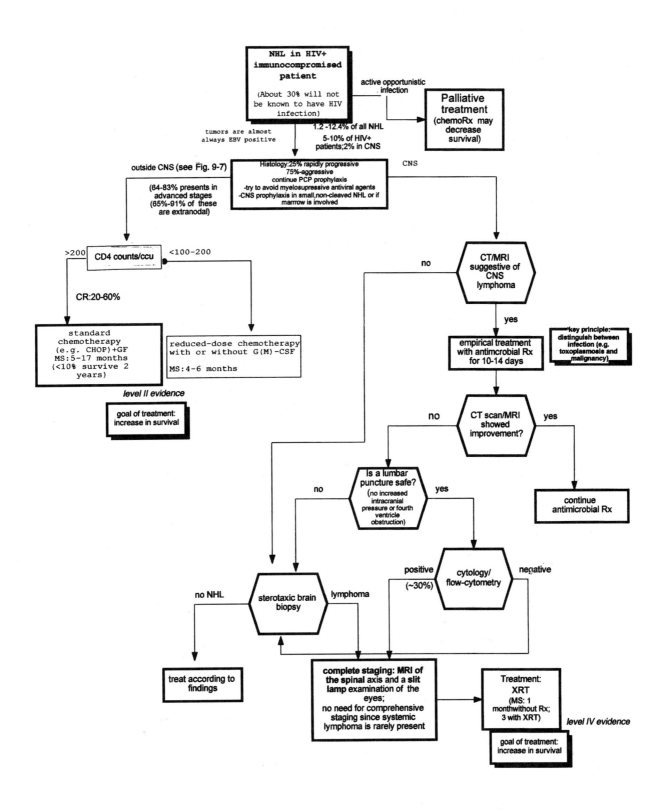

NHL in HIV+ immunocompromised patient

(About 30% will not be known to have HIV infection)

active opportunistic infection

Palliative treatment (chemoRx may decrease survival)

tumors are almost always EBV positive

1.2 -12.4% of all NHL
5-10% of HIV+ patients;2% in CNS

outside CNS (see Fig. 9-7)

Histology:25% rapidly progressive
75%-aggressive
continue PCP prophylaxis
-try to avoid myelosupressive antiviral agents
-CNS prophylaxis in small,non-cleaved NHL or if marrow is involved

CNS

(64-83% presents in advanced stages (65%-91% of these are extranodal)

>200   CD4 counts/ccu   <100-200

CR:20-60%

CT/MRI suggestive of CNS lymphoma

no

standard chemotherapy (e.g. CHOP)+GF MS:5-17 months (<10% survive 2 years)

reduced-dose chemotherapy with or without G(M)-CSF

MS:4-6 months

yes

empirical treatment with antimcrobial Rx for 10-14 days

key principle: distinguish between infection (e.g. toxoplasmosis and malignancy)

level II evidence

goal of treatment: increase in survival

no   CT scan/MRI showed improvement?   yes

continue antimicrobial Rx

Is a lumbar puncture safe? (no increased intracranial pressure or fourth ventricle obstruction)

no   yes

positive (~30%)   cytology/ flow-cytometry   negative

no NHL   sterotaxic brain biopsy   lymphoma

treat according to findings

complete staging: MRI of the spinal axis and a slit lamp examination of the eyes;
no need for comprehensive staging since systemic lymphoma is rarely present

Treatment: XRT (MS: 1 monthwithout Rx; 3 with XRT)

level IV evidence

goal of treatment: increase in survival

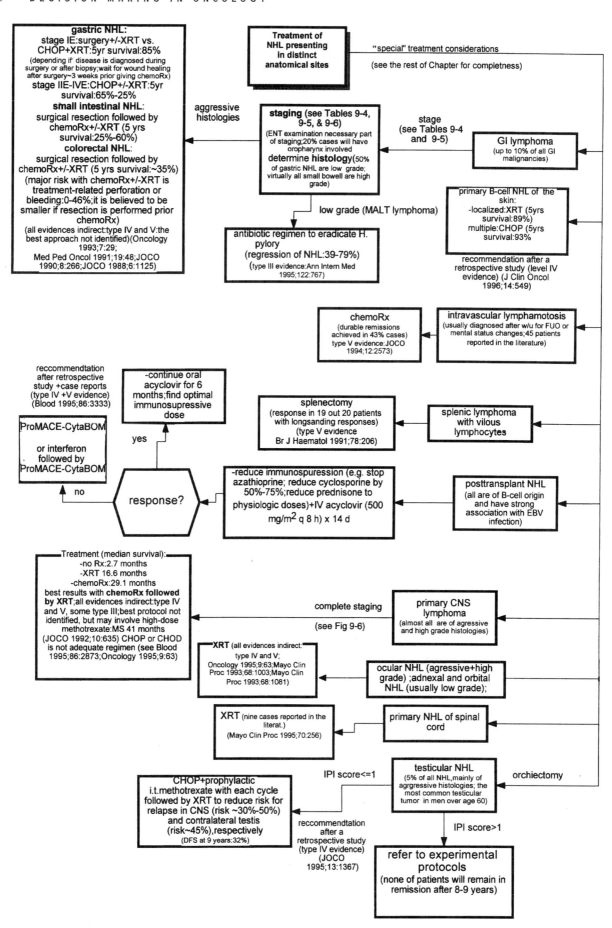

gastric NHL:
stage IE:surgery+/-XRT vs.
CHOP+XRT:5yr survival:85%
(depending if disease is diagnosed during surgery or after biopsy;wait for wound healing after surgery~3 weeks prior giving chemoRx)
stage IIE-IVE:CHOP+/-XRT:5yr survival:65%-25%
small intestinal NHL:
surgical resection followed by chemoRx+/-XRT (5 yrs survival:25%-60%)
colorectal NHL:
surgical resection followed by chemoRx+/-XRT (5 yrs survival:~35%)
(major risk with chemoRx+/-XRT is treatment-related perforation or bleeding:0-46%;it is believed to be smaller if resection is performed prior chemoRx)
(all evidences indirect:type IV and V:the best approach not identified)(Oncology 1993;7:29;
Med Ped Oncol 1991;19:48;JOCO 1990;8:266;JOCO 1988;6:1125)

Treatment of NHL presenting in distinct anatomical sites

"special" treatment considerations

(see the rest of Chapter for completness)

aggressive histologies

staging (see Tables 9-4, 9-5, & 9-6)
(ENT examination necessary part of staging;20% cases will have oropharynx involved
determine **histology**(50% of gastric NHL are low grade; virtually all small bowell are high grade)

stage (see Tables 9-4 and 9-5)

GI lymphoma
(up to 10% of all GI malignancies)

low grade (MALT lymphoma)

antibiotic regimen to eradicate H. pylori
(regression of NHL:39-79%)
(type III evidence:Ann Intern Med 1995;122:767)

primary B-cell NHL of the skin:
-localized:XRT (5yrs survival:89%)
multiple:CHOP (5yrs survival:93%

recommendation after a retrospective study (level IV evidence) (J Clin Oncol 1996;14:549)

chemoRx
(durable remissions achieved in 43% cases)
type V evidence:JOCO 1994;12:2573)

intravascular lymphamotosis
(usually diagnosed after w/u for FUO or mental status changes;45 patients reported in the literature)

reccommendtation after retrospective study +case reports (type IV +V evidence) (Blood 1995;86:3333)

-continue oral acyclovir for 6 months;find optimal immunosupressive dose

yes

ProMACE-CytaBOM
or interferon followed by ProMACE-CytaBOM

splenectomy
(response in 19 out 20 patients with longsanding responses)
(type V evidence Br J Haematol 1991;78:206)

splenic lymphoma with vilous lymphocytes

no

response?

-reduce immunospuression (e.g. stop azathioprine; reduce cyclosporine by 50%-75%;reduce prednisone to physiologic doses)+IV acyclovir (500 mg/m^2 q 8 h) x 14 d

posttransplant NHL
(all are of B-cell origin and have strong association with EBV infection)

Treatment (median survival):
-no Rx:2.7 months
-XRT 16.6 months
-chemoRx:29.1 months
best results with **chemoRx followed by XRT**;all evidences indirect:type IV and V, some type III;best protocol not identified, but may involve high-dose methotrexate:MS 41 months
(JOCO 1992;10:635) CHOP or CHOD is not adequate regimen (see Blood 1995;86:2873;Oncology 1995;9:63)

complete staging

(see Fig 9-6)

primary CNS lymphoma
(almost all are of agressive and high grade histologies)

XRT (all evidences indirect: type IV and V;
Oncology 1995;9:63;Mayo Clin Proc 1993;68:1003;Mayo Clin Proc 1993;68:1081)

ocular NHL (agressive+high grade) ;adnexal and orbital NHL (usually low grade);

XRT (nine cases reported in the literat.)
(Mayo Clin Proc 1995;70:256)

primary NHL of spinal cord

IPI score<=1

testicular NHL
(5% of all NHL,mainly of aggressive histologies; the most common testicular tumor in men over age 60)

orchiectomy

CHOP+prophylactic i.t.methotrexate with each cycle followed by XRT to reduce risk for relapse in CNS (risk ~30%-50%) and contralateral testis (risk~45%),respectively
(DFS at 9 years:32%)

reccommendtation after a retrospective study (type IV evidence) (JOCO 1995;13:1367)

IPI score>1

refer to experimental protocols
(none of patients will remain in remission after 8-9 years)

FIGURE 9-7 *Management of extranodal lymphoma (special sites non-Hodgkin's lymphoma NHL). Reasoning principles are based on understanding the natural history of disease, the tumor burden upon presentation (stage of disease), a specific anatomic site, probabilities of response, outcomes (cure, disease-free and overall survival), and risk of specific types of treatment. The goals vary from cure to prolongation of survival (depending on location). Note, these special sites NHL are largely characteristic of aggressive and rapidly progressive high-grade lymphomas; low-grade lymphomas, for example, do not involve the testes or central nervous system. However, gastric and lung MALT NHL are usually low-grade lymphoma. Since extranodal NHL are relatively rare entities, evidences to support particular treatments are usually based on indirect data (level IV and V). (For doses and treatment protocols see Appendix 9.)*

SUGGESTED READINGS

Armitage JO: Treatment of non-Hodgkin's lymphoma. N Engl J Med 328:1029, 1993

Harris NL, Jaffe ES, Stein H et al: A revised European-American classification of lymphoid neoplasms: a proposal from the international lymphoma study group. Blood 84:1361–1392, 1994

Horning SJ: Treatment approaches to the low-grade lymphomas. Blood 83:881–884, 1994

Johnson PWM, Rohatiner AZS, Whelan JS et al: Patterns of survival in patients with recurrent follicular lymphoma: a 20-year study from a single center. J Clin Oncol 13:140–147, 1995

Longo DL: What is the deal with follicular lymphomas? J Clin Oncol 11:202–208, 1993

Peterson BA: The role of transplantation in non-Hodgkin's lymphoma. J Clin Oncol 12:2524–2526, 1994

Shipp MA: Prognostic factors in aggressive non-Hodgkin's lymphoma: who has "high-risk" disease? Blood 83:1165–1173, 1994

Vose JM: Treatment for non-Hodgkin's lymphoma in relapse? What are alternatives? N Engl J Med 333:1565–1566, 1995

Wingo PA, Tong T, Bolden S: Cancer Statistics, 1995. Ca J Clinicians 45:30, 1995

10 T-Cell Lymphoma

Benjamin Djulbegović

Incidence: 4.2 cases/million/year in 1984; about 1,000 new cases are diagnosed each year; average age at diagnosis is 50 years, and most patients are over age of 30

Goal of treatment: Improvement of the quality of life

Prognosis (stage-dependent):

Plaque-only skin disease: median survival > 12 years

Cutaneous tumors, erythroderma, node or blood involvement, but no visceral disease: median survival 5 years

Visceral involvement or node effacement: median survival 2.5 years

INCIDENCE

The most common cutaneous T-cell lymphoma (CTCL) are (1) mycosis fungoides (MF), and (2) Sézary syndrome (SS), an erythrodermic variant associated with a leukemic phase of the disease (typical cerebriform cells of SS are usually found in the buffy coat). Other T-cell diseases that can present with skin involvement are listed in Table 10-1, and on occasion can be confused with MF and SS. The incidence of MF and SS in the United State has more than tripled from 1.3 cases/million/year in 1969 to 4.2 cases/million/year in 1984. About 1,000 new cases are diagnosed each year. The average age at diagnosis is 50 years, and most patients are over 30. The highest incidence is seen in black men and the lowest in white women.

DIAGNOSIS

The diagnosis of CTCL is often suspected when long-lasting, poorly classified dermatosis becomes resistant to topical steroids. (Usual preceding diagnosis to CTCL is atopic eczema, seborrheic dermatitis, or psoriasis.) A histologic confirmation of diagnosis of MF/SS is often reached after many nonspecific biopsies. Pathognomonic histopathologic findings consist of dermal infiltrates with atypical lymphocytes and *Pautrier's microabscesses*. Although these histopathologic signs have high specificity, they have poor sensitivity, and are often absent. Occasionally, gene rearrangement studies might be necessary to prove clonality of the process. Most of the cases of MF/SS are of the T-helper phenotype (CD4+).

MF and SS are disorders with a chronic course, and survival strongly correlates with a tumor burden. Staging is, therefore, essential in the clinical management of these patients. Figure 10-1 shows a staging system, recommended staging procedures and survival according to the stage of disease. It is thought that MF initially involves the skin and with time disseminates to lymph nodes, the spleen, the liver, or other visceral organs. In general, patients who are a good risk have only skin plaque lesions and a median survival of more than 12 years. The disease in patients at intermediate risk has spread to nodes or blood but without visceral involvement or node effacement; these patients have a median survival of about 5 years. Poor-risk patients have

TABLE 10-1 T-CELL LYMPHOMA WITH CUTANEOUS INVOLVEMENT

CTCL	Comments
Mycosis fungoides	Most common cutaneous T-cell lymphona
Sézary syndrome	Most common
Adult T-cell lymphoma/leukemia	Associated with the retrovirus HTLV-l; most HTLV-I infected patients remain asymptomatic, but about 2% to 4% have progressive disease characterized by visceral involvement, immunodeficiency, skeletal abnormalities, and hypercalcemia. The neoplastic T cells express high levels of IL-2 receptors. Figure 10-2 show recommendation for the treatment of this disease, after two studies (level III evidence) showed likely improvement in the prognosis of this deadly disorder.
Lymphomatoid papulosis[a]	Clinically benign disorder characterized by clonal rearrangement of T-cell receptor genes. It can be diagnosed only through careful history in which the characteristic waxing and waning of the skin lesions is identified through proper communications between pathologists and clinicians. If diagnosis is based only on histology, the disorder can be frequently misdiagnosed as lymphoma, melanoma, or carcinoma. Cummulative risk that disease will transform into aggressive lymphoma is estimated to be 80% at 15 years (level IV evidence). Patients who develop lymphoma respond well to cytotoxic therapy and can be cured.
Pagetoid reticulosis	An extremely rare generalized form.
Granulomatous slack-skin disorder	Differential diagnosis includes sarcoidosis and tuberculoid leprosy.
Large T-cell non-Hodgkin's lymphoma	Prognosis and treatment not different from B-cell NHL (see Chapter 9).
Angioimmunoblastic lymphadenopathy[b]	Subacute illness with generalized lymphadenopathy, organomegaly, skin rash, and hypergammaglobulinemia; about 30% of patients report drug allergies.
Large-granular lymphocyte leukemia[c]	Usually presents with neutropenia, mild rheumatic complaints, and positive rheumatoid factor.
T-cell chronic lymphocytic leukemia[d]	Rare condition; does not respond well to standard treatment shown in Chapter 6.

[a]*Ann Intern Med 122:210, 1995.*

[b]*Am J Hematol 20:301, 1985.*

[c]*Blood 82:1, 1993.*

[d]*Blood 86:1163, 1995.*

visceral involvement or node effacement, and their median survival is about 2.5 years. Infection, usually from the skin (*Staphylococcus aureus* and *Pseudomonas aeruginosa*), is the major cause of death (50%).

TREATMENT

Disseminated disease is found in about 50% of patients at initial presentation if staging is done by routine laboratory and imaging studies. A bone marrow biopsy is positive in about 20% of cases and is usually done only in patients in the advanced stages. An abdominal CT is not helpful in the early stages of disease. If, however, molecular biology techniques are employed in looking for clonal T-cell-gene rearrangement, then disseminated disease can be detected in more than 90% of patients. This has formed a rationale for early aggressive treatment of cutaneous T-cell lymphoma. Unfortunately,

a randomized trial comparing aggressive chemotherapy as an initial treatment with conservative treatment did not improve the prognosis of these patients. Therefore, until new modalities are developed, one should probably favor *topical treatment for localized disease and systemic chemotherapy for disseminated disease* (Fig. 10-2).

Like other low-grade lymphoma (see Chapter 9), CTCL cannot be cured. There is no evidence that any modality can lead to prolongation of survival. The goal of treatment is to improve the quality of life. Given the nature of this devastating disease, this outcome of the treatment can be as important as prolongation of survival, and every attempt should be made to control the disease for as long as possible.

What treatment and in which sequence to choose? In the management of CTCL fourteen different modalities of treatment and at least 57 different specific therapies have been described. Very few

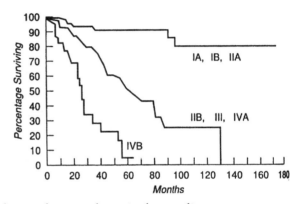

Staging Systems for Mycosis Fungoides

T stage
T1: Limited plaque, less than 10% body surface area
T2: Generalized plaque, 10% or greater of body surface area
T3: Cutaneous tumor (one or more)
T4: Erythroderma (generalized)

Adenopathy
Ad +: Palpable adenopathy
Ad −: No palpable adenopathy

Lymph node class (biopsy)
LN1: Reactive node
LN2: Dermatopathic node, small clusters of convoluted cells
LN3: Dermatopathic node, large clusters of convoluted cells
LN4: Lymph node effacement

Visceral
V+: Positive visceral biopsy
V−: Negative visceral biopsy

Stages*
IA: T1; Ad−; LN1, LN2, V−
IB: T2; Ad−; LN1, LN2, V−
IIA: T1, T2; Ad + ; LN1, LN2; V−
IIB: T3; Ad ±; LN1, LN2; V−
III: T4; Ad ±; LN1, LN2, V−
IVA: T1-T4; Ad ±; LN3 or LN4; V−
IVB: T1-T4; Ad±; LN1-LN4; V+

Blood
B+: Positive blood smear
B−: Negative blood smear

Modified Staging Evaluation of Mycosis Fungoides and the Sézary Syndrome*

Positive skin biopsy
Skin examination for T class
Node examination
  Adenopathy
  Biopsy
Peripheral blood smear and cell size
Visceral biopsy (marrow, liver if node examination or peripheral blood smear was positive)
Prognostic groups
  Low risk
    T1 or T2; LN1, LN2; negative peripheral blood smear; negative visceral biopsy
  Intermediate risk
    Not encompassed by low or high
  High risk
    LN4 or positive visceral biopsy

*T1-T4 = T stages of skin disease (38); LN1-LN4 = grade 1 to 4 lymph node histopathologic findings (35).

FIGURE 10-1 *Staging system, recommended procedures and survival according to stages of disease in mycosis fungoides/Sézary syndrome. Recommendation based on level IV evidence. (From Sausville EA, Eddy JL, Makuch RW et al: Ann Intern Med 109:372–382, 1989, with premission.)*

randomized trials have been performed. Given the rarity of CTCL, it is not surprising that most data are not of the highest quality (usually level IV or V) (see Chapter 1). This is a likely reason for the many practice variations that are current in the management of CTCL; Figure 10-2, therefore, represents one possible strategy, based on my interpretation of relative benefit/risk ratios of all treatments currently available and the quality of data used to assess these ratio (Tables 10-2 and 10-3).

SUGGESTED READINGS

Bunn PA, Hoffman SJ, Norris D, Golitz LE, Aeling JL: Systemic therapy of cutaneous T-cell lymphomas (mycosis fungoides and the Sézary syndrome). Ann Intern Med 121:592–602, 1994

Kaye FJ, Bunn PA, Steinberg SM et al: A randomized trial comparing combination electron-beam radiation and chemotherapy with topical therapy in the initial treatment of mycosis fungoides. N Engl J Med 321:1784–1790 1989
Kemme DJ, Bunn PA: State of the art therapy of mycosis fungoides and Sézary syndrome. Oncology 6:31–48, 1992
Kuzel TM, Roenigk HH, Rosen ST: Mycosis fungoides and the Sézary syndrome: a review of pathogenesis, diagnosis and therapy. J Clin Oncol 9:1298–1313, 1991
Sausville EA, Eddy JL, Makuch RW et al: Histopathologic staging at initial diagnosis of mycosis fungoides and the Sézary syndrome: definitions of three distinctive prognostic groups. Ann Intern Med 109:372–382 1989
Young RC: Mycosis fungoides: The therapeutic search continues. N Engl J Med 321:1822–1823, 1989

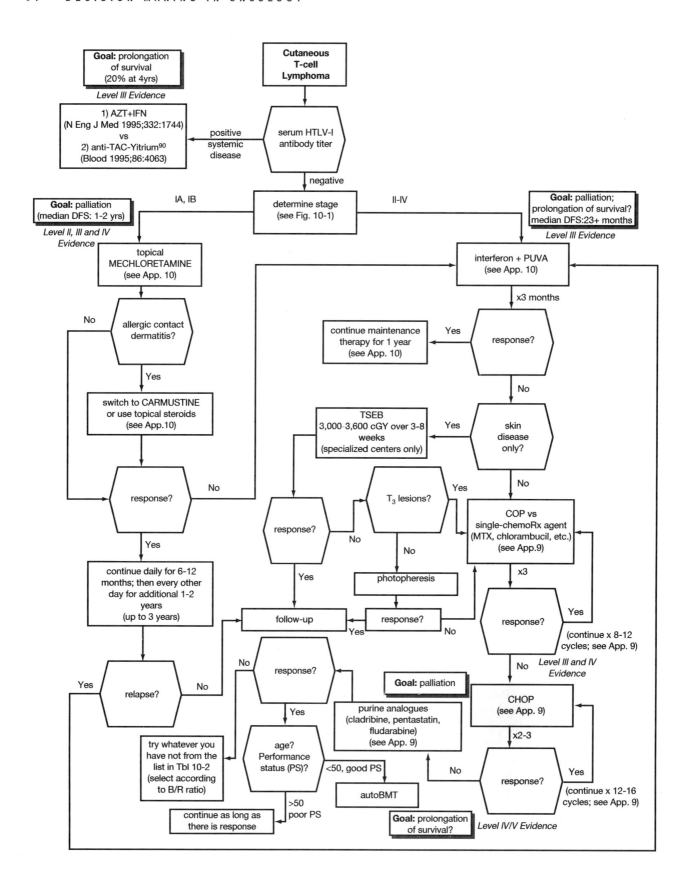

FIGURE 10-2 *An algorithm for the treatment of mycosis fungoides/Sézary syndrome. A rationale for the recommended strategy is based on information that initial aggressive chemotherapy does not improve the prognosis of these patients but causes greater toxicity (see also Table 10-3). Therefore, according to the risk/benefit principles, the sequences of the palliative therapies remain the treatment of choice in this long-lasting, but deadly, disease. The goal of the treatment is, therefore, improvement in the quality of life of patient. Initial decision about the choice of sequential topical therapy is based on level II evidence; further choices are mainly of level IV and V evidence, and some of level III evidence. Note that within these management principles a construction of a different treatment scenario is quite possible (see text for details; see Appendix 10 for doses and practical details on the management). DFS, disease-free survival; auto BMT, autologous bone marrow transplant; TSEB, total skin electron beam; AZT, ziduvidine; IFN, interferon; PUVA, psoralen + UV light A; MTX, methotrexate; TAC, T-activated cells; CHOP, cyclophosphamide, doxorubicin, vincristine, prednisone; App., Appendix.*

TABLE 10-2 COMPETITIVE TREATMENT ALTERNATIVES FOR CUTANEOUS T-CELL LYMPHOMA

Treatment Class[a]	Benefit: Risk Estimate[b]
Topical treatment	
Topical chemotherapy (mechlorethamine, carmustine)	Good
Psoralen + ultraviolet A light (PUVA)	Good
Total skin electron beam therapy	Fair
Photopheresis	Poor
Systemic therapy	
Single-agent chemotherapy (methotrexate, cyclophosphamide, chlorambucil, vincristine, etoposide, doxorubicin, cisplatin, prednisone, etc.)	Good
Combination chemotherapy (COP, CHOP, CAVE, CBP, BAM, VAB-CMP, etc.)	Fair
Interferons (α,β,γ)	Good
Purine analogues (pentostatin, cladribine, fludarabine)	Fair
Retinoids	Good
Cyclosporine	Poor
Monoclonal antibodies	Fair
Immunoconjugates	Fair
Thymopentin	?
Acyclovir	Poor
Auto-BMT	Fair (?)

[a] *At least 57 different specific therapies were described; very few randomized trials were performed comparing one treatment strategy with another; similarly, few controlled trials exist on comparison of different treatment agents within same treatment class.*

[b] *Most data are of low quality and precise quantiative benefit/risk estimate is not possible (see also Table 10-3).*

TABLE 10-3 BENEFITS/RISKS OF PREFERRED MANAGEMENT ALTERNATIVES FOR CUTANEOUS T-CELL LYMPHOMA AS SHOWN IN FIG. 10-2

Type of treatment	Outcomes						
	Complete Remission (CR) (%)	Disease Free Survival (DFS) (%)	Overall Survival (OS) (%)	Toxicity (%)	Type of Evidence	References	Comment

Decision Point # 1: Should combined therapy be used early in the course of the treatment of T-NHL?

A randomized trial (type II evidence) showed that early aggressive therapy with radiation and chemotherapy does not improve the prognosis for patients with T-NHL (stages I-IV) as compared with conservative approach beginning with sequential therapies (N Engl J Med 1989;321:1784)

Type of treatment	Complete Remission (CR) (%)	Disease Free Survival (DFS) (%)	Overall Survival (OS) (%)	Toxicity (%)	Type of Evidence	References	Comment
Total skin electron beam (TSEB) + ChemoRx	38% (CR+PR=90%)	10% at 3 years (median: 12.9 months)	Median: 7.6 years	36% severe toxicity (4% developed AML)	Level II	N Engl J Med 1989;321:1784	For stages I-IV; although results do not differ between aggressive and conservative treatment they are stage-dependent (survival varies from >80% at 5 years for stage I/II disease to less than 40% for stage IVB; see Fig. 10-1)
Mechlorethamine followed by PUVA, followed by TSEB; oral methotrexate in IVB stage	18% (CR+PR=65%)	10% at 3 years (median: 21.3 months)	Median: 6.3 years	Hypersensitivity (43%); about 15% patients can not tolerate topical treatment	Level II and III	N Engl J Med 1989; 321:1784; J Clin Oncol 1988; 6:1177	

Decision Point # 2: What is the best topical treatment for skin disease?

Many therapeutic strategies that exists have never been compared in randomized trials (except for PUVA + retinoids vs. PUVA) (Ann Intern Med 1994;121:592).
Most data are of level III, IV and V, and personal preferences, experience, availability of some equipment usually dictates the choice and sequence of treatment options shown in the Fig. 10-1. With data available, it is conceivable to construct the algorithm in many different ways.

Type of treatment	Complete Remission (CR) (%)	Disease Free Survival (DFS) (%)	Overall Survival (OS) (%)	Toxicity (%)	Type of Evidence	References	Comment
Mechlorethamine	0%-61% (T3 lesion); 26%-68% (T2); 51%-80% (T2)	Median DFS: 5-15 months (stage I: 16%; stage II: 6%; stage III: 11% at 8 yrs) Median time to relapse: 3.6 years	73%-89% at 5 years (median: 12 years when visceral disease is excluded)	Hypersensitivity (35%); increased incidence of skin cancers	Level III, IV (see also above)	J Clin Oncol Oncol 1991; 9:1298 J Clin Oncol 1987; 5:1796	Stages IV B excluded from survival statistics;

Treatment	Response rate	Duration of response	Survival	Side effects	Level of evidence	References	Comments
PUVA (psoralen + UV-A light)	58%–84%	9–53 months	Not reported	Mild nausea, vomiting, pruritus, sunburn-like changes, skin amyloidosis (psoralen); skin cancers (psoralen)	Level III, IV	J Clin Oncol 1991; 9:1298 Oncology 1992; 6:31	No CR are seen in patients with T3 lesions. In randomized study with etritonate + PUVA vs. PUVA no difference in responses were noted (Acta Dermatol Venereol 1989;69:536)
Total skin electron beam therapy	80%–90%	50% at 3 years (limited disease) 25% at 3 years (generalized disease)	MS: 10 years (T1 lesions: 41% 15 yrs survival; T3 lesions: 32% 15 yrs survival)	Acute radiodermatitis (72%); Decreased ability to sweat (84%); alopecia (100%); abnormal lacrimation similar to psoralen	Level III and IV	Oncology 1992; 6:31	Expensive equipment; available in specialized centers only
Photopheresis (extracorporeal photochemotherapy)	20% (CR+PR:57%)	Median: 48 months	MS: ~60 months from diagnosis (48 months from the treatment start)		Level IV and V	J Clin Oncol 1991; 9:1298 Oncology 1992;6:31 Ann Intern Med 1994;121:592	Studies difficult to interpret; many patients treated with other therapies while undergoing photopheresis; poor response in tumor-stage of the disease; many authors consider photopheresis experimental at this time
Topical carmustine	86% (T1 stage); 48% (T2); (21%) T4 (median time to CR: 11.5 weeks)	18% at 5 years	Median survival: 9.4 years (77% at 5 years)	Mild bone marrow depression (7.4%) hypersensitivity (6.6%) erythema (~100%)	Level IV	J Am Acad Dermatol 1990;22:802	Can be used in patients allergic to mechlorethamine

Continues

TABLE 10-3 *(Continued)*

Decision Point # 3: When should systemic therapy be indicated? What agents should be used as a first line treatment?

Although early administration of systemic therapy does not change the natural history of T-NHL, numerous type III and IV evidences favors the use of chemotherapy **in advanced disease or disease refractory to topical treatment**. There were no randomized trials comparing combination chemotherapy (Crx) with single-agent chemo-regimens. Type II evidence suggest that no particular combination is superior to another. With any approach, no cure is possible, and it is not clear whether any therapy leads to prolongation of survival. However, chemoRx clearly improves the quality of life of patients with CTCL and frequently leads to CR of this chronic debilitating disease. Since highest response rate was reported for inteferon + PUVA (Stages: IB-IVB) this treatment is included earlier in the algorithm than chemoRx, despite lower level of evidence for its true effectiveness (level III evidence).

Type of treatment	Outcomes				Type of Evidence	References	Comment
	Complete Remission (CR) (%)	Disease Free Survival (DFS) (%)	Overall Survival (OS) (%)	Toxicity (%)			
Single-agent chemotherapy (methotrexate, cyclophophamide, chlorambucil, vin cristine, etoposide, doxorubicin, prednisone, cisplatin, etc.)	33% (CR+PR:62%)	Median: 3–22 months	5–6 years	Usually well tolerated but mucositis, myelo-supression, nausea/vomiting, etc. has been described	Level III, IV, and V (based on 528 patients treated in stages II–IV)	J Clin Oncol 1991; 9:1298 Oncology 1992;6:31 Ann Intern Med 1994;121:592	No randomized studies comparing one agents versus another has been reported; therefore, it cannot be assessed that one single agent is preferred to another; most data exists for methotrexate
Combination chemotherapy (COP, CHOP, CAVE, CVBP, CBP, etc)	38% (CR + PR:81%)	Median: 5–41 months	5–7 years	Mucositis, myelo-supression, nausea/vomiting	Level II, III, IV (based on 331 patients treated in stages II–IV)	J Clin Oncol 1991;9:1298 Oncology 1992;6:31 Ann Intern Med 1994;121:5920	There were no randomized trials comparing combination chemotherapy (Crx) with single-agent chemoregimens. Two randomized trials compared one combination chemoRx with another; no difference in response rates were noted. With any approach, no cure is possible, and it is not clear whether any therapy leads to prolongation of survival.

Treatment	Response	Duration		Toxicity	Level of evidence	References	Comments
Interferons (IFN)	15% (CR + PR): 52%	Median: 4–28 months	Not reported (NR)	Flu-like syndrome (> 90%); pancytopenia neurological abnormalities	Level III and IV evidence	Oncology 1992;6:31 Ann Intern Med 1994; 121:592	Stage IB-IVB; optimal dose and duration not known but 3MU 3x week for 1 year is believed to be the right time and dose
Interferon + PUVA	80% (CR + PR: 93%)	Median duration of response: > 13 months (3–15+)	Not reported	Fever, malaise (93%) leukopenia (40%) photosensitivity (26%)	Level III	J Natl Cancer Inst. 1990;82:203	St. IB-IVB (only one patient with IVB; no CR noted); highest and longest CR reported so far; IFN in doses 18 MU tiw seems to be optimal dose
IFN + retinoids	11–14% (CR + PR: 43%–60%)	Median: 12 months	NR	Similar to IFN alone	Level III and IV	J Clin Oncol 1991; 9:1298 Oncology 1992;6:31 Ann Intern Med 1994;121:592	Stages II-IV; no randomized trials are performed to determine if this combination is superior to single modality alone, but single-arm studies do not suggest major advantage.
Retinoids	19% (CR + PR: 50%)	Median: 4–13 months	NR	Mild mucocutaneous dryness	Level III and IV	J Clin Oncol 1991; 9:1298 Oncology 1992;6:31 Ann Intern Med 1994;121:592	Activity of retinoids appear to be similar to to that of single-agent chemoRx or IFN

Continues

TABLE 10-3 (Continued)

Decision Point # 4: What to do when standard treatment options fail?
Numerous therapeutic strategies were reported in the literature. All data for their effectiveness are indirect (level IV and V evidence).
Below are summarized benefit/risks for some therapeutic alternatives listed in Table 10-2.

Type of treatment	Outcomes				Type of Evidence	References	Comment
	Complete Remission (CR) (%)	Disease Free Survival (DFS) (%)	Overall Survival (OS) (%)	Toxicity (%)			
Pentostatin	6% (CR+PR:41–62%)	Median: 1.3–66+ months	NR	Myelosupression; life-threatening infections: 15% (fatal: 6%); nausea/ vomiting, cardiotoxicity	Level IV, V	J Clin Oncol 1994; 12:258 8 Ann Intern Med 1994;121:592	Best responses noted in MF and not in SS; few data exist for the use as a first line therapy.
Cladribine	5%–19% (CR+PR:41%)	Median: 4-11 months (median from time of diagnosis:57 months)	NR	Fever/infections (38%)	Level IV, V some level III	J Clin Oncol 1994; 84:733 Ann Intern Med 1994;121:592 Blood 1996;87:906	Small series; few data exist for the use as a first line therapy.
Fludarabine	8% (CR+PR:36%)	Median: 1.3–8 months	NR	Myelosupression, infections, neurotoxicity	Level IV, V	Ann Intern Med 1994;121:592	Small series; few data exist for the use as a first line therapy.

Agent	Response	MS	Survival	Toxicity	Level	Reference	Comments
Cyclosporine	0% (CR + PR:32%)	Median: 2.4–3.5 months	NR	Immunosupression, renal & liver toxicity	Level V	Ann Intern Med 1994;121:592	Benefit/risk ratio does not justify the use of cyclosporine at this time
Acyclovir	0%	Median: 1 months	NR	Renal toxicity, myelosupression	Level V	Ann Intern Med 1994;121:592	Should be considered experimental at this time.
Thymopentin	8% (CR + PR:75%)	Median: 22 months	NR	NR	Level V	Ann Intern Med 1994;121:592	Biological activity of this pentapeptide is not clear at this time
Monoclonal antibody (MAb)+ immunoconjugates	CR + PR:0–45%	Brief response for MAb; some long-lasting responses noted for immuno-conjugates (3–29+ months)	NR	NR	Level IV/V	Ann Intern Med 1994;121:592	DAB$_{389}$-IL2 (diphteria toxin fused with IL-2) has most promising activity
AutoBMT	83%	33% at 1 year	NR	5%–10% mortality	Level IV/V	ω	Highly experimental approach; may be considered in younger patients with advanced, responsive disease and good performance status

Abbreviations: MS, median survival; MU, million units; T/W, three times a week.

11 Plasma Cell Disorders

Sead Beganović
Benjamin Djulbegović

Incidence: 4.3 cases per 100,000/year

Median age of diagnosis: Men 69; women 71

Median survival: 24–30 months

10-year survival: 3%

5-year survival: 27%

Goal of Treatment: Prolongation of survival

Most common causes of death: Sepsis

Hypercalcemia

Hemorrhage

Renal failure

M protein found in the serum or urine
during the course of disease: 99%

Elevated erythrocyte
sedimentation rate: 90%

Anemia: 67%

Skeletal lytic lesion: 60% of patients at presentation

Bone pain: 60% of patients at presentation

Hypercalcemia: 25% of patients at presentation

Renal insufficiency: 25% of patients at presentation

Amyloidosis: 10%–15%

Most important causes
of renal failure — Bence Jones proteinuria,
or hypercalcemia, or both,
in 95% of patients

Most common risk factors: Old age, ionizing radiation

MULTIPLE MYELOMA

Multiple myeloma (MM) is a disease characterized by the neoplastic proliferation of a single clone of plasma cells. Its incidence is about 3 to 5 per 100,000 population; it is the most common hematologic malignancy in blacks, with an incidence of about 9.6/100,000. Overall, it composes about 1% of all malignancies and about 10% of all hematologic malignancies. *MM should be suspected in any patient older than 40 years with unexplained anemia, renal dysfunction, or bone lesion* (only 2% of patients younger than 40 years suffer from myeloma). The clinical suspicion is confirmed by matching findings with diagnostic criteria (if-then rule; see Ch. 1). *If more than 10% of immature plasma cells (the most specific test, virtually 100%) + M protein in serum/urine + osteolytic lesions are found, then* MM is the diagnosis. This diagnostic rule, which is derived from the classical diagnostic triad (plasma cells + M protein + lytic lesions), is valid in most patients; criteria for diagnosis of patients presenting with less classic findings are shown in Table 11-1.)

About 60% of patients will produce a monoclonal IgG protein; 20%, IgA; 10% will be light-chain excretors only (Bence Jones proteins); and the rest will be accounted for by IgD, IgE, and IgM monoclonal productions. Serum protein electrophoresis (SPE) will detect M-spike in about 75% of patients, but immunoelectrophoresis (IPE) of serum and urine proteins (UPE) will detect 98% to 99% of cases (1%–2% of patients are nonsecretors). In other words, *negative IPE and UPE exclude MM with a probability of 98% to 99%.* Bone surveys will show lytic lesions in about 80% of patients. Magnetic resonance imaging (MRI) is a more sensitive

TABLE 11-1 DIAGNOSTIC CRITERIA FOR PLASMA CELL DISORDERS

Multiple Myeloma	
	Major Criteria:
	I. Plasmacytoma on tissue biopsy
	II. Bone marrow plasmacytosis with >30% plasma cells
	III. M protein: IgG >35 g/L, IgA >20 g/L, κ-or λ-light-chain
	excretion on urine electrophoresis > 1 g/24 hours (in the absence of amyloidosis)
	Minor criteria:
	A. Bone marrow plasmacytosis with 10% to 30% plasma cells
	B. Detection of an M protein in the serum or urine, but less than levels in III above
	C. Lytic bone lesion
	D. Residual normal IgM <500 mg/L, IgA <1g/L, or IgG < 6 g/L
	The diagnosis of multiple myeloma requires a minimum of one major and one minor criterion or three minor criteria that must include A + B. Combination of I and A is not diagnostic.
Monoclonal gammopathy of undetermined significance	Bone marrow plasma cells < 5%
	Asymptomatic patient
	M protein <3 g/dL
	Normal bone x-ray
	Normal hemoglobin and serum calcium
	No Bence-Jones proteinuria
	β-2 Microglobulin <3 mg/L
	Creatinine normal
Indolent myeloma	No symptoms or signs of disease
	No recurrent infections
	Serum IgG <7 g/dL or IgA <5 g/dL
	No bone lesions or < 3 lytic lesions
	Karnofsky performance status >70%
	Hemoglobin >10 mg/dL
	Normal serum calcium
	Serum creatinine <2.0 mg/dL
	Labeling index <1%
Smoldering myeloma	As an indolent mutiple myeloma +
	Bone marrow plasma cells 10%–30%
	No bone lesions

and specific test for detection of skeletal abnormalities, but at this time is generally not considered cost effective; most authors believe that radionuclide scan is inferior to x-ray and should not be ordered.

While diagnosis of MM is relatively easy, the treatment may be burdened with considerable difficulties. Stage of disease, performance status, presence of complications, and other prognostic factors may help tailor treatment for the individual patient (see Tables 11-1 to 11-3 and Fig. 11-1).

GOAL OF TREATMENT

At this time, MM is not considered curable. The goal of treatment for most patients with MM is prolongation of survival with good quality of life. This means that for a "typical" myeloma patient, a realistic goal is to achieve complete remission (CR) or partial remission (PR) that can be sustained for a long time with reasonable quality of life.

CLINICAL DECISIONS

The major *clinical decisions* in the treatment of myeloma follow.

1. Who should be treated? Every symptomatic patient with MM (including stage I) should be treated. Asymptomatic stage I patients and patients with smoldering or indolent MM do not require treatment. The rationale for deferring treatment for asymptomatic patients is based on the results of a

TABLE 11-2 STAGING SYSTEM AND PROGNOSTIC FACTORS FOR PATIENTS WITH MULTIPLE MYELOMA

Stage	5-Year Survival
Stage I, all of the following:	25% to 40%
Hb >10gldL	
Ca <12 mg/dL	
Normal x-ray or solitary lytic lesion	
IgG <5g/dl or IgA <3 g/dL	
Urine light chain <4 g/24 hours	
β_2-Microglobulin <4 mg/dL	
Stage II:	15% to 30%
Hb 8.5–10g/dL	
IgG 5–7 g/dL or IgA 3–5 g/dL	
β_2-Microglobulin 4–6 mg/dL	
Stage III, one or more of the following:	10% to 25%
Hb <8.5 g/dL	
IgG >7 g/dL or IgA >5 g/dL	
Calcium > 12 mg/dL	
Urinary κ or λ > 12 g/24 hours	
More than 3 bone lytic lesions	
β_2-Microglobulin >6 mg/dL	
Substage: A-creatinine ≤2 mg/dL	
B-creatinine >2 mg/dL	

Abbreviations: Hb, hemoglobin; Ca, calcium

randomized trial that showed no difference in survival between patients treated immediately and those for whom treatment was deferred.

2. How to treat? Patients with *solitary myeloma* of the bone (5% of all patients) should be treated with

TABLE 11-3 GENERAL TREATMENT APPROACH TO PATIENTS WITH MULTIPLE MYELOMA

Characteristics of Disease	Suggested Treatment Option
Majority of new cases of MM	MP
High C-reactive protein Elevated β_2-microglobulin Low serum albumin Low platelet count High plasma-cell thymidine-labeling index	Discuss with patient risks and benefits of BMT
Patients <65 years with stage II or III disease with good performance status and without organ failure	Consider combination therapy (for example, VMCP/BVAP) followed by high dose consolidation therapy + autologous BMT
Patient with renal failure or hypercalcemia	VAD
Extreme marrow hypofunction pancytopenia	Start with steroid pulses alone
Aggressive, rapidly progressive, MM	Combination therapy: VMCP/VBAP VAD VMCP

Abbreviations: BMT, bone marrow transplantation; MM, multiple myeloma; MP, mephalan prednisone; VAD, vincristine, Adriamycin (doxorubicin) dexamethasone; VMCP/BVAP, vincristine, melphalan, cyclophosphamide, prednisone, carmustine, doxorubicin, prednisone.

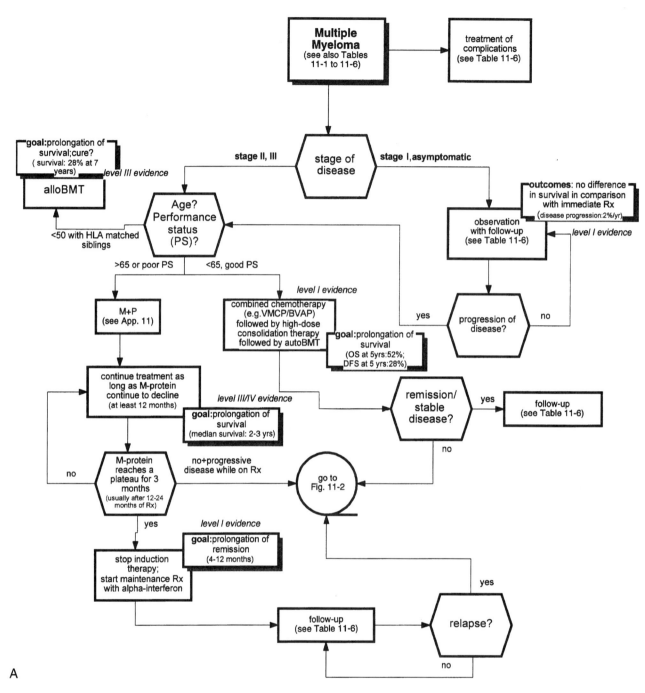

FIGURE 11-1 *(A & B) Management of multiple myeloma (MM). Assessment of a require-ment for the treatment represents a key reasoning principle in the management of MM. The goal of the treatment in MM is prolongation of survival. Treatment selection depends on estimate of benefit/risk ratios of alternative therapies that are currently available in the management of MM (see also Tables 11-3 to 11-5). Presented is strategy based mainly on level I/II evidence; treatment of relapsed/refractory MM is mainly based on level IV evidence. For dosage and other practical details of the management, see Appendix 11. M, melphalan; P, prednisone; V, vincristine; A, adriamycin; D, dexametha-sone; C, cyclophosphamide; B, carmustine; Rx therapy.*

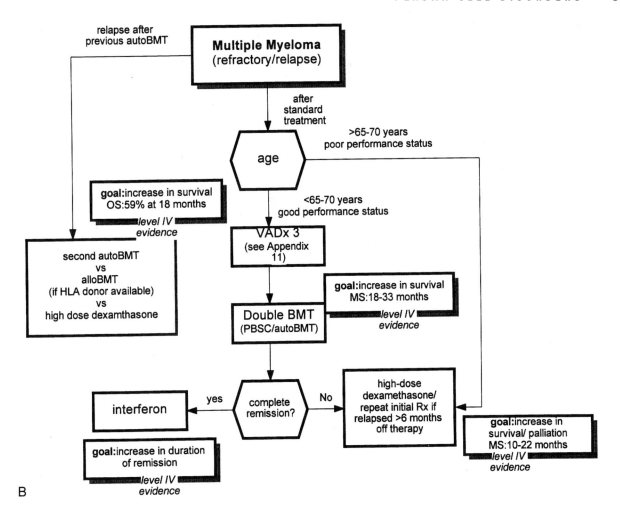

B

irradiation in the range of 4,000 to 5,000 rads. Lesions, however, remain solitary in about 15% of patients and, therefore, careful follow-up is indicated (see below; Table 11-4).

Extramedullary plasmacytoma (3% of patients) can be controlled by irradiation and/or surgical resection.

Patients with *symptomatic overt myeloma* should be treated with chemotherapy.

3. What is the best first-line chemotherapy?

Age of patients, stage of disease, presence of complications, organ dysfunction, and performance status are major factors that can influence treatment decisions in patients with MM. With all these factors, MP (melphalan + prednisone) is probably still standard treatment for most patients. Time to treatment failure (relapse disease progression, or death) with MP regimen is generally 12 to 18 months. A large number of trials that have compared MP regimen with more complex protocols, such as VBMCP or VMCP/VBAP, have produced conflicting results. An explicit answer to what is the best induction regimen for MM cannot be given. However, early high dose therapy followed by autologous bone marrow transplantation (autoBMT) has shown higher survival for patients treated with high dose therapy compared with those receiving standard treatment. In a recent prospective randomized study five-year probability of progression-free survival (PFS) was 28% for patients receiving high-dose treatment versus 10% for patients receiving conventional treatment; five-year probability of overall survival was 52% in the high-dose arm versus 12% for standard chemotherapy. A review of data on multiple modalities in the management of MM suggests the possibility of a dose-response relationship, which creates a rationale for early aggressive treatment.

It appears that patients in CR have much better chances for long-term survival after administration of high-dose consolidation treatment than patients with PR. However, achieving CR in patients with

TABLE 11-4 BENEFITS/RISKS OF PREFERRED MANAGEMENT ALTERNATIVES FOR AS SHOWN IN FIG. 11-1

Type of Treatment	Complete Remission (%)	Disease-Free Survival (%)	Overall Survival (%)	Mortality (%)	Type of Evidence	References	Comment
			Outcomes				

Decision Point 1: What is the best first line treatment for MM?

([Melphalan + prednisone] vs [combined chemotherapy] vs high-dose chemo therapy, followed by autoBMT)

Two meta-analyses (J Clin Oncol 1992;10:334; Blood 1991;78:114a) (level I evidence) integrated numerous randomized trials whose individual results produced conflicting evidence to show that overall results suggest no difference between two regimens. However, recent level I evidence (N Engl J Med 1996;335:91) demonstrated survival and DFS advantage for the use of autoBMT in patients younger than 65 years old in comparison with crx (see below under Decision Point 3).

Type of Treatment	Complete Remission (%)	Disease-Free Survival (%)	Overall Survival (%)	Mortality (%)	Type of Evidence	References	Comment
MP	42	NR (not reported)	Median 2-year: 45%–87%	~ 0-1% mortality 16% (severe + lethal toxicity)	Level I	J Clin Oncol 1992;10:334; Blood 1991; 78:114	It should be noted that many authors believe that crx is superior to MP and advocate its use as a first line therapy (Mayo Clin Proc 1994;69:781)
Crx	50	NR	50%–71%	~ 0%-1% mortality 17% (severe + lethal toxicity)	Level I	Blood 1991; 78:114	

Decision Point 2: Is maintenance treatment (with IFN) indicated in MM?

Level I evidence showed no increase in survival with MP as a maintenance therapy (Blood 1978;51:1005; Br J Cancer 1988;57:94–99; Hematol Oncol 1988;6:145). Results with IFN produced conflicting data, with some randomized studies showing increase in survival (N Engl J Med 1990;322:1430; J Clin Oncol 1995;13:2354), but other studies failing to, show survival advantage (J Clin Oncol 1994;12:2405; Ann Intern Med 1996;124:212) (grade C evidence). Several studies, however, demonstrate increase in median remission time by 4-12 months (level II evidence).

Type of Treatment	Complete Remission (%)	Disease-Free Survival (%)	Overall Survival (%)	Mortality (%)	Type of Evidence	References	Comment
IFN	Not available	Median duration of stable disease: 12–20 months (control:5.7–16 months)			Grade C evidence	J Clin Oncol 1995;13:235 Ann Intern Med 1996;124:21	Some authorities believe that increase in response time is sufficient to recommend IFN as a maintenance therapy (Ann Intern Med 1996; 124:264)

Decision Point 3: Who should be transplanted and when?

Level II, III, and IV evidences have suggested that both allogeneic and autologous BMT can prolong survival in comparison with standard therapy (N Engl J Med 1991;325:1267; Blood 1994;84:386a; Blood 1995;86:124a). AlloBMT may be considered in patients younger than 55 years old with low tumor burden who responded to first-line treatment (level IV evidence) (J Clin Oncol 1995;13:1312). Level I evidence (N Engl J Med 1996;335:91) support the use of autoBMT in patients younger than 65 years old.

alloBMT	60	34 at 6 years	28 at 7 years	29	Level III	J Clin Oncol 1995;13:1312	It is not clear wheher alloBMT can cure MM at this time; high mortality for alloBMT
autoBMT	22 + 16 (PR) (vs 5 + 9 for crx)	28 at 5 years (vs 10 for Crx)	52 at 5 years (vs. 12 for crx)	~3	Level I	Blood 1995; 86:124a; N Eng J Med 1996; 335:91	In various studies, response rate up to 35% was seen; mortality of autoBMT is up to 5%

Decision point 4: What is the best salvage treatment?

All evidence for recommended strategies in Fig 11-1B are indirect (level III and IV) (J Clin Oncol 1988;6:889). The role of myeloablative therapy is currently being evaluated, with, overall poor results in refractory diseases but with some responses noted in patients with primarily resistant disease transplanted during first year of therapy (level IV and V evidence), (Blood 1994;84:4278, Blood 1996;88:838, Bone Marrow Transplant 1995;16:7).

High-dose steroids	21 (response rate)	Median: 12–26 months	Median survival: 22 months (for responders)	10 steroid-induced psychosis	Level IV	Ann Intern Med 1986;105:811	
VAD	41–65		Median survival: 22 months (for responders)	22 (severe + lethal toxicity)	Level IV	Ann Intern Med 1986;105:811; Mayo Clin Proc 1994;69:7787	
Myeloablative therapy (melphalan 200 mg/m²) (Double transplant with PBSC ┃ auto-BMT rescue)	24%–43%	Median: 18–37 months	Median survival: 18–37 months	7	Level IV	Blood 1994;84: 950; Mayo Clin Proc 1994; 69:778; Blood 1996,82:838	Lower β_2-microglobulin, and CRP, age <50, normal LDH, primary unresponsive disease (vs resistant relapse) <12 months from diagnosis to transplant are factors associated with better response rate

Abbreviations: HDM, high-dose melphalan; ; MP, melphalan and prednisone; TBI, total body irradiation; CRP-C, reactive protein; VBAD,vincristine, carmustine, Adriamycin, dexamethasone; autoBMT, autologous BMT; PBSC, peripheral blood stem cells; P, prednisone; M, melphalan; NR, not reported; CRX, combined chemotherapy.

MM could be difficult. Preliminary results of some recent studies suggest that chances for achieving CR may depend on dose intensity. In the prospective randomized trial mentioned previously, only 5% of patients treated with vincristine, melphalan, cyclophosphamide, prednisone, carmustine, vincristine Admamycin, prednisone (VMCP/BVAP) achieved CR compared with 22% of patients treated with high-dose therapy followed by autoBMT (consisting of high-dose melphalan and total-body irradiation with bone marrow rescue). Similarly, in a report from the University of Arkansas, 14% of patients achieved CR after induction therapy; after first autoBMT, CR increased to 24%, and after second autoBMT, CR increased to 43%. Therefore, it appears a sufficient amount of good quality data has been generated at this time to enable us to recommend high-dose chemotherapy followed by autoBMT as a first-line therapy in patients younger than 65 with good performance status in advanced stages of MM (see Fig. 11-1). Patients older than 65 years with poor performance status and organ failure are generally not suitable candidates for high-dose chemotherapy.

4. How to follow treatment effects? M-spike (as determined by IPE or SPE if M-spike is visible) highly correlates with tumor mass and is a primary test to follow. β_2-microglobulin is also said to correlate even better with tumor mass and should be determined at frequent intervals (q 2–3 months). Recently, levels of C-reactive protein and interleukin-6 (IL-6) were shown to correlate with tumor mass and prognosis even better, but there are no data on usefulness of these markers in the monitoring of treatment effects. M-protein reduction does not always correlate with survival duration. A 70% reduction in M protein is not necessarily better than 30% reduction, because practically all responses achieved with current therapy are partial (except, perhaps, for high-dose chemotherapy, which appears to be able to produce some true CRs). In general, there are no uniformly accepted criteria for remission, and definition of complete remission may actually depend on how carefully one looks for residual disease. Table 11-5 shows recommendations for treatment monitoring in MM.

5. Is maintenance treatment (with interferon) indicated in the management of multiple myeloma? An important goal of treatment in myeloma patients is to prolong duration of remission with reasonable quality of life and few side effects. Has maintenance therapy any role in achieving this goal? Randomized studies that evaluated MP as a maintenance therapy showed no increase in survival. There is a theoretical possibility that myeloma patients who respond to chemotherapy without achieving stable plateau phase might benefit from additional chemotherapy. However, no studies are reported to confirm this hypothesis.

What is a rational treatment approach for the stable, plateau-phase patient? Not enough information is available to answer this question. Interferon has been demonstrated to prolong response duration and plateau phase duration but not survival. Results of several studies have shown that median remission time was prolonged by 4 to 12 months with interferon compared with no treatment. Some authors believe that this increase in duration of response is sufficient to recommend interferon as a standard maintenance treatment (see Table 11-4), which is also our preference.

6. Can BMT cure disease? Only about 5% of myeloma patients are eligible for allogeneic bone marrow transplantation (alloBMT) because of

TABLE 11-5 **TREATMENT MONITORING IN MUTIPLE MYELOMA**

Test	Frequency of administration
Complete blood count	Before each treatment
Calcium, creatinine, and uric acid	Every 1–2 months
Serum protein electrophoresis	Every 2 months
24-hour urine collection for total protein and light-chain analysis	Every 2–3 months
Beta-2 microglobulin	Every 2 months
Skeletal x-ray survey	Every 6–12 months or when clinically indicated
Marrow aspirate	In the case of pancytopenia (to distinguish between multiple myeloma and treatment effect)
Liver function	Every 6 months

(From Djulbegović B, Hendler F, Beganovic S: Mutiple myeloma. pp. 177–180. In Djulbegović B [ed]: Reasoning and Decision Making in Hematology. Churchill Livingstone, New York, 1992, with permission.)

TABLE 11-6 COMPLICATIONS IN MULTIPLE MYELOMA

Complication	Comment	General guidelines for treatment

Infection	Leading cause of death: 20%–50%
	 Febrile patients requires hospitalization
		Non-neutropenic patient:
		   S. pneumonia
		   H. pneumonia
		 Neutropenic patient:
		   S. aureus
		   Gram-negative bacteria

Hypercalcemia	Occurs in 25% of myeloma patients Suspect hypercalcemia in patient with vomiting, nausea, constipation, polyuria, polydipsia, weakness, confusion, or stupor	New presenting patients: hydration + VAD Other patients: Saline 120–150 ml/h + furosemide + prednisone 40–100 mg/d If calcium remains high after rehydration and diuresis, give biphosphonates, such as pamidronate disodium (pamidronate 90 mg as 4-hour infusion)

Renal insufficiency	Occurs in 50% of myeloma patients	Prevention: maintenance of high urine output: 3 L/24 hr
		 Renal insufficiency:
		   Fluid and mineral correction,
		   Furosemide to maintain urine flow rate of
		   100 ml/h VAD
		 Hemodialysis when required
		 If renal function dos not improve or renal failure is acute, plasmapheresis

Bone pain/spinal compression	MRI is the best test and can identify imminent cord compression before symptoms develop	Radiation therapy:, 2000 rads/5 days or 800 rads in one dose
Anemia	Keep hemoglobin >10 g/dl	(1) Erythropoietin 150 U/kg 3 times a week. Increase dose if no response is noted after 3 weeks of therapy. Increase to 250 U/kg if there is no response in next 3 weeks (2) No response to erythropoietin: Aqueous testosterone 50–100 mg IM q month or fluoxymesterone 5 mg PO tid
Hyperviscosity	Plasmapheresis should be started regardless of viscosity level if patient is symptomatic	Plasmapheresis
Myeloma-associated skeletal disease	Biphosphonates (clodronate and pamidronate) are effective in long-term control of osteolysis; pamidronate was shown to decrease skeletal complications (pathologic fracture, bone pain, spinal cord compression) in comparison with placebo (24% vs. 41%) (N Engl J Med 1996; 334:488) (Level II evidence) in stage III MM	Oral clonodronate 1600 mg/d or Pamidronate 90 mg as 4-hour infusion every 4 weeks × 9 (Administer in 500 mls of 5% Dextrose)

Abbrevation: VAD, vincristine, Adriamycin, dexamethasone.

advanced age and the lack of suitable donors. In addition, transplant-related mortality for alloBMT ranges from 15% to 40%. The overall survival rate for 162 myeloma patients (from the European Group for Blood and Marrow Transplantation registry) after alloBMT was 28% at 7 years. In the same registry of 162 patients who underwent alloBMT, only 9 patients remain in CR more than 4 years after allografting. On the other hand, as discussed above, early high-dose therapy followed by autoBMT has shown higher survival for patients treated with high-dose therapy compared with those receiving standard treatment. Transplant-related mortality for autografting is generally less than 5%. The best chances for long-term survival are in patients in CR at the time of BMT. However, it is difficult to achieve CR and eradicate malignant clones in the myeloma patient, even with high-dose therapy. There is no proof that even a second course of high-dose therapy can eradicate the malignant

TABLE 11-7 IMPORTANT INFORMATION ABOUT WALDENSTROM'S MACROGLOBULINEMIA

Anemia caused by plasma expansion	70% of patients
Hyperviscosity syndrome	70% of patients at some stage of the disease
Bleeding	70% of patients
Bone marrow suppression	70% of patients
Neutropenia	30% of patients
Thrombocytopenia	30% of patients
Lymphadenopathy or splenomegaly	20%–40% of patients
Cryoglobulin monoclonal IgM (type I)	15% (less than 5% symptomatic)
Signs of hyperviscosity syndrome	IgM around 40 to 50 g/L

clone. Therefore, at this time no evidence exists that BMT (or any other treatment modality) can cure MM. However, BMT (allogeneic and autologous) clearly prolong survival of these patients.

7. Who should be transplanted? Despite the lack of definitive proof that BMT can cure MM, this therapy might be indicated in certain subsets of patients. For a patient who is less than 55 years of age and who has an HLA-matched sibling, physicians should discuss risks and benefits of alloBMT. AutoBMT can be generally tolerated by patients up to 65 years of age. Patients with good performance status and without organ failure are generally the best candidates for autoBMT. As mentioned above, transplant-related mortality for alloBMT can be up to 40% and for autoBMT is generally less than 5% (see Table 11-4).

8. What is the prognosis in patients with MM? MM is not curable. The overall median survival is about 2 to 3 years but can range from about 15 months (stage IIIB) to 62 months (stage IA). Five-year survival depends on stage (i.e., estimated myeloma cell mass) and can range from 25% to 40% (stage 1) to 10% to 25% (stage III). Strategies for treatment of MM are shown in Figure 11-1 and Table 11-3. Treatment of complications is as important as treatment of the disease itself (Table 11-6).

WALDENSTROM'S MACROGLOBULINEMIA

Waldenstrom's macroglobulinemia (WM) is a relatively indolent lymphoproliferative disorder with monoclonal IgM production. Clinical course, cellular characteristics (CD5-, CD10-, and CD20-positive cells), and response to therapy (fludarabine) have some similarities with chronic lymphocytic leukemia. Intrinsic viscosity of IgM is high relative to IgG and IgA, and patients with macroglobulinemia are especially prone to develop hyperviscosity. Signs of hyperviscosity syndrome occur at an IgM concentration of about 4.0 to 5.0 g/dL. Ocular and neuro-

logic disturbances and other components of hyperviscosity syndrome rarely occur if relative viscosity is less than 4 but one should bear in mind that symptomatic threshold varies among patients. Therapy of WM is not curative, and patients are usually observed until clinical manifestations that require treatment develop. Table 11-7 shows the most important facts about WM, and Table 11-8. shows general guidelines for its management.

AMYLOIDOSIS

Primary systemic amyloidosis, also called AL amyloidosis, is a rare disease characterized by production of free light chains by a relatively small population of monoclonal plasma cells in the bone marrow. Depending on the appearance and number of plasma cells in the bone marrow, concentration of M protein in the serum or urine, and the presence of skeletal lesions, disease can be classified as AL amyloidosis or AL amyloidosis with multiple myeloma. Chemotherapy cannot completely eradicate monoclonal plasma cells, and median survival for this disease is 14 to 24 months. The summary of important facts about AL amyloidosis is presented in Table 11-9.

SUGGESTED READINGS

Alexanian R, Dimopoulos M: The treatment of multiple myeloma. N Engl J Med 330:484–489, 1994

Alexanian R, Dimopoulos MA, Hester J et al: Early myoablative therapy in multiple myeloma. Blood 84:4278–1282, 1994

Alexanian R, Weber D Whither interferon for myeloma or other hematologic malignancies? Ann Intern Med 124:264–265, 1996

Anderson C: Who benefits from high-dose therapy for multiple myeloma? J Clin Oncol 13:1291–1296, 1995

Attal M, Harousseau JL, Stoppa AM et al: A prospective, randomized trial of autologous bone marrow transplantation and chemotherapy in multiple myeloma. N Eng J Med 335: 91–7, 1996

Baldini A, Guffanti BM, Cesana M et al: Role of different hematologic variables in defining the risk of malignant transformation in monoclonal gammopathy. Blood 87:912–918, 1996

Blade J, Lopez-Guillermo A, Bosh F et al: Impact of response to treatment on survival in multiple myeloma: results in a series of 243 patients. Br J Haematol 88:117–121, 1994

Cunningham D, Paz-Ares L, Gore ME et al: High-dose melphalan for multiple myeloma: long-term follow-up data. J Clin Oncol 12:764–768, 1994

TABLE 11-8 **GENERAL GUIDELINES FOR MANAGEMENT OF PATIENTS WITH WALDENSTROM'S MACROGLOBULINEMIA**

median survival	*6 Years*	
Symptomatic patient with overt lymphoma	Chlorambucil + prednisone	Response rate, 57% Median survival, 5 years
	CHOP	Response rate, 65% Median survival, 7.3 years
	Fludarabine or CDA	Response rate, 79% Median survival: no data
Treatment of hyperviscosity syndrome	Plasmapheresis Goal; serum viscosity <4 Additional chemotherapy	
Symptomatic cryoglobulinemia or neuropathy without lymphoma	Plasmapheresis followed by chemotherapy Goal: reduce IgM for at least 3 months	

Abbreviations: CDA, 2-clorodeoxyadenosine; CHOP, cyclophosphamide, doxorubicin, vincristine, prednisone.

(Data from Dimopoulos and Alexanian and Giles.[15])

TABLE 11-9 **IMPORTANT INFORMATION ABOUT AL AMYLOIDOSIS**

Median survival	*24 months*
Median age of diagnosis	62 years
Nephrotic syndrome	30%–40% of patients at presentation
Congestive or restrictive cardiomyopathy	17%–25% of patients at presentation
Sensimotor peripheral neuropathy	15% of patients at presentation
Protein electrophoresis	45% localized band or spike 25% hypogammaglobulinemia
Serum or urine monoclonal protein	90% Single most useful screening method
Treatment	5-year survival 20% with melphalan + prednisone Possibility of longer survival with intensive treatment? 4'-iodo-4' deoxydoxorubicin (I-DOX) could be the prototype of new class of drugs that reverse amyloid deposition; its effect should be investigated further

Dimopoulos MA, Alexanian R: Waldenstrom's macroglobulinemia. Blood 83:1452–1459, 1994

Dimopoulos MA, O' Brien S, Kantarjian H et al: Treatment of Waldenstrom's macroglobulinemia with nucleoside analogues. Leukemia Lymphoma 11:105–108, 1993

Djulbegović B, Hendler F, Beganovic S: Mutiple myeloma. pp. 177–180. In Djulbegovic B (ed): Reasoning and Decision Making in Hematology. Churchill Livingstone, New York, 1992

Fermand JP, Chevret S, Ravaud P et al: High-dose chemoradiotherapy and autologous blood stem cell transplantation in multiple myeloma: result of a phase II trial involving 63 patients. Blood 82:2005–2009, 1993

Gahrton G: Autologous stem-cell transplantation in multiple myeloma. Wien Med Wochenschr 145:52–54, 1995

Garthon G, Tura S, Ljungman P et al: Prognostic factors in allogeneic bone marrow transplantation for multiple myeloma. J Clin Oncol 13:1312–1322, 1995

Giles F: Mutiple myeloma and Waldenstrom's macroglobulinemia. pp. 274–282. In Brain MC, Carbone PP: Current Therapy in Hematology Oncology. Mosby, St. Louis, 1995

Harrousseau JL, Milpied N I aporte JP et al: Double-intensive therapy in high-risk multiple myeloma. Blood 79:2827–2833, 1992

Kyle RA: Multiple myeloma and other plasma cell disorders. pp. 1354–1374. In Hoffman R et al: Hematology. Churchill Livingstone, New York, 1995

Oken M: Standard treatment of multiple myeloma. Mayo Clin Proc 69:781–786, 1994

Tricot G, Jagannath S, Vesole DH et al: The lapse of multiple myeloma after autologous transplantation: survival after salvage therapy. Bone Marrow Transplant 6:7–11, 1995

Vesole DH, Tricot G, Jagannath S et al: Autotransplants in multiple myeloma: what have we learned? Blood 88:838–847, 1996.

12 Nonmelanoma Skin Cancers

Zoran Potparić
Biljana Baškot

Incidence: 200/100, 000; commonest cancer in the United States

Goal of treatment: Cure in >95% of cases, palliation in metastatic disease

Main modality of treatment: Surgery with various techniques

Prognosis (5-year survival):

Basal cell carcinoma (BCC):	99%
BCC + metastases:	10%
Squamous cell carcinoma (SCC):	95%
SCC + metastases:	26%

More than 600,000 new cases of nonmelanoma skin cancer are diagnosed annually making it the most common cancer in the United States. Skin tumors are usually located on sun-exposed areas and are most common in individuals of fair complexion. Sun-damaged skin with actinic keratoses, senile lentigines, spider angiomas, telangiectasias, and dry and wrinkled skin is typical for those with high risk for skin cancer. Sunlight, in particular, the ultraviolet-B spectrum, is considered to have a major role in the development of all kinds of skin cancer. Radiation, immunosuppression, organ transplantation, chronic inflammatory, and scarring processes also predispose to skin cancer. Patients with xeroderma pigmentosum, Gorlin syndrome (basal cell nevus syndrome), and epidermodysplasia verruciforme have an increased risk of developing skin cancer.

Basal cell carcinoma (BCC) is by far the most commonly reported human malignancy. It accounts for 65% to 80% of all cases of nonmelanotic skin cancers, while squamous cell carcinoma (SCC) accounts for 10% to 20%. The incidence of new cases is constantly rising; there is a 20% increase of BCC and SCC in the United States in the last decade. Less common types of nonmelanotic skin cancer are sebaceous carcinoma, dermatofibrosarcoma protuberans, Merkel cell carcinoma, angiosarcoma, leiomyosarcoma, or malignant fibrous histiocytoma. Lymphomas may often present solely in the skin (see Chapters 9 and 10) as well as metastases from systemic carcinomas such as breast, prostate, renal cell, or melanoma.

DIAGNOSIS AND CLINICAL COURSE

Similar to nonmalignant lesions, skin cancers may appear as papules, nodules, or patches of erythema with scales. Often skin cancers present with ulceration, crusting, pigmentation, cystic collection, hypopigmentation, and scarring. BCC is typically characterized by pearly, slightly translucent, waxy papules with telangiectasias, and well-defined border. It may also present as a flat, hypopigmented and sclerotic plaque called the *morphea form* with ill-defined, usually hyperpigmented border. SCC is usually a poorly defined flesh-colored to red nodule, with a hyperkeratotic crust or ulceration. In the lower lip, SCC may appear as a nonhealing ulcer, white plaque, or rapidly growing nodule. Both BCC and SCC may form hyperkeratotic cutaneous horns.

Actinic keratosis is very often misdiagnosed as a skin cancer. Clinically, it presents as crusted or scaly papule, usually multiple, on the sun-exposed regions of fair-skinned individuals. If solitary and large, actinic keratosis is similar to SCC into which it can evolve if not treated. *Keratoacanthoma*, which appears on sun-exposed areas of face and extremities, is commonly seen in long-term renal transplant patients. The clinical appearance, size, and rapid growth may make it indistinguishable from SCC without biopsy.

The biologic behavior of skin cancer varies. While a BCC is typically a slow-growing lesion, a typical SCC grows rapidly over a period of several months. Penetration of BCC into deep tissue planes occurs infrequently and metastases are quite rare. Deep tissue penetration and metastatic rate around 2%, are characteristic of SCC. A large, long-lasting, recurrent BCC and SCC in the head and neck, have significantly increased risk of penetration and metastases. Dermatofibrosarcoma protuberans, leiomyosarcoma, sebaceous carcinoma, and eccrine carcinoma are all locally aggressive. Eccrine carcinoma has a high rate of regional metastasis.

TREATMENT

The goal of treatment is cure in localized disease but palliation in those rare patients who have metastatic disease.

Therapy for the primary nonmelanotic skin cancers depends on type, size, location, involvement of the vital structures, age, general health, and patient's cosmetic concerns. Treatment modalities include surgical excision, cryotherapy, radiation therapy, and topical application of 5-fluorouracil (5-FU). Effects of intralesional injection of interferon and methotrexate, photodynamic therapy and laser surgery are currently being studied. The goal of the treatment with all these modalities is cure.

Surgical excision and repair is the most commonly employed modality. It is safe, well-controlled, and inexpensive. Essential in planning surgical excision is the consideration of adequate surgical margins. In the case of BCC, excision of 1 to 2 mm of normal skin around the tumor margins results in 94% to 95% cure rate. Wider margins are required to treat BCC greater than 2 cm in diameter and morphea form tumors because they may extend beyond clinically evident margins. Surgical margins for SCC are more difficult to estimate because the lesion is often poorly demarcated. Generally 3 to 5 mm around the visible tumor and accompanying erythema are chosen. *Sebaceous carcinoma* is treated by wide 5 to 6 mm excision from the margins of normal skin or mucosa. *Dermatofibrosarcoma protuberans* is well known for high (40%–50%) recurrence rate even with margins as wide as 2 to 3 cm. *Leiomyosarcoma* must be removed with 4 to 5 cm margin of normal skin and deep to the muscular fascia.

Recurrence rates for all nonmelanoma skin cancers are in the range of 4% to 50%. They depend on treatment, histologic type, and tumor localization. The reported rate of metastatic BCC ranges from 0.0028% to 0.55%. The interval from onset of primary tumor to the time of metastasis is 1 to 45 years, with a median of 9 years. The sites of metastases are the lymph nodes, lung, bone, skin, and liver. The 1-year and 5-year survival rates for metastatic BCC are approximately 20% and 10%, respectively. Metastatic rate for SCC ranges from 0.3% to 17.3%. SCC metastasize in 85% via the lymphatic route to regional lymph nodes. The 5-year and 10-year survival rates for such cases are 26% and 16%, respectively. The other 15% SCC metastasize to the lung, liver, bone, brain, and mediastinum. When metastasis occurs, it usually does so within 3 years of the initial therapy, and within 2 years in more than 90% of cases; 75% of the metastatic cases are associated with previous unsuccessful treatment. Evidence of metastasis and local recurrence often appears simultaneously.

Overall, recurrence rate after primary excision of BCC and SCC is 5% to 6%. BCC greater than 2 cm, morphea form, SCC greater than 1 cm, tumors with poorly differentiated cytologic features and invasion into deep layers are more predisposed to recurrence. However, only 35% of BCC with positive margins recur. The recurrence rate for other skin tumors is greater. Unless there are absolute contraindications to further surgery, all primary skin malignancies with positive margins should be reexcised.

Cure rate is up to 99% if excision is accomplished by Mohs micrographic surgery. With this technique tissue is excised and microscopically examined in stages. This allows almost all the margins to be examined for presence of tumor cells. The technique is time-consuming and it is now almost exclusively used for excision of BCC and SCC with high risk of recurrence, recurrent tumors, or in the treatment of tumors with high recurrence rate such as dermatosarcoma protuberans and eccrine carcinoma.

Alternatives to surgical excision are radiotherapy, electrodesiccation with curettage, cryosurgery, laser surgery and photodynamic therapy. With all these techniques, however, there is no tissue obtained for histologic examination of the margins. Wound healing is provided by secondary intention and scar contracture. Patients with multiple small superficial BCC may benefit from the treatment with topical 5-FU, which affects only primarily atypical cells, including those of actinic keratosis; surrounding normal skin is spared. The recurrence rate is higher than that obtained by other modalities.

The goal of treatment of advanced and metastatic nonmelanoma skin cancer is palliation and improved quality of life. Combined chemotherapy and radiation or chemotherapy alone may be used for palliation. This recommendation is, however, based on indirect evidences (level IV/V evidences) as the vast majority of skin cancers do not metastasize and the numbers are too small to carry out experimental protocols. In patients that have previously received radiation, cisplatin-based chemotherapy is recommended in combination with 5-FU or mitomycin C with reported response rates from 53% to 90% (see also Appendix 12).

FOLLOW-UP AND PREVENTION

Follow-up is mandatory for every patient with history of prior skin cancer, since the patient who has had one skin cancer has 36% chance of developing a second skin cancer in 5 years. The entire skin surface, with particular attention to sun-exposed surfaces should be examined in 6- to 12-month intervals. Treatment of precursor lesions such as seborrheic keratoses, actinic keratosis, and Bowen's disease is still controversial. Treatment similar to one performed for skin cancer is suggested.

Decreasing sun exposure is thought to decrease the number of skin cancers. Chronic cumulative exposure should be minimized with adequate clothing and use of sunscreens with a sun protection factor (SPF) of 15 or more, as recommended by The Skin Cancer Foundation. Sunburns should be avoided as well as exposure to artificial sources of UV radiation for tanning.

Figure 12-1 shows the recommended approach to the management of nonmelanoma skin cancers. Recommended strategy for primary treatment is based on solid nonexperimental evidence (level III) and for treatment of metastatic cancer on case reports and small retrospective series (level V and IV evidence). Appendix 12 shows details on surgical biopsy of nonmelanoma skin cancer along with the

TABLE 12-1 CLINICAL AND PATHOLOGIC TUMOR, NODE, METASTASIS (TNM) CLASSIFICATION, STAGE GROUPING, AND HISTOPATHOLOGIC GRADING FOR SQUAMOUS CELL CARCINOMA (SCC) AND BASAL CELL CARCINOMA (BCC) EXCLUDING VULVA, PENIS, AND EYELID[a]

Stage	Definition
Primary tumor (T)	
TX	Primary tumor cannot be assessed
T0	No evidence of primary tumor
Tis	Carcinoma in situ
T1	Tumor 2 cm or less in greatest dimension
T2	Tumor more then 2 cm but less than 5 cm
T3	Tumor more then 5 cm
T4	Tumor invades deep extradermal structures (cartilage, muscle, bone)
Regional lymph nodes (N)	
NX	Regional lymph nodes cannot be assessed
N0	No regional lymph node metastasis
N1	Regional lymph node metastasis
Distant Metastasis (M)	
MX	Distant metastasis cannot be assessed
M0	No distant metastasis
M1	Distant metastasis
Histopathologic grade (G)	
GX	Grade cannot be assessed
G1	Well-differentiated tumor
G2	Moderately well-diferentiated tumor
G3	Poorly differentiated tumor
G4	Undifferentiated tumor

Stage Grouping			
Stage 0	Tis	N0	M0
Stage I	T1	N0	M0
Stage II	T2	N0	M0
	T3	N0	M0
Stage III	T4	N0	M0
	Any T	N1	M0
Stage IV	Any T	Any N	M1

[a]*A TNM classification similar to one used for mucosal SCC has been adopted by the American Joint Committee on Cancer for Carcinoma of the Skin. The classification depicted in this table is applicable only to SCC and BCC arising from skin areas other than vulva, penis, and eyelids. This classification applies to both clinical and pathologic staging. Clinical staging requires inspection and palpation of both tumor and the regional lymph nodes. If tumor fixation to the underlying bony structures or distant metastasis is suspected, imaging studies should assist in clinical staging. Pathologic staging requires complete resection of involved tissue, confirmation of lymph node involvement, and histologic classification via microscope examination.*

practical recommendations on type of chemotherapy in the management of nonmelanoma skin cancer. Table 12-1 shows staging system for BCC and SCC. Note that the main use of the system is to help determine localized versus metastatic disease.

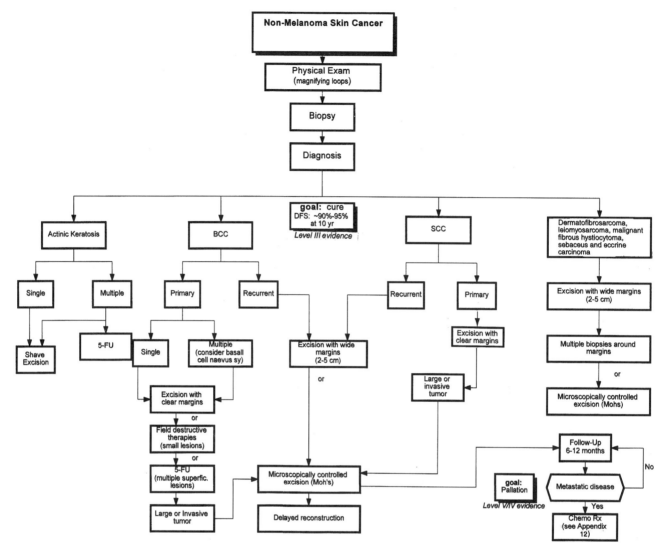

FIGURE 12-1 *The approach to management of the patients with nonmelanoma skin cancer is largely dependent on tumor histology and size. Most nonmelanoma skin cancers are localized tumors that rarely metastasize. Consequently the goal in the management of these tumors is curative surgical resection (90% to 95% at time). The goal of treatment of metastatic and advanced skin tumors is palliation and preservation of quality of life. Recommended strategy for primary treatment is based on solid nonexperimental evidence (level III) and for treatment of metastatic cancer on case reports and small retrospective series (level V and IV evidences) (see Appendix 12).*

SUGGESTED READINGS

Engel A, Johnson ML, Haynes SG: Health effect of sunlight exposure in the United States. Results from the first National Health and Nutrition Examination Survey, 1971–74. Arch Dermatol 124:72–79, 1988

Goldberg H, Tsalik M, Bernstein Z, Haim N: Cisplatin-based chemotherapy for advanced basal and squamous cell carcinomas. Harefuah (Israel) 127:217, 1994.

Haydon RC: Cutaneous squamous carcinoma and related lesions. Otolaryngol Clin North Am 26:57–71, 1993

Khansur T, Allred C, Little D, Anand V: Cisplatin and 5 fluoro-racil for metastatic squamous cell carcinoma from unknown primary. Cancer Invest 13:263, 1995

Luxenberg MN, Guthrie TH: Chemotherapy of basal cell and squamous cell carcinoma of the eyelids and periorbital tissues. Ophthalmology 93:504, 1986

Marks R: An overview of skin cancers: incidence and causation. Cancer 75:607–612, 1995

Olbricht SM: Treatment of malignant cutaneous tumores. Clin Plast Surg 20:167–180, 1993

Rowe DE, Carroll RJ, Day CL: Prognostic factors for local recurrence, metastasis, and survival rates in squamous cell carcinoma of the skin, ear, and lip. J Am Acad Dermatol 26:976–990, 1992

Wahlen SA, Slater JD, Wagner RJ, Wang WA et al: Concurrent radiation therapy and chemotherapy in the treatment of primary squamous cell carcinoma of the vulva. Cancer 75:2289, 1995

Wolf DJ, Zitelli JA: Surgical margins for basal cell carcinoma. Arch Dermatol 123:340–344, 1987

13 Malignant Melanoma

Geetha Joseph
Hiram C. Polk

Incidence: 12/100,000; incidence increasing in white population 7,000–8,000 deaths per year

Goal of treatment: Cure in node-negative patients, cure/prolongation of survival in node-positive patients and palliation in metastatic disease

Main modality of treatment: Surgery in all stages (if feasible); surgery + adjuvant chemoimmunotherapy in node-positive/deep primary disease; surgery or local or systemic chemotherapy for metastatic disease

Prognosis (10-year survival):

Stage I: 90% (47% of cases)

Stage II: 52% (38%)

Stage III: 33% (13%)

Stage IV: 10% (2%)

Malignant melanoma, which is diagnosed in 32,000 people annually in the United States and accounts for 7,200 deaths a year, is a cancer of the pigment-producing cell in the skin. Unfortunately, the incidence of melanoma (12 per 100,000) is increasing despite public education regarding risk factors and is estimated to be as high as 1 in 90 by the year 2000.

Risk factors for development of melanoma include fair complexion with red or blond hair, more than 20 nevi, dysplastic nevus syndrome, and severe sunburns, especially in childhood.

The symptoms are usually minor and include change in size or color of a mole, itching, ulceration, or bleeding.

Staging and classification of melanomas based on growth patterns are found in Table 13-1.

GOALS OF TREATMENT

The aims of melanoma treatment are: (1) *cure*: early detection with resultant surgical cure. The main modality of treatment is surgery; resection of isolated recurrences may also be curative; (2) *prolongation of survival*: adjuvant therapy of high risk disease in an attempt to improve overall survival; and (3) *palliation* with local or systemic chemotherapy to possibly improve disease-free or overall survival or palliate symptoms.

CURE

The treatment of localized melanoma is surgical. Numerous trials have examined surgical margins needed for cure. For melanomas less than 1 mm thick, a 1-cm margin is recommended, resulting in

119

TABLE 13-1 STAGING AND CLASSIFICATION OF MELANOMAS[a]

Classification of malignant melanomas
 Superficial spreading
 Lentigo maligna melanoma
 Acral lentiginous melanoma
 Mucosal lentiginous melanoma
 Nodular melanoma

Staging of melanoma (Clark's levels)

I	Melanoma confined to the epidermis
II	Melanoma infiltrates the papillary dermis without filling it
III	Plugs the papillary dermis and compresses the reticular dermis without infiltrating it.
IV	Infiltrates the reticular dermis
V	Infiltrates the subcutaneous fat tissue

American Joint Committee on Cancer (AJCC) Staging

IA	Localized melanoma < 0.75 mm or level II (T1, N0, M0)
IB	Localized melanoma 0.76–1.5 mm or level III (T2, N0, M0)
IIA	Localized melanoma 1.5–4.0 mm or level IV* (T3, N0, M0)
IIB	Localized melanoma > 4 mm or level V (T4, N0, M0)
III	Limited node metastases—only one regional node basin/<5 in-transit metastases (any T, N1, M0)
IV	Advanced regional metastases (any T, N2, M0) or distant metastases (any T, any N, M1, M2)
Note:	When thickness and level do not coincide with T classification, thickness takes precedence.

TNM staging

pT	Tumor after excision; N: regional nodes; M: distant metastases
pTX	Primary tumor cannot be assessed
pTis	In situ melanoma (Clarks level I)
pT1	Tumor <0.75 mm thick invading papillary dermis (Clark's level II)
pT2	Tumor >0.75 mm but < 1.5 mm thick and/or invading papillary—reticular dermis interface (Clark's level III)
pT3	Tumor >1.5 mm but <4 mm and /or invading reticular dermis (Clark's level IV)
pT4	Tumor >4 mm and/or invading subcutaneous tissue (Clark's level V) and/or satellites within 2 cm of primary
Note:	In case of discrepancy between tumor thickness and level, the pT category is based on the less favorable finding)
NX	Regional lymph nodes cannot be assessed
N0	No regional node metastasis
N1	Metastasis 3 cm or less in any regional node
N2	Metastasis > 3 cm in any regional node and/or in-transit metastases
(Note:	In transit melanoma involves skin/subcutaneous tissues >2 cm from primary but not beyond regional nodes)
MX	Metastases cannot be assessed
M0	No distant metastases
M1	Distant metastases

[a] Based on growth features.

---

a local recurrence of less than 1%. For lesions 1 to 4 mm thick a margin of 2 to 3 cm is adequate resulting in 1.7% local recurrence. The goal of surgical resection of the primary site is curative, and in 85% of patients, surgical therapy is actually curative. The role of elective lymph node dissection has not been clearly defined and shows no consistent survival benefit in randomized studies to date. For high-risk patients, the use of sentinel node mapping may help minimize morbidity related to node dissection and identify patients who will benefit from other adjuvant therapy.

PROLONGATION OF SURVIVAL

Adjuvant therapy of high-risk melanoma has been attempted with vaccines and nonspecific immunostimulants (BCG; *C. parvum*) but has been ineffective largely because of variable immunogenicity of these agents. Patients with positive delayed-type hypersensitivity responses (DTH) to a polyvalent melanoma cell vaccine (MCV) had significant prolongation of survival. Prophylactic/adjuvant isolated limb perfusion studies in high-risk patients (>1.5 mm) has not shown a survival benefit. Recently, a large intergroup study has demonstrated the efficacy of α-interferon in the adjuvant setting for melanomas deeper than 4 mm, and node-positive disease, with prolongation of disease-free and overall survival. The toxicity of the therapy is, however, significant, and this option may not be feasible for older and debilitated patients.

PALLIATION

Systemic Chemotherapy The treatment of unresectable metastatic melanoma is unsatisfactory. Despite many clinical trials using multiple chemotherapeutic agents, the overall response rate rarely exceeds 30% with less than 5% complete responses. Recently, in single institution studies, the use of biochemotherapy combining the most active drugs (cisplatin, vinblastine, DTIC, BCNU, tamoxifen) with IL-2 and α-interferon has been reported to have a complete response rate of 12% to 25%. Polyvalent MCV has also been tested in patients with metastatic disease and has shown some survival benefit in those with positive DTH reactions. We advocate recruitment of patients to clinical trials to improve results in this population.

Local Chemotherapy About 10% of melanomas that are larger than 1.5 mm will spread regionally giving rise to in-transit melanoma (Table 13-2). Treatment of in-transit melanoma involving an

TABLE 13-2 ESTIMATED RISK OF NODAL AND DISTANT METASTASES BASED ON DEPTH OF INVASION OF MELANOMA

Depth	Risk of Nodal Mets 3 yr (%)	Risk of Distant Mets 5 y(%)
<0.76 mm	2	3
0.76–1.5 mm	25	8
1.51–4.0 mm	57	15
>4.0 mm	62	72

Abbreviations: mets, metastasis.

TABLE 13-3 FOLLOW-UP SCHEDULE FOR MALIGNANT MELANOMA

Follow-up I	Physical examination every 3 months for 1 year, every 4 months for 1 year, then every 6 months
Follow-up II	Every 2 months for 1 year, every 3 months for 1 year, then every 6 months
Follow-up III	Same as II + annual chest radiograph: CT scans of previously affected site if necessary every 4–6 months 2 times, then as needed

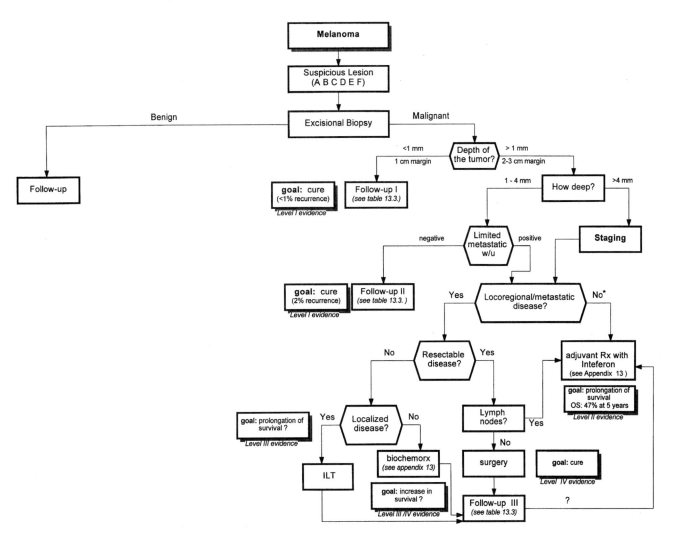

FIGURE 13-1 *Management of melanoma. The goal of treatment of melanoma is cure in localized melanoma, prolongation of survival in node-positive disease, and palliation in metastatic disease. Surgery is the main modality of treatment for melanoma, with 85% of all melanomas cured with this approach alone. The recommended strategy is based on level I evidence for extent of surgery and solid nonexperimental evidence on the curative role of surgery in localized melanoma. Level II evidence supports prolongation of survival with adjuvant therapy and level III/IV evidence exists for local and systemic chemotherapy. A, asymmetry of lesion; B, border irregularity; C, color variation; D, diameter > 6 mm; E, enlargement; F, family history; NEG, negative; POS, positive; adj Rx, adjuvant therapy; limited w/u, staging by physical examination of regional nodes; staging-chest radiograph, CT of abdomen and head; IFN, α-interferon; OS, overall survival; DFS, disease-free survival; ILT, isolated limb perfusion; biochemo, biochemotherapy. *Sentinel node dissection (experimental).*

extremity also includes isolated limb perfusion therapy (ILT). The use of hyperthermia and melphalan for ILT has shown 50% responses. The use of tumor necrosis factor coupled with γ-interferon and melphalan has resulted in 80% to 90% complete responses, but whether this will improve overall survival remains to be seen.

Detection of Recurrences During Follow-up (Table 13-3) Metastatic melanoma can be systemic or localized (in transit). Metastatic melanoma, when feasible, should also be surgically resected with curative intent, although this is not possible very often.

In view of the dismal response to therapy for metastatic melanoma, the focus has shifted to preventive measures aimed at educating the public about the use of sun screens and routine surveillance for skin changes. The ABCDEF strategy for workup of suspicious skin lesions and early diagnosis is stressed. As many as 10% of patients with melanoma will develop a second melanoma, which underscores the need for continued follow-up.

SUGGESTED READINGS

Alex JC, Weaver DL, Fairbank JT et al: Gamma probe guided lymph node localization in malignant melanoma. Surg Oncol 2:303, 1993

American Joint Committee on Cancer: In Beahrs OH, Henson DE, Hutter RVP, Kennedy BJ (eds): Manual for Staging of Cancer. 4th Ed. JB Lippincott, Philadelphia, 1992:145

Barth A, Hoon DSB, Foshag LJ et al: Polyvalent melanoma cell vaccine induces delayed-type hypersensitivity and in vitro cellular immune response. Cancer Res 54:3342, 1994

Fraker DL, Alexander HR, Andrich M, Rosenberg SA: Treatment of patients with melanoma of the extremity using hyperthermic isolated limb perfusion with melphalan, tumor necrosis factor and interferon gamma: results of a TNF dose escalation study. J Clin Oncol 14:479, 1996

Intergroup study on intermediate thickness melanomas.

Kirkwood JM, Strawderman MH, Ernstoff MS et al: Interferon α-2b adjuvant therapy of high-risk resected cutaneous melanoma: the Eastern Cooperative Oncology Group Trial EST 1684. J Clin Oncol 14:7, 1996

Legha S, Buzaid AC, Ring S et al: Improved results of treatment of metastatic melanoma with combined use of biotherapy and chemotherapy. Proc ASCO 13:394, 1994

Lienard D, Eggermont AMM, Schraffordt Koops H et al: Isolated perfusion of the limb with high dose tumor necrosis factor-alpha, interferon gamma, and melphalan for stage III melanoma: results of a multicenter pilot study. Melanoma Res 4:21, 1994

Morton DL, Foshag LJ, Hoon DSB et al: Prolongation of survival in metastatic melanoma following active specific immunotherapy with a new polyvalent melanoma vaccine. Ann Surg 216:463, 1992

Polk HC Jr. Individual treatment for malignant melanoma. J Surg Oncol 40:46, 1989

Richards J, Mehta N, Ramming K, Skosey P: Sequential chemoimmunotherapy in the treatment of metastatic melanoma. J Clin Oncol 10:1338, 1992

Veronesi U, Cascinelli N, Adamus J et al: Thin stage I primary cutaneous malignant melanoma: comparison of excision with margins of 1 or 3 cm. N Engl J Med, 318:1159, 1988

14 | Laryngeal Cancer

Srdjan Denić

Incidence: 12,600 new cases annually (USA)

Goal of treatment: Cure palliation

Treatment modality: Surgery or radiation therapy, early tumors. Combined surgery and radiation therapy, or chemotherapy combined with radiation therapy without or with surgery in advanced tumors.

Prognosis: A 5-year overall survival varies between 30% and 90%

PREVENTION

Most head and neck tumors are preventable with abstinence from tobacco and alcohol use. Wine use predisposes less to cancer than distilled alcohol products. Of patients who have had head and neck cancer 5% annually will develop a second primary tumor of the head and neck, lung, or esophagus. Vitamin A derivatives and analogues (retinoids) reduce the frequency of a second primary cancer but do not influence tumor recurrence rate. Because of retinoid toxicity, the safe and effective dose for prevention of a second primary cancer awaits additional studies.

DYSPLASIA

Dysplasia is a precancerous lesion that may evolve into carcinoma or may be associated with car-)cinoma at a different place in a mucosal field. Dysplasia is characterized by pleomorphic cells, an increased number of mitoses, and prominent nuclei. When dysplasia involves the full thickness of epithelium, it is called *carcinoma in situ*. Leukoplakia and erythroplakia are descriptive clinical terms of a condition that may or may not show dysplasia when examined under the microscope. Dysplasia is a potentially reversible lesion.

TUMOR TYPE AND GROWTH DYNAMICS

Squamous cell carcinoma makes up 95% of all malignant tumors of the larynx. The *supraglottic carcinomas* (above the true vocal cords) tend to be less well differentiated, more advanced at the time of diagnosis, and they often metastasize to the lymph nodes (20%–50% of all cases). The latter characteristics make the treatment of clinically negative neck desirable for most patients. Bilateral neck metastases are common in epiglottic as well as in all other supraglottic cancer patients with clinically positive necks (20%–40%). The *glottic carcinomas* (tumors of the true vocal cords) are smaller at the time of diagnosis because of early symptoms. Early cancer of the vocal cords rarely metastasizes to the lymph nodes, and treatment of the clinically negative neck is not generally recommended. Loss of vocal cord mobility is a sign of their involvement and a staging parameter in both glottic (T2) and supraglottic (T3) tumors (Table 14-1). Stage by stage, glottic carcinomas have a better prognosis than supraglottic carcinomas. *Subglottic* carcinomas are rare.

MULTIDISCIPLINARY APPROACH

The management of head and neck tumor presents a special challenge because of the combination of the following factors:

Proximity and relatively small size of the soft tissue and bone involved

Need for tumor-free margins

Treatment interference with vital functions (breathing, eating, and speaking)

Cosmetically the head and neck are more important than other organs

Patients often present with poor oral and dental hygiene

In addition to a surgeon, radiation therapist, and medical oncologist, most patients will require

TNM DEFINITIONS
TX – No information
T0 – No evidence of tumor
Tis – Carcinoma in situ

Supraglottis
T1 – Tumor in the single subsite and normal vocal cords
T2 – Tumor in more than one subsite (including glottis) and normal vocal cords
T3 – Tumor limited to larynx with fixed vocal cords or invades postcricoid area, pyriform sinus, or pre-epiglottic tissue
T4 – Tumor invades through the thyroid cartilage and/or to other tissue beyond the larynx

Glottis
T1 – Tumor limited to vocal cords with normal mobility
T2 – Tumor extends into supraglottis or subglottis; impaired vocal cord mobility
T3 – Tumor limited to larynx with fixed vocal cords
T4 – Tumor invades through the thyroid cartilage and/or to other tissue beyond the larynx

Subglottis
T1 – Tumor limited to subglottis
T2 – Tumor extends to vocal cords with abnormal or normal mobility
T3 – Tumor limited to larynx with fixed vocal cords
T4 – Tumor invades through the thyroid cartilage and/or to other tissue beyond the larynx; larynx with fixed vocal cords

NX – No information
N0 – No tumor present
N1 – Tumor in a single LN ≤3 cm
N2a – Tumor in single ipsilateral LN, 3–6 cm
N2b – Tumor in multiple ipsilateral LNs, none > 6 cm
N2c – Tumor in bilateral/contralateral LNs, none > 6 cm
N3 – Tumor in LNs, > 6 cm
MX – No information
M0 – No distant metastasis
M1 – Distant metastasis

TABLE 14-1 MANAGEMENT OF LARYNGEAL CARCINOMA BY STAGE

Anatomic Level	T	N	M	AJCC Stage	Survival (%)[a] 3 Years	5 years
Any	Tis	0	0	0		
Supraglottis	1	0	0	1		80
	2	0	0	II	60	
	3	0	0	III	60	
	1–3	1	0			
	4	≤ 1	0	IV	25	
	any	2, 3	0			
	any	any	1			
Glottis	1	0	0	I		90
	2	0	0	II		80
	3	0	0	III	65	60
	1–3	1	0			
	4	≤ 1	0	IV		30
	any	2,3	0			
	any	any	1			
Subglottis	1	0	0	I		
	2	0	0	II		35
	3	0	0	III		
	1–3	≤ 1				
	4	≤ 1	0	IV		
	any	2,3	0			
	any	any	1			
Any				Recurrent		

Abbreviations: AJCC, American Joint Committee on Cancer; C, curative; cGy, centigray; CR, complete response; CT, chemotherapy; d, day; I, investigational; LN, lymph nodes; P, palliative; PR, partial response; RT, radiotherapy; yr, year; wk, week.

[a]*Survival data are rounded and include salvage treatment; differences in survival within a single stage could be significant.*

the services of a dentist, dedicated nurse, social worker, and rehabilitation specialist.

TREATMENT

The untreated head and neck carcinomas are sensitive to radiation therapy and chemotherapy. The combination of cisplatin and fluorouracil produces 60% to 90% overall response and 15% to 50% complete response rate; usually this does not translate into better survival when the drugs are given in the neoadjuvant or adjuvant setting. Neoadjuvant chemotherapy administered to patients with advanced disease does improve organ preservation and thus may improve quality of life. Concomitant chemotherapy and radiation therapy increases survival at the cost of increased toxicity and is considered an investigational

		TREATMENT	
Evidence Level	Goal	Standard Choice	Comment
	C	•RT or •Surgery	
II, IV	C,I	•RT (including neck) or	RT preferred—better voice preservation
		•Supraglottic laryngectomy + unilateral/bilateral selective neck dissection or	If resection margins positive, add RT
			If LNs positive, treat neck bilaterally
		•Total laryngectomy + unilateral/bilateral selective neck dissection	< = Patient with COPD may not tolerate supraglottic laryngectomy
	C, P, I	•Total laryngectomy + bilateral neck dissection ± RT or	If resection margins positive, add RT
			If LNs positive, treat neck bilaterally
		•RT (including neck) or	< = Surgery reserved for salvagexe
I, II		•Neoadjuvant CT + RT ± Laryngectomy or	< = Preserves organ function in ~55% of cases but does not increase survival
I, II		•Concurrent CT and RT ± surgery	< = Improved survival, more toxicity
	P, I	•CT or •RT	
III, IV	C, I	•RT or	RT preferred—better voice preservation
		•Cordectomy or •Laser treatment or	< = Superficial tumor; selected patients
		•Laryngectomy (partial/total)	< = Preferred in anterior commisure tumor
	C, I	•RT or •Laryngectomy (patial/total)	RT preferred in smaller T2
	C, P, I	•Laryngectomy + selective neck dissection or	If lymph nodes positive, add RT
		•RT (including neck) or	< = In selected patients or surgery refused
I, II		•Neoadjuvant CT + RT ± Laryngectomy	< = Preserves organ function in ~55% of cases but does not increase survival
I, II		•Concurrent CT and RT ± surgery	Improved survival, more toxicity
	P, I	•CT or •RT	
IV, V	C, I	•RT or	Rare tumor
		•Surgery	Surgery if RT not feasible
	C, P, I	•Laryngectomy + thyroidectomy + tracheoesophageal lymphadenectomy + RT or	
		•RT	RT if surgery not feasible
	P, I	•CT or •RT	
	C, P, I	•Surgery or	Salvage is better with smaller tumors
		•RT	Re-irradiation could be considered
		•CT	Surgery or RT not feasible

	USA 1994			**WORLD**
	TOTAL	MALE	FEMALE	
New Cases	12,600	9,800	2,700	500,000
Deaths	3,800	3,000	800	
Case-Fatality	30%			

SCREENING RECOMMENDATION

• None

DIAGNOSIS

Pre-test probability of cancer is increased in patients with:
- hoarseness > 3 weeks (± history of smoking)
- lump or pain in neck > 3 weeks (± history of smoking)
- disphagia, aspiration
- prior cancer of head and neck

Tests
- indirect laryngoscopy (e.g., *movement of vocal cords—> staging*)
- direct laryngoscopy + multiple biopsies
- CT scan (*5mm cuts from base of tongue to upper trachea*) or MRI (*better tumor-muscle differentiation*) of larynx
  [if LN(s) > 1 CM or HETEROGENOUS ENHANCEMENT IS PRESENT ON CT SCAN then FINDING IS CONSISTENT WITH METASTASIS]
- CXR (*COPD, synchronous lung cancer, metastases*);
- Pulmonary function tests
- if ALKALINE PHOSPHATASE ↑ then BONE SCAN
- if DISPHAGIA then CONSIDER BARIUM SWALLOW
- if RADIOTHERAPY ANTICIPATED then TSH, T4

PREVENTION

• Stop cigarette smoking
*After cessation of smoking,
the risk starts to decrease after 5 years*

• Stop alcohol consumption

• Chemoprevention with retinoids
Check if still in the investigational phase

MOLECULAR GENETICS

Chromosome Deletion	Suppressor Gene
9p (65%)	
3p	
17p (55%)	p53* (50%)
13q	

*Could be used to assess presence of micrometastases in post-resection margins (Brennan JA, et al. N Engl J Med 1995;332:429.)

TREATMENTS

RADIATION THERAPY

EXTERNAL, CURATIVE INTENT
(Cobalt or 4MeV linear accelerator)

• TD = 6,000 – 7,000 cGy (180-200 cGy/day X 5 d/wk)
RR (local control) depends on the stage, tumor volume and anatomical level of cancer

if GLOTTIC TUMOR then 200 cGy FRACTION PREFERRED
if RT IS LENTEN or PATIENT SMOKES DURING RT then POORER CONTROL/SURVIVAL

SURGERY

LARYNGECTOMY

Total ...
Hemi ... • Horizontal (Supraglottic)
        • Vertical
          - Lateral
          - Frontal
Partial ...
Cordectomy

NECK DISSECTION

Radical (classic)—> enlarged LNS (e.g., N2-3)
Modified Radical—> enlarged LNS (e.g., N1)
Selective—> negative LNS (N0)
    a- Supraomohyoid
    b- Posterolateral
    c- Anterior compartment
    d- Lateral
Extended radical—> enlarged LNS

CHEMOTHERAPY

NEOADJUVANT

• Cisplatin 100 mg/m^2 IV day 1
  5-Fluorouracil 1000 mg/m^2 CIV qd X 5
  Cycle: 4 wks; No. of cycles: is 1-3 and depends on the response; RR ≤ 70%
if NO RESPONSE TO CHEMOTHERAPY then LARYNGECTOMY
if MAJOR RESPONSE TO CHEMOTHERAPY then RT
if NO CR AFTER RT then LARYNGECTOMY

PALLIATIVE

• Methotrexate 40–60 mg/m^2 IV q wk; *RR ≤ 30%*, or
• Cisplatin 100 mg/m^2 IV d 1 q 3 wks; *RR ≤ 30%*,
  or
• regimen as for neoadjuvant chemotherapy above;
  or
• other combination chemotherapy regimens

POST-TREATMENT STAGING

- Laryngoscopy ± biopsy
- MRI or CT scan (*MRI may better distinguish between tumor, normal tissue, and benign post-radiation effects; if pre-treatment CT was used then ability to compare films is decreased*)

FOLLOW UP

Salvage of an earlier detected recurrence is higher
- Indirect laryngoscopy   q 2 months X 1 year, then
                           q 3 months X 1 year, then
                           q 6 months X 1 year, then
                           q 12months X lifetime
- if RECURRENCE SUSPECTED then CT SCAN OR MRI
- Other tests triggered by positive pertinent findings

FIGURE 14-1 *Management points in laryngeal cancer. cGy, centigray; CIV, continuous intravenous; COPD, chronic obstructive lung disease; CR, complete response; CT, computed tomography; CXR, chest x-ray; d, day; LN, lymph nodes; MR, magnetic resonance imaging; PR, partial response; RR, response rate; RT, radiation therapy; wk, week. See Appendix 14.*

treatment at the time of this writing (Table 14-1). Recurrent carcinomas of the head and neck are not sensitive to chemotherapy; cisplatin and methotrexate each produce up to a 30% response rate of a few months duration. In the patients with recurrent tumors, the combination of cisplatin and fluorouracil, when compared with cisplatin and fluorouracil alone, produces a higher response rate but does not improve survival (Fig. 14-1).

SUGGESTED READINGS

Johnson A, Laryngeal cancer: variations in treatment. Lancet 344:1173–1774, 1994

Vokes EE, Weichselbaum RR, Lippman SM, Hong WK: Head and neck cancer. N Engl J Med 328:184–194, 1993

The Department of Veterans Affairs Laryngeal Cancer Study Group. Induction chemotherapy plus radiation compared with surgery plus radiation in patients with advanced laryngeal cancer. N Engl J Med 324:1685–1690, 1991

Lippman SM, Benner SE, Hong WK; Cancer chemoprevention. J Clin Oncol 12:851–873, 1994

15 Oropharyngeal Cancer

Srdjan Denić

Incidence: 29,600 new cases were estimated for 1994 in the United States

Goal of treatment: Cure/spalliation

Treatment modality: Surgery or radiotherapy for early tumors; combined surgery and radiotherapy for advanced tumors; neoadjuvant chemotherapy combined with radiation therapy ± surgery may be used in some patients

Prognosis: Survival or local control at 5 years varies widely depending on the stage and site (between 15% and 95%)

INCIDENCE AND FATALITY

Around 30,000 new cases of and 8,000 deaths from carcinoma of the lip, tongue, mouth, buccal cavity and oropharynx are expected annually in the United States.

PRIMARY PREVENTION

Most tumors are preventable by abstinence from tobacco and alcohol use. Risk of oral cancer in a person who smokes two packs of cigarettes per day is 12 times that of a nonsmoker. It may take 16 years of tobacco abstinence for cancer risk to decrease to the level of nonsmoker. Wine use predisposes less to cancer then distilled alcohol products.

DYSPLASIA

Dysplasia is characterized by pleomorphic cells, increased number of mitoses and prominent nuclei. When dysplasia involves the full thickness of epithelium, it is called *carcinoma in situ*. Leukoplakia and erythroplakia are descriptive clinical terms that may or may not have dysplasia when examined under the microscope. Dysplasia is a pre-cancerous lesion that may evolve into carcinoma or may be associated with carcinoma at different places in a mucosal field. Dysplasia is potentially reversible lesion.

MULTIDISCIPLINARY APPROACH

Management of head and neck tumor presents a special challenge due to the combination of following factors: proximity and relatively small size of soft and bone tissue involved; need for tumor-free margins; treatment interference with vital functions (breathing, eating, and speaking); cosmetic importance of the head and neck is bigger then that of other organs; often there is poor oral and dental hygiene. In addition to the surgeon, radiotherapist, and medical oncologist, most patients will require the services of a dentist, dedicated nurse, social worker, and rehabilitation specialist.

TREATMENT

The untreated head and neck carcinomas are sensitive to radiation therapy and chemotherapy. Combination of cisplatin and fluorouracil produce 60% to 90% overall response and 15% to 50% complete

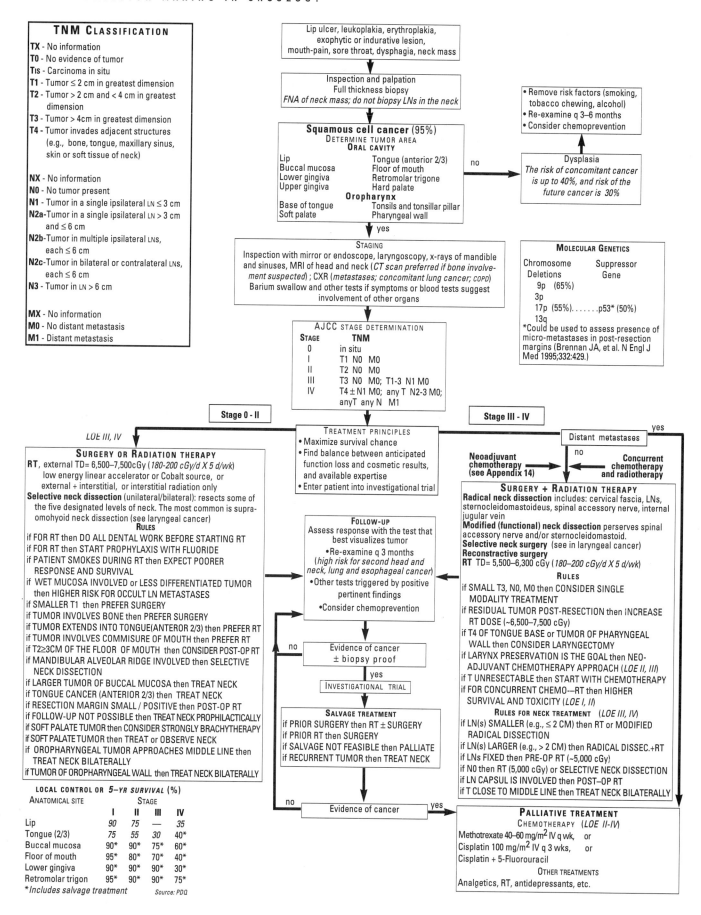

TNM CLASSIFICATION

TX - No information
T0 - No evidence of tumor
TIS - Carcinoma in situ
T1 - Tumor ≤ 2 cm in greatest dimension
T2 - Tumor > 2 cm and < 4 cm in greatest dimension
T3 - Tumor > 4cm in greatest dimension
T4 - Tumor invades adjacent structures (e.g., bone, tongue, maxillary sinus, skin or soft tissue of neck)

NX - No information
N0 - No tumor present
N1 - Tumor in a single ipsilateral LN ≤ 3 cm
N2a-Tumor in a single ipsilateral LN > 3 cm and ≤ 6 cm
N2b-Tumor in multiple ipsilateral LNs, each ≤ 6 cm
N2c-Tumor in bilateral or contralateral LNs, each ≤ 6 cm
N3 - Tumor in LN > 6 cm

MX - No information
M0 - No distant metastasis
M1 - Distant metastasis

Lip ulcer, leukoplakia, erythroplakia, exophytic or indurative lesion, mouth-pain, sore throat, dysphagia, neck mass

Inspection and palpation
Full thickness biopsy
FNA of neck mass; do not biopsy LNs in the neck

Squamous cell cancer (95%)
DETERMINE TUMOR AREA
ORAL CAVITY

Lip — Tongue (anterior 2/3)
Buccal mucosa — Floor of mouth
Lower gingiva — Retromolar trigone
Upper gingiva — Hard palate

Oropharynx
Base of tongue — Tonsils and tonsillar pillar
Soft palate — Pharyngeal wall

no →

• Remove risk factors (smoking, tobacco chewing, alcohol)
• Re-examine q 3–6 months
• Consider chemoprevention

Dysplasia
The risk of concomitant cancer is up to 40%, and risk of the future cancer is 30%

↓ yes

STAGING
Inspection with mirror or endoscope, laryngoscopy, x-rays of mandible and sinuses, MRI of head and neck *(CT scan preferred if bone involvement suspected)* ; CXR *(metastases; concomitant lung cancer; COPD)*
Barium swallow and other tests if symptoms or blood tests suggest involvement of other organs

MOLECULAR GENETICS

Chromosome Deletions	Suppressor Gene
9p (65%)	
3p	
17p (55%)	p53* (50%)
13q	

*Could be used to assess presence of micro-metastases in post-resection margins (Brennan JA, et al. N Engl J Med 1995;332:429.)

AJCC STAGE DETERMINATION

STAGE	TNM
0	in situ
I	T1 N0 M0
II	T2 N0 M0
III	T3 N0 M0; T1-3 N1 M0
IV	T4 ± N1 M0; any T N2-3 M0; anyT any N M1

Stage 0 - II

Stage III - IV

TREATMENT PRINCIPLES
• Maximize survival chance
• Find balance between anticipated function loss and cosmetic results, and available expertise
• Enter patient into investigational trial

Distant metastases — yes →

no ↓

Neoadjuvant chemotherapy (see Appendix 14) → ← Concurrent chemotherapy and radiotherapy

LOE III, IV

SURGERY OR RADIATION THERAPY
RT, external TD= 6,500–7,500cGy *(180-200 cGy/d X 5 d/wk)* low energy linear accelerator or Cobalt source, or external + interstitial, or interstitial radiation only
Selective neck dissection (unilateral/bilateral): resects some of the five designated levels of neck. The most common is supra-omohyoid neck dissection (see laryngeal cancer)

RULES
if FOR RT then DO ALL DENTAL WORK BEFORE STARTING RT
if FOR RT then START PROPHYLAXIS WITH FLUORIDE
if PATIENT SMOKES DURING RT then EXPECT POORER RESPONSE AND SURVIVAL
if WET MUCOSA INVOLVED or LESS DIFFERENTIATED TUMOR then HIGHER RISK FOR OCCULT LN METASTASES
if SMALLER T1 then PREFER SURGERY
if TUMOR INVOLVES BONE then PREFER SURGERY
if TUMOR EXTENDS INTO TONGUE(ANTEROR 2/3) then PREFER RT
if TUMOR INVOLVES COMMISURE OF MOUTH then PREFER RT
if T2≥3CM OF THE FLOOR OF MOUTH then CONSIDER POST-OP RT
if MANDIBULAR ALVEOLAR RIDGE INVOLVED then SELECTIVE NECK DISSECTION
if LARGER TUMOR OF BUCCAL MUCOSA then TREAT NECK
if TONGUE CANCER (ANTERIOR 2/3) then TREAT NECK
if RESECTION MARGIN SMALL / POSITIVE then POST-OP RT
if FOLLOW-UP NOT POSSIBLE then TREAT NECK PROPHILACTICALLY
if SOFT PALATE TUMOR then CONSIDER STRONGLY BRACHYTHERAPY
if SOFT PALATE TUMOR then TREAT or OBSERVE NECK
if OROPHARYNGEAL TUMOR APPROACHES MIDDLE LINE then TREAT NECK BILATERALLY
if TUMOR OF OROPHARYNGEAL WALL then TREAT NECK BILATERALLY

FOLLOW-UP
Assess response with the test that best visualizes tumor
• Re-examine q 3 months *(high risk for second head and neck, lung and esophageal cancer)*
• Other tests triggered by positive pertinent findings
• Consider chemoprevention

no ← **Evidence of cancer ± biopsy proof**

↓ yes

INVESTIGATIONAL TRIAL

SALVAGE TREATMENT
if PRIOR SURGERY then RT ± SURGERY
if PRIOR RT then SURGERY
if SALVAGE NOT FEASIBLE then PALLIATE
if RECURRENT TUMOR then TREAT NECK

no ← **Evidence of cancer** → yes

SURGERY + RADIATION THERAPY
Radical neck dissection includes: cervical fascia, LNs, sternocleidomastoideus, spinal accessory nerve, internal jugular vein
Modified (functional) neck dissection perserves spinal accessory nerve and/or sternocleidomastoid.
Selective neck surgery (see in laryngeal cancer)
Reconstractive surgery
RT TD= 5,500–6,300 cGy *(180–200 cGy/d X 5 d/wk)*

RULES
if SMALL T3, N0, M0 then CONSIDER SINGLE MODALITY TREATMENT
if RESIDUAL TUMOR POST-RESECTION then INCREASE RT DOSE (~6,500–7,500 cGy)
if T4 OF TONGUE BASE or TUMOR OF PHARYNGEAL WALL then CONSIDER LARYNGECTOMY
if LARYNX PRESERVATION IS THE GOAL then NEO-ADJUVANT CHEMOTHERAPY APPROACH *(LOE II, III)*
if T UNRESECTABLE then START WITH CHEMOTHERAPY
if FOR CONCURRENT CHEMO---RT then HIGHER SURVIVAL AND TOXICITY *(LOE I, II)*

RULES FOR NECK TREATMENT *(LOE III, IV)*
if LN(s) SMALLER (e.g., ≤ 2 CM) then RT or MODIFIED RADICAL DISSECTION
if LN(s) LARGER (e.g., > 2 CM) then RADICAL DISSEC.+RT
if LNs FIXED then PRE-OP RT (~5,000 cGy)
if N0 then RT (5,000 cGy) or SELECTIVE NECK DISSECTION
if LN CAPSUL IS INVOLVED then POST–OP RT
if T CLOSE TO MIDDLE LINE then TREAT NECK BILATERALLY

LOCAL CONTROL OR *5–YR SURVIVAL* (%)

ANATOMICAL SITE	STAGE			
	I	II	III	IV
Lip	90	75	—	35
Tongue (2/3)	75	55	30	40*
Buccal mucosa	90*	90*	75*	60*
Floor of mouth	95*	80*	70*	40*
Lower gingiva	90*	90*	90*	30*
Retromolar trigon	95*	90*	90*	75*

*Includes salvage treatment — Source: PDQ

PALLIATIVE TREATMENT
CHEMOTHERAPY *(LOE II-IV)*
Methotrexate 40–60 mg/m² IV q wk, or
Cisplatin 100 mg/m² IV q 3 wks, or
Cisplatin + 5-Fluorouracil

OTHER TREATMENTS
Analgetics, RT, antidepressants, etc.

FIGURE 15-1 *Management of carcinoma of the oral cavity and oropharynx. Surgical and radiation treatment recommendations are empirical, although very few control trials have been performed. The rules vary greatly in acceptability, and the ones listed should be considered strongly. The rules do change in time, and may differ between geographic areas and individual physicians. AJCC, American Joint Committee on Cancer; cGy: centigray; COPD, chronic obstructive lung disease; CT, computed tomographic scan; CXR, chest x-ray; d, day; FNA, fine needle aspirate; LN, lymph node(s); LOE, level of evidence; MRI, magnetic resonance imaging; RT, radiation therapy; wk, week. (See also Appendix 14.)*

response rate. This, most of the time, does not translate into better survival when the drugs are given in the neoadjuvant or adjuvant setting. Neoadjuvant chemotherapy administered to the patients with advanced disease do improve organ preservation and thus may improve quality of life; this seems to be more achievable in laryngeal than in other head and neck carcinomas. The recurrent carcinomas of head and neck are not sensitive to chemotherapy; cisplatin and methotrexate each produce up to 30% response rate of a few months' duration. In patients with recurrent tumors, the combination of cisplatin and fluorouracil, when compared to cisplatin and fluorouracil alone, produces higher response rate but does not improve survival. Concomitant chemotherapy and radiotherapy increases survival at the cost of increased toxicity.

CHEMOPREVENTION

Vitamin A derivatives and analogues (retinoids) reduce frequence of second primary cancer but do not influence tumor recurrence rate. Because of retinoid toxicity , the safe and effective dose for prevention of second primary cancer awaits additional studies (Fig. 15-1).

SUGGESTED READINGS

Jacobs C, Lyman G, Velez-Garcia E, Sridhar KS, Knight W, Hochster H et al: A phase III randomized study comparing cisplatin and fluorouracil as single agents and in combination for advanced squamous cell carcinoma of the head and neck. J Clin Oncol 10:257–263, 1992

Lippman SM, Benner SE, Hong WK: Cancer chemoprevention. J Clin Oncol 12:851–873, 1994

Merlano M, Vitale V, Rosso R, Benasso M, Corvo R, Cavallari M et al: Treatment of advanced squamous-cell carcinoma of the head and neck with alternating chemotherapy and radiotherapy. N Engl J Med 327:1115–1121, 1992

Vokes EE, Weichselbaum RR, Lippman SM, Hong WK: Head and neck cancer. N Engl J Med 328:184–194, 1993

16 Hypopharyngeal Cancer

Srdjan Denić

Incidence: 2,500 new cases annually

Goal of treatment: Cure/palliation

Treatment modality: Surgery or radiation therapy for early tumors. Combined surgery and radiation therapy for advanced tumors.

Prognosis: A 5-year overall survival varies between 60% and 80%

PRIMARY PREVENTION

Most tumors are preventable by abstinence from use of tobacco and alcohol. Wine use predisposes less to cancer than distilled alcohol products. Plummer Vinson syndrome, an iron deficiency state, is a risk factor for hypopharyngeal carcinoma.

DYSPLASIA

Dysplasia is characterized by pleomorphic cells, increased number of mitoses, and prominent nuclei. When dysplasia involves the full thickness of epithelium, it is called *carcinoma in situ*. Leukoplakia and erythroplakia are descriptive clinical terms of conditions that may or may not involve dysplasia when examined under the microscope. Dysplasia is a precancerous lesion that may evolve into carcinoma or may be associated with carcinoma at a different place in a mucosal field. Dysplasia is a potentially reversible lesion. Multiple areas of dysplasia and cancer are common in the hypopharynx.

TUMOR TYPE AND DYNAMICS

The pyriform sinus is the site for squamous cell carcinoma in 75% of cases (Fig. 16-1). Because of the late appearance of symptoms, usually after the cancer has spread to the lymphatic system in the hypopharynx, the tumor is advanced at the time of diagnosis; cervical lymphadenopathy is present in 50% of patients, and distant metastases will eventually develop in 25% of them. Tumors of the posterior pharyngeal wall and postcricoid site have a high frequency of bilateral lymph node metastases. Squamous cancer of the hypopharynx often grows under the mucosa and produces "skip" metastases and frequently occult lymph node metastases. Multiple tumors appear simultaneously in up to 20% of patients.

MULTIDISCIPLINARY APPROACH

Management of head and neck tumor presents a special challenge because of the combination of the following factors:

Proximity and relatively small size of the soft tissue and bone involved

Need for tumor-free margins

Treatment interference with vital functions (breathing, eating, and speaking)

Cosmetically, the head and neck are more important than other organs

Poor oral and dental hygiene are often present

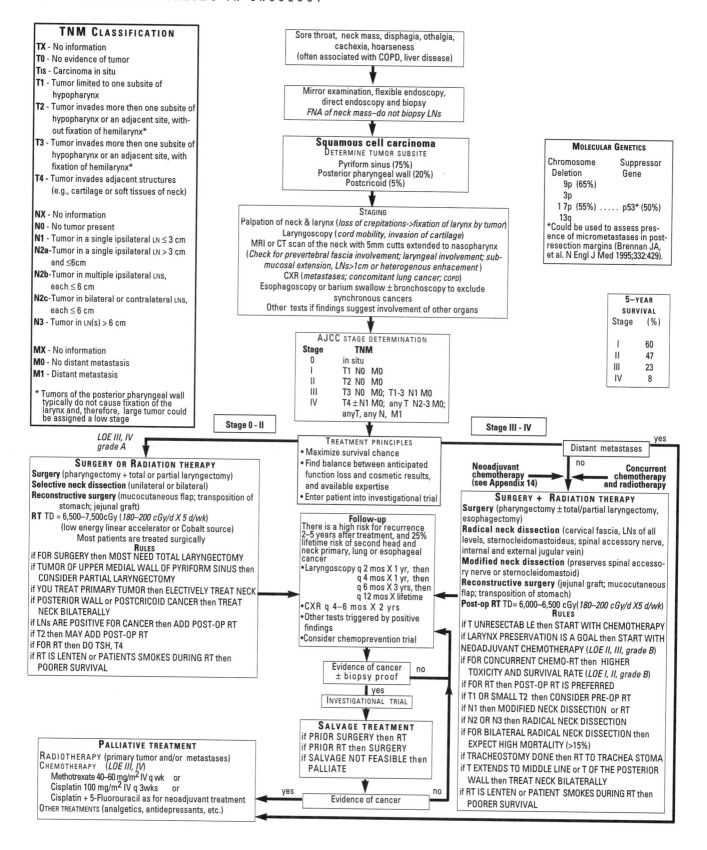

TNM CLASSIFICATION

TX - No information
T0 - No evidence of tumor
TIS - Carcinoma in situ
T1 - Tumor limited to one subsite of hypopharynx
T2 - Tumor invades more then one subsite of hypopharynx or an adjacent site, without fixation of hemilarynx*
T3 - Tumor invades more then one subsite of hypopharynx or an adjacent site, with fixation of hemilarynx*
T4 - Tumor invades adjacent structures (e.g., cartilage or soft tissues of neck)

NX - No information
N0 - No tumor present
N1 - Tumor in a single ipsilateral LN ≤ 3 cm
N2a-Tumor in a single ipsilateral LN > 3 cm and ≤6cm
N2b-Tumor in multiple ipsilateral LNs, each ≤ 6 cm
N2c-Tumor in bilateral or contralateral LNs, each ≤6 cm
N3 - Tumor in LN(s) > 6 cm

MX - No information
M0 - No distant metastasis
M1 - Distant metastasis

* Tumors of the posterior pharyngeal wall typically do not cause fixation of the larynx and, therefore, large tumor could be assigned a low stage

---

Sore throat, neck mass, disphagia, othalgia, cachexia, hoarseness
(often associated with COPD, liver disease)

Mirror examination, flexible endoscopy, direct endoscopy and biopsy
FNA of neck mass–do not biopsy LNs

Squamous cell carcinoma
DETERMINE TUMOR SUBSITE
Pyriform sinus (75%)
Posterior pharyngeal wall (20%)
Postcricoid (5%)

STAGING
Palpation of neck & larynx (*loss of crepitations->fixation of larynx by tumor*)
Laryngoscopy (*cord mobility, invasion of cartilage*)
MRI or CT scan of the neck with 5mm cuts extended to nasopharynx
(*Check for prevertebral fascia involvement; laryngeal involvement; submucosal extension; LNs>1cm or heterogenous enhancement*)
CXR (*metastases; concomitant lung cancer; COPD*)
Esophagoscopy or barium swallow ± bronchoscopy to exclude synchronous cancers
Other tests if findings suggest involvement of other organs

AJCC STAGE DETERMINATION
Stage	TNM
0	in situ
I	T1 N0 M0
II	T2 N0 M0
III	T3 N0 M0; T1-3 N1 M0
IV	T4 ± N1 M0; any T N2-3 M0; anyT, any N, M1

MOLECULAR GENETICS
Chromosome Deletion	Suppressor Gene
9p (65%)	
3p	
17p (55%)	p53* (50%)
13q	

*Could be used to assess presence of micrometastases in post-resection margins (Brennan JA, et al. N Engl J Med 1995;332:429).

5–YEAR SURVIVAL
Stage	(%)
I	60
II	47
III	23
IV	8

Stage 0 - II

LOE III, IV grade A

Stage III - IV

Distant metastases — yes →

TREATMENT PRINCIPLES
• Maximize survival chance
• Find balance between anticipated function loss and cosmetic results, and available expertise
• Enter patient into investigational trial

Neoadjuvant chemotherapy (see Appendix 14) — no — Concurrent chemotherapy and radiotherapy

SURGERY OR RADIATION THERAPY
Surgery (pharyngectomy + total or partial laryngectomy)
Selective neck dissection (unilateral or bilateral)
Reconstructive surgery (mucocutaneous flap; transposition of stomach; jejunal graft)
RT TD = 6,500–7,500cGy (*180–200 cGy/d X 5 d/wk*)
(low energy linear accelerator or Cobalt source)
Most patients are treated surgically
RULES
if FOR SURGERY then MOST NEED TOTAL LARYNGECTOMY
if TUMOR OF UPPER MEDIAL WALL OF PYRIFORM SINUS then CONSIDER PARTIAL LARYNGECTOMY
if YOU TREAT PRIMARY TUMOR then ELECTIVELY TREAT NECK
if POSTERIOR WALL or POSTCRICOID CANCER then TREAT NECK BILATERALLY
if LNs ARE POSITIVE FOR CANCER then ADD POST-OP RT
if T2 then MAY ADD POST-OP RT
if FOR RT then DO TSH, T4
if RT IS LENTEN or PATIENTS SMOKES DURING RT then POORER SURVIVAL

SURGERY + RADIATION THERAPY
Surgery (pharyngectomy ± total/partial laryngectomy, esophagectomy)
Radical neck dissection (cervical fascia, LNs of all levels, sternocleidomastoideus, spinal accessory nerve, internal and external jugular vein)
Modified neck dissection (preserves spinal accessory nerve or sternocleidomastoid)
Reconstructive surgery (jejunal graft; mucocutaneous flap; transposition of stomach)
Post-op RT TD= 6,000–6,500 cGy(*180–200 cGy/d X5 d/wk*)
RULES
if T UNRESECTABLE then START WITH CHEMOTHERAPY
if LARYNX PRESERVATION IS A GOAL then START WITH NEOADJUVANT CHEMOTHERAPY (*LOE II, III, grade B*)
if FOR CONCURRENT CHEMO-RT then HIGHER TOXICITY AND SURVIVAL RATE (*LOE I, II, grade B*)
if FOR RT then POST-OP RT IS PREFERRED
if T1 OR SMALL T2 then CONSIDER PRE-OP RT
if N1 then MODIFIED NECK DISSECTION or RT
if N2 OR N3 then RADICAL NECK DISSECTION
if FOR BILATERAL RADICAL NECK DISSECTION then EXPECT HIGH MORTALITY (>15%)
if TRACHEOSTOMY DONE then RT TO TRACHEA STOMA
if T EXTENDS TO MIDDLE LINE or T OF THE POSTERIOR WALL then TREAT NECK BILATERALLY
if RT IS LENTEN or PATIENT SMOKES DURING RT then POORER SURVIVAL

Follow-up
There is a high risk for recurrence 2–5 years after treatment, and 25% lifetime risk of second head and neck primary, lung or esophageal cancer
• Laryngoscopy q 2 mos X 1 yr, then q 4 mos X 1 yr, then q 6 mos X 3 yrs, then q 12 mos X lifetime
• CXR q 4–6 mos X 2 yrs
• Other tests triggered by positive findings
• Consider chemoprevention trial

Evidence of cancer ± biopsy proof — no →
↓ yes
INVESTIGATIONAL TRIAL

SALVAGE TREATMENT
if PRIOR SURGERY then RT
if PRIOR RT then SURGERY
if SALVAGE NOT FEASIBLE then PALLIATE

PALLIATIVE TREATMENT
RADIOTHERAPY (primary tumor and/or metastases)
CHEMOTHERAPY (*LOE III, IV*)
Methotrexate 40–60 mg/m² IV q wk or
Cisplatin 100 mg/m² IV q 3wks or
Cisplatin + 5-Fluorouracil as for neoadjuvant treatment
OTHER TREATMENTS (analgetics, antidepressants, etc.)

Evidence of cancer — yes / no

FIGURE 16-1 *Management of carcinoma of the hypopharynx. Surgical and radiation treatment recommendations are empirical, although few controlled trials have been performed. The rules of practice in general are ambiguous, considering the same condition may be managed in various ways by different physicians. Physicians' interpretation and choice of the rules are based primarily on their experience (cases seen, conferences attended, journals read, protocols used). AJCC, American Joint Committee on Cancer; cGy, centigray; COPD, chronic obstructive lung disease; CT, computed tomography; CXR, chest x-ray; MRI, magnetic resonance imaging; FNA, fine needle aspirate; RT, radiation therapy; LN, lymph node; LOE, level of evidence; wk, week; mos, months; yr, year. (See also Appendix 14.)*

In addition to a surgeon, radiation therapist, and medical oncologist, most patients will require the services of a dentist, dedicated nurse, social worker, and rehabilitation specialist.

TREATMENT

Untreated head and neck carcinomas are sensitive to radiation therapy and chemotherapy. The combination of cisplatin and fluorouracil produce 60% to 90% overall response and 15% to 50% complete response rate, but usually this does not translate into better survival when the drugs are given in the neoadjuvant or adjuvant setting. Neoadjuvant chemotherapy administered to patients with advanced disease does improve organ preservation and thus may improve quality of life. This treatment modality is considered investigational although it is supported by the level II grade B evidence. (Fig. 16-1). Concomitant chemotherapy and radiation therapy improve patient survival—at the cost of increased toxicity. All patients with carcinoma of the hypopharynx and clinically negative neck, do require neck treatment; the probability of occult cancer in these patients is above the suggested treatment threshold of 20%. Recurrent carcinomas of the head and neck are not sensitive to chemotherapy; cisplatin and methotrexate each produce a 30% response rate of a few months' duration. In patients with recurrent tumors, the combination of cisplatin and fluorouracil, when compared with cisplatin and fluorouracil alone, produces a higher response rate but does not improve survival.

CHEMOPREVENTION

Vitamin A derivatives and analogues (retinoids) reduce the frequency of a second primary cancer but do not influence the tumor recurrence rate. Because of the toxicity of retinoids, the safe and effective dose for prevention of a second primary cancer awaits additional studies.

SUGGESTED READINGS

Browman GP: Evidence-based recommendations against neoadjuvant chemotherapy for routine management of patients with squamous cell head and neck cancer. Cancer Invest 12:662–671, 1994

El-Sayed, Nelson N: Adjuvant and adjunctive chemotherapy in the management of squamous cell carcinoma of the head and neck region: a meta-analysis of prospective and randomized trials. J Clin Oncol 12:838–847, 1996

Vokes EE, Weichselbaum RR, Lippman SM, Hong WK: Head and neck cancer. N Engl J Med 328:184–194, 1993

17 Nasopharyngeal Cancer

Srdjan Denić

Prevalence: 0.2% of all cancers in the United States and 18% in China

Incidence: Very small

Goal of treatment: Cure

Treatment modality: Radiation therapy or combined chemotherapy and radiation therapy

Prognosis: A 5-year overall survival varies between 20% and 80%

EPSTEIN-BARR VIRUS

Epstein-Barr virus (EBV) is integrated in the genome of tumor cells and could be detected with polymerase chain reaction (PCR) (Table 17-1). Most patients have IgA and IgG antibodies against viral capsid (VC) and early antigen (EA) of EBV (Table 17-1). Antibody studies are important for the understanding of tumorigenesis, development of screening recommendations in endemic areas (South China, North Africa, and Northern America [natives]), diagnosis of carcinoma of neck without obvious primary site, and follow-up of treated patients.

TUMOR TYPE AND DYNAMICS

Most tumors are undifferentiated carcinomas that lack early symptoms and result in advanced disease in most patients. The tumor metastasizes to the lymph nodes on both sides of the neck, grows into the rest of the pharynx and nose, and invades bone locally. Distant metastases are commonly detected in a locally advanced cancer. A keratinizing neoplasm less often has distant metastases but has a more aggressive local growth.

TESTS

For evaluation of the locoregional extent of disease, magnetic resonance imaging (MRI) appears to be a

TABLE 17-1   RULES FOR THE MANAGEMENT OF NASOPHARYNGEAL CARCINOMA

If suspicion is high and nasopharyngeal mucosa is normal, then do blind biopsy of mucosa

If histologic diagnosis is in question, then do polymerase chain reaction on tumor tissue for Epstein-Barr virus genome

If uncertain about the best staging test, then do magnetic resonance imaging of head and neck

If uncertain about serology tests, then order IgG and IgA for viral capsid antigen and earl antigen of Epstein-Barr virus

If T≥3 or N≥1, then do bone scan, liver ultrasound, chest x-ray ± bone marrow biopsy

If neck is clinically negative, then irradiate it anyway

If neck is clinically positive then irradiate it with a higher dose

If residual neck disease is present after radiation therapy, then resect

little better test then computed tomographic scan. The probability of distant metastases increases dramatically in locally advanced disease (stages III and IV). The chest x-ray, bone scan, liver ultrasound, and bone marrow biopsy are most likely to detect distant metastases.

TREATMENT

Because of the location of tumor in a bony chamber behind the center of the face, surgery is not an

137

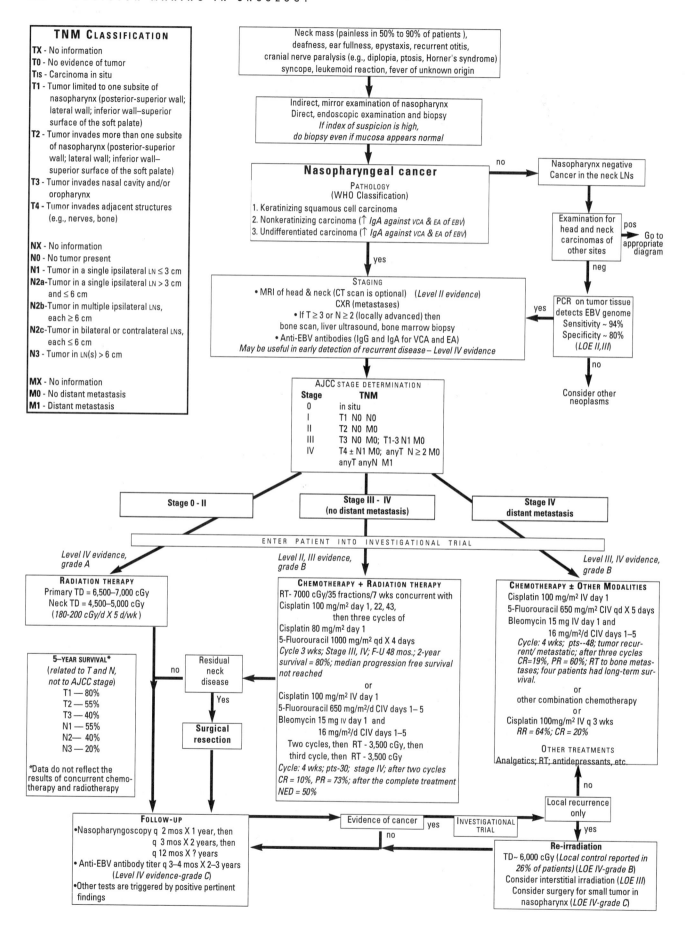

FIGURE 17-1 *Management of nasopharyngeal carcinoma. Radiotherapy is the main treatment modality for early disease. Combination of chemotherapy and radiation therapy is the treatment of choice for advanced disease. AJCC, American Joint Committee on Cancer; cGy, centigray; CIV, continuous intravenous infusion; CR, complete response; CT, computed tomographic scan; CXR, chest x-ray; d, day; EA, early antigen; EBV, Epstein-Barr virus; F-U, follow-up; LN, lymph nodes; mos, months; LOE, level of evidence; MRI, magnetic resonance imaging; NED, no evidence of disease; PCR, polymerase chain reaction; Pts, patients; RR, response rate; RT, radiation therapy; TD, total dose; yr, year; VCA, viral capsid antigen; wk, week. (See also Appendix 14.)*

option. Nasopharygeal carcinoma is sensitive to radiation therapy and chemotherapy (Fig. 17-1). Localized and small disease is curable with radiation therapy (Fig. 17-1 & Table 17-1). Combined chemo-

therapy and radiation therapy significantly improve the survival of patients with stage III and IV cancer. Surgery is not needed for metastatic disease to the neck because radiation therapy control locoregional metastases well; residual disease after radiation, however, need to be resected. Locally recurrent cancer in selected patients could be irradiated again. Metastatic disease could be managed with a single-drug (cisplatin, methotrexate) or combination chemotherapy.

SUGGESTED READINGS

Azli N, Armand JP, Rahal M et al: Alternating chemoradiotherapy with cisplatin and 5-fluorouracil plus bleomycin by continuous infusion for locally advanced undifferentiated carcinoma nasopharyngeal type. Eur J Cancer 28:1792–1797, 1992

Boussen H, Cvitkovic E, Wendling JL et al: Chemotherapy of metastatic and/or recurrent undifferentiated nasopharyngeal carcinoma with cisplatin, bleomycin, and fluorouracil. J Clin Oncol 9:1675–1681, 1991

Cvitkovic E, Bachouchi M, Boussen H et al: Leukemoid reaction, bone marrow invasion, fever of unknown origin, and metastatic pattern in the natural history of advanced undifferentiated carcinoma of nasopharyngeal type: a review of 255 consecutive cases. J Clin Oncol 11:2434–2442, 1993

18 | Paranasal Sinus Cancer

Srdjan Denić

Incidence: 1:100,000 people

Goal of treatment: Cure/palliation

Treatment modality: Surgery, surgery combined with radiation therapy, or radiation therapy alone

Prognosis: A 5-year survival depends on the stage of tumor and varies between 11% and 99%

PREVALENCE, RISK FACTORS, ANDCHEMOPREVENTION

The estimated annual incidence of the carcinoma of nose and paranasal sinuses is one in 100,000 people; two-thirds are carcinomas of the maxillary sinus. Nasal cavity adenocarcinoma is associated with exposure to nickel (refinery fumes) and wood dust (carpentry, furniture industry). Carcinoma of the maxillary sinus was induced with now-abandoned radioactive contrast material Thorotrast. Smoking is not strongly associated with nasal and paranasal sinus carcinomas. The risk of the second respiratory tract cancer is not high and chemoprevention may have less importance in these tumors.

TUMOR TYPE AND DYNAMICS

Squamous cell carcinoma is the most common histologic type (80%). The second in frequency is tumor of the salivary gland. Inverted papilloma is a rare benign tumor that is specific for this anatomic location. It has a marked tendency toward local recurrence and may ultimately require radiation therapy for growth control. Maxillary sinus carcinoma is typically advanced by the time of diagnosis. Metastases to the submandibular, preparotid, and other lymph node-bearing areas are not com-

mon, and therefore prophylactic neck dissection is not advised. Cancer of the paranasal sinuses recur locally, and most recurrences happen within two years of treatment.

MULTIDISCIPLINARY APPROACH

Almost all cancers require multidisciplinary approach (Fig. 18-1). Management of the paranasal sinus tumor, however, presents a particular challenge owing to a combination of the following factors: proximity and relatively small size of soft and bone tissue involved; need for tumor-free margins; treatment interference with vital functions (breathing, eating, and speaking); cosmetic importance of the head and neck is greater than for other organs; oral and dental hygiene is often poor. In addition to the surgeon, radiation therapist, and medical oncologist, most patients will require the services of a dentist, dedicated nurse, social worker, and rehabilitation specialist.

TREATMENT

Most patients are treated with the combination of tumor resection and radiation therapy. There is no role for neoadjuvant chemotherapy outside clinical trial. Intra-arterial chemotherapy has produced

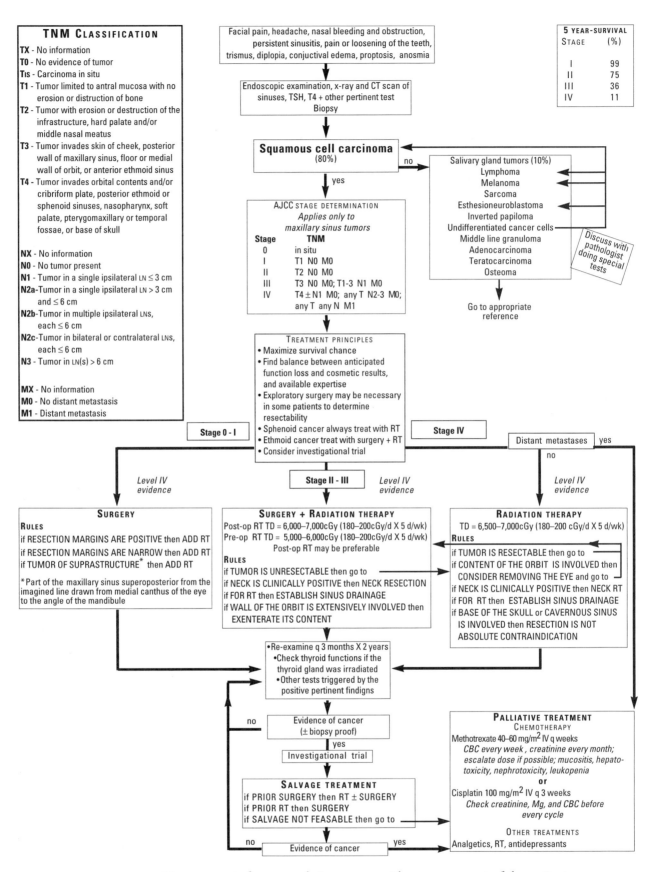

TNM Classification

TX - No information
T0 - No evidence of tumor
Tis - Carcinoma in situ
T1 - Tumor limited to antral mucosa with no erosion or distruction of bone
T2 - Tumor with erosion or destruction of the infrastructure, hard palate and/or middle nasal meatus
T3 - Tumor invades skin of cheek, posterior wall of maxillary sinus, floor or medial wall of orbit, or anterior ethmoid sinus
T4 - Tumor invades orbital contents and/or cribriform plate, posterior ethmoid or sphenoid sinuses, nasopharynx, soft palate, pterygomaxillary or temporal fossae, or base of skull

NX - No information
N0 - No tumor present
N1 - Tumor in a single ipsilateral LN ≤ 3 cm
N2a-Tumor in a single ipsilateral LN > 3 cm and ≤ 6 cm
N2b-Tumor in multiple ipsilateral LNs, each ≤ 6 cm
N2c-Tumor in bilateral or contralateral LNs, each ≤ 6 cm
N3 - Tumor in LN(s) > 6 cm

MX - No information
M0 - No distant metastasis
M1 - Distant metastasis

Facial pain, headache, nasal bleeding and obstruction, persistent sinusitis, pain or loosening of the teeth, trismus, diplopia, conjuctival edema, proptosis, anosmia

Endoscopic examination, x-ray and CT scan of sinuses, TSH, T4 + other pertinent test
Biopsy

Squamous cell carcinoma
(80%)

→ no → Salivary gland tumors (10%)
Lymphoma
Melanoma
Sarcoma
Esthesioneuroblastoma
Inverted papiloma
Undifferentiated cancer cells
Middle line granuloma
Adenocarcinoma
Teratocarcinoma
Osteoma

Discuss with pathologist doing special tests

Go to appropriate reference

5 YEAR-SURVIVAL

STAGE	(%)
I	99
II	75
III	36
IV	11

yes ↓

AJCC STAGE DETERMINATION
Applies only to maxillary sinus tumors

Stage	TNM
0	in situ
I	T1 N0 M0
II	T2 N0 M0
III	T3 N0 M0; T1-3 N1 M0
IV	T4 ± N1 M0; any T N2-3 M0; any T any N M1

TREATMENT PRINCIPLES
• Maximize survival chance
• Find balance between anticipated function loss and cosmetic results, and available expertise
• Exploratory surgery may be necessary in some patients to determine resectability
• Sphenoid cancer always treat with RT
• Ethmoid cancer treat with surgery + RT
• Consider investigational trial

Stage 0 - I   **Stage IV**   Distant metastases → yes

Stage II - III   no ↓

Level IV evidence   *Level IV evidence*   *Level IV evidence*

SURGERY

RULES

if RESECTION MARGINS ARE POSITIVE then ADD RT
if RESECTION MARGINS ARE NARROW then ADD RT
if TUMOR OF SUPRASTRUCTURE* then ADD RT

*Part of the maxillary sinus superoposterior from the imagined line drawn from medial canthus of the eye to the angle of the mandible

SURGERY + RADIATION THERAPY
Post-op RT TD = 6,000–7,000cGy (180–200cGy/d X 5 d/wk)
Pre-op RT TD = 5,000–6,000cGy (180–200cGy/d X 5 d/wk)
Post-op RT may be preferable

RULES
if TUMOR IS UNRESECTABLE then go to
if NECK IS CLINICALLY POSITIVE then NECK RESECTION
if FOR RT then ESTABLISH SINUS DRAINAGE
if WALL OF THE ORBIT IS EXTENSIVELY INVOLVED then EXENTERATE ITS CONTENT

RADIATION THERAPY
TD = 6,500–7,000cGy (180–200 cGy/d X 5 d/wk)

RULES
if TUMOR IS RESECTABLE then go to
if CONTENT OF THE ORBIT IS INVOLVED then CONSIDER REMOVING THE EYE and go to
if NECK IS CLINICALLY POSITIVE then NECK RT
if FOR RT then ESTABLISH SINUS DRAINAGE
if BASE OF THE SKULL or CAVERNOUS SINUS IS INVOLVED then RESECTION IS NOT ABSOLUTE CONTRAINDICATION

• Re-examine q 3 months X 2 years
• Check thyroid functions if the thyroid gland was irradiated
• Other tests triggered by the positive pertinent findigns

no ← Evidence of cancer (± biopsy proof)

yes ↓

Investigational trial

SALVAGE TREATMENT
if PRIOR SURGERY then RT ± SURGERY
if PRIOR RT then SURGERY
if SALVAGE NOT FEASABLE then go to

no ← Evidence of cancer → yes

PALLIATIVE TREATMENT
CHEMOTHERAPY
Methotrexate 40–60 mg/m² IV q weeks
CBC every week , creatinine every month; escalate dose if possible; mucositis, hepato-toxicity, nephrotoxicity, leukopenia
or
Cisplatin 100 mg/m² IV q 3 weeks
Check creatinine, Mg, and CBC before every cycle

OTHER TREATMENTS
Analgetics, RT, antidepressants

FIGURE 18-1 *Management of paranasal sinus cancer. The management of the patient needs to be individualized, although all treatment data presented here are empirical. cGy, centigray; CT, computed tomographic scan; d, day; LN, lymph node(s); RT, radiation therapy; TD, total dose; yr, year; wk, week. (See also Appendix 14.)*

good responses in advanced tumors but is not standard treatment. Due to the rarity of this malignancy, treatment results are not collected in a sufficiently controlled manner. All sphenoid sinus carcinoma and nonresectable ethmoid sinus carcinomas are treated with radiation therapy.

SUGGESTED READINGS

Schantz SP, Harrison LB, Ki Hong W: Tumors of the nasal cavity and paranasal sinuses, nasopharynx, oral cavity, and oropharynx. pp. 592–597. In DeVita VT, Hellman S, Rosenberg SA (eds): Cancer: Principles and Practice of Oncology 4th Ed. JB Lippincott, Philadelphia, 1993

Zaharia M, Salem L, Travezan R et al: Post-operative radiation therapy in the management of cancer of the maxillary sinus. Int J Radiat Oncol Biol Phys 17:967–971, 1989

19 | Salivary Gland Cancer

Jeffrey M. Bumpous

Incidence/Prevalence: 1:100,000 overall; 6:100,000 in age group > 80 years

Goals of treatment:

Surgery: Cure, local and regional control

Irradiation: Adjunctive for cure and local and regional control palliation

Chemotherapy: Clinical trials, palliation

Main modality of treatment: Surgery +/– adjunctive irradiation

Prognosis: (by histology)

Histology	Survival (%)		
	5 yr	*10 yr*	*15 yr*
Acinic cell	76–100	63–100	
Mucoepidermoid			
Low grade	76–95		
High grade	31–49		
Adenoid cystic	50–87	29–67	25–26
Adenocarcinoma	76–85	34–65	
Malignant mixed	31–65	23–36	
Squamous cell carcinoma	5–50	0–18	

Salivary gland malignancy represents a relatively small but important aspect of head and neck cancer. Head and neck cancer represents approximately 5% of the new cancer reported yearly in the United States; salivary gland malignancy represents only 7% of all head and neck malignancy. This rate of occurrence translates into an incidence of 1.1/100,000/year. There is no apparent sex predilection for salivary malignancy as a whole; however, for certain specific types (i.e., acinic cell carcinoma) a predilection may exist. The peak incidence occurs in persons greater than 60 years of age. The incidence in the population over the age of 80 increases to 6.0/100,000/year. Salivary gland malignancies may arise from the major salivary glands (parotid, submandibular, sublingual) or from one of thousands of minor salivary glands throughout the upper aerodigestive tract. Parotid gland tumors are responsible for 90% of all salivary neoplasms. However, a parotid mass is less likely to be malignant than submandibular, sublingual, and minor salivary tumors.

Tumors arising from salivary gland tissue may manifest in a variety of histologic types. Table 19-1 lists the major types of malignant salivary gland tumors. *The most common parotid malignancies in*

145

TABLE 19-1   MALIGNANT PAROTID TUMORS

Histologic Type	Rate of Occurrence[a] (%)
Mucoepidermoid carcinoma	15.7
Adenoid cystic carcinoma	10.0
Adenocarcinoma	8.0
Malignant mixed tumor	5.7
Acinic cell carcinoma	3.0
Squamous cell carcinoma	1.9
Other (i.e., melanoma, lymphoma)	1.3

[a]Reflects the percentage of tumor type out of all parotid malignancies, both benign and malignant.

descending order of occurrence are mucoepidermoid carcinoma, adenoid cystic carcinoma, and adenocarcinoma. In contrast, the most common malignancy in the submandibular, sublingual, and minor salivary glands is adenoid cystic carcinoma.

Three factors have been implicated in the etiopathogenesis of salivary gland malignancy: (1) *Ionizing radiation* may significantly increase the risk of these tumors. Childhood survivors of the atom bomb in Japan have an 11-fold increase in the incidence of these tumors compared with the normal population. (2) Prolonged exposure to wood dust results in an increased development of adenocarcinoma from the minor salivary glands in the sinonasal area. (3) Genetic factors certainly are involved. Up to one third of the patients with a salivary malignancy have a positive family history of the same. Additionally, there is an increased incidence of salivary gland malignancy in the Eskimo population.

CLINICAL EVALUATION

Appropriate diagnosis and staging are important in developing a logical therapeutic strategy. Since parotid masses are the most commonly encountered, a diagnostic and treatment strategy for these malignancies is outlined in Figure 19-1 and will be described in more detail. *Because 80% of parotid masses are benign, it is incumbent upon the clinician to have a strategy to appropriately segregate the 20% of malignant lesions* and therefore proceed to the most efficacious therapy. In addition to a detailed history eliciting some of the aforementioned etiologic risk factors, several pieces of clinical information should heighten the practitioner's suspicion of malignancy. *A mass that is painful continually and in which the pain bears no relationship to eating is suspicious for malignancy.* The pain resulting from sialoadenitis generally increases with eating. Pain is reported in up to 29% of parotid and up to 50% of

submandibular gland malignancies. Pain may be present because of a predisposition of certain of these tumors for perineural invasion. The absence of pain does not under any circumstance rule out the possibility of malignancy. *Other factors that indicate malignancy are a rapid pattern of growth, evidence of neuropathy (facial nerve palsy), and associated cervical lymphadenopathy.*

In the evaluation of the patient with a salivary mass, two adjuncts to history and physical examination are often helpful. Fine needle aspiration biopsy (FNAB) can be quite simply done and is often informative. Studies performed in centers with an experienced cytopathologist have been able to distinguish benign from malignant salivary gland tumors in 87% to 93% of the cases. However, establishing a precise diagnosis is less certain, varying from 23% to 87% accuracy. Unfortunately, most errors result in misreading malignant lesions as benign. Computed tomography and magnetic resonance imaging can be very helpful in determining the extent of the tumors, perineural invasion, caranial base involvement, and associated lymphadenopathy. Plain films, sialography, and nuclear imaging add little to the diagnostic work-up. After establishing a diagnosis of malignancy, staging may be performed. The primary staging system employed is that established by the American Joint Commission on Cancer (AJCC) in 1992. Table 19-2 outlines the staging system. Stage based on this schema correlates well with the outcome (see Treatment and Prognosis). The likelihood of distant metastatic disease at the time of presentation is generally low but varies greatly with stage, histologic type, and response to prior treatment.

TREATMENT AND PROGNOSIS

Once the diagnosis of a malignant salivary gland lesion has been established, the treatment plan must be designed. Two treatment schemes will be discussed. Treatment of the primary, previously untreated, and potentially resectable lesion is discussed first (Fig. 19-1). Treatment of the recurrent or technically unresectable lesion is discussed second (Fig. 19-2).

The mainstay of treatment of salivary gland malignancies has been surgery with or without adjuvant radiation therapy regardless of histologic diagnosis. The extent of surgery and the application of radiation therapy have largely been based on histologic diagnosis, pathologic factors, and to a large extent clinical judgment. The role of chemotherapy in the treatment of these malignancies is less well defined, largely because of the paucity of these tumors cou-

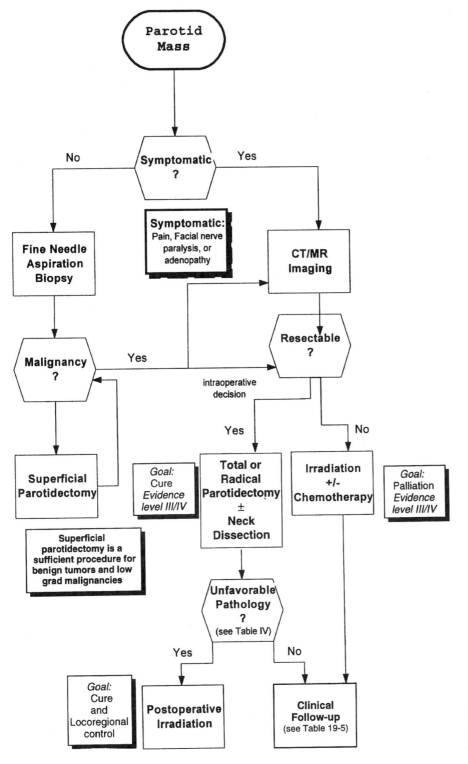

FIGURE 19-1 *Management of the parotid tumor based on type III and IV evidence.*

pled with the numerous histologic types. Table 19–3 outlines the most recent and pertinent chemotherapeutic trials in the treatment of advanced and recurrent salivary gland malignancy with an emphasis on the outcome.

COMPLETE RESECTION

In our first scenario (the newly diagnosed, primary, resectable salivary gland malignancy), the major principal in treatment involves the complete resection of the tumor as well as treatment of the

TABLE 19-2   AJCC STAGING OF SALIVARY GLAND CANCER[a]

T (Primary tumor)

T1	Tumor 2 cm or less in dimension
T2	Tumor greater than 2 cm but less than 4 cm
T3	Tumor greater than 4 cm but not more than 6 cm
T4	Tumor greater than 6 cm
	(All T stages may be subdivided into (a) no local extension or (b) local extension (i.e., nerve, skin, adjacent soft tissue, and bone)

N (Nodal stage)

N0	No evidence of regional node involvement
N1	Single ipsilateral node less than 3 cm
N2	Node(s) greater than 3 cm but less than 6 cm
	a. Single ipsilateral node between 3 and 6 cm
	b. Multiple ipsilateral nodes all less than 6 cm
	c. Bilateral or contralateral node(s) less than 6 cm
N3	Node (s) greater than 6 cm in greatest diameter

M (Tumor metastasis)

Mx	Presence of distant metastasis undetermined
M0	No known distant metastasis
M1	Distant metastasis present

[a]*American Joint Commission on Cancer. Manual for Staging. 4th Ed. Lippincott-Raven, Philadelphia, 1992, p. 49.*

regional lymphatics in the N+ neck or in the "at risk" N0 neck. In general this involves a superficial parotidectomy or total parotidectomy, depending on the location of the tumor. Resection of the facial nerve, which clinically separates the superficial from the deep lobe of the parotid, should be performed if the nerve is clinically or grossly involved. Proximal perineural spread along the facial nerve may necessitate partial temporal bone resection or dissection into the mastoid to secure negative margins. If the nerve is adjacent to the tumor but not clinically involved, most surgeons contend that the nerve may be spared and the operative field then treated with postoperative irradiation. Neural reconstructive techniques as well as static procedures have improved greatly the cosmetic results in patients who have undergone facial nerve resection. Therefore, under no circumstance in which nerve involvement is questionable should it be preserved. In general, the cervical lymphatics should be addressed with a comprehensive neck dissection (radical or modified radical) in the clinically involved neck. The N0 neck should only be addressed for histopathologic tumors with a high rate of occult nodal involvement, including high grade mucoepidermoid carcinoma and squamous cell carcinoma. Neck dissection should be performed in all resectable submandibular and sublingual carcinomas to secure a resection margin.

Adenocarcinomas, adenoid cystic carcinoma, and acinic cell carcinomas have a low rate of occult

TABLE 19-3   SUMMARY OF PERTINENT CHEMOTHERAPY TRIALS IN ADVANCED AND RECURRENT SALIVARY GLAND CANCER

Reference	Regimen	Patient Number	Response Rate (%)	Median Survival (Overall)	Median Survival (Responders)
Airoldi et al. (1994)	CDDP (Jones et al. [1993]) Adriam (Hicks et al. [1993]) Poly (Spiro and Spiro, [1989])	27	mono: CR,0 PR, 23 PR, 23 CR, 9.1 PR,36.3	8 months	14 months
Jones et al. (1993)	Epirubicin + 5-FU vs CDDP	16 (Airoldi et al. [1994]) (Licitra et al. [1991])	Epi/5 FU-0 CDDP-11	NR	NR
Licitra 1991	CDDP	31	18	14 months	NR
Dimery et al. (1991)	5-FU, doxorubicin, cyclophosphamide, and CDDP	16	50 (1CR/7PR)	18 months	NR
Belani, Eisenberger & Gray (1988)	Cyclophosphamide, doxorubicin, and CDDP	8	63 (3CR/2PR)	NR	NR
Creagan et al. (1988)	CDDP	34	38 (2CR/11PR)	15 months	18 months

Abbreviations: Adriam, Adriamycin; CDDP, cisplatin; CR, complete response; 5-FU, 5-fluorouracil; NR, not reported; poly, CDDP + epirubicin + 5-FU + cyclophosphamide; PR, partial response; mono, monotherapy.

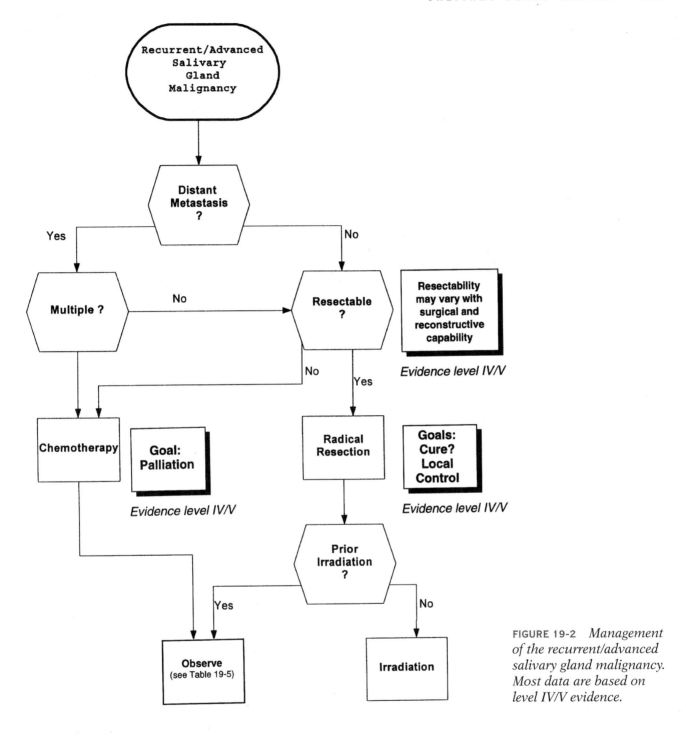

FIGURE 19-2 *Management of the recurrent/advanced salivary gland malignancy. Most data are based on level IV/V evidence.*

nodal involvement and therefore do not require neck dissection for the N0 neck. In treating the N0 neck a modified or selective approach should be undertaken to preserve important neurovascular structures where possible (i.e., spinal accessory nerve). The application of postoperative radiation therapy is based on stage, tumor histology, resection margins, involvement of regional lymphatics, evidence of perineural invasion, and to a certain extent clinical judgment. Substantial improvement in local and regional control (65 vs. 85%) and survival has been appreciated with the addition of postoperative radiation therapy in stage III and IV parotid tumors. Tumors that demonstrate perineural invasion have commonly spread further along the nerve than the surgeon may appreciate;

therefore, this is regarded as an indication for adjuvant radiation. The prognosis is multifactorial. Table 19-4 outlines indicators of a poor prognosis.

UNRESECTABLE MALIGNANCY

In the treatment of the locally advanced ("unresectable") and recurrent salivary gland malignancy, well-designed prospective clinical trials with adequate control and numbers are lacking. Therefore, information must be gleaned from the clinical impressions of experienced surgeons and oncologists as well as a few small clinical trials. *Great care should be given to declaring a salivary gland malignancy "unresectable."* Improved techniques in cranial base surgery and head and neck reconstruction have greatly extended the limits of resectability.

EXTENDED RESECTIONS

Extended resections (i.e., cranial base resections) have demonstrated lower rates of recurrence and trends toward improved survival in other areas of the head and neck (i.e., the paranasal sinuses). The efficacy of such extended surgeries in the treatment of salivary gland malignancies is not presently known. In general, the role of chemotherapy has been largely palliative in the management of advanced or recurrent salivary malignancies. The response rate to chemotherapy varies greatly, depending on the regimen employed, and ranges from 18% to 63%. There is a trend for improved response rates in multiagent regimens that include cisplatin compared with single-agent therapy. The median survival of patients with advanced and recurrent salivary gland malignancies who receive chemotherapy ranges from 8 to 15 months and is

TABLE 19-4   POOR PROGNOSTIC FACTORS IN
SALIVARY CANCER

Stage
Histologic type
   High-grade mucoepidermoid carcinoma
   Adenoid cystic carcinoma (solid pattern)
   Adenocarcinoma (high grade)
   Squamous cell carcinoma
Regional lymphadenopathy
Clinical and/or pathologic evidence of perineural invasion
   Location
   Submandibular gland
   Sublingual gland
   Minor salivary gland (worst location)
Distant metastasis
Local and regional recurrence

---

slightly higher in the responding patients. One notable exception with regard to survivorship in advanced and recurrent disease is *adenoid cystic carcinoma*. Distant metastases eventually occur in approximately 50% of patients with adenoid cystic carcinoma. Patients with a solid histopathologic pattern and evidence of perineural invasion are at higher risk for distant disease. Distant metastases in adenoid cystic carcinoma tend to be pulmonary. Oddly, *patients with distant metastatic disease may live for a prolonged period (years) despite the presence of distant disease*. Distant metastatic disease may also manifest many years after presentation of the index tumor, making 5-year survival statistics less meaningful in adenoid cystic carcinoma. High-grade mucoepidermoid carcinoma and squamous cell carcinoma of the salivary glands that are advanced or recurrent are almost uniformly fatal despite treatment. Some evidence suggests that adenocarcinomas may in general be more responsive to chemotherapy compared with other histologic subtypes. Acinic cell carcinomas account for only 7% of salivary malignancies and in general have a more indolent course. Late recurrences have been reported, and lifetime follow-up is therefore indicated.

CONCLUSIONS

Salivary gland malignancies are rare and will therefore be infrequently encountered in a given oncology practice. Additionally, few adequately designed and numbered prospective trials are available for guidance in the treatment of advanced and recurrent salivary gland malignancy. In general, early appropriate diagnosis with discretionary use of FNAB and imaging techniques (computed tomography and magnetic resource imaging, aggressive surgical resection, and application of postoperative radiation therapy by defined guidelines afford the best opportunity for local and regional control and survival. Chemotherapy is for the most part a palliative treatment for advanced and recurrent disease. However, response rates as impressive as 63% certainly are cause for enthusiasm and further clinical investigation. Ideally a large multicenter clinical trial is the vehicle for appropriately evaluating the role of chemotherapy in the management of advanced salivary malignancy. Advanced stage, histologic type, evidence of regional nodal involvement, and the presence of perineural invasion portend for a poorer prognosis and a higher rate of local and regional recurrence. Advances in surgical technique, radiation therapy, chemotherapy, and

TABLE 19-5   **STRATEGY FOR CLINICAL FOLLOW-UP IN PATIENTS WITH SALIVARY GLAND MALIGNANCY**

1. Clinical follow-up should consist of a complete head and neck examination and a comprehensive cranial nerve examination every 3 months after initial treatment for the first 2 years and annually after that. Rationale: Approximately 80% of recurrences overall will appear in the first 2 years of follow-up. Timely diagnosis of recurrence may allow the patient to have treatment with the goal of an increased disease-free interval.

2. Indications for radiologic imaging in follow-up:
   a. Chest x-ray: indicated annually for patients with adenoid cystic carcinoma because 50% of these patients will develop metastases, with the most common site being the lungs.
   b. Computed tomography, or magnetic resource imaging as both may be indicated when the primary tumor is deeply seated (deep lobe of the parotid) and therefore inaccessible to palpation (indicated every 6 months for the first 2 years, then annually) or when new onset of pain, mass, adenopathy, or cranial neuropathy occurs.

biological therapy may afford new opportunities for enhanced control and survival for patients with advanced and recurrent salivary gland cancers (see Table 19-5 for follow-up).

SUGGESTED READINGS

Airoldi M, Brando V, Giordano C et al: Chemotherapy for recurrent salivary gland malignancies: experience of the ENT department of Turin University. Oto-Rhino-Laryngol 56:105–111, 1994

Anderson J, Beenken S, Crowe R et al: Prognostic factors in minor salivary gland cancer. Head & Neck 17:480–486, 1995

Batsakis J: Tumors of the major salivary glands. pp. 1–37. In Batsakis J (ed.): Tumors of the Head and Neck. Williams & Wilkins, Baltimore, 1974

Belani C, Eisenberger M, Gray W: Preliminary experience with chemotherapy in advanced salivary gland neoplasms. Med Pediatr Oncol 16:197–202, 1988

Creagan E, Woods J, Rubin J, Schaid D: Cisplatin-based chemotherapy for neoplasms arising from salivary glands and contiguous structures in the head and neck. Cancer 62:2313–2319, 1988

Dimery I, Legha S, Shirinian M, Hong W: Fluorouracil, doxorubicin, cyclophosphamide, and cisplatin combination chemotherapy in advanced or recurrent salivary gland carcinoma. J Clin Oncol 8:1056–1062, 1990

Hicks J, El-Naggar A, Flaitz C et al: Histocytologic grading of mucoepidermoid carcinoma of major salivary glands in prognosis and survival: a clinicopathologic and flow cytometric investigation. Head & Neck 17:89–95, 1995

Joe V, Westesson P: Tumors of the parotid gland: MR imaging characteristics of various histologic types. AJR 163:433–438, 1994

Jones A, Phillips D, Cook J, Helliwell T: A randomised phase II trial of epirubicin and 5-fluorouracil versus cisplatinum in the palliation of advanced and recurrent malignant tumour of the salivary glands. Br J Cancer 67:112–114, 1993

Kim K, Sung M, Chung P et al: Adenoid cystic carcinoma of the head and neck. Arch Otolaryngol Head Neck Surg 120:721–726, 1994

Licitra L, Marchini S, Spinazze S et al: Cisplatin in advanced salivary gland carcinoma. A phase II study of 25 patients. Cancer 68:1874–1877, 1991

Rice D, Spiro R: General management guidelines. pp. 1–15. In Rice D, Spiro R (eds): Current Concepts in Head and Neck Cancer. American Cancer Society, 1988

Rice D, Spiro R. Carcinoma of the major salivary glands. pp. 29–39. In Rice D, Spiro R (eds): Current Concepts in Head & Neck Cancer. American Cancer Society, 1988

Schramm V, Srodes C, Myers E. Cisplatin therapy for adenoid cystic carcinoma. Arch Otolaryngol 107:739–741, 1981

Spiro R, Spiro J: Cancer of the salivary glands. pp. 645–668. In Myers E, Suen J (eds): Cancer of the Head and Neck. 2nd Ed. Churchill Livingstone, New York, 1989

20 | Cancer of the Unknown Primary Site

Shawn D. Glisson

Prevalence: 5% to 10% of all cancer patients

Goal of treatment: Palliation; less frequently for cure

Main modality of treatment: Chemotherapy and/or radiation therapy; occasionally surgery

Prognosis: 4–8 months for the group as a whole

Cancer of the unknown primary site (UPS) is a relatively common clinical condition, accounting for at least 5% of cancer diagnoses. Since early diagnosis is not possible by definition, screening is impossible. Unfortunately, the very nature of this category of tumors is one of early metastatic spread. Not surprisingly, the results of surgery, radiation therapy, and chemotherapy often have been disappointing (Table 20-1). Despite this assessment, an attempt should be made to determine the nature of the malignancy. The goal should be the identification of those malignancies that can be treated.

Since the diagnosis of UPS is one of exclusion, an adequate diagnostic workup (i.e., H+P, CBC, UA, C18, CXR, CT Abd/Pelvis) is the first step. Other tests, such as computed tomographic scan of the chest, endoscopy, and intravenous urography are expensive and should be considered only when clinically indicated. The type of UPS tumor is the initial determinant for what kind of workup should follow. There are basically three different pathologic reports that may return when a UPS tumor is biopsied (Table 20-2).

The poorly differentiated neoplasm presents a challenge in that there are some tumors that are treatable (Fig. 20-1A). Once a diagnosis is made by immunocytochemistry, treatment may begin. While waiting for the pathologist to do the appropriate studies, certain clinical presentations should prompt the physician to rule out certain malignancies (Table 20-3).

Adenocarcinoma accounts for almost two-thirds of all UPS tumors. Common metastatic sites are liver, lung, and bone. The most common primary sites are the lung and pancreas (Fig. 20-1B). Other GI sites are also common. Adenocarcinoma from breast, prostate, and ovary are infrequently found to be UPS tumors.

As a group, those who have UPS adenocarcinoma have a median survival of only 3 or 4 months, although not all patients will have such a poor prognosis. For example, peritoneal carcinomatosis in women should be treated as a stage IV ovarian cancer. CA 125 levels may be elevated. The most effective treatment has been shown to be a cisplatin-based chemotherapy. The results have been encouraging, since 39% in one study had a complete response, and the median survival was 23 months for the entire group.

Those patients who are found to have UPS adenocarcinoma only in an axillary lymph node usually may be regarded as having a stage II breast cancer. CA 15-3 may be elevated. A modified radical masectomy should be performed with chemotherapy to follow. The patient should be treated with curative intent in many instances. Hormonal therapy is indicated if the tumor is positive for estrogen and progesterone receptors.

Men who have widespread bony metastasis are likely to have prostate carcinoma. The metastatic lesions will usually be blastic. A prostate-specific antigen (PSA) and/or PAP provides evidence for this UPS tumor. Hormonal therapy may provide palliation.

153

TABLE 20-1   FACTORS FOR FAVORABLE OUTCOME[a]

1.   Predominant tumor location in the retroperitoneum or peripheral lymph nodes
2.   Tumor limited to one or two metastatic sites
3.   Normal carcinoembryonic antigen level
4.   Normal lactose dehydrogenase level
5.   No history of cigarette use

[a] *Based on 220 patients compiled at Vanderbilt.*

TABLE 20-2   TYPES OF UPS TUMORS (BASED ON LIGHT MICROSCOPY)

Poorly differentiated neoplasm (including poorly differentiated carcinoma and poorly differentiated adenocarcinoma

Well-differentiated and moderately well-differentiated adenocarcinoma

Squamous cell carcinoma

TABLE 20-3   TUMOR MARKERS USEFUL IN SELECTED PATIENTS WITH UPS

Clinical Situation	Need to Rule Out	Serum or Urine Marker
Young male/female with mediastinal or retroperitoneal mass(es)	Extragonadal germ cell tumor	AFP, BhCG
Young male/female with pelvic mass(es)	Neuroblastoma, pheochromocytoma	HVA, VMA
Female with adenocarcinoma in an axillary node	Breast cancer	CA 15-3, CEA
Female with ascites	Ovarian cancer	CA 125
Male with metastases to lungs +/− bones	Prostate cancer	PSA
Males/female with a single or multiple masses in the liver	Hepatocellular cancer	AFP, CEA

TABLE 20-4   EVALUATION OF PATIENTS WITH CARCINOMA OF AN UNKNOWN PRIMARY SITE TO IDENTIFY THOSE WHOSE TUMORS MAY BE TREATABLE

Carcinoma	Clinical Evaluation	Pathologic Studies	Special Subgroups	Therapy	Prognosis
Adenocarcinoma (well differentiated or moderately well differentiated)	Abdominal CT: serum PSA in men, mammography in women	PSA stain in men; status of ERs and PRs in women	Women with axillary-node involvement	Treat as primary breast cancer	Poor for entire group (median survival 4 months); better for subgroups
			Women with peritoneal carcinomatosis	Surgical cytoreduction + chemotherapy effective in ovarian cancer	
			Men with blastic bone metastases, high serum PSA, or PSA tumor staining	Hormonal therapy for prostate cancer	
			Patient with single peripheral nodal site of involvement	Lymph-node dissection ± radiotherapy	
Squamous carcinoma	Panendoscopy for cervical-node presentation; pelvic + rectal examination, anoscopy for inguinal presentation	None	Cervical adenopathy	Radiation therapy ± neck dissection	5- year survival, 25%–50%
			Inguinal adenopathy	Inguinal-node dissection ± radiation therapy	Potential long-term survival
Poorly differentiated carcinoma or adenocarcinoma	Chest, abdominal CT; serum hCG, AFP	Immunoperoxidase staining (see Fig. 20-1), electron microscopy, chromosomal analysis	Atypical germ-cell tumors (identified by chromosomal abnormalities only)	Treatment for germ-cell tumor	Treatment results similar to those for extragonadal germ-cell tumor
			Neuroendocrine tumors	Cisplatin-based therapy	10%–20% cured with therapy; high overall response rate
			Predominant tumor location in retroperitoneum, peripheral nodes	Cisplatin, etoposide, and bleomycin	

Abbreviations: CT, computed tomography; PSA, prostate-specific antigen; ER, estrogen receptor; PR, progesterone receptor, hCG, human chorionic gonadotropin; and AFP, α-fetoprotein; HVA, homovanillic acid; VMA, vanillymandelic acid. (From Hainsworth JD, Greeco AF: Treatment of patients with cancer of unknown primary site. N Engl J Med 329:257–263, 1993, with permission.)

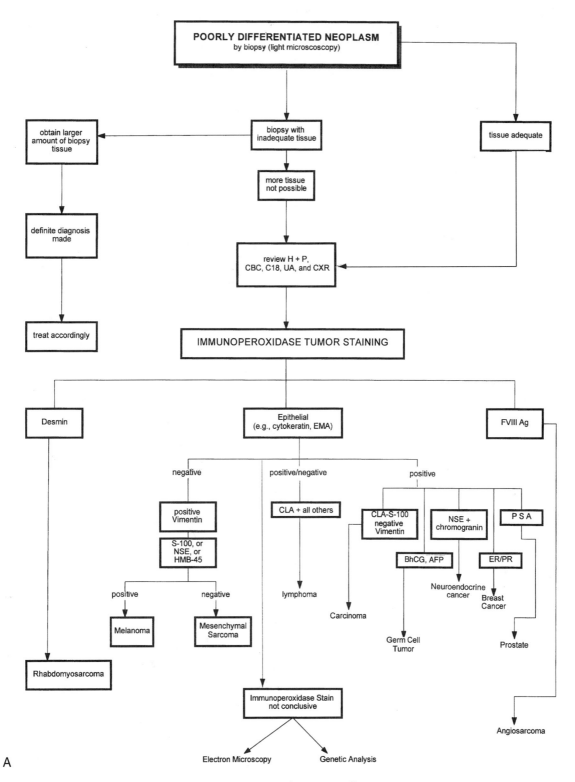

A

FIGURE 20-1 *(Continued).*

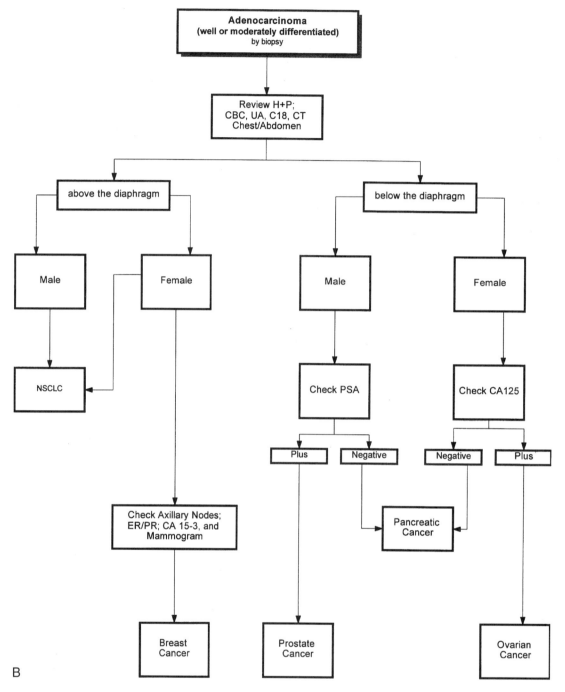

FIGURE 20-1 *(Continued).*

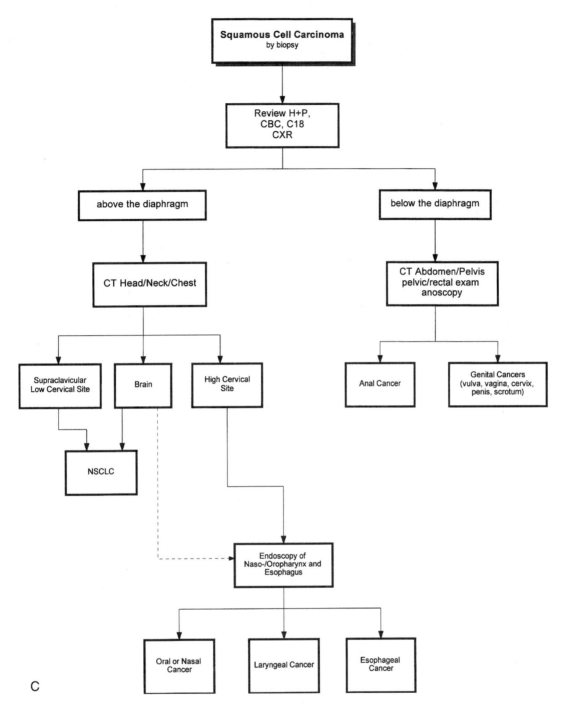

FIGURE 20-1 *(A–C) (Continued). Diagnostic workup of patients presenting with cancer of an unknown primary. Initial categorization is based on light microscopy (adenocarcinoma, poorly differentiated neoplasm, squamous cell cancer); further subcategorization is dependent on result of immunochemical, molecular biologic, cytogenetic and electron microscopy techniques. A key reasoning principle is based on the fact that within this seemingly uniform category of cancer of unknown primary sites, there are subgroups of patients who are pathologically and clinically distinct.) The goal of treatment is identification of those malignancies that can be treated (see Table 20-4). Recommended strategy is based on solid (level II) nonexperimental evidence. CLA, common leukocyte antigen; NSE, neuron-specific enolase; EMA, epithelial membrane antigen.*

Survival is poor for those with adenocarcinoma not found with a likely ovarian, breast, or prostate carcinoma. Cisplatin appears to have no role in the treatment of these tumors. The most effective therapy appears to be FAM (5-FU, doxorubicin, mitomycin C). Median survival could be increased from 3 months to 11 months using this regimen.

Squamous cell carcinoma is the least common UPS tumor. The most common site of origin is dependent on whether the metastasis is above or below the diaphragm (Fig. 20-1C). Those tumors found above the diaphragm will be either NSCLC or upper aerodigestive tract carcinoma. When no primary site is found, local treatment should be given to the involved neck. Local treatment with surgery and radiation, with or without chemotherapy, have shown similar results (i.e., 30% to 70% 5-year survival).

In general, all patients with poorly differentiated carcinoma or poorly differentiated adenocarcinoma of UPS should be considered for a trial of cisplatin-based chemotherapy (e.g., cisplatin, etoposide, bleomycin) (see Appendix 15). This serves to identify patients with responsive tumors (after 1 or 2 courses of chemotherapy). If response is noted, therapy should be continued for a total of four courses. Table 20-4 shows summary data on the management of patients with carcinoma of unknown primary site.

SUGGESTED READINGS

Bitran J, Ultmann J: Malignancies of undetermined primary origin. Dis Mon 38:221–260, 1992

Greco FA, Hainsworth JD: Cancer of Unknown Primary Site: Principles and Practice of Oncology. 4th Ed.

Goldberg RM, Smith FP, Ueno W et al: Fluorouracil, adriamycin, and mitomycin in the treatment of adenocarcinoma of unknown primary. J Clin Oncol 4:395–399, 1986

Hainsworth JD, Grecco AF: Treatment of patients with cancer of unknown primary site. N Engl J Med 329:257–263, 1993

Lembersky B, Thomas L: Metastases of unknown primary site. Med Clin North Am 80:153–171, 1996

Strand CM, Grosh WW, Baxter J et al: Peritoneal carcinomatosis of unknown primary site in women. Ann Intern Med 111:231–217, 1989

21 Management of Small-Cell Lung Cancer

Shawn D. Glisson

Incidence: 14/100,000

Significance: About 35,000 new cases in the United States annually

Goal of treatment: Increase life by 3 to 4 times the natural history of disease; cure is rare

Main modality of treatment: Chemotherapy; chemotherapy with radiation therapy in limited disease; there is presently no role for surgery outside of controlled studies

Small-cell lung cancer (SCLC) with its variants accounts for roughly 20% of all lung cancers. As in non-small-cell lung cancer NSCLC, cigarette smoking is by far the greatest risk factor for developing this malignancy. Uranium and radon gas exposure also constitute independent risk factors. Unlike NSCLC, however, SCLC is considered a systemic disease even in the earliest stage. Even though the diagnostic work-up is the same (Fig. 21-1), it is largely because of this distinction that SCLC is approached differently from NSCLC.

DIAGNOSIS

SCLC is harder to diagnose that NSCLC. The most important factor in making the diagnosis of SCLC is an adequate tissue sample. For example, a small needle biopsy may cloud the issue since crushed NSCLC cells may appear as SCLC. Even with an adequate tissue block, pathologists may not agree on the diagnosis. For all practical purposes, if an experienced pathologist believes that there is a definite SCLC component to a tumor, the patient should be considered to have SCLC. The significance of the various SCLCs is not completely known.

The clinical presentation of SCLC is similar to NSCLC (Table 21-1). SCLC usually presents with hilar and mediastinal adenopathy. It is less typical for an SCLC to present peripherally, with a pleural effusion, or with chest wall involvement. Unfortunately, metastatic spread of SCLC is usually present at the time of diagnosis. Clinically detectable distant metastases are present in about two thirds of patients with SCLC at diagnosis. However, these distant metastases are usually asymptomatic unless brain metastasis has occurred.

Paraneoplastic syndromes are not uncommon (Table 21-2). The syndrome of inappropriate anti-diuretic hormone (SIADH) secretion (11% of patients), Cushing's syndrome (2.4% of patients), and the Eaton-Lambert syndrome are most commonly associated with SCLC.

The main goal of staging SCLC is to find those patients who may be treated with local therapies (Table 21-3) along with chemotherapy. Chemother-

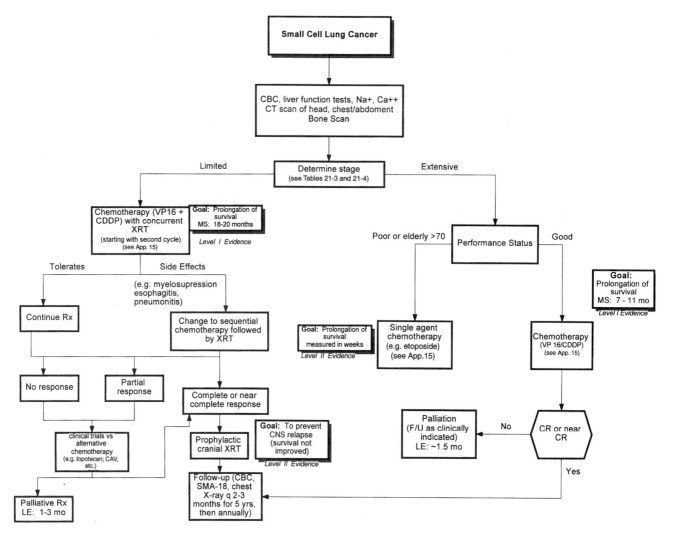

FIGURE 21-1 *Management of small-cell lung cancer (SCLC). SCLC is systemic malignancy and disseminates early in its course in most patients. Understanding this systemic nature of SCLC is the key reasoning principle in the management of this malignancy. Determination of the stage is important deciding about including radiation therapy in the management of limited SCLC. Currently, SCLC is only very rarely cured and the goal of treatment is prolongation of survival, which is usually measured in months rather than years. Recommended strategy is based on level I and II evidence for initial treatment choice. Recommendations for follow-up are based on common practice (level V evidence).*

TABLE 21-1 CLASSIFICATION OF SMALL-CELL LUNG CANCER

Small cell carcinoma (formerly oat cell) 90%
Mixed small cell and large cell variant
Combined small-cell lung cancer and non-small-cell lung cancer

Those patients with mixed small and large cell types generally have shorter survival than those with small-cell carcinoma. Those with combined may present with surgically resectable disease.

apy remains the mainstay of treatment for SCLC, since approximately 80% of patients will produce objective tumor response to chemotherapy. For patients with limited-stage disease, the addition of radiation therapy to the thorax modestly improves local control and survival benefit. The cost of these benefits, however, is an increase in toxic reactions.

Other reasons to stage the disease accurately are to ascertain prognosis and to monitor disease

TABLE 21-2 PARANEOPLASTIC SYNDROMES RELATED TO SMALL CELL LUNG CANCER

Endocrine

Hypercalcemia (ectopic adrenal hormone)

Cushing's syndrome

SIADH (sepndrome of inappropriate antiduiretic hormone)

Carcinoid syndrome

Gynecomastia

Hypercalcitonemia

↑ Growth hormone

↑ Prolactin follicle-stimulating hormone/luteinizing hormone

Hypoglycemia

Hypothyroidism

Neurologic

Encephalopathy

Subacute cerebellar degeneration

Progressive multifocal leukoencephalopathy

Peripheral neuropathy

Polymyositis

Autonomic neuropathy

Eaton-Lambert syndrome

Optic neuritis

Skeletal

Pulmonary hypertrophic osteoarthropathy

Hematologic

Anemia

Leukemoid reactions

Thrombocytosis

Thrombocytopenia

Eosinophilia

Pure red cell aplasia

Leukoerythroblastosis

Disseminated intravascular coagulation (DIC)

Trousseau's syndrome

Murantic endocarditis

Dermatologic

Hyperkeratosis (acquired ichthyosis and Bazex disease)

Dermatomyositis

Acanthosis nigricans

Hyperpigmentation

Erythema gyratum repens

Hypertrichosis lanuginosa → ↑ Urinary level of free cortisol

Leukoerythroblastosis

DIC

Trousseau's syndrome

Murantic endocarditis

Lanuginosa acquista

Leser-Trélat syndrome

Pachydermoperiostitis → R/O lung abscess and benign tumor

Other

Secretion of vasoactive

Intestinal peptide with diarrhea

Hyperamylasemia

Nephrotic syndrome

Hypouricemia

TABLE 21-3 STAGING OF SMALL-CELL LUNG CANCER

| Limited: | Tumor confined to one hemithorax and the regional lymph nodes |
| Extensive: | Tumor not confined to one hemithorax or to the regional lymph nodes |

These definitions are based on the clinical judgment as to whether all detectable tumor can be encompassed within a tolerable radiation therapy port.

response to treatment. The clinical course of SCLC without treatment is a median survival of 5 weeks for those with limited disease and 12 weeks for those with extensive disease. Combination chemotherapy given either with or without chest irradiation improves survival rate fourfold to fivefold in both limited and extensive disease.

The basic work-up for staging is essentially the same as in NSCLC (Table 21-4). The only exception may be the need for a bilateral bone marrow biopsy and aspiration if there is an abnormality in the complete blood count. This should be done in those who are to receive stage-dependent treatment (i.e., treatment for limited disease), as 10% to 12% may have bone marrow involvement. If the bone marrow is positive for SCLC, then the patient would be staged as having extensive disease.

Treatment must include systemic chemotherapy because the disease process is systemic early in its course in most patients (Table 21-5). Surgery has not been shown to be effective in the treatment of SCLC. Radiation therapy is effective in the treatment of limited-stage SCLC. It may also be used in the treatment of CNS involvement.

TABLE 21-4 STAGING PROCEDURES FOR SMALL-CELL LUNG CANCER

Complete history and physical examination

Chemoradiation therapy and computed tomography (and CT) scan of the chart to assist in portal design if chest irradiation (other than palliative) is to be used; use fiberoptic bronchoscopy if no evaluable tumor is found on chest film

Liver function tests with CT Abd. Use liver biopsy if abnormality is detected and information is needed for selected therapy

Bone scan

Brain CT

Complete blood count: if abnormality, then bilateral bone marrow biopsy and aspiration if information is needed for selected therapy

TABLE 21-5 INFLUENCE OF MODERN COMBINATION CHEMOTHERAPY ON SURVIVAL AMONG PATIENTS WITH SMALL-CELL LUNG CANCER

	Survival	
Era	Limited Disease	Extensive Diseases
Prechemotherapy		
Supportive care (median)	3 months	1.5 months
Surgery (5-year)	<1%	—
Radiation therapy (5-year)	1%–3%	—
Chemotherapy		
Single agent (median)[a]	6 months	4 months
Combination		
Median	10–14 months	7–11 months
5-year	2%–8%	0–1%
Combination with chest irradiation		
Median	12–16 months	7–11 months
5-year	6%–12%	0–1%

[a]Some recent results suggest that longer median survival may be possible in selected patients.

(From Ihde DC et al: Chemotherapy of lung cancer. N Eng J Med 327:1438, 1992, with permission.)

SUGGESTED READINGS

Healey EA Abner A: Thoracic and cranial radiotherapy for limited-stage small cell lung cancer. Chest 107:249S–254S, 1995

Hirsch FR et al: Histopathologic classification of small cell lung cancer: changing concepts and terminology. Cancer 62:973–977, 1988

Histopathologic classification of small cell carcinoma of the lung: comments based on an interobserver examination. Cancer 50:1360–1366, 1982

Ihde DC: Chemotherapy of lung cancer. N Engl J Med 327:1434–1441, 1992

Ihde DC et al: Small cell lung cancer pp. 723–758. In DeVita VT Jr (ed): Cancer: Principles & Practice of Oncology. 4th Ed. 1993

Johnson DH et al: Cisplatin and etoposide plus concurrent thoracic radiotherapy administered once versus twice daily for limited-stage small cell lung cancer (abstract). Proc Am Soc Clin Oncol 13:333, 1994

Murray N, Coy P, Pater JL et al: Importance of timing for thoracic irradiation in the combined modality treatment of limited-stage small-cell lung cancer. Oncol 11:336–344, 1993

Perry MC, Eaton WL, Propert KJ et al: Chemotherapy with or without radiation therapy in limited small-cell carcinoma of the lung. 316:912–918, 1987

Pignon JP, Arriagada R N Engl J Med Ihde DC et al: A meta-analysis of thoracic radiotherapy for small-cell lung cancer. N Engl J Med 327:1618–1624, 1992

Warde P, Payne D: Does thoracic radiation improve survival and local control in limited-stage small cell carcinoma of the lung? J Clin Oncol 10:890–895, 1992

22 Management of Non-Small-Cell Lung Cancer

Shawn D. Glisson

Incidence: 56/100,000

Significance: Number 1 cause of cancer death in the United States

Goal of treatment: Curative intent in the early stages; palliation in the late stages

Main modality of treatment: Surgery with curative intent (or x-ray treatment for poor performance status) in the early stages, chemotherapy in the later stages

Prognosis: 13% five-year survival overall

Stage dependent: Stage I, 50% five-year survival

Stage II, 30%

Stage IIIa, 10–15%

Stage IIIb, <5%

Stage IV, <2%

Non-small-cell lung cancer (NSCLC) accounts for roughly 80% of all lung cancers, making NSCLC the most common cause of cancer death in the United States. There will be at least 135,000 new cases each year in this country throughout the 1990s. Cigarette smoking is by far the greatest risk factor for developing NSCLC, accounting for 90% of the lung cancer in men and 75% to 80% in women. To a lesser extent, passive smoking, asbestos, radon, bis(chloromethyl)ether, polycyclic aromatic hydrocarbons, chromium, nickel, and inorganic arsenic compounds have also been associated as independent risk factors. Dietary and genetic risk factors have not yet been conclusively determined.

There are at least three distinct histologic types of NSCLC (Table 22-1). Adenocarcinoma (AC) is now the most common type of NSCLC in the United States, accounting for 40% of all lung cancers. It usually arises peripherally and may present as a solitary pulmonary nodule or as a rapidly progressive disease invading many lobes. It generally has a poorer prognosis than squamous cell carcinoma (SCC), which accounts for 30% of all lung cancers. SCC is slow growing and usually arises in the proximal bronchi. Because SCC tends to exfoliate, it may be detected by sputum cytology at an early stage. Large cell carcinoma (LCC) accounts for the remaining 15% of NSCLC.

On the basis of past studies, screening for lung cancer is not recommended. Initial common presenting symptoms are usually vague (Table 22-2). Paraneoplastic syndromes may occur (Table 22-3). When lung cancer is suspected, a chest x-ray should be obtained as it remains the best diagnostic procedure. For any suspicious findings, computed tomo-

TABLE 22-1 HISTOPATHOLOGY OF NON-SMALL-CELL LUNG CANCER

Adenocarcinoma (in 40% of all lung cancer)
  Acinar
  Papillary
  Bronchoalveolar
  Solid tumor with mucin
Squamous cell (epidermoid) carcinoma (in 30% of all lung cancer)
  Spindle cell variant
Large cell carcinoma (in 15% of all lung cancer)
  Giant cell
  Clear cell
Adenosquamous carcinoma

TABLE 22-2 COMMON PRESENTING SYMPTOM OF NON-SMALL-CELL LUNG CANCER

General
  Fatigue (84%)
  Decreased activity (81%)
  Weight loss (54%–68%)
  Malaise (26%)
  Lymphadenopathy (23%)
  Fever (21%)
  Asymptomatic (12%)
  Loss of taste for cigarettes
  Dizziness (4%)
Skeletal
  Bone Pain (25%)
  Clubbing (20%)
Neurologic
  Horner's Syndrome
    Enophthalmos
    Meiosis
    Ptosis
  Ulnar pain/shoulder pain
  Hoarseness/dysphagia
Cardiovascular
  Superior vena cava syndrome (4%)
  Tamponade/CHF/arrhythmia
Gastroenterologic
  Hepatomegaly (21%)
  Dysphagia
Resplratory
  Endobronchial/central tumor growth
  Cough
  Dyspnea (obstructive)
  Chest pain (dull)
  Sputum production
    Hemoptysis (25%)
    Wheeze/stridor
  Peripheral tumor growth
    Cough (71%–74%)
    Pyspma (restrictive) (58%–59%)
    Chest pain (sharp) (48%–49%)
Chest x-ray

graphic scan of the chest is required to evaluate the extent of disease.

Before a diagnosis of NSCLC can be made, tissue must be examined (Fig. 22-1). If a tumor is located centrally, it may be diagnosed, in about 80% of cases, with three morning sputums preserved in Saccamano solution. SCC tumors are more frequently diagnosed than are other histologic types. If SCC is diagnosed by sputum cytology, the clinician may move on to staging the tumor. If AC is diagnosed, the clinician must remember that some viral illnesses may produce dysplasia that may be confused with AC. If there is any question about the diagnosis, a more invasive procedure, such as bronchoscopy, should be performed.

Since the staging of NSCLC has important therapeutic and prognostic implications, care must be taken to define the extent of disease accurately. Extrapulmonary symptomatology usually suggests either extensive disease or a paraneoplastic syndrome. Outside of pleural and pulmonary spread, bone, brain, adrenal glands, pericardium, and liver are the most common sites of metastatic spread. Clinical staging is based on physical examination and radiographic and laboratory studies. Pathologic staging is based on examination of surgically removed tissue and is much more reliable. Staging is based on the TNM classification system proposed in 1986 which has become the universal standard (Table 22-3).

Treatment options are based on staging (Fig. 22-2). Surgical resection is possible for those patients with disease limited to the hemithorax without extension to the pleura and not associated with enlarged lymph nodes. This includes those patients with stage I, II, and some IIIa NSCLC. Before resection, careful preoperative assessment of the patient's pulmonary reserve is critical. A 3% to 5% mortality may be expected with lobectomy, but this is age related. Patients with poor pulmonary reserve may be considered for segmental or wedge resection of the primary tumor. Those who are considered inoperable may undergo radiation therapy with curative intent. Neoadjuvant and adjuvant chemotherapy trials are being conducted, and all eligible patients should be enrolled.

Those patients with unresectable stage IIIa and IIIb disease present a greater treatment dilemma. Ideally, those patients with good performance status would be entered into neoadjuvant chemotherapy/radiation therapy trials in an attempt to make

TABLE 22-3 STAGING OF NON-SMALL-CELL LUNG CANCER

Primary tumor (T)

TX:	Primary tumor cannot be assessed or tumor proven by the presence of malignant cells in sputum or bronchial washings but not visualized by imaging or bronchoscopy
T0:	No evidence of primary tumor
Tis:	Carcinoma in situ
T1:	A tumor that is 3.0 cm or less in greatest diameter, surrounded by lung or visceral pleura, and without evidence of invasion more proximal than the lobar bronchus (i.e., not in the main bronchus)[a]
T2:	A tumor with any of the following features of size or extent: >3.0 cm in greatest dimension Involving the main bronchus, 2.0 cm or more distal to the carina Invading the visceral pleura Associated with atelectasis or obstructive pneumonitis that extends to the hilar region but does not involve the entire lung
T3:	A tumor of any size with direct extension to the chest wall (including superior sulcus, diaphragm, mediastinal pleura, parietal pericardium; a tumor in the main bronchus less than 2.0 cm distal to the carina but without involvement of the carina; associated atelectasis or obstructive pneumonitis of the entire lung
T4:	A tumor of any size that invades any of the following: mediastinum, heart, great vessels, trachea, esophagus, vertebral body, carina; or a tumor with a malignant effusion[b]

Nodal involvement (N)

NX:	Regional lymph nodes cannot be excluded
N0:	No regional lymph node metastasis
N1:	Metastasis in ipsilateral peribronchial and/or ipsilateral hilar lymph nodes, including direct extension
N2:	Metastasis in ipsilateral mediastinal and/or subcarinal lymph node(s)
N3:	Metastasis in contralateral mediastinal, contralateral hilar, ipsilateral or contralateral scalene, or supraclavicular lymph node(s)

Distant metastasis (M)

MX:	Presence of distant metastasis cannot be assessed
M0:	No distant metastasis
M1:	Distant metastasis (beyond the ipsilateral supraclavicular nodes)
Occult Stage:	TX, N0, M0
Stage 0:	Tis, N0, M0
Stage I:	T1, N0, M0
	T2, N0, M0
Stage II:	T1, N1, M0
	T2, N1, M0
Stage IIIa	T1, N2, M0
	T2, N2, M0
	T3, N0, M0
	T3, N1, M0
	T3, N2, M0
Stage IIIb:	Any T, N3, M0
Stage IV:	T4, any N, M0

a The uncommon superficial tumor of any size with its invasive component limited to the bronchial wall, which may extend proximal to the main bronchus, is also classified as T1.

b In the few patients for whom multiple cytopathologic examinations of pleural fluid are negative for tumor, i.e., fluid is non-bloody and is not an exudate, and clinical judgment dictates that the effusion is not related to the tumor; the effusion should be excluded as a staging element and the patient should be staged as T1, T2, or T3.

an unresectable tumor resectable. Such trials are currently in progress. Irradiation plus cisplatin-based chemotherapy is considered optimal treatment. The 3-year survival rate for those patients treated with chemotherapy plus chest irradiation was 19% to 26% versus those who received irradiation alone (13% to 17%). Studies are currently tak-ing place that indicate that carboplatin/paclitaxel may give a survival advantage over cisplatin/etoposide, which are the current standard chemotherapeutic agents.

Patients who are found to have stage IV disease are usually not considered candidates for resection. The only exception to this may be those who pre-

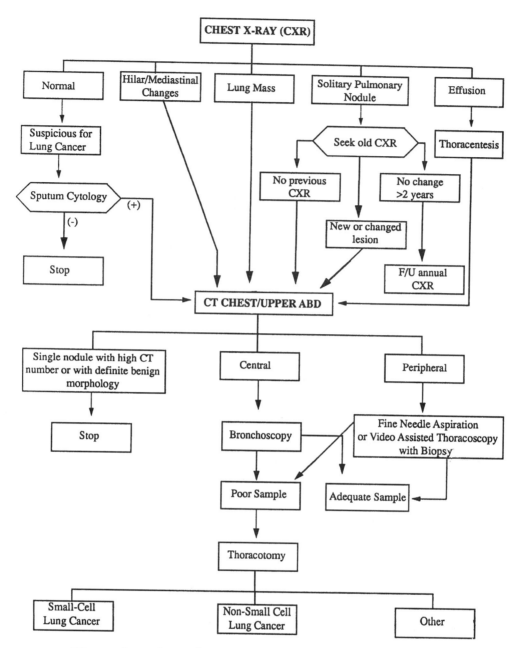

FIGURE 22-1 *Diagnostic work-up of patients with suspected lung cancer. Recommendations are based on solid nonexperimental evidence. CT, computed tomography.*

sent with a single pulmonary nodule and a single central nervous system metastatic lesion. This would include those patients who develop a cranial metastatic lesion within 60 days after the removal of a stage I or II lesion from the chest. Various studies indicate that these patients have a 5-year survival of 10% or more with resection.

Those patients with unresectable metastatic disease with good performance status should be considered for chemotherapeutic randomized tri-

als. Presently a platinum-based chemotherapeutic regimen is the standard treatment (see Appendix 15). More studies are needed with new agents. This is clear because while patients who received chemotherapy versus best supportive care lived longer, the survival advantage is measured only in weeks. On the other hand, surgical resection for a patient with a T1-2 N0 tumor with negative resected margins has a 40% to 50% 5 year survival rate.

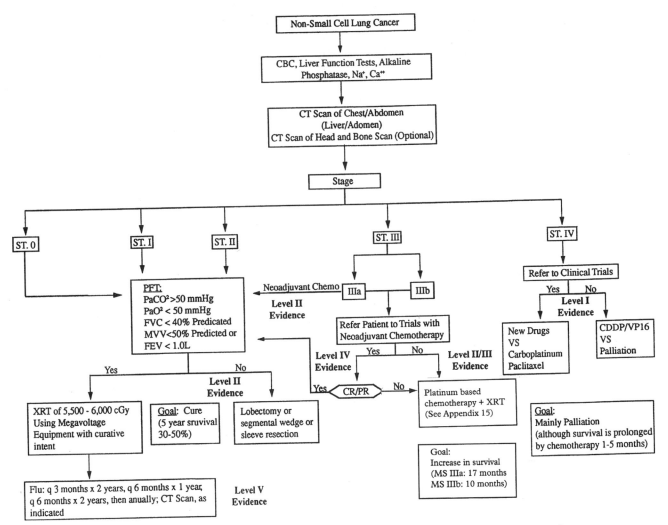

FIGURE 22-2 *Management of non-small-cell lung cancer (NSCLC). Determination of resectability represents the key reasoning principle in the management of patients with NSCLC. Goal of treatment is cure in early stages (I and II) and slight prolongation of survival for the rest of patients. Since lung cancer is the number one cause of cancer death in the United States, and the treatment in advanced stages is so unsatisfactory, every effort should be made to enter patients into clinical trials with new promising treatment modalities. Recommended strategy is based on level II evidence for the role of surgery in the treatment of early stages and on level I and II for the treatment of advanced stages. Current recommendation for neoadjuvant therapy is of level II evidence in stage IIIa and level IV in stage IIIb and for follow-up of level IV and V. Note that no effective salvage treatment exists, although for some localized recurrence, effective surgical salvage might exist (see text). CBC, complete blood count; PFT, pulmonary function tests; CT, computed tomography; MS, median survival.*

SUGGESTED READINGS

Cohen MH: Signs and symptoms of bronchogenic carcinoma. pp. 85–94. In Straus MJ (ed): Lung Cancer: Clinical Diagnosis and Treatment. New York, 1977

Ginsberg et al: Cancer of the lung. pp. 673–723 Lippincott-Raven. In DeVita VT, Jr (ed): Cancer: Principles & Practice of Oncology. 4th Ed. Philadelphia, 1993

Mentzer S: Thoracoscopy and video-assisted thoracic surgery in the treatment of lung cancer. Chest 107:2985–3018, 1995

Rosell R et al: A randomized trial comparing preoperative chemotherapy plus surgery with surgery alone in patients with non-small cell lung cancer. N Engl J Med 330:153–158, 1994

23 Esophageal Cancer

Rambabu Tummala
Sheron R. Williams

Incidence: The annual age-adjusted incidence rates of esophageal cancer range from less than 5 cases per 100,000 population among whites to as high as 14 cases per 100,000 population among American blacks. They represent less than 1% of all new cancer cases but account for 2% of all cancer deaths. It is also the seventh most common cause of cancer death among blacks.

Goals of treatment: Cure in early-stage disease and prolongation of survival with effective palliation of symptoms in advanced disease.

Main modality of therapy: Surgery for early stage disease and multimodality therapy for locally advanced disease.

Prognosis: 5-year survival is as follows:

Stage 0, 75%

Stage I, 50%

Stage IIa, 40%

Stage IIb, 20%

Stage III, 15%

Stage IV, 0%

Cancer of the esophagus is the ninth most common cancer in the world and ranks seventh among the causes of death from cancer. It is most often seen in developing countries. In the United States, the American Cancer Society estimates that in 1996 about 12,300 new cases (<1% of all new cancer cases) will be diagnosed with about 11,200 deaths (2% of all cancer deaths) from this disease. Even though esophageal cancer is three times less common than rectal carcinoma, its mortality exceeds that of rectal cancer. Its incidence varies from country to country, with the lowest rates among the white Americans and the highest rates in certain regions of China and Iran. Because of the changing economic climate and habits, the incidence of esophageal cancer is declining in China and is increasing in central and eastern Europe.

The incidence of esophageal cancer increases with age and is two to four times more common in men than in women. Of the two major histologies, squamous cell carcinoma is about five times more common in black men than in white men. However, the incidence of adenocarcinoma in white men is increasing at a rate of nearly 10% per year, faster than any other cancer. There is a marked increase in the number of cases of adenocarcinoma involving the lower third of esophagus or gastroesophageal junction. It is now estimated that the incidence of adenocarcinoma equals or exceeds that of squamous cell carcinoma. Esophageal cancer is the seventh most common cause of cancer death among blacks, with a black/white ratio in mortality exceeding sixfold for those younger than 55 years.

RISK FACTORS

The major causes of squamous cell carcinoma of the esophagus in the United States are tobacco use and alcohol consumption. Both of them increase the risk in a synergistic fashion. A recent population-based, case-control study from National Cancer Institute (NCI) reported that the excess risk of squamous cell carcinoma of the esophagus in black men could not be explained by differences in tobacco and alcohol use alone, suggesting a role for other environmental factors or differences in genetic susceptibility accounting for the racial disparity. Epidemiologic studies indicate a role for dietary factors in the etiology, with a twofold increase in the risk of esophageal cancer with low intake of fruits and vegetables. Jun-Yao Li and colleagues randomized patients with dysplasia of the esophagus to either mineral and vitamin supplementation, particularly with the combination of β-carotene, vitamin E, and selenium or a placebo. This trial suggests little initial benefit in cancer incidence or mortality with the above supplementation. Other factors, including asbestos, ionizing radiation, and drinking hot beverages, are reported to increase the risk of esophageal cancer.

The reasons for the increasing incidence of adenocarcinoma are poorly understood. However, a recent case-control study from NCI suggests a role for obesity and a low fiber intake in its etiology. Prior history of hiatal hernia and duodenal ulcer is also reported to increase the risk of adenocarcinoma of the esophagus.

The risk factors for squamous cell carcinoma include achalasia (highest risk of cancer in the first year after diagnosis of achalasia), tylosis, lye strictures (risk is increased 40 years after caustic injury), and esophageal webs (with Plummer-Vinson syndrome). Barrett esophagus is the single most important risk factor for adenocarcinoma of the esophagus, 59% to 86% of tumors arising from Barrett mucosa. This is a columnar cell-lined esophagus. For adult patients with Barrett esophagus, the annual risk of cancer development is approximately 0.8%. For these reasons, at least biannual screening endoscopy is recommended for all patients with *Barrett esophagus* with no evidence of either dysplasia or carcinoma. Any lesion with severe dysplasia should be resected and followed by regular endoscopic surveillance.

CLINICAL PRESENTATION

Dysphagia and weight loss are the initial symptoms in the majority of patients with esophageal cancer. Because of the distensibility of the esophagus, the symptom of dysphagia does not develop until the disease is locally advanced. Other presentations include odynophagia, aspiration pneumonia, Horner syndrome, painful bony metastasis, and palpable cervical adenopathy. The symptoms of advanced disease are shown in Table 23-1.

DIAGNOSIS

Any patient with a history of dysphagia and weight loss should have a workup to exclude esophageal cancer. A history and physical examination may show adenopathy, Horner syndrome or evidence of metastatic disease. A chest x-ray may show evidence of metastatic disease in the lungs. The diagnosis is primarily based on upper gastrointestinal endoscopy and biopsy, which can be performed as a primary procedure or following barium contrast examination. An eosophagogram may show the extent of esophageal and/or other intrathoracic structural involvement. Both endoscopic biopsies and cytologic brushings are required for definitive diagnosis. Endoscopic biopsies are diagnostic in 70% of cases, whereas the brushings are diagnostic in 90% of cases. Both of them are complementary to each other and together are diagnostic in 95% of cases.

STAGING

The present TNM staging system is based on pathologic staging and may not be accurate in patients who are not initially managed with surgery. Table 23-2 represents the TNM classification. Accurate staging is important for determining the resectability of a primary tumor, by careful exclusion of locally advanced and metastatic disease, and to follow and compare the response to various treatment modalities. Staging studies include a complete his-

TABLE 23-1   SYMPTOMS OF ADVANCED ESOPHAGEAL CANCER

Symptoms	Patients With Symptoms (%)
Dysphagia	80–96
Weight loss	42–46
Pain	6–20
Cachexia	6
Cough/hoarseness	3–4
Tracheoesophageal fistula	1–13

(Adapted from Roth JA, Lichter AS, Putnam JB, Forastiere AA: Cancer of esophagus. p. 781. In DeVita VT, Jr, Hellman S, Rosenbemg SA [eds]: Cancer: Principles and Practice of Oncology. Lippincott-Raven, Philadelphia, 1993.)

tory and physical examination, chest x-ray, barium swallow, esophagogastroscopy, computed tomography (CT) scanning of the chest and abdomen, and bronchoscopy in patients with lesions at or above the carina. Recent advances like endoscopic ultrasonography (EUS) and minimally invasive surgery (thoracoscopy and laparoscopy) improve the overall accuracy of staging.

TABLE 23-2   TNM CLASSIFICATION AND STAGING OF ESOPHAGEAL CANCER

Primary tumor (T)
TX	Primary tumor cannot be assessed
T0	No evidence of primary tumor
Tis	Carcinoma in situ
T1	Tumor invades lamina propria or submucosa
T2	Tumor invades muscularis propria
T3	Tumor invades adventitia
T4	Tumor invades adjacent structures

Regional lymph nodes (N)
NX	Regional lymph nodes cannot be assessed
N0	No regional lymph node metastasis
N1	Regional lymph node metastasis

Distant metastasis (M)
MX	Presence of distant metastasis cannot be assessed
M0	No distant metastasis
M1	Distant metastasis

Stage grouping
Stage 0	Tis	N0	M0
Stage I	T1	N0	M0
Stage IIA	T2	N0	M0
	T3	N0	M0
Stage IIB	T1	N1	M0
	T2	N1	M0
Stage III	T3	N1	M0
	T4	Any N	M0
Stage IV	Any T	Any N	M1

EUS is a relatively new technique in staging and is a good tool for detection of depth of tumor invasion. In a recent review of endosonographic staging, T. Rosch reported an overall accuracy rate of 84% for T stage (total 1,154 procedures) and 77% for N stage (total 1,035 procedures) in patients who underwent surgery. The accuracy of EUS (confirmed after surgery) was reported as T1, 80.5%; T2, 76%; T3, 92%; T4, 86%; N0, 69%; and N1, 89%. The use of EUS is confined to locoregional disease because of its limited accuracy to diagnose metastasis in celiac lymph nodes, distant peritoneum, liver, and lungs. Conventional EUS is also not very reliable for differentiating mucosal versus submucosal invasion, when considering any form of local therapy for mucosal lesions. EUS may also under- or overstage, particularly T2 disease, and tracheobronchial involvement is also difficult to diagnose by this technique. Stenotic lesions, however, can be traversed after stepwise dilatations with comparable accuracy in staging to nonstenotic lesions. T. Rosch also showed, by comparison of the pooled data in the literature, the higher accuracy of EUS when compared to CT scan (compared to surgical staging) for both T (85% vs. 58%) and N (75% vs. 54%) staging. CT scan, however, is more accurate for staging celiac nodes (82%), liver disease (98%), aortic and pericardial invasion (94%), and tracheobronchial involvement (97%). Thus, CT and EUS are complementary to each other. Three studies have compared MRI with CT scans and found no difference in predicting mediastinal invasion.

Recent advances in thoracoscopy have allowed more accurate staging of mediastinal disease. It allows evaluation of the entire thoracic esophagus, periesophageal nodes and the aortopulmonary window nodes. Occult pleural and pulmonary metastasis can be identified. Thoracoscopy also allows direct visualization of the adventitia of the esophagus and can identify local spread of the disease. Regional lymph nodes can be sampled. M. J. Krasna and colleagues demonstrated in a prospective, multiinstitutional pilot study that a satisfactory thoracoscopic lymph node staging can be achieved in 95% of the patients. Of the patients undergoing resection, 88% were accurately staged by thoracoscopy. This allowed accurate staging of thoracic lymph node status and better definition of the T status. Similarly, staging laparoscopy or minilaparotomy provides greater accuracy in the evaluation of regional and celiac lymph nodes, as well as peritoneal and liver metastases. Staging laparoscopy combined with thoracoscopy can asses lymph nodes on either side of the diaphragm and provides additional information in those patients in whom EUS can not be performed.

Bronchoscopy is generally advised in all patients with tumors in the upper or middle third of the esophagus. However, G. J. Argyros and associates noted a low yield of bronchoscopy in the evaluation of asymptomatic patients. He found it of value in patients with pulmonary symptoms of cough and/or hemoptysis or an abnormal chest radiograph. A bone scan should be obtained in patients with bone pain, along with plain films of the corresponding bones. G. C. O'Sullivan and coworkers recently found, by flow cytometry, micrometastases in the bone marrow samples of 20% to 30% of patients with gastroesophageal adenocarcinoma undergoing curative resection. However, the clinical significance of this finding is not clear at the present time.

The term "superficial" carcinoma refers only to the extent of the primary tumor, defined as in situ carcinoma or invasive carcinoma limited to the submucosa, independent of the lymph node status. "Early" esophageal cancer is a superficial carcinoma without lymph node metastasis. Tis (carcinoma in situ) and T1 tumors comprise less than 20% of esophageal cancer in the United States, with less than 3% confined to the mucosa alone. Once the tumor invades the submucosa, vascular invasion is seen in 56% of cases with lymph node metastasis in 32%. This subset of patients with submucosal invasion has a low 5-year survival compared to those with only mucosal involvement (55% vs 88%). A study from Japan reported lymph node metastasis in 10% of mucosal and 45% of submucosal lesions. These indicate the rapid involvement of lymph nodes even with early stage disease.

PROGNOSTIC FACTORS

Earlier studies indicated that the length of the primary lesion predicts survival. However, recent studies indicate that the depth of tumor invasion is a better prognostic indicator, irrespective of the length of the tumor. Patients with lymph node involvement have a poor prognosis. The number of lymph nodes involved is an additional prognostic indicator. Patients with involvement of less than 4 nodes have a better survival than those with more than 4 nodes in four different series. Weight loss of more than 10% at diagnosis also carries a poor prognosis. Recently, the tumor supressor gene called p53 is shown to be associated with a poor prognosis. M. Sarbia and colleagues in their retrospective analysis of patients with squamous cell carcinoma found that both vascular and lymphatic invasion are independent prognostic factors. Neural invasion, however, was not associated with any difference in survival rates. M. D. Lieberman and colleagues from their retrospective analysis of 258 patients, noted no prognostic value for the histologic type of tumor.

THERAPY

An *understanding of the natural history* of esophageal cancer is essential in planning a logical approach to therapy. Various autopsy studies indicate evidence of residual local and/or metastatic disease in 75% to 94% of cases. *Lymph nodes* are involved in 42% to 75% of cases, *the liver in* 14% to 47%, and *lungs in* 15% to 52% of cases. These studies reveal a predominance of both local and distant failure with few cases of isolated local or distant failure only. These data show that esophageal cancer is a metastatic disease at the time of death. Failure to recognize this early in the treatment plan will lead to failure, if therapy is aimed at local disease only. The above series also report a higher incidence of comorbid conditions, like alcohol-related liver disease and extensive atherosclerosis. A coexisting secondary primary tumor was found in 3.5% to 27% of cases.

It is also important to note that most of the data presented here include only a minority of patients with adenocarcinoma. Earlier studies included mostly cases of squamous cell carcinoma, and recent reports do include both of these histologies. It is not yet clear whether there is any difference in their natural history or response to therapy. The *aim of therapy* is cure for early stage, improving the disease-free and overall survival in advanced disease, with effective palliation of symptoms and improving the quality of life. Most of the multimodality clinical trials are limited by small number of patients, lack of uniformity in chemotherapy regimens, doses, and schedules of chemotherapy agents, and radiation therapy.

SINGLE-MODALITY THERAPY

Surgery Resection of the esophagus remains the standard approach for patients with local or locoregional disease that is resectable, outside of a clinical trial. It is effective both as a potentially curative and palliative procedure. Comparison of the end results is often difficult because of the variety of operative techniques and inadequate staging information. Curative resection is feasible in only 50% of cases, with a median survival of about 11 months in patients with resected tumors. The 5-year survival is stage-dependent and ranges from 68% to 85% for stages I–II to 15% to 28% for stages III–IV patients undergoing Lewis esophagectomy. Both local and distant failure are common after resection. Surgical mortality has declined in the past 10 years and is well below 10% in most major centers.

Endoscopic Mucosal Resection This technique is used in Japan to treat squamous cell carcinoma involving the mucosa alone, if the lesion is flat and less than 2 cm in size. The 5-year disease-specific survival rate is over 90%, with a recurrence rate of about 5%. Comparison of the results of esophagectomy to mucosal resection in superficial cancer, shows similar 5-year survival rates.

Radiation Therapy This is often used as a primary therapy for patients who are medically unfit for surgery or whose tumors are technically unresectable. When radiation is given with an intent to cure, results are poor, with a median survival of 6 to 12 months and a 5-year survival of equal or less than 10%. It is equally effective against both adeno- and squamous cell carcinoma. Review of clinical failure patterns indicate the persistence or recurrence of tumor at the primary site in 56% to 85%, relapse in neck or mediastinum in 10% to 43%, and distant metastasis in 36% to 50% of cases. Recently, H. Nishio and coworkers reported the clinical results of a retrospective study of 788 patients with M0 esophageal carcinoma who received more than 60 Gy. A complete response was obtained in 35% of patients with a 5-year survival of 23% in this subgroup of patients. M. Mukai and coworkers reported impressive results in a pilot study using a combination of radiation (average total dose is 61.1 Gy) and local administration of OK-432 (lyophilized powder of the Su strain of *Streptococcus pyogene)* in patients without distant metastases. Complete response was obtained in 70% of cases with a 5-year survival of 45% in those with complete remission. These higher results needs further examination in future trials. There are no prospective randomized studies comparing surgery to radiation as a single modality of therapy. There is no evidence that radiation alone can achieve local control equal to that of surgery.

THE VALUE OF ADJUVANT TREATMENT

Preoperative Radiation Therapy The potential advantages include increased resectability and decreased chance of tumor spread at the time of surgery. The tumor may also be more radiosensitive due to better oxygenation prior to surgery. Out of the five randomized studies of preoperative radiation versus surgery alone, only two reports demonstrated a significant decrease in locoregional failure rate in the radiation therapy arm. W. Mei and colleagues noted a decrease in local recurrence from 13% to 4% in their series of 206 patients, while M. Gignoux and colleagues reported a decrease from 67% to 46% in 229 patients. However, there is no clear advantage of overall survival or resectability.

Postoperative Radiation Therapy The advantages include accurate staging with surgery and the ability to treat areas at risk for recurrence. Out of the three randomized studies, only P. Teniere and associates showed a significant reduction in locoregional failure with postoperative radiation (35% vs. 10%) in the subgroup of patients with negative nodes after curative resection. M. Fok and coworkers, in their randomized study, reported no advantage of adjuvant therapy in patients with curative resection. However, among the group who underwent palliative resection, the local failure rate significantly decreased from 46% to 20% with postoperative radiation. An increase in the incidence of gastric complications (M. Fok and colleagues) and fibrotic strictures (H. U. Zieren and colleagues) was noted with the adjuvant therapy. There was also no survival advantage in any of the studies.

T. Lizuka and collaborators reported in his randomized study an improvement in 4-year survival (20% vs. 33%) and median survival (13 months vs. 22 months) in patients who received postoperative radiation compared to those with both preoperative and postoperative radiation. This study is, however, criticized for inclusion of a higher percentage of patients with large tumors in the preoperative and postoperative radiation arm.

Preoperative Chemotherapy Several phase II trials involving cisplatin-based regimens have reported 40% to 60% clinical responses, but with few pathologic complete responses. There are four randomized studies reported in the literature comparing preoperative chemotherapy to surgery. J. A. Roth and coworkers, reported a response rate of 47% and a pathologic CR of 6% in the chemotherapy arm. The median survival was improved in responders (>20 months) compared to nonresponders (6.2 months) and those treated with surgery (8.6 months). P. M. Schlag and coworkers reported a similar response of 47% and a median survival of 8 months with chemotherapy compared to 9 months with surgery. In another randomized study, P. M. Schlag showed an improved median survival in patients responding to chemotherapy (13 months) compared to nonresponders (5 months). He, however, reported considerable number of infections and pulmonary complications with a high postoperative mortality rate (19% vs. 10%) in the preoperative chemotherapy arm. In conclusion, preoperative chemotherapy neither influence the resectability nor the overall survival of patients with localized esophageal cancer. There is a trend toward improving median survival in chemotherapy responsive patients.

A phase III intergroup study comparing presurgical and postsurgical chemotherapy to surgery alone is still accruing patients. T. Lizuka and colleagues comparing postoperative chemotherapy to curative surgery alone in a randomized study and the final outcome is still pending. Recently, X. Pouliquen and associates, reported the results of their multicenter, randomized trial comparing combination chemotherapy after palliative surgery to palliative surgery alone. There is no difference in overall survival between the two groups, and the chemotherapy arm has significant toxicity. D. Kelsen and associates, compared the effectiveness of preoperative chemotherapy to preoperative radiotherapy with postoperative crossover in patients with positive nodes in a randomized study. There are no significant differences in resectability, operative mortality, or survival between the two groups.

MULTIMODALITY THERAPY

Chemoradiotherapy Combined With Surgery
This design is based on the success of therapy for treatment of anal cancer. The goal is to control both local and systemic disease at the same time. Cisplatin, 5-fluorouracil, and vinblastine are the commonly used drugs. Several phase II trials with preoperative Chemoradiation therapy reported a response rate of 40% to 70% and a complete pathologic response in up to 42% of patients. The median survival ranged from 12 to 29 months. There is substantial morbidity, with a therapy related mortality as high as 15%. The best results are reported by A. A. Forastiere and colleagues by using a more aggressive chemoradiation regimen. Two-year overall survival is 57% with a reported 5-year survival of 60% in patients with a complete pathologic response. These results, however, were not duplicated in a randomized trial. Using the same chemoradiation protocol, S. Urba and colleagues reported a randomized study comparing concurrent chemoradiation with subsequent surgery to surgery alone (transhiatal esophagectomy) for locoregional disease. Complete pathologic

responses were seen in 28% of patients has but there was no difference in the estimated 2-year survival between the two groups. Improved survival was reported with tumors less than 5 cm in size and those with a complete pathologic response. Grades III–IV neutropenia was noted in 78% of patients with grades III–IV thrombocytopenia in 32% of cases. M. Gignoux and colleagues, in his randomized study comparing concurrent chemoradiation followed by surgery to surgery alone in stage I or II squamous cell carcinoma of the esophagus reported a median survival of 20 months for both groups. There was no increase in surgical mortality or morbidity in the combined therapy arm. This study, however, is criticized for not using aggressive preoperative chemoradiation. E. LePrise and colleagues reported no survival advantage in another randomized study where radiation therapy was not given concurrently with chemotherapy. This study is criticized for using only a low total dose of radiation (20 Gy). Because of the limitations with the above randomized studies, and high rates of pathologic response, further trials are ongoing.

K. Kitamura and colleagues evaluated the role of hyperthermia in a randomized study of 66 patients who were treated with preoperative chemoradiation. He noted better local control and improved long-term survival (3-year survival: 50% vs. 24%) in the group treated with hyperthermia. This needs to be confirmed in larger trials. There are no randomized studies evaluating the role of postoperative chemoradiation. Phase II trials, however, are encouraging.

Chemoradiation Therapy Alone as Primary Management
Because of the concern with high morbidity and mortality associated with esophagectomy at some centers, and the advances in chemotherapy and radiation, nonsurgical treatment is being evaluated for locoregional disease. There are four randomized studies comparing concurrent chemoradiation to radiation therapy alone as the primary choice of therapy. Of these, the landmark study was published in 1992 by A. Herskovic and co-workers, from Radiation Therapy Oncology Group. Patients with local disease were randomized into either definitive radiotherapy (64 Gy) or four cycles of combined cisplatin (75 mg/m² on day 1) and 5-flurouracil (1,000 mg/m² per day for 4 days), two cycles during and two after radiotherapy (50 Gy). This trial was stopped early after an interim analysis showed a significant difference in median survival (12.5 vs. 8.5 months) and 2-year survival (38%

vs. 10%), favoring the chemoradiation arm. A significant decrease in local, and distant relapse was also noted. This, however, was associated with higher toxicity. Because of the higher local failure rates in both groups, subsequent trials are focusing on giving higher doses of radiation therapy and adding brachytherapy. Another important question that has not been answered yet, is whether combined therapy is superior to surgery alone.

Palliative Therapy The goals of treatment of advanced esophageal cancer is palliation of symptoms. Esophagectomy or bypass surgery usually results in reasonable palliation of dysphagia in more than 70% of cases with a median survival range of 5 to 8 months. This is unfortunately associated with a mortality ranging from 10% to 20% and is now used in patients who are operated with curative intent but found to have extensive disease intraoperatively. Radiation alone is effective for relief of dysphagia in 50% to 76% of cases, lasting for 5 to 10 months. However, radiation therapy may be complicated by stricture formation in more than a third of the cases. This is still preferable to surgery because it is noninvasive with less morbidity. Endoscopic palliation includes esophageal dilation, prostheses, electrocautery, laser excision, and gastrostomy. Infiltrating tumors require stenting, while polypoid tumors require debulking. Recanalization of inoperable tumors can be obtained in over 90% of cases with laser therapy. The risk of perforation with laser therapy is about 2% of the treatment episodes. Single-agent chemotherapy has response rates of 15% to 20% with no indication of survival benefit. Symptomatic benefit is also brief. Cisplatin-based combination therapy has response rates of 11% to 54%, but the duration of response is brief, ranging from 3 to 6 months. Currently, taxol is being investigated, both in locally advanced and in metastatic disease. Chemoradiation is also used as palliative therapy.

FOLLOW-UP

Review of autopsy studies indicate that local failure occurs as often as distant disease as a cause of treatment failure. Distant nonnodal disease is present in 40% to 65% of cases, where as 15% to 40% die only with local recurrence.

Symptoms of local recurrence are difficult to diagnose, and follow-up studies are useful. CT scans are of limited value to diagnose anastomotic recurrence. Similarly, upper endoscopy is not diagnostic if the recurrent tumor is submucosal or extramural in location. Recent reports indicate that EUS has a sensitivity of 96% and a specificity of 85% in detecting anastomotic recurrence in symptomatic patients. Early diagnosis may lead to further therapy to improve the survival.

Diagnosis of metastatic disease is associated with poor prognosis. There are no studies in the literature about further follow-up of the patients with esophageal cancer after primary therapy. If the primary therapy is surgery only, follow-up with EUS (upper endoscopy if EUS is unavailable) may help to identify local recurrence early and plan for further therapy. Most of the oncologists follow the patients with esophageal cancer with complete history and physical examination (every 3 months) upper endoscopy (every 3–6 months), and CT scans of the chest, including the upper abdomen (every 3–6 months).

RECOMMENDATIONS

There is no consensus as the standard therapy of choice in the management of esophageal cancer. The following are the guidelines, and therapy should be individualized depending on the stage of diagnosis, age of the patient, performance status, and the associated comorbid conditions.

1. *Severe dysplasia with or without Barrett esophagus and with or without aneuploidy*: Chemoprevention protocols, if available; frequent endoscopic surveillance; surgical resection followed by surveillance.

2. *Carcinoma in situ*: Consider surgical resection; consider endoscopic resection in high-risk patients for surgery if the tumor is flat and less than 2 cm in size.

3. *T1 or T2 primary with N0M0*: Surgical resection is the first choice; chemoradiation for medically unfit patients.

4. *T2 or T3 primary with N1M0*: Any protocols if available; surgery if preoperative staging shows minimal adenopathy; chemoradiation for the medically unfit or for those with major adenopathy in preoperative staging.

5. *T4 primary with any N and M0*: Any protocols if available; chemoradiation or palliative therapy.

6. *Metastatic disease*: Palliative care only; chemotherapy or radiation or a combination of both.

Figures 23-1 and 23-2 summarize the diagnostic workup and management of esophageal cancer. Appendix 16 shows details of treatment protocols and the preceding text offers follow-up recommendations.

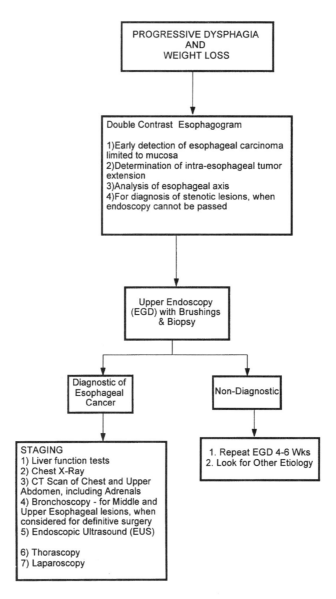

FIGURE 23-1 *The principle in diagnosis is to have both brushings and biopsy to enhance the sensitivity of EGD (endoscopic gastroduodenoscopy). The important step in staging is accuracy for defining better treatment strategy and to exclude patients with metastatic disease when curative thearpy is considered. If the chest x-ray is suggestive of metastatic disease, further workup is not recommended. If EUS (endoscopic ultrasound) is not available, thoracoscopy provides similar kind of data. Laparoscopy is helpful for staging disease below the diaphragm. The quality of evidence for EUS and CT scan staging is level I.*

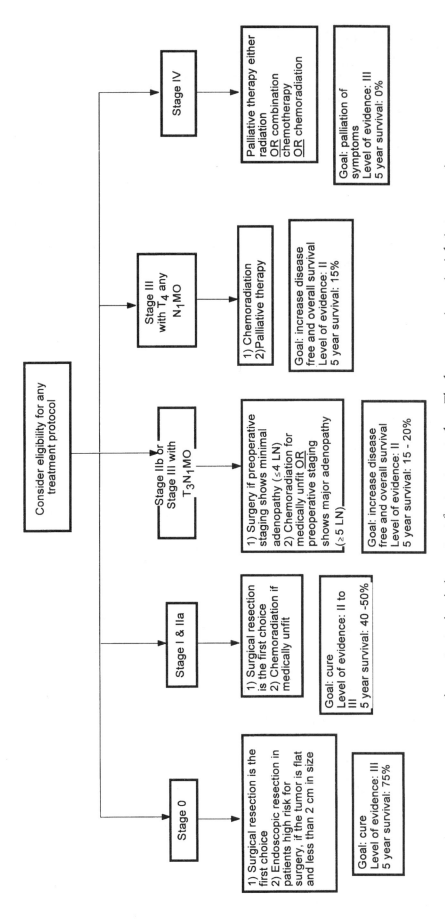

FIGURE 23-2. *Accurate staging is important for treatment plan. The key reasoning principle is to recognize that esophageal carcinoma is a metastatic disease at diagnosis and to understand the failure patterns with single-modality therapy. The treatment recommendations are based on quality of evidence of level II to III. See Appendix 16 for details on actual treatment protocol.*

177

SUGGESTED READINGS

Anderson LL, Lad TE: Autopsy findings in squamous cell carcinoma of the esophagus. Cancer 50:1587–1590, 1982

Argyros GJ, Torrington KG: Fiberoptic bronchoscopy in the evaluation of newly diagnosed esophageal carcinoma. Chest 107:1447–1449, 1995

Brown LM, Hoover RN, Greenberg RS et al: Are racial differences in squamous cell esophageal cancer explained by alcohol and tobacco use? J Natl Cancer Inst 86:1340–1492, 1994

Brown LM, Swanson CA, Gridley G et al: Adenocarcinoma of the esophagus: role of obesity and diet. J Natl Cancer Inst 87:104–109, 1994

Coia LR, Sauter ER: Esophageal cancer. Curr Probl Cancer July/August: 196–247, 1994

Fok M, Sham JST, Choy D et al: Postoperative radiotherapy for carcinoma of the esophagus: a prospective, randomized controlled trial. Surgery 113:138–147, 1993

Forastiere AA, Orringer MB, Perez-Tamayo C et al: Preoperative chemoradiation followed by transhiatal esophagectomy for carcinoma of the esophagus; final report. JCO 111:1118–1123, 1993

Gignoux M, Roussel A, Paillot B: The value of preoperative radiotherapy in esophageal cancer. Results of a study of the EORTC. World J Surg 11:426–432, 1987

Gignoux M, Triboulet JP, Tiret E et al: Randomized phase III clinical trial comparing surgery alone vs. preoperative combined radiochemotherapy in stage I–II epidermoid cancer of the thoracic esophagus. Preliminary analysis. Proc Annu Meet Am Soc Clin Oncol 13:A197, 1994

Herskovic A, Martz K, Al-Saraf M et al: Combined chemotherap and radiotherapy compared with radiotherapy alone in patients with cancer of esophagus. NEJM 326:1593–1598, 1992

Kelsen DP, Minsky BD, Smith M et al: Preoperative therapy for esophageal cancer; A randomized comparision of chemotherapy vs. radiation therapy. JCO 8:1352–1361, 1990

Kitamura K, Kuwano H, Watanabe M et al: Prospective randomized study of hyperthermia combined with chemoradiotherapy for esphgeal carcinoma. J Surg Oncol 60:55–58, 1995

Krasna MJ, Reed CE, Jaklitsch MT, Cushing D, Sugarbaker DJ: Thoracoscopic staging of esophageal cancer: a prospective, multiinstitutional trial. Cancer and Leukemia Group B Thoracic Surgeons. Ann Thorac Surg 60:1337–1340, 1995

LePrise E, Etienne P, Meunier B, Maddern G: A randomized comparison of chemotherapy, radiation therapy and surgery vs. surgery for localized squamous cell carcinoma of the esophagus. Cancer 73:1779–1784, 1994

Lizuka T, Ide H, Kakegawa T et al: Preoperative radioactive therapy for esophageal carcinoma; Randomized evaluation trial in eight institutions. Chest 93:1054–1058, 1988

Mei W, Xian-Zhi G, Weibo Y et al: Randomized clinical trial on the combination of preoperative irradiation and surgery in the treatment of esophageal carcinoma; Report on 206 patients. Int J Radiat Oncol Biol Phys 16:325–327, 1989

Mukai M, Kubota S, Morita S, Akanuma A: A pilot study of combination therapy of radiation and local administration of OK-432 for esophageal cancer. Cancer 75:2276–2280, 1995

Philip PA, Ajani JA: Has combined modality therapy improved the outlook in carcinoma of esophagus. Oncol 8:37–42, 1994

Pouliquen X, Levard H, Hay JM et al: 5-Fluoruracil and cisplatin therapy after palliative surgical resection of squamous cell carcinoma of the esophagus. A multicenter randomized trial. Ann Surg 223:127–133, 1996

Rosch T: Endosonographic staging of esophageal cancer: a review of literature results. Gastrointestinal Endosc 5:537–547, 1995

Roth JA, Pass HI, Flanagan MM, et al: Randomized trial of preoperative and postoperative adjuvant therapy with cisplatin, vindesine and bleomycin for carcinoma of the esophagus. J Thorac Cardiovas Surg 96:242–248, 1988

Roth JA, Putnam JB: Surgery for cancer of esophagus. Seminars in Oncology 21:453–461, 1994

Schlag P: Randomized trial of preoperative chemotherapy for squamous cell carcinoma of the esophagus. Acta Oncol 27:811–814, 1988

Schlag PM: Randomized trial of preoperative chemotherapy for squamous cell carcinoma of the esophagus. Arch Surg 127:1446–1450, 1992

Sugarbaker DJ, Jaklitsch MT, Liptay MJ: Thoracoscopic staging and surgical therapy for esophageal cancer. Chest 107(supp 6):218s–223s, 1995

Teniere P, Hay JM, Fingerhut A et al: Postoperative radiation therapy does not increase survival after resection for squamous cell carcinoma of the middle and lower esophagus as shown by a multicenter controlled trial. Surg Gynecol Obstet 173:123–130, 1991

Thompson WM, Halvorsen RA Jr. Staging esophageal carcinoma II: CT and MRI. Semin Oncol 21:447–452, 1994

Urba S, Orringer M, Turrisi A et al: A randomized trial comparing transhiatal esophagectomy to preoperative concurrent chemoradiation followed by esophagectomy in locoregional esophageal carcinoma (meeting abstract). Proc Annu Meet Am Soc Clin Oncol 14:A475, 1995

24 | Stomach Cancer

Leela Bhupalam

Incidence: 7.9/100,000/year

Main modality of treatment: Surgery, chemotherapy, and radiation

Goal of treatment: Prolongation of survival and palliation

Prognosis: 5-year survival:

Stage 0, 90%

Stage I, > 50%

Stage II, 29%

Stage III, 13%

Stage IV, 3%

EPIDEMIOLOGY, ETIOLOGY, AND RISK FACTORS

Gastric cancer is the seventh leading cause of cancer death in the United States. In 1994, cancer of the stomach had an expected incidence of 24,000 and expected cancer death rate of 14,000. The age-adjusted gastric cancer death rate has decreased dramatically since 1930 from 28 per 100,000 to 2.3 per 100,000 in females and from 38 to 5.2 per 100,000 in males. The annual incidence of gastric cancer has decreased from 35 per 100,000 in 1935 to 7.9 per 100,000 in the last decade. The incidence of stomach cancer is highest in Japan, South America, Eastern Europe, and the Middle East. In Japan, incidence is as high as 100 per 100,000. Despite the increased incidence in Japan the mortality rate over the last 25 years has decreased, possibly as a result of mass screening. Death rate remains high in Chile, Costa Rica, and the former Soviet Union. In the United States, environmental factors, chiefly dietary, are suspected as a cause for the lower incidence.

Gastric cancer occurs twice as often in men as in women. Its incidence increases with age, increasing in the fourth decade and peaking in the seventh decade in men. In the United States there has been an increase in incidence of proximal gastric cancer over the last 10 to 15 years. The proximal tumors have poorer prognosis stage by stage compared with the distal cancers. The national Cancer Institute (NCI) Surveillance, Epidemiology, and End Results program (SEER) data base from 1976 to 1987 reported that a shift to proximal cancer occurred with an annual increase in proximal gastric lesions of 4.3% in white men, 4.1% in white women, 3.6% in black men, and 5.6% in black women. Factors that are associated with increased incidence of gastric cancer have been diet, environmental factors, and several other factors shown in Table 24-1.

PATHOLOGY

About 95% of all malignant gastric neoplasms are adenocarcinomas. Other rare histologies include squamous cell carcinomas, adenoacanthoma, carcinoid syndrome, leiomyosarcoma, and lymphoma. The largest percentage of gastric cancers still arise

179

TABLE 24-1   RISK FACTORS FOR GASTRIC CANCER

Precursor Conditions

1. Chronic atrophic gastritis, intestinal metaplasia, achlorhydria
2. Pernicious anemia (2- to 3-fold increase in risk of stomach cancer)
3. Partial gastrectomy for benign disease (relative risk 1.3 to 3, but the risk is increased only 15 to 20
    years after resection
4. *Helicobacter pylori* infection (3- to 6-fold increase in risk of intestinal type of gastric cancer and can-
    cer of distal stomach)
5. Ménétrier's disease
6. Gastric adenomatous polyps (malignant potential is directly related to the size of the polyp and the
    degree of dysplasia)
7. Barrett's esophagus (0.8% risk per year, mainly adenocarcinoma of cardia or distal esophagus)

Genetic and Environmental Factors

1. Family history of gastric cancer (first degree relatives, either parent or sibling have a 2- to 3-fold
    increase in risk of developing the disease)
2. Blood group type A (risk appears to be more pronounced for diffuse lesion than intestinal type;
    subsequent epidemiologic studies have not confirmed this finding; if any risk, is extremely small)
3. Hereditary nonpolyposis colon cancer syndrome
4. Low socioeconomic status
5. Low consumption of fruits and vegetables
6. Consumption of salted, smoked, or poorly preserved food
7. Diets low in animal fat and protein, high in complex carbohydrates, low in vitamins A and C, food
    contaminated with aflatoxin
8. Nitrates in drinking water
9. Occupational risks in coal miners, rubber workers, and asbestos and nickel refining
10. Cigarette smoking (1.5- to 3-fold increase in risk of gastric cancer)

(Adapted from Fuchs CS, Mayer RJ: Gastric cancer. N Engl J Med 333:32–41, 1995, and Alexander HR,
Kelsen DP, Tepper JE: Cancer of the stomach. pp. 819–820. In: deVita VT, Hellman S, Rosenberg SA (eds);
Cancer: Principles and Practice of Oncology. 4th Ed. Lippincott-Raven, Philaldelphia, 1993, with permission.)

in the antrum or distal stomach (40%); they are least common in the body of the stomach (25%) and are intermediate in frequency in the fundus and esophagogastric junction (35%). Table 24-2 shows the pathologic classification of gastric cancer.

MODES OF SPREAD

Gastric cancer can spread by direct extension, lymphatically, and hematogenously.

SYMPTOMS AND SIGNS

Table 24-3 summarizes symptoms present at initial diagnosis. On physical examination, there may be evidence of metastatic disease (e.g., palpable epigastric mass). Other signs that occasionally can be found include ascites, jaundice, supraclavicular adenopathy (Virchow's node), left axillary adenopathy (Irish's node), hepatomegaly, periumbilical (Sister Mary Joseph's node), large ovarian mass (Krukenberg's tumor), or large peritoneal implant in the rectum (Blumer's shelf) that can produce

symptoms of obstruction. A patient can present with anemia (85%); guaiac-positive stools (50%), and elevated carcinoembryonic antigen (50%)

DIAGNOSTIC PROCEDURES

Diagnostic procedures follow.

Stool examination for occult-blood

Barium study using double-contrast techniques. A positive diagnosis of 5- to 10-mm lesions can be made in about 75% of patients. Characteristic radiologic signs of malignant lesions relate to their irregular margins and rugal folds that do not radiate from the ulcer.

Endoscopy with biopsy. Multiple biopsies are important. First biopsy yields the correct diagnosis in 70% of cases. Three additional biopsies increase the yield to greater than 95%. Seven biopsy specimens result in a yield greater than 98%. Seven biopsies combined with cytology increase the diagnostic yield to close to 100%. Current recommendations

TABLE 24-2 PATHOLOGY OF GASTRIC CANCER

Gastric carcinomas are categorized by microscopic and gross pathologic features. There are two classifications:

Lauren Classification
Intestinal variant
  Arises in precancerous areas such as gastric atrophy or intestinal metaplasia in the stomach
  More common in men than women
  Incidence is higher in older population
  Dominant where gastric carcinoma is epidemic, suggesting an environmental cause.
Diffuse type
  Occurs in younger patients
  Women are affected more than men
  Occurs in endemic areas

Borrmann's Classification
I. Polypoid or fungating
II. Ulcerating lesions with surrounding elevated borders
III. Ulceration with invasion into gastric wall
IV. Diffusely infiltrating (linnitus plastica)
V. Unclassifiable

are for at least four biopsy specimens seen at endoscopy with one cytologic specimen submitted for diagnosis. If the cytologic specimen is not collected, then seven biopsy specimens should be obtained.

TABLE 24-3 SYMPTOMS PRESENT AT INITIAL DIAGNOSIS[a]

Symptom	Patients (%)
Weight loss	61.6
Abdominal pain	51.6
Nausea	34.3
Anorexia	32.0
Dysphagia	26.1
Melena	20.2
Early satiety	17.5
Ulcer-type pain	17.1
Swelling, lower extremities	5.9
Previous history	
Gastric ulcer	25.5
Duodenal ulcer	7.5
Pernicious anemia	5.9
Gastric polyps	3.5
Polyps in large bowel	3.0
Achlorhydria	1.8
Polyposis, small bowel	1.4

[a]1982 and 1987 studies combined. Total number of new patients, 18,365.

(From Wanebo HJ, Kennedy BJ, Chmiel J et al: Cancer of the stomach: a patient care study by the American College of Surgeons. Ann Surg 218:583–592, 1993, with permission.)

Computed tomography (CT) is the most helpful procedure for detecting evidence of metastatic spread to liver, ovaries, and peritoneal surfaces. *CT helps in determining distant metastasis but is not helpful in determining local invasion into the gastric wall and gastric lymph nodes*, for which it has 61% specificity and 67% sensitivity. About 50% of patients have more extensive disease found at laparotomy than predicted by preoperative CT.

Endoscopic ultrasound allows highly accurate staging of the depth of invasion of primary tumor (T stage) and is more accurate that CT for *lymph node status*, which is *the key factor in prognosis for patients with local regional disease*. In gastric cancer ultrasound accurately stages and detects nodal metastasis in 83% and 66% of cases, respectively. Detection of distant metastasis is 85% accurate but is only 33% sensitive, because endoscopic ultrasound has limited view of distant structures. A prospective study showed that in 50 patients with a localized gastric cancer, endoscopic ultrasound was superior to CT or magnetic resonance imaging (MRI) in assessing the T (tumor) and N (nodal) stage. Because the entire abdomen cannot be examined with ultrasonic endoscopy, sensitivity cannot approach that of CT scanning in detecting distant metastases.

Laparotomy is a primary procedure for staging and assessment of resectability. Studies have shown that using laparotomy for staging does not increase the mortality rate and provides the best information for effecting cure or palliation.

Carcinoembryonic Antigen (CEA) levels greater than 5 ng/dL are reported in 40% to 50% of patients with metastatic gastric carcinomas. CEA has no role in diagnosis of gastric cancer but may be important in postoperative follow-up.

SCREENING

Early detection would improve the prognosis of gastric cancer in the United States because surgery has a high cure rate with lesions limited to the mucosa and submucosa. But the incidence of early gastric cancer in the United States is less than 5%. While mass screening is useful in Japan to detect early cancers, defined high-risk populations do not exist in the United States to justify the expense of widespread screening. Individual physicians should use upper GI series and endoscopy to screen patients who have occupational or precursor risk factors or patients with persistent dyspepsia or gastroesophageal symptoms.

PROGNOSIS

The two most important prognostic features are: depth of invasion (T-stage) and lymph node status (N-stage). Table 24-4 shows factors affecting prognosis in gastric cancer.

TREATMENT

GOAL OF TREATMENT

The goal of treatment of gastric cancer is cure in early stages and palliation in late stages. There are three modes of treatment: surgery, radiation, and chemotherapy. Gastric cancer is relatively resistant to radiation therapy. For patients with locally recurrent metastatic disease, moderate doses of external beam radiation are used to palliate symptoms but not to improve survival. Prospective controlled trials have failed to demonstrate a survival benefit for patients receiving radiation therapy alone after curative resection.

TREATMENT OF LOCALIZED GASTRIC CANCER

The only potentially curative modality for localized gastric cancer is surgery. The goals of surgery are to provide safe removal of all tumor and produce the least morbidity and mortality (Fig. 24-1). The extent

TABLE 24-4   FACTORS AFFECTING PROGNOSIS IN STOMACH CANCER

Stage of disease (see Table 24-5)

Lymph node status

Size of primary tumor > 4 cm

Proximal tumor

Histologically diffuse, undifferentiated, signet-ring cell types

Diffused variant (has 5-year survival of 10% compared with intestinal type, which has a 5-year survival of 23%)

Aneuploid tumors have worst prognosis. P53 mutations are associated with aneuploid tumors.

Overexpression of c-erb B-2 protein is associated with significantly poorer prognosis

Location of the tumor predicts outcome; 96% of proximal tumors are found to be aneuploid, and only 50% of distal tumors are aneuploid. Rate of survival 5 years after resection is approximately 20 to 25% in distal tumors, 10% in patients with proximal tumors, and 5% for those whose entire stomach is involved

(Data from Fuchs CS, Mayer RJ: Gastric Cancer. N Engl J Med; 333:32–41, 1995; and Alexander HR, Kelsen DP, Tepper JE: Cancer of the stomach. pp. 819–820. In: deVita VT, Hellman S, Rosenberg SA [eds]: Cancer: Principles and Practice of Oncology. 4th Ed. Lippincott-Raven, Philadelphia, 1993.)

of resection depends on location of tumor. For patients with distal tumors, partial gastrectomy with resection of adjacent lymph nodes appears to be sufficient. For patients with proximal lesions, large midgastric lesions, or disease involving the entire stomach, total gastrectomy is necessary. Routine splenectomy is not advocated for tumors not adhering to the spleen and has been associated with a higher complication rate and no clearer survival benefit (Tables 24-4 and 24-5).

The data from the National Cancer Center in Japan suggests substantially improved stage-specific survival compared with data from the United States (Table 24-6). The improved survival may be the result of population-based screening, although some observers suggest that they reflect the use of more aggressive surgical procedures in Japan. Retrospective studies from Japan suggest that extended lymphadenectomy can improve survival. Two small, prospective trials, however, failed to demonstrate a benefit of extensive lymphadenectomy, which was associated with substantial morbidity. The potential difference in stage-specific survival between Japan and Western countries may be explained, in part, by the higher incidence of proximal and diffuse-type tumors in Western societies. Furthermore, the less extensive nodal dissection employed in the United States probably results in an underestimation of the full extent of disease, thereby generating lower rates of stage-specific survival. The value of radical lymph-node resection continues to be debated and is currently being evaluated in randomized, controlled trials.

The Norwegian stomach cancer trial prospectively studied the incidence of postoperative complications and mortality in more than 1,000 patients undergoing surgery for gastric cancer. Postoperative mortality was 8.3% and was highest in patients receiving proximal resection (16%) and lower in those with total gastrectomy (8%), subtotal gastrectomy (10%), or distal resection (7%). Postoperative complication rates were highest in proximal resection (52%), followed by total gastrectomy (38%), subtotal resection (28%), and distal resection (19%). Factors related to postoperative complications were advancing age, male sex, no antibiotic prophylaxis, and splenectomy.

After curative resection, even patients without nodal metastasis (T3 N0) have a 50% chance of dying in 5 years. A lymph node metastasis is an ominous prognostic sign; 80% to 90% of patients in the United States fall into this category. *Adjunct chemotherapy* is considered to be additional treatment for patients who have undergone potentially curative resection. *Single agents* that are active in

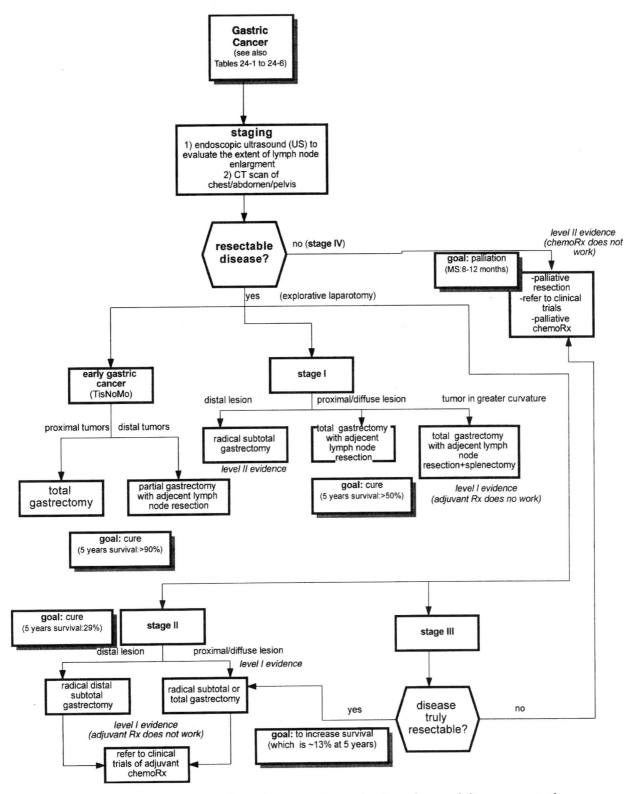

FIGURE 24-1 *Management of gastric cancer. Determination of resectability represents the key reasoning principle in the management of patients with gastric cancer. Goal of treatment is cure in early stages and palliation in advanced stages. Recommended strategy is based on solid level I and level II evidences; numerous studies have convincingly demonstrated that adjuvant radiation and chemotherapy do not lead to increase in survival. Dismal prognosis in gastric cancer can only be improved by finding more new drugs that are more effective than the ones so far studied. For details on treatment regimens see Appendix 17. F/U, follow up; MS, median survival; CT, computed tomography; Rx, therapy.*

TABLE 24-5   AMERICAN JOINT COMMITTEE ON CANCER STAGING OF GASTRIC CANCER, 1988

Primary Tumor (T)

TX   Primary tumor cannot be assessed

T0   No evidence of primary tumor

Tis   Carcinoma in situ

T1   Tumor invades lamina propria or submucosa

T2   Tumor invades muscularis propria

T3   Tumor invades adventitia

T4   Tumor invades adjacent structures

Regional Lymph Nodes (N)

NX   Regional lymph node(s) cannot be assessed

N0   No regional lymph node metastasis

N1   Metastasis in perigastric lymph node(s) within 3 cm of edge of primary tumor

N2   Metastasis in perigastric lymph node(s) more than 3 cm from edge of primary tumor, or in lymph nodes along left gastric, common hepatic, splenic, or celiac arteries

Distant Metastasis (M)

MX   Presence of distant metastasis cannot be assessed

M0   No distant metastasis

M1   Distant metastasis

Stage Grouping

Stage 0	Tis	N0	M0
Stage IA	T1	N0	M0
Stage IB	T1	N1	M0
	T2	N0	M0
Stage II	T1	N2	M0
	T2	N1	M0
	T3	N0	M0
Stage IIIA	T2	N2	M0
	T3	N1	M0
	T4	N0	M0
Stage IIIB	T3	N2	M0
	T4	N1	M0
Stage IV	T4	N2	M0
	Any T	Any N	M1

(From Alexander HR, Kelsen DP, Tepper JE: Cancer of the stomach. pp. 819–820. In deVita VT; Hellman S, Rosenberg SA (eds); Cancer: Principles and Practice of Oncology. 4th Ed. Lippincott-Raven, Philaldelphia, 1993, with permission.)

TABLE 24-6   SURVIVAL AFTER RESECTION OF GASTRIC CARCINOMA AMONG PATIENTS AT U.S. AND JAPANESE CENTERS

Stage of Disease	United States (1982–1987)[a]		Japan (1971–1985)[b]	
	No. of Cases (%)	5-Year Survival (%)	No. of Cases (%)	5-year Survival (%)
I	2,004 (18.1)	50.0	1,s453 (45.7)	90.7
II	1,796 (16.2)	29.0	377 (11.9)	71.7
III	3,945 (35.6)	13.0	693 (21.8)	44.3
IV	3,342 (30.1)	3.0	653 (20.6)	9.0

[a]The number of cases is based on data on 11,087 patients who underwent pathologic stage at 700 U.S. hospitals; age-adjusted survival is based on the 10,237 patients who underwent gastric resection.

[b]The number of cases and age-adjusted survival are based on data on 3,176 patients wl underwent gastric resection at the National Cancer Center Hospital, Tokyo, Japan.

(From Suchs CS, Mayer RJ: Review article in gastric carcinoma. N Engl J Med 333:32–42, 1995, with permission.)

gastric cancer are 5-FU (5-fluorouracil), mitomycin, cisplatinum, doxorubicin, carmustine, semustine, methotrexate, and trimethrexate. 5-FU has a response rate of 20%. Complete responses with single agents are rare, and partial regressions are brief. Combination chemotherapy regimens that were tested in stomach cancer include FAMTX (5-fluorouracil, doxorubicin, methotreaxte), EAP (etoposide, doxorubicin, platinum), FAP, FAM (5-fluorouracil, doxorubicin, mitomycin C), ELF (etoposide, leukovorin, 5-FU). Response rate with FAM is 30% to 40%. EAP has a response rate of 64%, but subsequent trials with this regimen showed a lower response rate and increased toxicity.

Administration of chemotherapy shortly after completing the resection in patients at high risk of recurrence of disease has been assessed as a means of eradicating clinically undetectable micrometastasis. Meta-analysis of fourteen randomized control trials, most of which were conducted in the United States and Europe, concluded that postoperative chemotherapy offers no survival benefit beyond that associated with curative resection. Therefore, administration of adjunct chemotherapy in patients who have undergone curative resection cannot be recommended as a routine practice.

TREATMENT OF ADVANCED DISEASE

Goal of treatment The goal of treatment in advanced disease is palliation. In the absence of ascites or extensive metastatic disease, patients who are believed to be surgically incurable should be considered for palliative gastric resection, which can be performed with acceptably low risk of morbidity and mortality. Although approximate median survival remains only 8 to 12 months after palliative resection, this procedure can provide relief from obstruction, bleeding, and pain. So, when resection is not possible, a bypass of the obstructing lesion can be performed. Endoscopic methods are available for palliation of symptoms. Laser ablation of tumor tissue can be effective, although relief appears to be transient. Use of plastic and expansible metal stents has been associated with a success rate higher than 85% among selected patients with gastroesophageal tumors or tumors of the cardia. In advanced gastric cancer no combination chemotherapy regimen has been found to be superior to 5-FU alone.

FOLLOW-UP

The issue of effective follow-up has never been systematically studied, and in practice large variation in follow-up strategies is seen. One of the reasons for this is that once cancer recurs, no effective treatment exists, which raises questions about the need for surveillance studies. Nevertheless, most physicians see patients every three months when they order routine laboratory data. Endoscopic studies are usually ordered once a year along with a CT scan of the abdomen or as patients' symptoms and signs dictate. The importance of the routine complete blood count is not so much to detect recurrence, but not to overlook anemia secondary to vitamin B_{12} deficiency that develops in most patients after total or distal gastrectomy. For this reason, all patients after distal or total gastrectomy are recommended to take supplemental B_{12} injections (1,000 µg intramuscularly every month).

SUGGESTED READINGS

Botet JF, Lightdale CJ, Zauber AG et al: Preoperative staging of esophageal cancer: comparison of endoscopic US and dynamic CT[1]. Radiology 181:419–425, 1991

Cullinan SA, Moertel CG, Wieand HS et al: Controlled evaluation of three-drug combination regimen versus 5-fluorouracil alone for therapy of advanced gastric cancer. J Clin Oncol 12:412–416, 1994

Dent DM, Madden MV, Price SK: Randomized comparison of R_1 and R_2 gastrectomy for gastric carcinoma. Br J Surg 75:110, 1988

Ekbom GA, Gleysteen JJ: Gastric malignancy: resection for palliation. Surgery 88:476–481, 1980

Graham DY, Schwartz JT, Cain GD, Gyorkey F: Prospective evaluation of biopsy number in the diagnosis of esophageal and gastric carcinoma. Gastroenterology 82:228–231, 1982

Green PH, O'Toole KM, Slonim B et al: Increasing incidence and excellent survival of patients with early gastric cancer. Experience in a United States medical center. Am J Med 85:658–661, 1988

Hallissey MT, Dunn JA, Ward LE: The second British Stomach Cancer Group Trial of adjuvant radiotherapy or chemotherapy in resectable gastric cancer: five-year follow-up. Lancet 343:1309–1312, 1994

Hermans J, Bonenkamp JJ, Boon NC et al: Adjuvant therapy after curative resection for gastric cancer. Meta-analysis of randomized trials. Clin Oncol 11:1441–1447, 1993

MacDonald JS: Southwest Oncology Group NCI high-priority clinical trial phase III randomized study of adjuvant chemotherapy with 5FU leucovorin in patients with resected gastric cancer. Summary last modified 3/95. SWOG 9008 Clinical trials, 8/1/91.

Robertson CS, Chung SC, Woods SD et al: A prospective randomized trial comparing R_1 subtotal gastrectomy with R_3 total gastrectomy for antral cancer. Ann SWRG 200:176–182, 1994

Suchs CS, Mayer RJ: Review article in gastric carcinoma. N Engl J Med 333:32–42, 1995

Uchino S, Hitoshi T, Maruyama K et al: Overexpression of c-erbB-2 protein in gastric cancer; its correlation with long-term survival of patients. Cancer 72:3179–3184, 1993

Wanebo HJ, Kennedy BJ, Chmiel J et al: Cancer of the stomach: a patient care study by the American College of Surgeons. Ann Surg 218:583–592, 1993

Wang KK, DiMagno EP: Endoscopic ultrasonography: high technology and cost containment. Gastroenterology 105:283–296, 1993

25 Pancreatic Cancer

Sheron R. Williams

Incidence/prevalence: 9.1/100,000

Goal of treatment: Prolongation of survival for resectable disease; palliation for advanced disease

Main modality of treatment: Multimodality approach for resectable disease (surgery, chemotherapy, and radiation therapy)

Prognosis (5-year survival): Approximately 8% in localized stage; 1.5% for advanced disease

Pancreatic cancer, the fifth leading cause of cancer death in the United States, represents approximately 2% of all cancers in men and women. In 1995 approximately 27,000 new cases were estimated, and 25,900 deaths were due to pancreatic cancer alone. The incidence of pancreatic cancer significantly increased from 1940 through 1970 and plateaued at approximately 28,000 new cases from the 1970s through the 1990s. African-Americans in the United States have a higher incidence than Caucasians. The median survival is 3 to 4 months, with five-year survival approximately 3 percent. Male/female ratio is approximately 1.3 to 1. The average age at diagnosis is in the sixth decade.

RISK FACTORS

Several risk factors are associated with pancreatic cancer: consumption of a high-fat diet, prior gastrectomy, chronic pancreatitis, diabetes mellitus, and occupational exposure to petroleum derivatives, DDT, and 2-napthylamine. There is no known etiology. Excessive alcohol use is not a significant risk factor, nor is caffeine use.

Histologic types are adenocarcinomas, adeno canthomas, squamous cell and papillary carcinomas, sarcomas, and lymphomas. *Adenocarcinomas* account for 95% of all exocrine pancreatic neoplasms. They are most often multicentric, and 75% are located in the head of the pancreas. Sarcomas and lymphomas are rare. *Papillary-cystic pancreatic carcinoma* a rare carcinoma, occurs most commonly in young women. It has a better prognosis than typical adenocarcinoma. This variety has a 40% to 50% five-year survival after surgical resection.

The most frequent site of metastasis is the regional lymph nodes. Visceral metastasis occurs commonly in the liver and lung, with bone metastasis less frequently. The initial symptoms may be anorexia, weight loss, progressive jaundice, and upper abdominal discomfort. These early symptoms are nonspecific, which may contribute to a delay in diagnosis. Many patients present late in the course of the disease. Physical findings are rarely found early in the course of the disease. Visceral metastasis is seen in about 50% of patients at the time of presentation.

DIAGNOSIS

Diagnosis is most commonly based on imaging studies of the abdomen (computed tomography [CT] or ultrasound). There is little role for magnetic resonance imaging (MRI) in pancreatic cancer. Endoscopic retrograde cholangiopancreatography (ERCP) is often used for patients with normal or atypical CT scans. ERCP may identify obstruction or encasement of pancreatic ducts, and cytology obtained may be diagnostic. Percutaneous aspiration of the pancreas has high sensitivity for diagnosis of pancreatic cancer. The complication rate is low, but "seeding" may occur. It should be avoided in patients with potentially resectable lesions, as should intraoperative biopsy of the pancreas. Intraoperative biopsy is associated with increased rate of pancreatitis, bleeding, fistula, and abscess formation. Angiography, endoscopic ultrasound, and immunoscintigraphy may help in making the diagnosis. Tumor markers CA-19-9, CEA, and serologic testosterone-to-dihydrotestosterone ratio may be increased in the presence of pancreatic cancer. They are nonspecific but may be used to support the diagnosis.

TREATMENT

Treatment is based on disease stage (Table 25-1). Usually patients are classified as *resectable* or *unresectable*. Tumor that is limited to the pancreas or that extends locally into the duodenum, bile duct, and parapancreatic tissue without lymph node invasion may be resectable. Median survival for stage I disease is approximately 1.5 years. Treatment failure after potentially curative surgery results in both local and metastatic recurrences.

Surgical procedure of choice for resection of tumors of the head of the pancreas is a *Whipple's procedure* or variation of this procedure. *Radiation therapy* is often used with the goals of palliation, local control, or perhaps prolongation of survival. In advanced cases it may be used to relieve pain. Current treatment for resectable disease involves a *multimodality approach* (i.e., surgery followed by adjuvant concurrent chemotherapy and radiation therapy). The Gastrointestinal Study Group showed that adjuvant chemotherapy with concurrent radiation therapy resulted in a two-year survival of 43% compared with a two-year survival of 18 percent when there was no further therapy after surgery. Adjuvant therapy is recommended in resectable patients for at least six additional months.

Treatment of locally advanced disease consists of external beam radiation and concurrent chemotherapy. The median survival for patients with locally advanced disease is 7 to 13 months and a two-year survival of 10% to 20 percent. Failure to control local disease reduces survival and is the cause of death in about 50 percent of patients.

For those patients with *advanced disease*, best supportive care is as important as chemotherapy. 5-Fluorouracil (5-Fu) is usually the agent of choice for palliative purposes, with reported response rates of about 28% (0%–67%). Combination chemotherapy adds no benefit over single agent therapy, but it does add to toxicity and cost. Recently, gemcitabine, a new nucleoside analogue, showed clinical benefits in treatment of pancreatic cancer. Preliminary data from a randomized trial comparing gemcitabine with 5-FU show improved response rates (23.8% vs 4.8%), median survival (5.65 vs 4.41 months) and one-year survival (18% vs 2%) in favor of gemcitabine. Fig 25-1 shows recommended strategies for diagnosis and treatment of pancreatic cancer. Management recommendations for initial treatment are based on data from randomized trials (level I and II evidence) and treatment of recurrent disease on preliminary level III evidence. (See Figure 25-1, Table 25-2, and Appendix 18 for specific/practical details about management of pancreatic cancer.)

TABLE 25-1 THE INTERNATIONAL TNM STAGING SYSTEM FOR EXOCRINE PANCREAS

Primary tumor (T)

TX	Primary tumor cannot be assessed
T0	No evidence of primary tumor
TI	Tumor limited to the pancreas
	T1a tumor ≤2 cm in greatest dimension
	T1b tumor >2 cm in greatest dimension
T2	Tumor extends directly to the duodenum, bile duct, or peripancreatic tissues
T3	Tumor extends directly to the stomach, spleen, colon, or adjacent large vessels

Regional lymph nodes (N)

NX	Regional lymph nodes cannot be assessed
N0	No regional lymph node metastasis
N1	Regional lymph node metastasis

Distant metastasis (M)

MX	Presence of distant metastasis cannot be assessed
M0	No distant metastasis
M1	Distant metastasis

Stage Grouping

Stage I	T1	N0	M0
	T2	N0	M0
Stage II	T3	N0	M0
Stage III	Any T	NI	M0
Stage IV	Any T	Any N	M1

(From Beahrs OH et al [eds]: The American Joint Committee on Cancer: Manual for Staging of Cancer. 4th Ed. Lippincott-Raven, Philadelphia. 1992, p 109, with permission.)

TABLE 25-2 FOLLOW-UP OF THE PATIENT WITH PANCREATIC CANCER

	1st and 2nd Years (Months)				3rd–5th Years (Months)	Thereafter (Months)	
	3	6	9	12	6	12	12
History							
Complete	×	×	×				
Appetite, weight	×	×	×	×			
Jaundice, itching	×	×	×	×			
Nausea, vomiting	×	×	×	×			
Abdominal pain	×	×	×	×			
Urine color	×	×	×	×			
Bowel function	×	×	×	×			
Diarrhea	×	×		×			
Physical							
Complete	×	×	×				
Abdominal mass	×	×	×	×			
Liver	×	×	×	×			
Jaundice	×	×	×	×			
Ascites	×	×	×	×			
Rectal	×	×	×	×			
Tests							
Chest x-ray				×		×	×
Complete blood count	×	×	×	×	×	×	×
Liver function	×	×	×	×	×	×	×
CT scan/ultrasound	×	×	×	×	×		

(Modified from Casper ES: pp. 44–46. In Fischer DS (ed): Follow-up of Cancer: A Handbook for Physicians. 4th Ed. Lippincott-Raven, Philadelphia, 1996, with permission.)

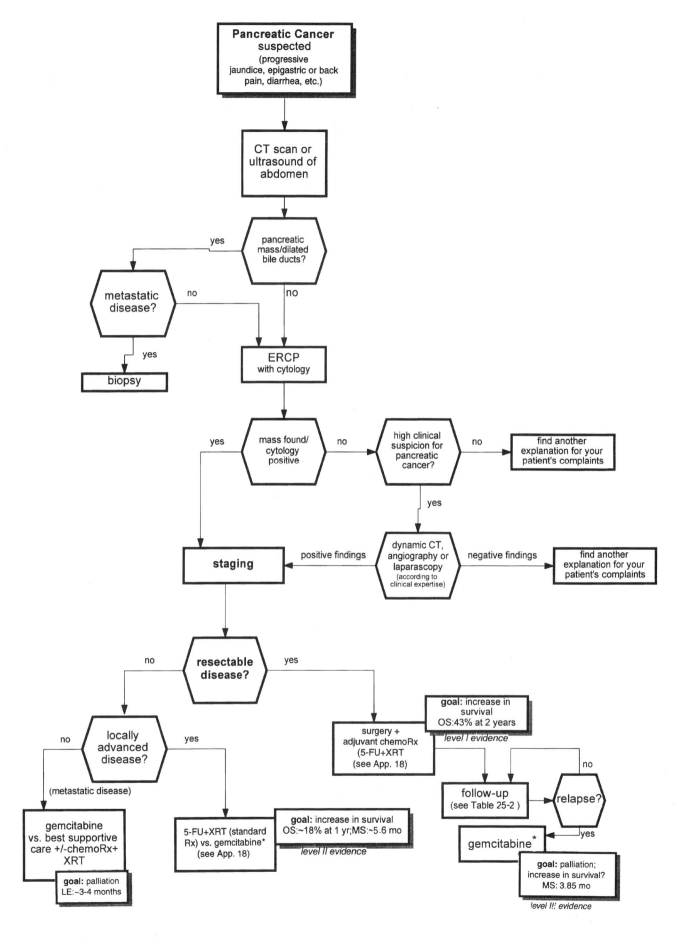

Pancreatic Cancer
suspected
(progressive jaundice, epigastric or back pain, diarrhea, etc.)

CT scan or ultrasound of abdomen

pancreatic mass/dilated bile ducts?

yes

metastatic disease?

no

yes

biopsy

no

ERCP with cytology

mass found/ cytology positive

no

high clinical suspicion for pancreatic cancer?

no

find another explanation for your patient's complaints

yes

yes

dynamic CT, angiography or laparascopy (according to clinical expertise)

positive findings

negative findings

find another explanation for your patient's complaints

staging

resectable disease?

no

yes

surgery + adjuvant chemoRx (5-FU+XRT (see App. 18)

goal: increase in survival OS:43% at 2 years
level I evidence

locally advanced disease?

no

(metastatic disease)

yes

follow-up (see Table 25-2)

relapse?

no

yes

gemcitabine*

goal: palliation; increase in survival? MS: 3.85 mo

level II evidence

gemcitabine vs. best supportive care +/-chemoRx+ XRT

goal: palliation LE:~3-4 months

5-FU+XRT (standard Rx) vs. gemcitabine* (see App. 18)

goal: increase in survival OS:~18% at 1 yr;MS:~5.6 mo

level II evidence

FIGURE 25-1 *Management of pancreatic cancer. Determination of resectability represents the key reasoning principle in the management of patients with pancreatic cancer. The goal of treatment is to increase of survival, which is, unfortunately, possible in only a minority of patients. Recommended strategy is based on level I evidence for the role of combined modality approach in resectable disease. Treatment of unresectable disease is mainly based on preliminary level II and III evidence of the role of gemcitabine in the management of pancreatic cancer. (See also Appendix 18 and Table 25-2 for further details on management.) CT, computed tomography; Rx, therapy; XRT, radiation therapy; ERCP, endoscopic retrograde cholangiopancreatography; MS, median survival; OS, overall survival; *, preliminary data from Eli Lilly and Co.*

SUGGESTED READING

Borg: Handbook of Cancer Diagnosis and Staging: A Clinical Atlas. John Wiley & Sons, New York, 1985

Cullinan SA et al: A comparison of three chemotherapeutic regimens in the treatment of advanced pancreatic and gastric carcinoma. JAMA 253:2061, 1995

DeVita VT. Cancer Principles and Practice. 4th Ed. Lippincott-Raven, Philadelphia, 1993

Fischer DS: Follow Up of Cancer. 4th Ed. Lippincott-Raven, Philadelphia, 1995

Gastrointestinal Tumor Study Group: Phase II studies of drug combinations in advanced pancreatic carcinoma: fluorouracil plus doxorubicin plus mitomycin C and two regimens streptozotocin plus mitomycin C plus fluorouracil. J Clin Oncol 4:1794–1798, 1986

Harvey: Cancer Surgery. WB Saunders, Philadelphia, 1995

Haskell CM (ed): Cancer Treatment. 4th Ed. WB Saunders, Philadelphia, 1985

Skeel RT, Lanchat NA: Handbook of Cancer Chemotherapy. 4th Ed. Little Brown, Boston, 1995, pp. 258–260

Smith FP: Fluorouracil, adriamycin and mitomycin (FAM) chemotherapy for advanced adenocarcinoma of the pancreas. Cancer 46:2014–2018, 1980

26 Biliary Tract Cancer

Koji Nakagawa
Michael Edwards
Geetha Joseph

Incidence: 1.9/100,000; rare in the United States

Goal of treatment: Cure in early stages, palliation in unresectable disease

Main modality of treatment: Surgery in resectable cases with radiation therapy in selected cases to improve survival, surgical/endoscopic/percutaneous stenting for palliation

Prognosis (5-year survival):   Resected 13% to 22%; unresectable <5%

Bile duct cancer, although not among the common tumors with an incidence of 1.1 in 100,000, still accounts for more than 4,000 deaths a year in the United States. Its location and anatomic relationships to vital structures requires specialized techniques for diagnosis, and it remains one of the most difficult cancers for diagnosis and treatment, even with the best of modern imaging techniques. In this chapter, intrahepatic bile duct cancer (cholangiocarcinoma) is not included, because clinically it is treated as a primary liver cancer.

The causes of this tumor are unknown, but bile duct cancer occurs more frequently in patients with a history of chronic ulcerative colitis, choledochal cyst, or infection with the fluke, *Clonorchis sinensis*. The relative risk for individuals with ulcerative colitis is about 30 times that in the general population. Clinical experience and pathologic evidence strongly support an association between primary sclerosing cholangitis (PSC) and bile duct cancer. This tumor tends to occur in the older age group, most patients being about 60 years old. Slightly more males than females are affected.

CLINICAL PRESENTATION

Patients with bile duct cancer come to medical attention because of *jaundice, abdominal pain, fever, and pruritus.* Weakness and weight loss may be marked. Biochemical changes in bile duct cancer are those of *obstructive jaundice*, with high serum bilirubin, alkaline phosphatase, and γ-glutamyl transpeptidase. Jaundice may be delayed if only one main duct is involved.

Most bile duct cancers are multicentric, slow-growing, and only locally invasive *adenocarcinomas*. Macroscopically 3 types are seen: papillary, nodular, and diffuse. *Papillary lesions* are usually seen at the sphincter of Oddi. The nodular type forms a localized mass which projects into the lumen of the bile duct. A sclerosing variant occurs commonly at the hilum, while the nodular type is most common in the middle third. The diffuse type is most common in the upper third and is difficult to distinguish from sclerosing cholangitis and has the worst prognosis. Histologically the tumor is usually a mucus-secreting adenocarcinoma (cholangiocarcinoma) (Table 26-1). Perineural invasion is common and has a negative impact on survival.

The clinical picture and treatment differ according to site. Three anatomic sites are recognized: *the upper third*, consisting of the common hepatic duct and the confluence of the right and left hepatic ducts (58% of lesions); the *middle third*, involving the common bile duct between the cystic duct and the upper border of the pancreas (17%); the *lower third*, from the upper border of the pancreas to the ampulla of Vater (18%). The remaining 7% involves the extrahepatic bile ducts diffusely. The tumor often spreads along the bile duct and may extend into the liver. Hematogenous hepatic metastases may occur with bile duct cancers of all sites. The local and distant metastases commonly involve the peritoneum, abdominal lymph nodes, diaphragm, or gallbladder.

DIAGNOSIS

Accurate characterization and staging of bile duct cancers are essential for decision making for the treatments. Staging of the tumor is usually aided by ultrasonography (US), computed tomography (CT) scan, endoscopic retrograde cholangiopancreatography (ERCP), and/or percutaneous transhepatic cholangiography (PTC) and angiography (Fig. 26-1).

US is particularly useful in the cholestatic patient because it is inexpensive and noninvasive. In the case of bile duct cancer, it shows dilated intrahepatic bile ducts, and the extrahepatic bile duct may be dilated down to a tumor. It can sometimes identify an echogenic tumor mass at the hilum.

CT scans show intrahepatic and/or extrahepatic biliary dilation; the tumor is however, difficult to demonstrate, since bile duct cancers are usually isodense with the liver. In many cases the CT scan is useful in assessing lymph node enlargement suggestive of regional metastasis. Magnetic resonance imaging (MRI) may be similarly useful but more expensive.

ERCP or PTC, or both, are essential for the characterization and staging of bile duct cancers, and should be performed in all patients with cholestasis and dilated intrahepatic ducts shown by US or CT scan. Cholangiography may confirm the diagnosis and show the size and level of the tumor, as well as the extent of the tumor along the biliary tree.

PTC is successful in over 90% of patients and is virtually diagnostic for proximal tumors. When right and left hepatic ducts are individually obstructed, puncture of both systems may be necessary to outline the obstruction. While most frequently successful, the disadvantage of PTC relative to ERCP is the discomfort associated with the transhepatic approach. ERCP is better tolerated and has a lower risk of bleeding, but its reliability is dependent on the experience of the endoscopist. Transpapillary cytology and biopsy at the time of ERCP may be performed. Endoscopic US is useful in assessing the extent of tumor at the lower end of the bile duct.

Angiography and venography are needed to evaluate vascular invasion, and are important for staging and determining resectability of the tumor. Screening for distant metastases that present late in the course of the disease, is done with chest x-ray and CT scans.

TNM staging should be used after surgery and pathologic examination of the resected specimen. Stages defined by TNM classification apply to all primary carcinomas arising in the extrahepatic bile ducts or in the cystic duct (Table 26-2).

TABLE 26-1   THE HISTOLOGIC CLASSIFICATION OF THE EXTRAHEPATIC BILE DUCT CANCERS

Carcinoma in situ
Adenocarcinoma
Papillary adenocarcinoma
Adenocarcinoma, intestinal type
Mucinous adenocarcinoma
Clear cell adenocarcinoma
Signet-ring cell carcinoma
Adenosquamous cell carcinoma
Squamous cell carcinoma
Small cell (oat cell) carcinoma
Undifferentiated carcinoma
Carcinoma, NOS

TREATMENT

CURATIVE SURGICAL RESECTION

Although therapeutic options for extrahepatic bile duct cancers include endoscopic or percutaneous intubation, surgery, radiation, and chemotherapy, surgical resection has been the only curative therapy (Fig. 26-1). Unfortunately, extrahepatic bile duct cancer is curable by surgery in fewer than 10% of all cases. However, it is now diagnosed more frequently and precisely with the development of modern diagnostic methods, which may provide for a better selection of patients and a resultant increase

TABLE 26-2   THE STAGES OF EXTRAHEPATIC BILE DUCT CANCERS BY TNM CLASSIFICATION

Stage	T	N	M
0	Tis	0	0
I	1	0	0
II	2	0	0
III	1,2	1	0
IVA	3	Any	0
IVB	Any	Any	1

Primary tumor (T)
  TX: Primary tumor cannot be assessed
  T0: No evidence of primary tumor
  Tis: Carcinoma in situ
  T1: Tumor invades the mucosa or muscle layer
    T1a: Tumor invades the mucosa
    T1b: Tumor invades the muscle area
  T2: Tumor invades perimuscular connective tissue
  T3: Tumor invades adjacent structure: liver, pancreas, duodenum, gallbladder, colon, stomach

Regional lymph node (N)
  NX: Regional lymph nodes cannot be assessed
  N0: No regional lymph node metastasis
  N1: Metastasis in cystic duct, pericholedochal and/or hilar lymph nodes (i.e., in the hepatoduodenal ligament)
  N2: Metastasis in peripancreatic (head only), periduodenal, periportal, celiac, and/or superior mesenteric lymph nodes

Distant metastasis (M)
  MX: Presence of distant metastasis cannot be assessed
  M1: No distant metastasis
  M2: Distant metastasis

in the cure rate. The main modality of treatment is surgery.

Prognosis and resectability depend on tumor location along the biliary tree, the extent of hepatic parenchymal involvement, and the invasion by the tumor of major blood vessels. Tumors arising in the distal bile duct are resectable in 25% to 30% of patients with a 1-year survival rate of 60% to 80% and a 5-year survival rate of 22%. The resectability rate is clearly better for distal than for more proximal lesions. The more frequent proximal bile duct cancer (Klatskin tumor) is more problematic. In a minority of cases, proximal bile duct cancer can be completely resected. The tumor is most frequently detected at an advanced stage, which precludes potentially curative resection. Often the tumor invades directly into the adjacent liver along the common bile duct, or into the hepatic artery or portal vein.

If the tumor extensively involves both lobes of the liver or involves the main portal vein or hepatic artery, the lesion is considered unresectable.

In comparison, if the tumor affects one lobe of the liver only, or only involves the portal vein and hepatic artery on the same side, the lesion may be resectable with partial hepatectomy. Involvement of the portal vein and hepatic artery do not necessarily preclude resection. Resections combined with major liver resection give a 5% to 8% operative mortality and a 13% to 17% 5-year survival rate. Pancreaticoduodenectomy is frequently helpful for lower third tumors.

Surgical resection of the tumor now can be performed with low mortality and, when possible, provides the longest and best palliation, and offers potential for cure. The key decision-making principle is to determine resectability of extrahepatic bile duct tumors.

In jaundiced patients, there should be preoperative consideration of percutaneous transhepatic catheter drainage or endoscopic placement of a stent for relief of biliary obstruction, if jaundice is severe.

Liver transplantation for locally advanced tumors gives poor results; recurrence of the tumor is usual.

PALLIATION

In the majority of patients with extrahepatic bile duct cancer, the tumor cannot be completely removed by surgery, and this can usually be determined by radiographic studies as outlined. Since these patients cannot be cured, a palliative procedure is needed. Jaundice and pruritus may be relieved by anastomosis of the bile duct to bowel or placement of bile duct stents by operative, endoscopic, or percutaneous techniques, which provides good quality survival.

The selection of the method is individualized, since there are no controlled trials. For tumors found at operation to be unresectable, operative biliary enteric bypass provides durable palliation. Nonoperative methods may be better for elderly patients or those with advanced disease, because they are less invasive.

In patients with unresectable proximal extrahepatic bile duct cancer treated by palliative procedures, the in-hospital mortality is 7% to 14% with a mean survival of 6 to 12 months. Occasional patients treated by incomplete resection with complete relief of biliary obstruction may survive several years.

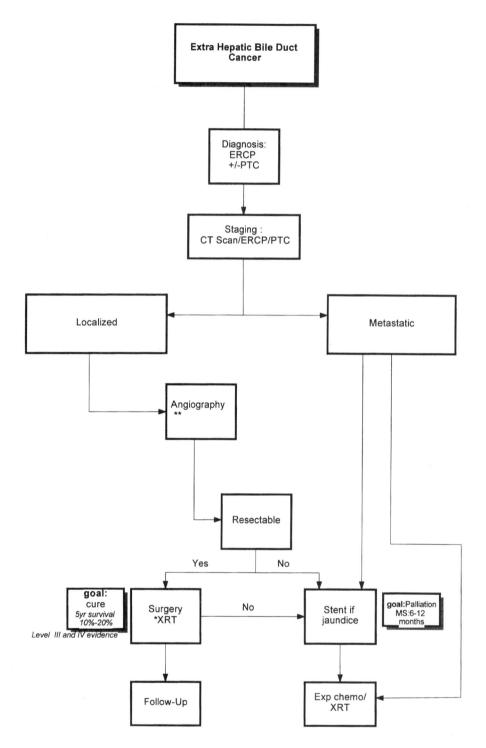

FIGURE 26-1   *Management of extrahepatic bile duct cancer. Determination of resectability represents a key decision-making principle in the management of extrahepatic bile duct cancer. The goal of treatment is cure in resectable cases, possible prolongation of survival with postoperative radiation in selected cases and palliation in unresectable or metastatic disease. The recommended strategy is based on nonexperimental evidence for the curative role of surgery in early disease and level III/IV evidence for prolongation of survival and palliation. *, consider radiation therapy for close margins. **, exclude major artery and portal vein involvement; EXP, experimental; chemo, chemotherapy; XRT, radiation; MS, median survival.*

RADIATION THERAPY

Several authors have suggested that radiotherapy may prolong survival after curative resection as well as after palliative procedures (level III evidence). However, the role of radiotherapy in the management of bile duct cancer remains controversial, and further data from randomized studies are necessary to confirm its beneficial effect. Experimental trials of intraoperative radiation and brachytherapy are warranted for small volume disease that is unresectable.

CHEMOTHERAPY

Generally cytotoxic drugs are ineffective, but fluorouracil, doxorubicin, and mitomycin have been reported to produce transient, partial remission in a small proportion of patients (level IV). There is no evidence favoring multiagent chemotherapy over single agent therapy. The combination of intra-arterial fluorodeoxyuridine (floxuridine) (FUDR) with conformational radiation therapy have shown promising results, but only small numbers of patients have been studied. Further studies of adjuvant and neoadjuvant chemotherapy in combination with radiation will be necessary to improve the prognosis, but, because of the rarity of these tumors, randomized trials will be difficult to perform.

FOLLOW-UP AND PROGNOSIS

Follow-up after curative resection is generally done every 3 months for 2 years, biannually for 3 years, and annually thereafter. Complete history and liver function tests may be helpful. Ultrasonography or CT scan can be done at 6-month intervals for the first 2 years and then annually. Few scientific data currently exist regarding optimal follow-up.

Death is most often due to hepatocellular failure and infection, usually suppurative cholangitis and septicemia. Massive invasion of the liver by tumor or extrahepatic metastases rarely causes death. Prognosis depends on the site of the tumor, which affects its resectability. Distal bile duct cancer has a better prognosis than a proximal one. The histologically differentiated do better than the undifferentiated. Polypoid cancers have the best prognosis.

SUGGESTED READINGS

Adam A, Benjamin IS: The staging of cholangiocarcinoma. 46:299, 1992

Bhuiya MR, Nimura K, Kamiya J et al: Clinico-pathologic studies on perineural invasion of bile duct carcinoma. Ann Surg 215:344, 1992

Blumgart LH, Hadjis NH, Benjamin IS et al: Surgical approaches to cholangiocarcinoma at confluence of hepatic ducts. Lancet i:66, 1984

Cameron JL, Pitt HA, Zinner MJ et al: Management of proximal cholangiocarcinomas by surgical resection and radiotherapy. Am J Surg 159:91, 1990

Dancygier H, Rosch T, Lorenz J et al: Preoperative staging of a distal common bile duct tumor by endoscopic ultrasound. Gastroenterology 69:219, 1988

Fritz P, Brambs HJ, Schraube P et al: Combined external beam radiotherapy and intraluminal high dose rate brachytherapy on bile duct carcinomas. Int J Radiol Oncol Biol Physics 29:855, 1994

Goldstein RM, Stone M, Tillery GW et al: Is liver transplantation indicated for cholangiocarcinoma? Am J Surg 166:768, 1993

Heson DE, Albores-Saavedra J, Corle D: Carcinoma of the extrahepatic bile ducts histologic types, stage of disease, grade and survival rates. Cancer 70:1498, 1992

Nordback IH, Pitt HA, Coleman J et al: Unresectable hilar carcinoma: percutaneous versus operative palliation. Surgery 115:597, 1994

Norton RA, Foster EA: Bile duct cancer. Ca 40:225, 1990

Parkin DM, Ohshima H, Srivatankul P, Vatanaspt V: Cholangiocarcinoma: Epidemiology, mechanisms of carcinogenesis and prevention. Cancer Epidemiol Biomarkers Prev 2:537, 1993

Polydorou AA, Cairns SR, Dowacett JF et al: Palliation of proximal malignant biliary obstruction by endoscopic endoprosthesis insertion. Gut 32:685, 1991

Robertson JR, Lawrence TS, Dworzanin IM et al: Treatment of primary hepatobiliary cancers with conformational radiation therapy and regional chemotherapy. J Clin Oncol 11:1286, 1993

Ros PR, Buck JL, Goodman ZD et al: Intrahepatic cholangiocarcinoma: radiologic-pathologic correlation. Radiology 167:689, 1988

Rosen CB, Nagorney DM, Wiesner RH et al: Cholangiocarcinoma complicating primary sclerosing cholangitis. Ann Surg 213:21, 1991

Shutze WP, Sack J, Aldrete JS: Long-term follow up of 24 patients undergoing radical resection for ampullary carcinoma. Cancer 66:1717, 1990

Tompkins RK, Saunders K, Roslyn JJ, Longmire WP: Changing patterns in diagnosis and management of bile duct cancer. Ann Surg 211:614, 1990

27 Hepatocellular Carcinoma

Koji Nakagawa
Geetha Joseph
Michael Edwards

Incidence: 2.7/100,000, rare in the United States

Goal of treatment: Cure in small localized tumors if resectable or transplant candidates (10%); prolongation of survival in localized unresectable tumors; palliation in multiple or metastatic tumors

Main modality of treatment: Liver resection or transplant in early stages; transcatheter arterial embolization (TAE) or percutaneous ethanol injections (PEI) for unresectable cases. Observation versus experimental chemotherapy in all others.

Prognosis (3-year survival):

Localized, resectable tumors:	56%–80%
Localized unresectable with transplant:	18%–30%
Localized unresectable with PEI/TAE:	38%–55%
Multiple or metastatic lesions:	<15%

INCIDENCE AND RISK FACTORS

Primary liver cancer (PLC), although uncommon in the United States (incidence 2.7 in 100,000), is the most common cause of cancer fatality in the world with the highest incidence in Africa and Asia. There are two main cell types: hepatocellular carcinoma (HCC) and intrahepatic cholangiocarcinoma (CCC) (for extrahepatic CCC, see Ch. 26). More than 70% of PLC are HCC. Overall surgical cure is possible in 5% to 10% of all patients (Table 27-1).

Risk factors for HCC include hepatitis B carrier state (relative risk 234:1), hepatitis C infection, alcoholic cirrhosis, and toxins such as polyvinyl chloride, aflatoxin, and hemochromatosis. Men are affected three times more than women, and the incidence increases with age independent of risk factors.

The main risk factors for CCC are different from HCC and include inflammatory bowel disease, *Clonorchis sinensis* infestation and sclerosing cholangitis.

DIAGNOSIS

Symptoms of PLC include anorexia, weight loss, abdominal pain, right upper quadrant mass, and ascites. As many as 30% of patients may be asymptomatic. Jaundice is not a usual feature. Biochemical changes in HCC are similar to those in hepatic cirrhosis and chronic hepatitis, with elevations of alkaline phosphatase and transaminases.

TABLE 27-1   THE HISTOLOGIC CLASSIFICATION OF THE ADULT PRIMARY LIVER CANCERS

Hepatocellular carcinoma
(liver cell carcinoma)
Hepatocellular carcinoma
(fibrolamellar variant)
Cholangiocarcinoma
(intrahepatic bile duct carcinoma)
Mixed hepatocellular cholangiocarcinoma
Undifferentiated carcinoma

Early diagnosis of PLC may result in more cases suitable for curative treatments and lead to longer survival. Accurate characterization and staging of PLC are essential for decision making for treatment. In most cases the diagnosis is suspected by a combination of imaging tools including ultrasonography (US), computed tomography (CT) scan, magnetic resonance imaging (MRI), and angiography (Fig. 27-1). However, the diagnosis must be confirmed by biopsy of the lesion, usually by percutaneous needle biopsy (Fig. 27-1). US is the best tool for screening primary liver cancer because it can be performed easily, is inexpensive, and is noninvasive. US also plays an important role in decision making because of its ability to demonstrate hepatic vascular anatomy, as well as tumors. The accuracy of US has increased with development of higher resolution, real-time scanners, and intraoperative applications.

Supportive data include elevation of *α-fetoprotein* (AFP), which is an α_1-globulin detected in more than *90% of patients with HCC*. Elevations of AFP may be seen in chronic hepatitis and cirrhosis but only 4% to 9% have levels higher than 400 ng/mL, while in 80% of patients with HCC the AFP level is higher than 400 ng/mL. Differentiation of HCC from CCC, metastatic disease, and benign adenomas is crucial. AFP elevations are rare in CCC and metastatic disease unless associated with metastatic nonseminomatous germ cell tumors. Chest x-ray and bone scans are indicated to exclude other primary tumors and metastases.

TREATMENT

Determining resectability is the key reasoning principle in the management of patients with PLC, since surgical resection of PLC has been the only curative therapy.

The goals of treatment of PLC are (1) cure, (2) prolongation of survival, and (3) palliation.

Determination of resectability of PLC mainly depends on (1) location and number of lesions, (2) extent of involvement, (3) underlying liver pathology making resection medically unfeasible, and (4) distant metastases (Fig. 27-1).

Surgical resection of the PLC is the best option and has a 3-year actuarial survival of 56% and a 24% recurrence at 1 year, with a 5% to 10% operative mortality. In areas where screening has detected tumors early (<2 cm), more than 80% of 3-year survivals have been reported. Fibrolamellar carcinoma and early TNM stages of HCC are highly represented among long-term survivors and the survival rates after surgical resection correlate well with TNM stages (Table 27-2). Unfortunately, only 5% to 10% of all patients with PLC are resectable for a variety of reasons. While up to 80% of a noncirrhotic liver can be removed with eventual recovery, the amount of the liver that can be resected is dependent on the hepatic reserve capacity in a cirrhotic liver. There are, however, no simple and well-established criteria for decision making regarding resectability and liver function. Generally, medical contraindications to partial hepatectomy include high bilirubin due to hepatocellular dysfunction, Child's class C cirrhosis (Table 27-3), elevation in the prothrombin time, and other organ dysfunction. Bilaterality of lesions, metastases outside the liver, major invasion of the inferior vena cava, portal vein, or adjacent structures are also contraindications. Ascites due to liver cirrhosis is not a contraindication to surgery, if it is controllable and cytologically benign.

Patients with unresectable tumors because of inadequate liver function or tumor location that requires more than trisegmentectomy may be eligible for liver transplantation. Solitary tumors have the best chance for cure. However, recurrence rates are as high as 65%, usually within two years and often within one year; two-year and five-year survivals are 30% and 18%, respectively. Patients with unresectable fibrolamellar carcinoma may be considered for liver transplantation.

PROLONGATION OF SURVIVAL

Unfortunately, there is no standard therapy for unresectable tumors. However, percutaneous ethanol injection (PEI) has been used in HCC but not CCC as local therapy for poor surgical candidates. PEI has been shown to prolong survival and should be considered for unresectable disease for three or fewer lesions smaller than 3 cm. Recurrence rates of 66% at 2 years (45% after surgery)

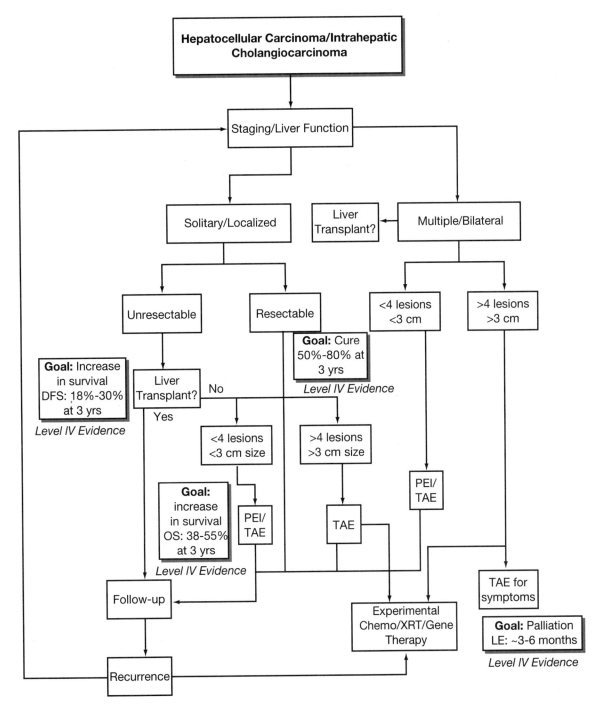

FIGURE 27-1 *Management of primary liver cancer (PLC). Determination of resectability represents a key reasoning principle in the management of PLC. The goal of treatment is cure in localized tumors and prolongation of survival in unresectable cases of HCC. The recommended strategy is based on solid nonexperimental evidence of the curative potential of surgery and level III/IV evidence for prolongation of survival with PEI/TAE. Strategies for CCC are limited to surgery for resectable disease based on solid nonexperimental evidence and experimental chemotherapy/radiation for unresectable disease based on level IV/V evidence. These options apply for CCC (intrahepatic cholangiocarcinoma). PEI, percutaneous ethanol injections; TAE, transcatheter arterial embolization; HCC, hepatocellular carcinoma; LE, life expectancy.*

TABLE 27-2   **THE STAGES OF THE ADULT PRIMARY LIVER CANCERS BY TNM CLASSIFICATION**

Stage	T	N	M
I	1	0	0
II	2	0	0
III	1,2	1	0
	3	Any	0
IVA	4	Any	0
IVB	Any	Any	1

Primary tumor (T)

   TX: Primary tumor cannot be assessed

   T0: No evidence of primary tumor

   T1: Solitary tumor 2.0 cm or less in greatest dimension without vascular invasion

   T2: Solitary tumor 2.0 cm or less in greatest dimension with vascular invasion; or multiple tumors limited to one lobe, or a solitary tumor more than 2.0 cm in the greatest dimension without vascular invasion

   T3: Solitary tumor more than 2.0 cm in greatest dimension with vascular invasion, or multiple tumors limited to one lobe, any more than 2.0 cm in greatest dimension, with or without vascular invasion

   T4: Multiple tumors in more than one lobe or tumor(s) involving a major branch of portal or hepatic vein

Regional lymph node (N)

   NX: Regional lymph nodes cannot be assessed

   N0: No regional lymph node metastasis

   N1: Regional lymph node metastasis

Note: The regional lymph nodes are hilar (i.e., those in the hepatoduodenal ligament, hepatic and periportal nodes). Regional lymph nodes also include those along the inferior vena cava, hepatic artery, and portal vein. Any lymph node involvement beyond these nodes is considered distant metastasis and should be coded as M1.

Distant metastasis (M)

   MX: Presence of distant metastasis cannot be assessed

   M0: No distant metastasis

   M1: Distant metastasis

TABLE 27-3   **MODIFIED CHILD CLASSIFICATION**[a]

Parameter	Score		
	1	*2*	*3*
Serum bilirubin (mg/100 mL)	1–2	2–3	>3
Albumin (g/L)	>35	28–35	<28
Prothrombin time (seconds prolonged)	1–4	4–6	>6
Encephalopathy (grade)	—	1–2	3–4
Ascites	Absent	Slight	Moderate

[a]*Group designation: A = 5–6 points; B = 7–9 points; C = 10–15 points.*

have been reported, but in solitary lesions smaller than 3 cm, survival is similar to surgery at 3 years (55%).

Transcatheter arterial embolization (TAE) has been used for unresectable HCC and occasionally as a preliminary to resection or for recurrence. After TAE, a favorable response (extensive necrosis with reduction of tumor area greater than 50%) is seen in more than 80% of patients with 38% 2-year survival. TAE may be a useful treatment modality in selected patients, but in the absence of controlled trials, the prolongation of survival after TAE remains controversial.

Many kinds of regional and systemic chemotherapies have been proposed for unresectable PLC and the use of intra-arterial chemotherapy via an indwelling pump has also been studied. Single-agent Adriamycin with a response rate of 20% has been used, but no survival benefit has been shown with this or other chemotherapy combinations. Tamoxifen has been used with marginal improvement in survival in one study. Unfortunately, there is to date no effective chemotherapy for PLC. Other therapies include cryosurgery, radiation therapy, immunotherapy, immunotargeting therapy, anticancer drug with lipiodol, and gene therapy. These therapies may be used in combination with other treatments, such as resection, TAE, and PEI. However, no controlled trials have been done to suggest survival advantage. Since further studies are needed to determine their effectiveness and usefulness, patients with PLC should be considered for experimental chemotherapy protocols.

PALLIATION

TAE may be used for a large HCC as palliative therapy by decreasing size of tumors, although TAE is thought to have no effect on prolongation of survival for large HCCs.

FOLLOW-UP AND PROGNOSIS

Follow-up strategies for resected patients to detect early relapse or new primary tumors should include monitoring AFP levels if initially elevated, along with ultrasonography, which is sensitive, noninvasive, and inexpensive. Few scientific data currently exist, however, regarding optimal follow-up.

Prognosis of patients with PLC in general has been dismal. The cause of death is usually liver failure, hemorrhage from esophageal bleeding or ruptured tumor, and infection.

Since early detection of PLC may change the prognosis of patients with PLC, which is dismal currently, screening of high-risk patients (PSC, hepatitis B carriers, hepatitis C, hemochromatosis) with AFP levels and ultrasound may be warranted. The use of interferon-wα in patients with hepatitis C-associated cirrhosis has decreased the incidence of HCC significantly.

SUGGESTED READINGS

Albert ME, Hutt MS, Wogan GN et al: Association between afla-toxin content of food and hepatoma frequency in Uganda. Cancer 28:253, 1971

Bruix J, Barrera JM, Calvet X et al: Prevalence of antibodies to hepatitis C virus in Spain patients with hepatocellular carci-noma and hepatic cirrhosis. Lancet 2:1004, 1989

Bruix J, Castell A, Montanya X et al: Phase II study of transarte-rial embolization in European patients with hepatocellular carcinoma: need for controlled trial. Hepatology 20:643, 1994

Castells A, Bruix J, Bru C et al: Treatment of small hepatocellu-lar carcinoma in cirrhotic patients: a cohort study comparing surgical resection and percutaneous ethanol injection. Hepa-tology 18:1121, 1993

Farmer DG, Rosove MH, Shaked AS et al: Current treatment modalities for hepatocellular carcinoma. Ann Surg 219:236, 1994

Farinati F, Salvagnini M, de Maria N et al: Unresectable hepato-cellular carcinoma: a prospective controlled trial with Tamox-ifen. J Hepatol, 11:297, 1990

Hardell L, Bengtsson NO, Jonsson U et al: Aetiological aspects of primary liver cancer with special regard to alcohol, organic solvents and acute intermittent porphyria: an epidemiological investigation. Br J Cancer 50:389, 1984

Iwatsuki S, Starzl TE, Sheahan DG et al: Hepatic resection ver-sus transplantation for hepatocellular carcinoma. Ann Surg 214:221, 1991

Kawasaki S, Makuuchi M, Kosuge T et al: Systematic subseg-mentectomy for hepatocellular carcinoma. pp. 235–242. In Tobe T, Kameda H, Ohto M et al (eds): Primary Liver Cancer in Japan. Tokyo: Springer-Verlag, 1992

Mazzaferro V, Regalia E, Doci R et al: Liver transplantation for the treatment of small hepatocellular carcinomas in patients with cirrhosis. N Engl J Med 334:693, 1996

Nishiguchi S, Kuroki T, Nakatani S, Morimoto H et al: Random-ized trial of effects of interferon-a on incidence of hepatocel-lular carcinoma in chronic active hepatitis C with cirrhosis. Lancet 346:1051, 1995

Parkin DM, Ohshima H, Srivatanakul P, Vatanaspt V: Cholangio-carcinoma: epidemiology, mechanisms of carcinogenesis and prevention. Cancer Epidemiol Biomarkers Prev 2:537, 1993

Penn I: Hepatic transplantation for primary and metastatic can-cers of the liver. Surgery 110:726, 1991

Sherock S, Dooley J: Disease of the Liver and Biliary System. 9th ed. pp. 503–531. Cambridge, MA: Blackwell Scientific Publications, 1993

Shiratori Y, Terano A et al: Percutaneous ethanol injection ther-apy for hepatocellular carcinoma: results in 146 patients. AJR 160:1023, 1993

Starzl TE, Twatsuki S, Shaw BW Jr et al: Treatment of fibro-lamellar hepatoma with partial or total hepatectomy and transplantation of the liver. Surg Gynecol Obstet 162:145, 1986

Taketa K. Alpha-fetoprotein: reevaluation in hepatology. Hepa-tology 12:1420, 1990

Venook AP: Treatment of hepatocellular carcinoma: too many options? J Clin Oncol 12:1323, 1994

Vilana R, Bruix J, Bru C et al: Tumor size determines the efficacy of percutaneous ethanol injection for the treatment of small hepatocellular carcinoma. Hepatology 16:353, 1992

Yeo CJ, Pitt HA, Cameron JL: Cholangiocarcinoma. Surg Clin North Am 70:1429, 1990

28 | Colon Cancer

Geetha Joseph
Wayne Tuckson

Incidence: 11/100,000 (18% of all cancer deaths; third leading cause of cancer deaths in the United States

Goal of treatment: cure in early stages (A and B); prolongation of survival in stage C; palliation in stage D colon cancer

Main modality of treatment: surgery in early stages; surgery + adjuvant chemotherapy in stage C; observation vs chemotherapy in stage D colon cancer.

Prognosis (5-year survival):

Stage A/B1:   85%–90%

Stage B2:   70%–75%

Stage C: 45%–60%

Stage D: 15%–20%

Annually there are 160,000 new patients diagnosed with colon cancer in the US (incidence 11 in 100,000). Also there are 58,000 deaths from colon cancer making it the third leading cause of cancer deaths (18% of cancer deaths). Resection for cure is possible in 70% to 75% of all patients; however, 50% still die from their disease.

Risk factors for the development of colon cancer include familial polyposis syndromes (familial adenomatous polyposis (FAP), familial cancer syndromes (hereditary nonpolyposis colon cancer), a family history of colon cancer, inflammatory bowel disease, and prior radiation treatment.

The *symptoms* of colon cancer include a change in bowel habits (12%), change in stool caliber, overt rectal bleeding, abdominal pain or distension (11%). Less commonly, patients present with complete bowel obstruction or perforation. Other patients present with nonspecific symptoms such as weight loss and anemia, the workup of which leads to the diagnosis of colon cancer. The value of *early detection* is underscored by the fact that asymptomatic patients have a 5-year survival of 71% compared to 49% for symptomatic patients.

The colon extends from the ileocecal valve to the junction of the rectum and sigmoid colon. It is easily visualized and accessible for diagnostic studies. The primary diagnostic modalities for colon cancer are endoscopy and contrast radiography. Endoscopy offers not only visualization but also removal of premalignant lesions and biopsy for tissue diagnosis.

Histologic subsets of colon cancer include adenocarcinoma (95%), carcinoid tumors, squamous cell carcinoma, lymphomas, and leiomyosarcoma.

PROGNOSTIC FACTORS FOR COLON CANCER

1. Depth of penetration of the bowel wall.

2. The presence and number of lymph nodes with metastases.

3. Histologic appearance, i.e., well differentiated versus poorly differentiated or mucinous.

Stage remains the single best prognostic factor in colon cancer. Other features such as perforation and obstruction significantly decrease survival. Size alone has not proven to be of prognostic significance. Laboratory parameters such as DNA ploidy, S phase and deletions of chromosome 18 are being evaluated as prognostic factors.

The key decision-making principle in colon cancer is determining resectability.

GOALS/STRATEGIES IN THE MANAGEMENT OF COLON CANCER

The goal of treatment in colon carcinoma is curative with surgery being the primary modality of therapy. The treatment options for confirmed colon cancer are (1) complete surgical resection and staging with curative intent at diagnosis and surgery for recurrences detected during follow up. (2) Prolongation of survival with adjuvant therapy to prevent or decrease recurrence and improve survival. Resection of recurrences detected during follow up. (3) Palliative therapy of unresectable primary tumors to improve quality of life.

CURE

Once the tissue diagnosis of colon cancer is made, definitive resection is undertaken unless accentuating events such as perforation, clinical bowel obstruction or contraindication to surgery is present. If required, temporizing measures including diverting colostomy/ileostomy can be done with subsequent definitive resection to follow.

The extent of the resection depends on both the location of the cancer and the presence of adjacent organ involvement. Cancer found in polyps is adequately treated by polypectomy if the margin of resection is free and the cancer is either well or moderately differentiated. Colon resection is required for positive margins or poorly differentiated cancers. Removal of the cancer and draining lymph nodes in the mesentery is recommended and is curative in 50% of patients. Removal of relevant intermediate lymph nodes should be done if needed as the goal of surgery is curative. Laparoscopic resection of colon cancer is not recommended currently. *Surgical staging* is based on the modified (Astler-Coller) Dukes' classification (see Table 28-1). To complete staging, computed tomography (CT) scan of the abdomen is recommended. Whether evaluation of the liver by CT scan is required preoperatively is not clear but a preoperative chest x-ray is required. Preoperative and postoperative measurement of carcinoembryonic antigen (CEA) levels are also recommended although its bearing on treatment is questionable.

Prolongation of Survival *Adjuvant therapy* is given in order to decrease recurrence and improve overall survival. The rational for postoperative therapy is that there is minimal tumor burden at this time.

Adjuvant therapy is not required for patients with Dukes' A or B1 stages who have an estimated 5-year survival of greater than 90% and 85%, respectively.

Dukes' B2 lesions have a 5-year survival of 70% to 75% while Dukes' C has 45% to 60%. Adjuvant therapy of B2 disease has not shown survival benefit although a trend favoring adjuvant therapy with 5-fluorouracil (5-FU) and levamisole was seen in the Intergroup trial. Prognostic factors identifying patients with B2 disease with increased risk of relapse are being identified in an effort to target this group for adjuvant trials. In one study, DNA

TABLE 28-1 MODIFIED ASTLER-COLLER STAGING SYSTEM CORRELATED WITH TNM (TUMOR, NODE, METASTASIS) STAGING SYSTEM

Dukes A-	Involving the submucosa (T1, N0, M0)
Dukes B1-	Invading the muscularis propria (T2, N0, M0)
Dukes B2-	Invasion through the muscularis propria into subserosal fat (T3, N0, M0)
Dukes B3-	Invasion of adjacent organs (T4, N0, M0)
Dukes C1-	Depth of invasion + lymph node involvement (T2, N1, M0, T2, N2, M0)
Dukes C2-	Same as B2 + nodes (T3-4, N1-2, M0)
Dukes C3-	Same as B3 + nodes (T4, N1-2, M0)
Dukes D-	Distant metastases

TABLE 28-2 FOLLOW UP

Physical examination every 4 months for 3 years, every 6 months for 2 years, then annually.
CBC, liver function tests, CEA at each visit (omit CEA after 5 years).
Colonoscopy at 6 months to 1 year after surgery, then every 3 years.
Chest x-ray annually.
CT scans or special studies as indicated by symptoms and CEA, etc.

Abbreviations: CEA, Carcinoembryonic antigen; CT, computed tomography

aneuploidy and high S phase (>20%) were been shown to be prognostic factors in predicting recurrence in B2 disease; 37% recurrence in aneuploid/high S phase tumors versus 20% in diploid low S phase tumors. Deletion of chromosome 18 in B2 tumors was associated with 5-year survival of 50% while the absence of this finding was associated with 90% 5-year survival. Although no definite conclusions can be reached, patients with B2 disease should be treated in clinical trials to establish a benefit for adjuvant therapy which cannot be recommended routinely.

The Intergroup trial did show both disease free and overall survival benefit for Dukes' C cancer with 5-FU and levamisole compared to observation or levamisole alone. There was a 41% reduction in relative recurrence rate and 33% reduction in relative risk of mortality compared to no treatment.

The optimum drug combination for adjuvant chemotherapy is being defined. 5-FU and leucovorin have been studied by 4 different groups in Dukes' B2 and C tumors and all 4 studies show significant improvements in disease-free survival and 3 show overall survival benefit with a trend toward improved survival in the fourth study. The use of a monoclonal antibody to colonic epithelial cell surface cytokeratin has shown benefit in disease-free and overall survival, and the effect of adding this antibody to 5-FU-based adjuvant therapy is being tested. Outside of a clinical trial, pending follow-up of 5-FU/leucovorin-based therapy, 5-FU/levamisole for 1 year should be used adjuvantly for Dukes' C adenocarcinoma of the colon.

Detection of Recurrences (Post-Treatment Follow-up Table 28-2)

Eighty percent of all recurrences occur in the first 2 years after surgery. Intensive follow-up at 3- to 4-month intervals during the first 3 years is therefore recommended. Thereafter, follow-up at 6-month intervals for 2 years and then annually are sufficient. The frequency of colonoscopic surveillance is debatable, but because of low rates of suture-line recurrence, after the initial postoperative evaluation, 3-year intervals are adequate to detect new primaries. Serial CEA measurements at these time points may identify a small population (3%) of patients who benefit from surgical resection of recurrent isolated metastatic disease, usually in the liver. Studies assessing the effect of intensive postoperative follow-up on overall survival have not shown a survival benefit associated with this strategy except in subgroup analysis. Whether patients with Dukes A and B1 lesions require less intensive follow-up is not known. Large trials are underway to better answer this question.

Resection of metastatic disease isolated to the liver has been associated with improved survival (34 month median, 25% to 30% 5-year survival) and is recommended when feasible. The number of lesions that can be resected is controversial but less than 3 lesions in the same lobe has the best prognosis. Liver metastases at diagnosis or within 1 year of diagnosis have a 27% to 30% 5-year survival compared to 42% when the metastases are detected greater than 1 year after diagnosis. Reresection of hepatic metastases can also be beneficial with 3-year survivals of 33%.

Palliation

Treatment of unresectable/metastatic colon cancer is palliative. Responses of 35% to 50% are reported with minimal prolongation of survival in some studies, with 5-FU and leucovorin compared to 5-FU alone. Meta-analysis of 9 randomized trials with 5-FU versus 5-FU and leucovorin in differing doses does not confirm a survival advantage. The optimal doses of 5-FU and leucovorin are unknown.*

The use of hepatic arterial infusional chemotherapy with fluorodeoxyuridine has been shown to prolong survival compared to no treatment or single agent 5-FU in a prospective trial. However, comparison with 5-FU/leucovorin has not been done. Additionally, placement of implantable pumps is limited to special centers and therefore not widely available.

*Irinotecan (CPT-11) has shown promise in metastatic disease with response rates of 23% in pretreated patients. Optimal dose and schedule is being determined.

TABLE 28-3 AMERICAN CANCER SOCIETY GUIDELINES FOR COLORECTAL CANCER SCREENING

From age 40—Annual DRE
From age 50—Annual fecal occult blood testing (FOBT) and DRE
Flexible sigmoidoscopy every 3–5 years

Abbreviations: DRE, digital rectal exam.

We recommend entering patients into trials of new agents to find a drug or combination of drugs that will enhance survival in metastatic colon cancer.

Unresectable primary tumor should be managed with a diverting colostomy/ileostomy if possible.

SCREENING

Early detection/screening for colon carcinoma is an important issue but the cost/benefit of screening will not be addressed in this chapter. The American Cancer Society recommendations for screening are found in Table 28-3. Patients at high risk with familial syndromes or inflammatory bowel disease should be screened more intensively (familial polyposis and nonpolyposis cancer syndromes, polyps, previous colon cancer)—screening should commence at an earlier age. In addition to FOBT and DRE, colonoscopy should be added at 1-to-2 year intervals. Figure 28-1 summarizes our recommendations for the management of colon cancer. Recommended strategies are formulated on high quality evidence (level I and II) except for surgery in recurrent/metastatic diseases for which supporting data are of level III evidence.

SUGGESTED READINGS

Advanced Colorectal Cancer Meta-Analysis Project: Modulation of fluorouracil by leucovorin in patients with advanced colorectal cancer: evidence in terms of response rate. J Clin Oncol 10:896, 1992

Ballantyne GH, Modlin IM: Postoperative followup for colorectal cancer: who are we kidding? [Editorial] J Clin Gastroenterol 10:359, 1988

Bruinvels DJ, Stiggelbout AM, Kievet J et al: Followup of patients with colorectal cancer: a meta-analysis. Ann Surg 219:174, 1993

Bulow S, Svendsen LB, Mellemgaard A: Metachronous colorectal carcinoma. Br J Surg 77:502, 1990

Erlichman C, Marsoni S, Seitz J et al: Event free and overall survival is increased by FUFA in resected B and C colon cancer: a prospective pooled analysis of 3 randomized trials, abstracted. Proc Am Soc Clin Oncol 13:562,1994

Francini G, Petrioli R, Lorenzini L et al: Folinic acid and fluorouracil as adjuvant therapy in colon cancer. Gastroenterology 106:899, 1994

Hughes K, Simon R, Songhorabodi S et al: Resection of the liver for colorectal carcinoma metastases: a multiinstitutional study of indications for resection: Registry of hepatic metastases. Surgery 103:278, 1988

Jen J, Kim H, Piantadosi S et al: Allelic loss of chromosome 18 and prognosis in colorectal cancer. N Engl J Med 331:213, 1994

Mayer RJ, O'Connell MJ, Tepper JE et al: Status of adjuvant therapy for colorectal cancer. J Nat Can Inst 81:1359, 1989

Mettlin C, Dodd GD: The American Cancer Society Guidelines for the cancer-related check up: an update. Ca 41:279, 1991

Moertel CG, Loprinzi CL, Witzig TE et al: The dilemma of stage B2 colon cancer: is adjuvant therapy justified, abstracted. Proc Am Soc Clin Oncol 9:108, 1990

Moertel CG, Fleming TR, MacDonald JS et al: An evaluation of the carcinoembryonic antigen (CEA) test for monitoring patients with resected colon cancer. JAMA 270:943, 1993

Moertel C, Fleming T, MacDonald J et al: Fluorouracil plus levamisole as effective adjuvant therapy after resection of stage II colon carcinoma: a final report. Ann Intern Med 122:321, 1995

Moertel CG, Fleming TR, MacDonald JS, Haller DG et al: Intergroup study of fluorouracil plus levamisole as adjuvant therapy for stage II/Dukes B2 colon cancer. J Clin Oncol 13:2936, 1995

NIH Consensus Conference: Adjuvant therapy for patients with colon and rectal cancer. JAMA 264:1444, 1990

Nordlinger B, Vaillant JC, Guiguet M et al: Survival benefit of repeat liver resections for recurrent colorectal metastases: 143 cases. J Clin Oncol 12:1491, 1994

O'Connell M, Maillard J, MacDonald J et al: An intergroup trial of intensive course 5FU and low dose leucovorin as surgical adjuvant therapy for high risk colon cancer, abstracted. Proc Am Soc Clin Oncol 12:552, 1993

Poon MA, O'Connell MJ, Moertel CG et al: Biochemical modulation of fluorouracil: evidence of significant improvement in survival and quality of life in patients with advanced colorectal carcinoma. J Clin Oncol 7:1407, 1989

Reithmuller G, Schneider-Gadicke E, Schlimok G et al: Randomized trial of monoclonal antibody for adjuvant therapy of resected Dukes' C colorectal carcinoma. Lancet 343:1177, 1994

Rosen CB, Nagorney DM, Taswell HF et al: Perioperative blood transfusions and determinants of survival after resection for metastatic colorectal carcinoma. Ann Surg 216:493, 1992

Rothenberg ML, Eckardt JR, Kuhn JG et al: Phase II trial of irinotecan in patients with progressive or rapidly recurrent colorectal cancer. J Clin Oncol 14:1128, 1996

Rougier P, Laplanche A, Huguier M et al: Hepatic arterial infusion of Floxuridine in patients with liver metastases from colorectal carcinoma: long term results of a prospective randomized trial. J Clin Oncol 10:1112, 1992

Steele G Jr: Follow-up plans after treatment of primary rectum and colon cancer. World J Surg 15:583, 1991

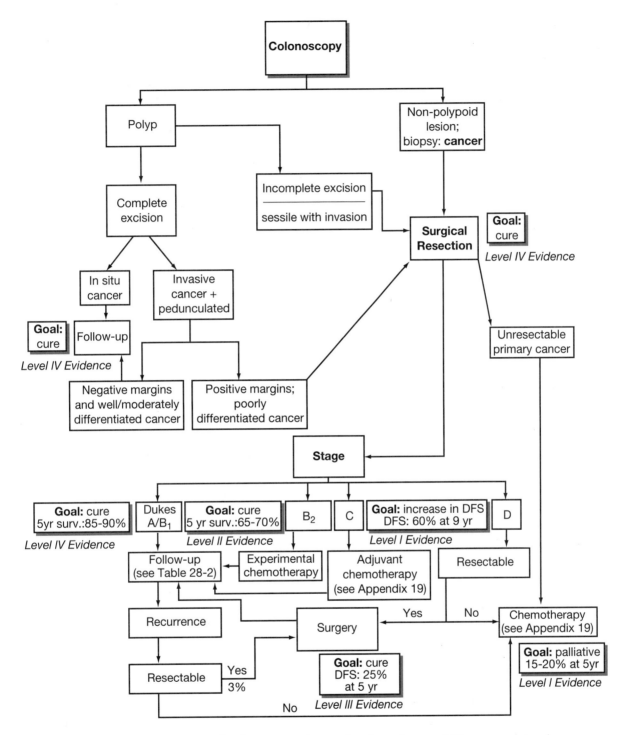

FIGURE 28-1 *Management of colon cancer. Determination of resectability represents a key reasoning principle in the management of colon cancer. The goal of treatment is cure in early stages (A, B), prolongation of survival in intermediate stage (C) and improvement in the quality of life in advanced stages (D). The recommended strategy is based on high-level experimental evidence (levels I and II) in the management of stage C, level IV in stage D, and solid nonexperimental evidence on the curative role of surgery in early stages of colon cancer. The role of surgery for metastatic disease is based on level III evidence. (See Appendix 19 for practical details on the management of colon cancer.)*

29 Rectal Cancer

Baby O. Jose

Incidence: 14/100,000/year

Goal of the treatment: Cure in early stages (A and B1); prolongation of survival in stages B2, B3, and C; palliation in stage D

Main modality of treatment: Surgery in early stages; surgery plus adjuvant radiation and chemotherapy in stage B2, B3, and C; observation versus chemotherapy in stage D of colon cancer

Prognosis (5 year survival):

Stage A: 88%–93%
Stage B: 71%–79%
Stage C: 29%–41%
Stage D: ~5%

Adenocarcinoma of colon and rectum is estimated to occur in 160,000 persons in the United States and causes approximately 60,000 deaths. The male to female ratio is almost equal. Patients with inflammatory disease of the bowel, familial polyposis, and Gardner's syndrome are at high risk for these cancers. Many etiologic factors, such as dietary fiber, fat intake, and bile acids, are studied in this disease.

SIGNS AND SYMPTOMS

The principal symptoms of rectal cancer include bleeding, changes in bowel habits, and change in the caliber of stool. On extensive disease, pain is associated with infiltration to the nerves. Digital rectal examination is important to diagnose and evaluate the extent of the disease. The recommended guidelines for further work-up, staging, management, and follow-up are shown in Figure 29-1. The current tumor, node, metastasis (TNM) staging is defined in Table 29-1.

SUGGESTED FOLLOW-UP GUIDELINES

A history and physical examination should be done every three months for the first two to three years, then every six months for the next two years. Follow-up CEA level, if elevated before surgery, is useful every three months for two to three years, then every six months for the next two years.

Yearly chest x-ray and liver profile need to be done for five years. Colonoscopy is recommended at six months to one year and then yearly for up to five years.

ADJUVANT THERAPY

The adjuvant therapy of rectal cancer has been defined by both randomized and nonrandomized studies. Twenty to forty percent of the patients with tumors extending through the bowel wall will get local recurrence. Forty to sixty percent of the patients with tumors extending through the bowel wall and with positive lymph nodes will get local/

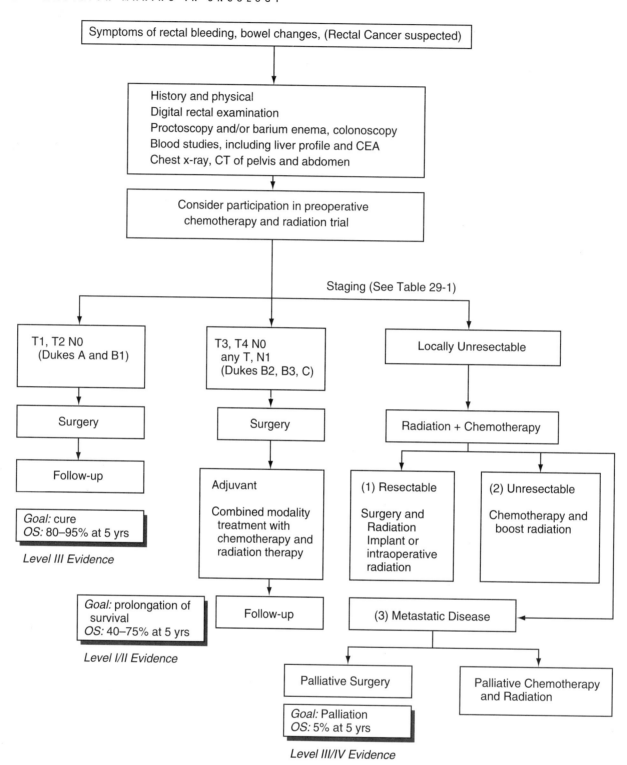

FIGURE 29-1 *Management of rectal cancer. The approach is stage-dependent. Goal of treatment in early stages (A and B1) is cure; goal of treatment in stages B2, B3, and C is prolongation of survival and in metastatic disease is palliation. Recommended strategy is based on level I and II evidence. Trials are underway to address issue of neoadjuvant treatment in rectal cancer (see text for details). (See also Appendix 20 for details on treatment; see Chapter 28 and Appendix 19 for treatment of metastatic colorectal cancer.) Abbreviations: OS, overall survival.*

TABLE 29-1 AMERICAN JOINT COMMITTEE ON STAGING SYSTEM FOR COLORECTAL CANCER

Primary tumor (T)

TX	Primary tumor cannot be assessed
T0	No evidence of primary tumor
Tis	Carcinoma in situ
T1	Tumor invades submucosa
T2	Tumor invades muscularis propria
T3	Tumor invades through the muscularis propria sub serosa or into nonperitonealized perirectal tissues
T4	Tumor perforates the visceral peritoneum or invades other organs or structures

Regional lymph nodes (N)

NX	Regional lymph nodes cannot be assessed
N0	No regional lymph node metastasis
N1	Metastasis in one to three pericolic or perirectal lymph nodes
N2	Metastasis in 4 or more pericolic or perirectal nodes
N3	Metastasis in any lymph node along the count of a lymph named vascular trunk

Distant metastasis (M)

MX	Presence of distant metastasis cannot be assessed
M0	No distant metastasis
M1	Distant metastasis

Stage grouping

Stage 0	TIS	N0	M0
Stage I	T1	N0	M0-Dukes-A
	T2	N0	M0-Dukes-B[1]
Stage II	T3	N0	M0-Dukes-B[2]
	T4	N0	M0-Dukes-B[3]
Stage III	Any T	N1	M0-Dukes-C
	Any T	N2, N3	M0
Stage IV	Any T	Any N	M

Abbreviations: T, primary tumor; N, regional lymph nodes; M, distant metastasis.

regional recurrence. The timing of the adjuvant treatment is being studied by ongoing preoperative and postoperative clinical trials.

PREOPERATIVE TREATMENT

A trial of concurrent preoperative irradiation (45 Gy), bolus 5-fluorouracil (5-FU), and low-dose leucovorin was done by the Europeon Organization for Research and Treatment of Cancer (EORTC) group. The study included 73 patients and showed acceptable toxicity and better results. Based on this data, (EORTC) is conducting a four arm randomized trial with preoperative radiation therapy (45 Gy) as the standard arm. This study will determine if 5-FU/leucovorin either preoperatively or postoperatively is superior to preoperative radiation therapy alone. Two other trials testing preoperative chemo-therapy and irradiation are intergroup 0147 Radiation Therapy Oncology Group [RTOG-9401] and National Surgical Adjuvant Breast and Bowel Project (NSABP) R-03. The regimen includes combination of 5-FU and leucovorin with irradiation up to a dose of 50.4 Gy either as preoperative or postoperative regimen.

POSTOPERATIVE TREATMENT

Multiple studies have reported on postoperative combined modality. The Gastrointestinal Tumor Study Group (GITSG) randomized 202 patients into postoperative radiation therapy, 5-FU/Me CCnu, radiation therapy plus 5-FU/MeCCnu, or surgery alone. Patients who received radiation therapy plus chemotherapy showed a survival benefit compared with surgery alone (54% vs. 27%, $P = .005$). Patients in the radiation therapy or chemotherapy alone arm showed no survival benefit compared with surgery alone. In the Mayo/North Central Cancer Treatment Group (NCCTG) trial, 204 patients were randomized to postoperative radiation therapy versus postoperative radiation therapy plus 5-FU/MeCCnu. Patients who had radiation therapy plus chemotherapy had a significant decrease in local failure (14% vs. 25%, $P = .036$) and distant failure (29% vs. 46%, $P = .011$), and an increase in five-year disease-free survival (DFS) (63% vs. 42%, $P = .016$) and overall survival (57% vs. 48% $P = 0.025$) compared with the radiation therapy control arm.

In the NSABP R-01 trial, 528 patients were randomized to postoperative MeCCNU, vincristine, 5-FU chemotherapy, radiation therapy, or surgery alone. For the total group there was a significant five year DFS (42% vs. 30%, $P = .006$) and overall survival (53% vs. 43%, $P = .05$) in patients who had chemotherapy. Patients who had radiation therapy had a better pelvic control rate (84% vs. 75%, $P = .06$) compared with surgery alone. In the subset analysis, this benefit with chemotherapy was shown only in males, not in females. In NSABP R-02, patients based on gender were randomized to MOF with or without radiation therapy or 5-FU/LV with or without radiation therapy. Men were randomized to all 4 arms, while women were randomized to 5-FU/LV with or without radiation therapy arms. The preliminary results show a significant decrease in local failure in the 2 arms with chemotherapy and radiation therapy (7% vs. 11%, $P = .045$) versus the two arms that had chemotherapy alone. In a large intergroup trial, radiation therapy with protracted venous infusion of 5-FU improved both local control and survival compared with radiation therapy and bolus FU.

An ongoing large, intergroup trial uses protracted FU during radiation therapy for all patients, with randomization to several forms of additional adjuvant chemotherapy before and after radiation therapy.

AVOIDANCE OF COMPLICATIONS

The side effects of surgery and adjuvant-combined treatment can be minimized by limiting the volume of small bowel in the pelvis by omental sling, by using multiple custom-made fields for radiation therapy, and by adjusting the dose of chemotherapy. With the ongoing trials, the guidelines in the management of rectal cancer should be more defined, and a better outcome is expected.

SUGGESTED READINGS

Abeloff MD, Armitage JO, Lichter AS, Niederhuber JE: Clinical Oncology. Churchill Livingstone, New York, 1995

Bosset J F et al: Eur J Cancer 29:476–486, 1993

DeVita VT Jr, Hellman S, Rosenberg SA: Cancer, Principles and Practices of Oncology. 4th Ed. Lippincott-Raven, Philadelphia, 1993

Fisher B, Wolmark N, Rockette H et al: Postoperative adjuvant chemotherapy or radiation therapy for rectal cancer: results for NSABP protocol R-01. J Natl Cancer Inst 80:21–29, 1988

Fuchs CS, Mayer RJ. Adjuvant chemotherapy for colon and rectal cancer. Semin Oncol 22:472–487, 1995

Gastrointestinal Tumor Group: Adjuvant therapy of colon cancer—results of a prospectively randomized trial. N Engl J Med 310:737–743, 1984

Gastrointestinal Tumor Group: Prolongation of the disease-free survival in surgically treated rectal carcinoma. N Engl J Med 312:1465–1472, 1985

Krook JE, Moertal CG, Gunderson LL: N Engl J Med 324:709–715, 1991

Minsky BD: Lower Gastrointestinal Malignancies. ASTRO, 1995

O'Connell M, Martenson J, Wieand H et al: Improving adjuvant therapy for rectal cancer by coming protracted-infusion, fluorouracil with radiation therapy after curative surgery. N Engl J Med 331:502–507, 1994

Perez CA, Brady, Luther W: Principles and Practices of Radiation Oncology. 2nd Ed. Lippincott-Raven, Philadelphia, 1992

Rockette H, Deutsch M, Petrelli N et al: Effect of postoperative radiation therapy when used with adjuvant chemotherapy in Dukes' B and C rectal cancer: results from NSABP R-02 (abstracted). Proc Am Soc Clin Oncol 13:193, 1994

Silverberg E, Boring CL, Squries TF: Cancer statistics, 1990. CA 40:9, 1990

30 Cancer of the Anal Region

Biljana Baškot

Incidence: 6/1,000,000 population in whites; highest incidence is among nonwhite females (9/1,000,000).

Goal of the treatment: Cure

Main modality of treatment: Combined radiation therapy and chemotherapy

Prognosis: Primary disease: 5 years' disease-free Survival: 65%–80%
Persistent/recurrent disease: 40%–50% disease-free survival

Carcinoma of the anus is an uncommon malignancy composing only 1% to 2% of all large bowel tumors, with its highest incidence among nonwhite middle-aged women (ratio of females to males, 2:1). Recent studies have shown increasing incidence among young homosexual men. According to surveillance, epidemiology, and end results (SEER) data, the average annual age-adjusted incidence rate is 0.6 cases per 100,000. Nonwhite females show the highest incidence of 9 per 1,000,000; the lowest incidence is among white and Hispanic males 5 per 1,000,000.

ETIOLOGY

Immunosuppression seems to be a major factor for increased risk of anal cancer, possibly through viral mechanisms. Current reports show an increased incidence of anal cancer among people who are positive for human immunodefiency virus HIV AIDS. Considerable evidence implicates human papilloma virus (HPV) (especially type HPV-16) in the pathogenesis of anal cancer, and it is known to

be associated with invasive squamous cell carcinoma. Other infections, such as *Chlamydia*, herpes simplex virus (HSV) type 2, and gonorrhea, are also associated with an increased incidence of anal cancer, as are chronic anorectal diseases (e.g., anal fistulas, fissures, abscesses, and leukoplakia) and several precancerous conditions (e.g., Paget's and Bowen's disease). Cigarette smoking and alcohol intake are also well known etiologic factors.

DIAGNOSIS

Every suspicious perineal lesion or one that fails to respond to standard treatment within one month should be biopsied. Full thickness biopsy should be done in the center and at the edges of the lesion. There is much confusion about classification of anal malignancies because of the complex anatomy of this region and lack of accurate and universally accepted anatomic definition of anal canal and anal margin. *Accurate localization and staging of the lesion is of primary importance for further management and prognosis.* Cancer of anal area may be

215

divided into (1) carcinoma of the anal canal and (2) carcinoma of the anal margin. The World Health Organization (WHO) accepts the following anatomic definition of anal cancer:

1. Anal canal neoplasms are lesions arising from the anorectal ring proximally (including the anal transitional zone) to the dentate line distally. 2. Anal margin neoplasms are lesions arising distal to the dentate line to the junction of perineal skin with the hair bearing skin of the buttocks. (See Fig. 30-1.)

HISTOLOGY

Most carcinomas are squamous cell or variants (epidermoid, mucoepidermoid, transitional, basaloid) or adenocarcinoma. *The variations in squamous cell histologies do not significantly impact on long-term survival or response to treatment.*

Adenocarcinoma small cell carcinoma, and melanoma are very rare histologic types characterized by an aggressive course and poorer prognosis than squamous cell cancers. They are treated and staged as squamous cell carcinoma. There are no comparative studies that would allow analysis of risks and benefits of different treatment options according to histologic subtypes.

STAGING

After confirmation of diagnosis, staging is important for proper management and to predict outcome. Table 30-1 shows the American Joint Committee on Cancer/International Union Against Cancer AJCC/UICC staging system for anal cancer. The complex structure of the area makes estimation of the size of the tumor and the depth of invasion difficult. Detailed examination under anesthesia is sometimes

necessary, and computed tomography (CT) of the pelvis is frequently used. A new modality used in pretreatment staging is transrectal ultrasonography (TRUS). This technique enables evaluation of tumor size, depth of invasion, and tumor volume. Some authors classify tumors by depth of invasion using TRUS as

1. UT1   Tumor of anal epithelium and subendothelial connective tissue (mucosa and submucosa)

2. UT2   Tumor of sphincter muscle/muscularis propria

3. UT3   Tumor penetrating sphincter muscle/muscularis propria

4. UT4   Tumor growing into surrounding organs of the pelvis

Two-thirds of T1–2 clinical tumors had TRUS evidence of anorectal muscular wall penetration (UT 3-UT4). TRUS is useful and should complement digital examination and CT of the pelvis in staging of anal cancer. It appears accurate in predicting response to therapy.

PROGNOSTIC FACTORS

Location of the Tumor   Cancer of the anal margin behaves like epidermoid skin cancer.

Histologic Type   No difference exists in survival for patients with various types of anal cancer, except for small-cell cancer and melanoma.

Tumor Size   Tumor size correlates well with clinical outcome. In some studies tumor thickness was a strong predictor of disease outcome; tumors 10 mm thick had 85% five-year survival in contrast to

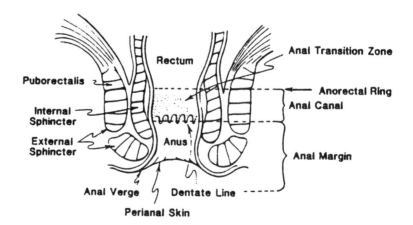

FIGURE 30-1 *Anatomy of the anus. Understanding anatomy of the anal area is an important reasoning principle in management of anal cancer. Accurate localization and staging of the lesion (see Table 30-1) is of key importance in the treatment of anal cancer. (From Cohen AM, Winawer SJ [eds]: Cancer of the Colon, Rectum and Anus. McGraw Hill, New York, 1995, with permission.)*

TABLE 30-1 AJCC/UICC STAGING SYSTEM FOR CARCINOMA OF THE ANAL CANAL AND ANAL MARGIN

Primary Tumor (T)

Tx	Primary tumor cannot be assessed
T0	No evidence of primary tumor
Tis	Carcinoma in situ
T1	≤ 2 cm in greatest dimension
T2	> 2 cm but ≤ 5 cm in greatest dimension
T3	> 5 cm in greatest dimension

Anal canal

T4	Invading adjacent structures: vagina, urethra, or bladder. Involvement of sphincter muscle alone is not classified as T4

Anal margin

T4	Invading deep extradermal structure: skeletal muscle or bone

Regional Lymph Node Involvement (N)

Nx	Regional lymph nodes cannot be assessed
N0	No regional lymph node involvement

Anal canal

N1	Metastases to perirectal lymph nodes
N2	Metastases to unilateral internal iliac and/or unilateral inguinal lymph nodes
N3	Metastases to perirectal and inguinal lymph nodes and/or bilateral internal iliac and/or bilateral inguinal lymph nodes

Anal margin

N1	Metastases to ipsilateral inguinal lymph nodes

Distant Metastases (M)

Mx	Distant metastases cannot be assessed
M0	No distant metastases
M1	Distant metastases present

STAGING

Stage 0	Tis	N0	M0
Stage I	T1	N0	M0
Stage II	T2	N0	M0
	T3	N0	M0
Anal canal			
Stage IIIA	T4	N0	M0
	T1–3	N1	M0
Stage IIIB	T4	N1	M0
	Any T	N1–3	M0
Anal margin			
Stage III	T4	N0	M0
	Any T	N1	M0
Both			
Stage IV	Any T	Any N	M1

Abbreviations: AJCC/UICC, American Joint Committee on Cancer/International Union Against Cancer.

tumors 21 to 30 mm thick whose five-year survival rate was only 25%. Although tumor size appears to be an important prognostic factor, the thickness and depth of invasion seems to be more predictive of final outcome of disease.

Depth of Invasion Depth of invasion seems to be an important independent prognostic variable, although it is not entirely clear whether tumor size or depth of invasion influences survival directly. For now, tumor size is easier to assess clinically. New modalities such as TRUS will help significantly in accurate staging and emphasize the importance of depth of invasion as a prognostic factor.

Lymph Node Involvement Lymph node involvement, especially inguinal, has been associated with poor prognosis. Inguinal node disease was found to parallel tumor size and to influence outcome directly.

DNA Ploidy DNA ploidy is an excellent predictor of the biologic behavior of tumors. Nondiploid tumors tend to be poorly differentiated, invasive, and associated with early metastases. Although not a widely accepted practice, flow cytometry might be a useful tool in staging and prognostication.

To summarize, the three most important prognostic factors are location, depth of invasion/tumor size, and lymph node status.

MANAGEMENT OF ANAL CANCER

TREATMENT OF PRIMARY DISEASE

The main modality of treatment of anal cancer is a *combination of chemotherapy and radiation therapy*. Goals of combined chemoradiation treatment is cure and preservation of anorectal function. Below are discussed management options in the treatment of anal cancer.

Primary Surgical Therapy Currently surgery is not the primary therapy of an anal cancer. It has been replaced by less mutilating and more successful approaches. However, lesions that are less than 2 cm in diameter may still be successfully treated by local excision with clear margins. Five-year survival of patients with small lesions treated by surgery alone ranges from 25% to 83%. This treatment modality has a high recurrence rate of 63% for anal margin and 91% for anal canal region. *Melanoma* of the anal canal is rare and aggressive. Tumor thickness and the patients' survival after treatment may not correlate. Most patients with melanoma of the anal canal have been treated with abdominoperineal resection (APR) with generally unsatisfactory results. Other treatment modalities have been sporadically used and showed less promise than surgery (see Ch. 13). *Small cell cancer* has a high propensity for

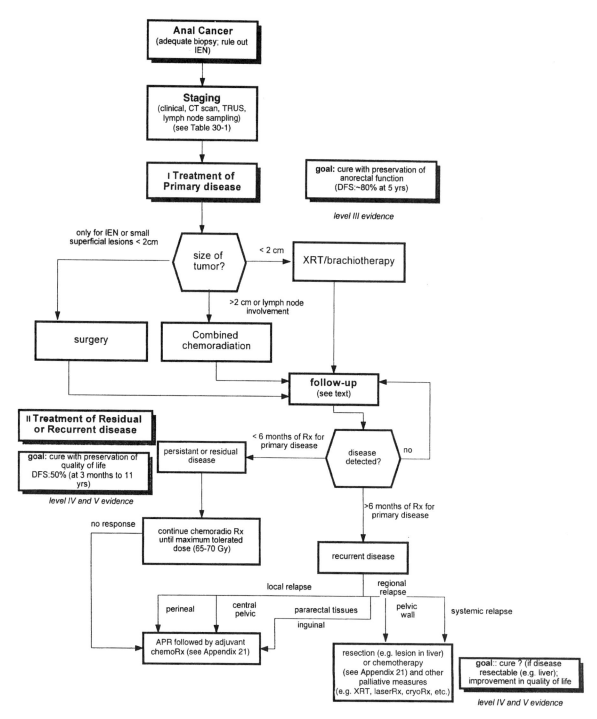

FIGURE 30-2 *Algorithm for the management of anal cancer. An approach to the management of patients with anal cancer largely depends on histology (squamous vs nonsquamous). In patients with nonmetastatic epidermoid cancer, the goal of treatment is cure with combined radiation and chemotherapy. In metastatic disease, the goal of the treatment is palliation. Recommended strategy for the treatment of primary disease is mainly based on level III evidence and for treatment of residual/recurrent disease on level IV and V evidence. IEN, intraepithelial neoplasia; APR, abdominoperineal resection; XRT, radiation therapy Rx, treatment; DFS, disease-free survival; TRUS, transrectal ultrasonography. (See also Appendix 21 for practical details on the management of anal cancer.)*

early remote metastases, consistent with features of lung cancer of the same histology and is treated and staged as small cell cancer.

Radiation Without Chemotherapy Over the past 20 years, several cooperative group studies consistently reported high cure rates with preservation of anorectal function using radiation alone or combined chemoradiation. The literature reports cure rates (in terms of 5-year survival) of about 70% with 90% preservation of anorectal function. Radiation modalities include interistitial and external beam irradiation.

Interstitial Irradiation Interstitial irradiation is used with best results in small primary cancers. It is infrequently used as the only method of treatment of tumors larger than 2 cm in diameter because of its inability to control growth of regional node metastases and the need for relatively high doses of irradiation, which are associated with unacceptably high side effects (the standard approach is a single-implant therapy 40–50 Gy over 3–4 days or 55 Gy over 7 days).

External Beam Irradiation External beam irradiation has frequently been used as a first-line treatment of anal cancer. It covers both the area of primary tumor and regional lymph nodes, delivering a relatively homogeneous dose. Radiation doses in the range of 50 Gy over 4 weeks to 65 Gy over 6 to 7 weeks are commonly prescribed. To avoid major side effects, the technique of direct perineal portal was introduced and conventional fractionation was modified so that the patient would have scheduled treatment breaks. There was no reduction in control or cure rates with these changes, and the higher doses of irradiation were better tolerated. Survival rates at 5 years in series that included smaller and larger tumors were 45% to 65%. Complications associated with external beam radiation could be acute, in the form of perineal skin dermatitis, irritation of anal and rectal mucosa with diarrhea and tenesmus. Chronic complications range from severe proctitis and rectal bleeding to milder problems, manifested only by telangiectasias or urgency of defecation. Overall anorectal function is preserved by about 65% in all patients and in about 85% of those whose cancer was eradicated by radiation. Despite apparent effectiveness of radiation therapy in the treatment of anal cancer, the management, of anal cancer has slowly evolved to combine chemotherapy with radiation therapy (chemoradiation).

Combined Chemoradiation Since 1974, chemoradiation has been successfully introduced and has shown the best results in cure rate, years of survival, quality of life, and preservation, of anorectal function. Nigro introduced the first such protocol, which combined radiation therapy with mitomycin (MMC) and continuous infusion of 5-fluorouracil (5-FU). Overall disease-free survival at 2 years after treatment ranged from 65% to 85%. This original protocol has been modified over the years. Doses of radiation were increased for better control of larger (4–5 cm) cancers, and a second 5-FU infusion, which was included in the initial protocol, was omitted. However, most of the protocols still use 5-FU and MMC as the chemotherapeutic agents of choice.

The optimum radiation dose and technique of chemotherapy are not yet known. Most data are derived from single-arm prospective studies (level III evidence). However, the Radiation Therapy Oncology Group (RTOG) completed a randomized trial in 1993 (level I evidence) that evaluated the merits of 5-FU with or without MMC with irradiation. Their initial report did not recognize a great advantage of the addition of MMC to the protocol. A recently published RTOG phase III randomized study showed that MMC in combination with 5-FU and radiotherapy favorably affects therapeutic response and disease-free survival (73% at 4 yrs) in all patients with squamous cell cancer of the anal canal except possibly those with very small primary tumors where high incidence of side effects (neutropenia) does not justify its use. However, no significant difference in overall survival was noted. (See Appendix 21.)

Other combined protocols using bleomycin or platinum were not based on randomized trials, and further studies are needed to compare them with widely used radiation + 5-FU + MMC treatment regimens.

Although many centers prefer chemoradiation to radiation alone, no completed randomized trials support this preference. A multicenter randomized study by United Kingdom Coordinating Committee for Cancer Research (UKCCCR) and European Organization for the Research and Treatment of Cancer (EORTC) is currently testing these two approaches against each other. Preliminary reports suggest that the addition of 5-FU and MMC improves local tumor control. The benefit was seen mostly with larger tumors. No significant difference was found in tumors up to 3 to 4 cm in diameter.

Today chemoradiation is considered first-line treatment for anal cancer, especially for lesions

TABLE 30-2 SELECTED RESULTS OF CONCURRENT RADIATION, 5-FLUOROURACIL, AND MITOMYCIN C

Reference	Chemotherapy		Radiation Grays/Fractions/Time	Primary Tumor Control		Regional Node Control	5-Year Survival
	5-FU[a]	Mitomycin C					
Leichman et al.	1000 mg/m^2/24 h IVI d 1–4 and d 29–32	15 mg/m^2 IVB d 1	30 Gy/15/d 1–21	31/34 (91%) (≤5 cm)	7/10 (70%) (>5 cm)	NS	80%, crude
Sischy et al.	1,000 mg/m^2/24 h IVI d 2–5 and d 28–31	10 mg/m^2 IVB d 1	40.8 Gy/24/d 1–35	22/26 (85%) (>3 cm)	32/50 (64%) (≥3 cm)	NA	73%, 3 years actuarial
Cummings et al.	1,000 mg/m^2/24 h IVI d 1–4 and d 43–46	10 mg/m^2 IVB d 1 and d 43	48–50 Gy/24–20/d 1–58 (split course)	25/27 (93%) (≤5 cm)	16/20 (80%) (>5 cm or T)	4/5	65%, actuarial
Schneider et al.	1000 mg/m^2/24 h IVI d 1–4 and d 29–32	10 mg/m^2 IVB d 1 and d 29	50 Gy/25–28/d 1–35 ± boost	21/22 (95%) (≤5 cm)	14/19 (74%) (>5 cm or T4)	3/4	77%, actuarial
Papillon and Montbarbon 1987	600 mg/m^2/24 h IVI (120 h) d 1–5	12 mg/m^2 IVB d 1	42 Gy/10/d 1–19 plus interstitial boost 20 Gy d 78	No data in original publication	57/70 (81%) (≥4 cm)	NS	NS
Tanum et al. 1991	1,000 mg/m^2/24 h IVI d 1–4	10–15 mg/m^2 IVB d 1	50–54 Gy/25–27/d 1–35	28/30(93%) (>5 cm or T4)	42/56 (75%) (≤5 cm)	NS	72% actuarial
Cummings et al 1984	1,000 mg/m^2/24 h IVI d 1–4	10 mg/m^2 IVB d 1	50 Gy/20/d 1–28	3/3 (>5 cm or T4)	11/13(85%) (≤5 cm)	3/3	75%, actuarial
Doci et al. 1992	750 mg/m^2/24 h IVI (120 h) d 1–5/d 43–47/ d 85–85	15 mg/m^2 IVB d 1/d 43/d 85	54–60 Gy/30–33/d 1–53 (split course)	28/38 (74%) (≤5 cm)	9/17 (53%) (>5 cm)	8/8	81%, actuarial

[a]All infusions 96 hours, except where shown.

Abbreviations: d, day(s); h, hour(s); IVI, continuous intravenous infusion; IVB, intravenous bolus injection; NS, not stated; NA, not applicable; T_4, invading adjacent organs.

(From Cohen AM, Winawer SJ (eds): Cancer of the Colon, Rectum and Anus. McGraw Hill, New York, 1995, with permission.)

larger than 4 to 5 cm in diameter. For large but fortuitously located tumors, good local control with cure is still possible. Current protocols give high 5-year disease-free survival rates (up to 80% with combined treatment modality) and high likelihood of preservation of anorectal function, which has a tremendous influence on the quality of life (see Table 30-2 for results of combined treatment for anal cancer; for treatment protocols and orders, see Appendix 21).

Chemoradiation also controls regional *lymph node metastases* quite well, and their presence at the time of diagnosis is not a contraindication for this treatment modality.

Recommendations for chemotherapeutic treatment of anal cancer with distant metastases is based on single case reports or prospective single-arm studies with small numbers of patients observed.

Risk of severe side effects is increased with combined treatment. The skin of the perineum and anorectum, bowel mucosa and bone marrow are principally affected. Severe toxicity with Nigro's traditional protocol is 5% to 10% and could be modified by altering daily and total dose of irradiation. Overall, anorectal function is lost in 5% to 10% of patients because of late toxicity manifested as anal ulcerations, strictures with rectal bleeding, and incontinence.

For HIV-positive patients with anal cancer, goals of treatment are practically the same as for other patients. AIDS patients, however, have a shorter life span because of their underlying disease and are prone to severe side effects to chemoradiation, so ultimately treatment results are less satisfactory.

THERAPY OF PERSISTENT AND RECURRENT LOCAL DISEASE

About 20% of patients will not respond to the initial therapy or their disease will recur. Persistent disease is defined as that detected within 6 months of treatment; recurrent disease is that discovered more than 6 months after treatment. It is believed that local recurrence is caused by regrowth of irradiated, chemotherapy-resistant cells six or more months after initial treatment. There are still controversies about whether a complete response to initial treatment should be proved by biopsy of the area of original tumor or whether this should be reserved only for palpable or visible residual disease (see Follow-up).

Residual disease is usually *treated by* continuance of chemoradiation to the maximum of therapeutic dose or systemic postirradiation chemotherapy (65–70 Gy). This treatment modality

should be tried before resorting to APR for surgical salvage.

Recurrences usually present as

1. Local disease occurring in the perineal area

2. Local/regional disease involving muscle, perirectal fat, adjacent lymph nodes (central pelvis)

3. Local/regional disease involving inguinal nodes

4. Local/regional disease involving the pelvic wall

5. Systemic disease with visceral metastases amenable only for palliative therapy with abdominoperineal resection

A *"salvage" APR* is the treatment of choice for patients with resectable local, central pelvic, and inguinal recurrent disease, with curative potential. The practical aim of this therapy is removal of all tumor with histologically negative margins and preparation of an area for possible further local treatment with brachytherapy, additional external irradiation, or adjuvant chemotherapy.

Inguinal node metastases can be confirmed by aspiration biopsy or local lymph node excision and treated by radical lymphadenectomy. *Lymph node dissection* is done if lymph nodes are the only place of metastatic disease, with the five-year survival rate estimated at 60%.

In general, chemoradiation for recurrent and metastatic disease is of low efficacy, with the possible exception of pelvic recurrence of anal cancer that was initially treated by APR.

Chemotherapy may be used in cases of advanced residual (primary chemoradiation failure), recurrent (especially after surgery), and metastatic anal cancer. Various combinations of 5-FU, MMC platinum, bleomycin, adriamycin have been employed with limited and short-lived responses. The very small number of cases treated in this fashion makes evaluation of this modality difficult. So far, the most active regimens proved to be (1) sequential MTX, 5-FU, and leucovorin; (2) 5-FU infusion with cisplatinum, (3) weekly low-dose adriamycin, and (4) 5-FU infusion with MMC (Appendix 21).

All these regimens need further investigation through multicenter randomized trials to prove their real efficacy in treatment of advanced anal cancer.

Goal of Therapy The goal of therapy in metastatic disease is palliation. However, in one small retrospective study, 2 of 24 patients (8.3%) were free of disease at 6 and 42 months, respectively, after surgery for resectable metastatic disease in the liver. This implies that even in metastatic disease, cure can be an achievable goal in subset of these patients.

Recommendations for chemotherapeutic treatment of anal cancer with distant metastases is based on single-case reports or prospective single-arm studies with a small number of patients observed. Patients with a good performance status should be entered into clinical trials.

Palliative Approaches Nonresectional, palliative approaches are indicated for patients not considered candidates for surgery and mainly involve electrocoagulation, cryotherapy, and laser therapy. Palliative treatment aims to preserve quality of life by relieving the pain and obstruction and lessening mucous discharge and bleeding and should be individually tailored.

FOLLOW-UP

Follow-up includes detailed history and examination, liver function tests every 2 to 3 months for the first 3 years, then semiannually for 10 years, preferably, by the same physician. Important to be included is chest-x-ray and abdominopelvic computed tomography annually for the first 3 years. Any new growth six or more months after completion of the main therapeutic trial should be biopsied and examined by a pathologist. However, no final consensus on the exact timing of biopsy exists at this time. Some authors advocate a biopsy 6 to 8 weeks after completion of treatment; others advise against blind biopsies, believing that cancer cells that can be detected this way are not viable cells.

SUGGESTED READINGS

Brunet R, Sadek H, Vignoud J et al: Cisplatin(P) and 5 fluorouracil (5FU) for the neoadjuvant treatment of epidermoid anal carcinoma (EACC). Proc ASCO 9:104, 1990

Chadha M, Rosenblatt EA, Malamud S, Pisch J, Berson A: Squamous-cell carcinoma of the anus in HIV-positive patients. Dis Colon Rectum 37:1994

Cho CC, Taylor CW, Padmanabhan A et al: Squamous cell carcinoma of the anal canal: management with combined chemoradiation therapy. Dis Colon Rectum 34:675–678, 1991

Cohen, AM, Winawer SJ, Friedman MA, Gunderson LL: Cancer of the Colon, Rectum and Anus. McGraw Hill, New York, 1995

Cummings BJ: Concomitant radiotherapy and chemotherapy for anal cancer. Semin Oncol 19(suppl 11):102–108, 1992

Cummings B, Keane T, Thomas G, Harwood A, Rider W: Results and toxicity of the treatment of anal canal carcinoma by radiation therapy or radiation therapy and chemotherapy. Cancer 54:2062–2068, 1984

Daling JR, Weiss NS, Hislop G et al: Sexual practices, sexually transmitted diseases, and the incidence of anal cancer. N Engl J Med 317:973–977, 1987

Doci R, Zucali R, Bombelli L et al: Combined chemoradiation therapy for anal cancer: a report of 56 cases. Ann Surg 215:150–156, 1992

Fisher WB, Herbst KD, Sims JE, Critchfield CF: Metastatic cloacogenic carcinoma of the anus: sequential responses to Adriamycin and cis-dichlorodiammineplatinum(II). Cancer Treat Rep 62:91–97, 1978

Flam M, John M, Pajak TF et al: Role of mitomycin (MMC) incombination with fluorouracil (5-FU) and radiotherapy, and salvage chemoradiation in the definitive nonsurgical treatment of epidermoid carcinoma of the anal canal: results of a phase III randomized intergroup study. J Clin Oncol 14:2527–2539, 1996

Flam MS, John MJ, Peters T et al: Radiation and 5-fluorouracil (5-FU) vs radiation, 5-FU, mitomycin C (MMC) in the treatment of anal canal carcinoma: preliminary results of a phase II randomized RTOG/ECOG intergroup trial. Poc ASCO 12:192, 1993

Goldman S, Glimelius B, Norming U et al: Transanorectal ultrasonography in anal carcinoma: a prospective study of 21 patients. Acta Radiol 29:337–341, 1988

Holland JM, Swift PS: Tolerance of patients with human immunodeficiency virus and anal carcinoma to treatment with combined chemotherapy and radiation therapy. Radiology 193:251–254, 1994

Holly E, Whittemore AS, Aston DA et al: Anal cancer incidence: genital warts, anal fissure or fistula, hemorrhoids, and smoking. J Natl Cancer Inst 81:1726–1731, 1989

Lonogo WE, Vernava AM, Wade TP et al: Recurrent squamous cell carcinoma of the anal canal. Predictors of initial treatment failure and results of salvage therapy. Ann Surg 220:40–49, 1994

Martenson James A, Gunderson MS: External radiation therapy without chemotherapy in the management of anal cancer. Cancer 71:1736–1740, 1993

Melbye M, Cote TR, Kessler L, Gail M, Biggar RJ, and the AIDS-Cancer Working Group. High incidence of anal cancer among AIDS patients. Lancet 343:636–639, 1994

Miller EJ, Quan SHQ, Thaler HT: Treatment of squamous cell carcinoma of the anal canal. Cancer 67:2038–2041, 1991

Nigro ND, Gunter Seydel H, Considine B et al: Combined preoperative radiation and chemotherapy for squamous cell carcinoma of the anal canal. Cancer 51:1826–1829, 1983

Nigro ND, Viatkevicius VK, Buroker T, Bradley GT, Considine B: Combined therapy for cancer of the anal canal. Dis Colon Rectum 24:73–75, 1981

Nigro ND, Viatkevicius VK, Considine B Jr: Combined therapy for cancer of the anal canal: a preliminary report. Dis Colon Rectum 17:354–356, 1974

Palmer JG, Scholefield JH, Coates PJ et al: Anal cancer and human papillomaviruses. Dis Colon Rectum 32:1016–1022, 1989

Papillon J: Rectal and Anal Cancers. Springer-Verlag, New York, 1982

Papillon J, Montbarbon JF: Epidermoid carcinoma of the anal canal: a series of 276 cases. Dis Colon Rectum 30:324–333, 1987

Quan SHQ, Magill GB, Leaming RH et al: Multidisciplinary preoperative approach to the management of epidermoid carcinoma of the anus and anorectum. Dis Colon Rectum 21:89–91, 1978

Salem PA, Habboubi N, Anaissie E et al: Effectiveness of cisplatin in the treatment of anal squamous cell carcinoma. Cancer Treat Rep 69:1985

Salmon RJ, Fenton J, Asselain B et al: Treatment of epidermoid anal canal cancer. Am J Surg 147:43–48, 1984

Scott NA, Beart RW Jr, Weiland LH et al: Carcinoma of the canal and flow cytometric DNA analysis. Br J Cancer 60:56–58, 1989

Shank B, Cohen AM, Kelsen D: Cancer of the anal region. In DeVita V, Hellman S, Rosenberg S (eds): Principles and Practice of Oncology. 4th Ed. Lippincott-Raven, Philadelphia, 1993

Shepherd NA, Scholefield JH, Love SB et al: Prognostic factors in anal squamous carcinoma: a multivariate analysis of clinical, pathological, and flow cytometric parameters in 235 cases. Histopathology 16:545–555, 1990

Smith DE, Shah KH, Rao AR et al: Cancer of the anal canal: treatment with chemotherapy and low-dose radiation therapy. Radiology 191:569–572, 1994

Strauss RJ, Fazio V: Bowen's disease of the anal and perianal area: a report and analysis of twelve cases. Am J Surg 137:231–234, 1979

Tanum G, Tveit K, Karlsen KO, Hauer-Jensen M: Chemotherapy and radiation therapy for anal carcinoma. Survival and late morbidity. Cancer 67:2462–2466, 1991

Touboul E, Schlienger MN, Buffat L et al: Epidermoid carcinoma of the anal canal. Results of curative-intent radiation therapy in a series of 270 patients. Cancer 73:1569–1579, 1994

Wilking N, Petrelli N, Herrera L, Mittelman A: Phase II study of combination bleomycin, vincristine and high-dose methotrexate (BOM) with leucovorin rescue in advanced squamous cell carcinoma of the anal canal. Cancer Chemother Pharmacol 15:300–302, 1985

Zimm S, Wampler GL: Response of metastatic cloacogenic carcinoma to treatment with semustine. Cancer 48:2575–2576, 1981

31 Thyroid Carcinoma

Jane M. Weaver
Michael B. Flynn

Incidence: 2.4–4.0 per 100,000/year (female/male 3:1)

Goal of the treatment: Cure (differentiated types)

Main modality of treatment: Surgery

Prognosis (10-year survival): ~90%

In the United States, approximately 13,000 new thyroid cancers are diagnosed each year. Over the last two decades the incidence has increased from 2.4 to 4.0 cases per 100,000 population. Prior irradiation of the head and neck may be a factor in this increase. About 1,000 persons die each year in the United States of thyroid carcinoma, most from medullary, anaplastic, or invasive follicular cancers.

Thyroid cancer is classified as differentiated, medullary, or anaplastic (Tables 31-1 and 31-2). Together these account for 99% of all thyroid cancer. The differentiated thyroid cancers originate from the follicular cell and include papillary, follicular, and Hürthle cell neoplasms. Medullary carcinomas arise in the calcitonin-producing C cells and may be found as part of the MEN IIa or MEN IIb syndromes. Other tumors found much less frequently include lymphoma, sarcoma, and squamous cell carcinoma. Tumor, node, metastasis (TNM) classification and American Joint Committee on Cancer AJCC staging of predominant thyroid malignancies is found in Table 31-3.

The goal in the management of a thyroid mass is to identify individuals who should undergo excisional biopsy and those who can be safely observed (Fig. 31-1). A small proportion of patients with thyroid mass are better managed by surgical excision without any other investigation. Certain elements of the history and physical examination should evoke a high index of suspicion, precluding the necessity of further work-up. Rapid growth, a hard nodule, signs of local invasion (fixation to adjacent structures, vocal cord paralysis, and enlarged regional lymph nodes) have correlated with malignancy rates greater than 70%. The association of a thyroid nodule with a history of low-dose irradiation to the neck carries a 40% chance of developing thyroid cancer. Family history of medullary or papillary cancer increases the likelihood that a thyroid nodule may be malignant. Patient preference may also lead directly to excisional biopsy.

For the majority of patients presenting with a thyroid mass, fine needle aspiration biopsy (FNAB) has become the initial diagnostic test of choice. It is safe, inexpensive, easy to perform, and leads to a better selection of patients for surgery than any other test. Detection of thyroid nodules by history, physical examination, radionuclide scanning, and ultrasound results in diagnosis of malignant disease in 10% to 20% of surgically excised nodules. FNAB has decreased by half the number of patients undergoing surgery and doubled the yield of carcinoma in surgical specimens. FNAB has reduced the need for ultrasound, radionuclide scans, and unnecessary surgery, thereby reducing the cost of care.

When an adequate specimen is obtained, three cytologic diagnoses are possible: benign, malignant,

TABLE 31-1 **CLASSIFICATION AND RELATIVE FREQUENCY OF THYROID CANCERS**

Classification	Incidence %
Differentiated	
Papillary	80
Follicular	10
Hürthle cell	3
Medullary	5
Anaplastic	1
Others	1

TABLE 31-2 **COMPARISON OF SURVIVAL WITH THYROID MALIGNANT TUMORS**

Histologic Type	5-year	Survival 10% year
Papillary	95	90
Follicular	90	70
Medullary	80	60
Anaplastic	Rare	—

TABLE 31-3 **STAGING OF THYROID CANCERS USING AMERICAN JOINT COMMISSION TNM CLASSIFICATION**

Primary Tumor (T)

TX	Primary tumor cannot be assessed
T0	No evidence of primary tumor
T1	Tumor 1 cm or less in greatest dimension, limited to the thyroid
T2	Tumor more than 1 cm but not more than 4 cm in greatest dimension, limited to the thyroid
T3	Tumor more than 4 cm in greatest dimension, limited to the thyroid
T4	Tumor of any size extending beyond the thyroid capsule

Regional Lymph Nodes (N)

NX	Regional lymph nodes cannot be assessed
N0	No regional lymph node metastasis
N1	Regional lymph node metastasis
N1a	Metastasis in ipsilateral cervical lymph node(s)
N1b	Metastasis in bilateral, midline, or contralateral cervical or mediastinal lymph node(s)

Distant Metastasis (M)

MX	Presence of distant metastasis cannot be assessed
M0	No distant metastasis
M1	Distant metastasis

Differentiated

	Under 45 Years	45 Years and Older
Stage I	Any T, Any N, M0	T1, N0, M0
Stage II	Any T, Any N, M1	T2, N0, M0
Stage III		T4, N0, M0
		Any T, N1, M0
Stage IV		Any T, Any N, M1

Medullary

Stage I	T1, N0, M0
Stage II	T2, N0, M0
	T3, N0, M0
	T4, N0, M0
Stage III	Any T, N1, M0
Stage IV	Any T, any N, M1

Undifferentiated
All cases are
    Stage IV—Any T, any N, any M

and indeterminate. Inadequate sampling may occur in up to 20% of specimens; however, repeat FNA will be diagnostic in half of these cases. Performed properly, inadequate sampling rates should be no higher than 5%. Accuracy of cytology ranges from 70% to 97%, depending on the experience of the individual performing the biopsy and the pathologist (Table 31-4). False-negative rates for FNAB range from 1% to 6%. False-positive rates have been reported as high as 8%. This represents the interpretive skill of the pathologist and should be in the 1% range. Reliability of FNAB depends heavily upon experience and collaboration of an interested pathologist. It must be emphasized that while FNAB provides useful information with a high degree of accuracy it will not unequivocally exclude a malignancy.

Some patients will require further evaluation before a decision regarding management. Repeat FNAB represents the best option when the initial cytologic diagnosis is equivocal. Additional sampling of the nodule may yield a more definitive diagnosis. While radionuclide scanning has little diagnostic value, it is useful to determine the functional status of the nodule. A "cold" solitary thyroid nodule that cannot be confirmed benign by cytology should be excised. When a thyroid nodule is to be followed clinically, ultrasound provides the most useful information for repeated examina-

tions. As well as differentiating solid from cystic lesions, it gives reliable, objective data regarding the size of the mass. Double-blind clinical trials have demonstrated no benefit of levothyroxine over placebo in suppressing growth of benign thyroid nodules. Suppressive therapy carries with it the risk of varying degrees of thyrotoxicosis as well as cardiovascular side effects. It is counterproductive to subject patients to these risks when thyroid-stimulating hormone (TSH) suppression has no proven benefit in this situation.

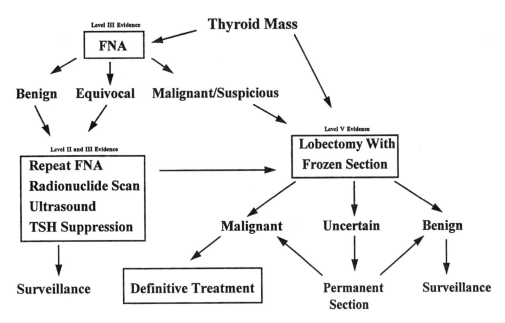

FIGURE 31-1 *Algorithm for management of thyroid mass. This approach is recommended to distinguish between individuals with a higher risk of malignancy requiring definitive diagnosis from those patients who can be safely observed. The approach depends heavily upon accurate fine needle aspiration biopsy.*

Observation of a thyroid mass involves a combination of patient education, physical examination, and ultrasound. The individual should be advised to return for examination if change in size or consistency is noted. Follow-up visits consist of interview, examination, and ultrasound scheduled at 3 and 9 months after initial evaluation and then by annual clinical examinations, assuming no change has occurred. A change in size (growth) or consistency is an indication for either repeat FNAB or excision for diagnosis.

A well-conducted anatomic dissection and excision of the thyroid lobe is the safest method of excisional biopsy, both from the standpoint of removing cancerous tumors and minimizing surgical morbidity. After removal of the thyroid lobe, the specimen is presented to the pathologist for frozen section analysis. Under optimal circumstances, 95%

TABLE 31-4 **RESULTS OF FINE NEEDLE ASPIRATION BIOPSY OF THE THYROID**

Author	Patients Biopsied	Sensitivity	Specificity	False Negative[a]	False Positive[a]
Grant (1989)	641	94	87	1	0
Dwarakanathan (1989)	354	99	57	4	6
Altavilla (1990)	2433	71	100	6	0
Giansanti (1989)	1886	78	95	1	6
Hamming (1990)	169	92	71	3	7
Pepper (1989)	104	83	47	1	—
Hall (1989)	795	95	63	1	3
Nishiyama (1986)	410	86	87	2	12
Belfiore (1989)	2327	—	—	3	—
Total/Average	9119	87		5	6

[a]*Inadequate specimens not included; false-negative and false-positive rates are therefore not supplementary to sensivity and specificity, respectively (see Ch. 1).*

accuracy rate should be anticipated. When benign disease is identified or rarely when the pathologist is unable to establish a diagnosis, the procedure should be terminated until the tissue can be analyzed further. If malignancy is identified, treatment will depend on the histologic type, extent of disease, and the experience of the surgeon.

SELECTION OF TREATMENT

SURGICAL RESECTION

The only potentially curative treatment for all varieties of thyroid cancer is surgical resection. The extent of resection of the thyroid and neighboring structures will depend on the histologic type of thyroid cancer, the extent of disease, and the experience and philosophy of the surgeon (Fig. 31-2).

Radioactive iodine, external radiation therapy, and TSH suppression using exogenous thyroid hormone all may have an adjunctive role. The effectiveness of these adjunctive treatments will vary depending upon the specific histologic type.

DIFFERENTIATED THYROID CANCER

When a differentiated thyroid cancer (papillary, mixed papillary, and follicular or follicular carcinoma) is identified on frozen section analysis, the extent of thyroid resection will be determined predominantly by stage of disease. With small primary tumors (1.5 cm), there is no significant difference in recurrence rate or survival after total thyroid lobectomy, subtotal thyroidectomy, or total thyroidectomy. Under these circumstances, the experience of the operating surgeon becomes an important factor

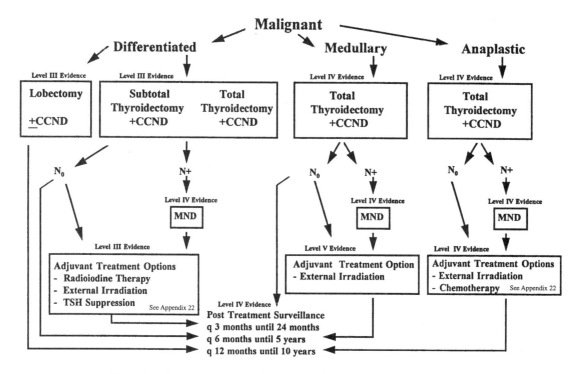

FIGURE 31-2 *Algorithm for management histologically proven thyroid cancer. Rationale for recommended treatment is based upon recognition that the histologic type of malignancy represents the best indicator of treatment outcome. For differentiated thyroid cancer, the extent of thyroidectomy will depend on the size and location of the primary tumor, evidence of extracapsular spread, or multicentricity. Because of local tumor aggressiveness, total thyroidectomy is recommended for both medullary and anaplastic carcinoma. Treatment recommendations are based upon level III and IV evidence. Goal of treatment for differentiated thyroid cancer and medullary thyroid cancer is curative; goal of treatment for anaplastic thyroid cncer is locoregional control of desease. CCND, central compartment neck dissection; MND, modified neck dissection. (See also Ch. 22.)*

in determining the extent of thyroidectomy. Subtotal and total thyroidectomy were recommended as a result of studies demonstrating multicentricity in a high proportion of thyroid cancers examined by whole-organ section. An important consideration in determining extent of thyroidectomy is postoperative morbidity. More experienced surgeons may favor total thyroidectomy as a definitive resection when the procedure can be carried out with minimum morbidity. Another consideration in determining the extent of thyroid excision is the prospect of postoperative radioiodine therapy. If radioiodine therapy is likely, total thyroidectomy is desirable to facilitate administration of the isotope. For less experienced surgeons, lobectomy or subtotal thyroidectomy may represent a better choice in terms of morbidity risk. Components of adequate surgical resection for differentiated thyroid cancer are shown in Table 31-5.

Rarely, thyroid malignancy will be identified on permanent section analysis of a specimen that was not recognized on frozen section analysis. Completion thyroidectomy is occasionally indicated for unfavorable histology (medullary or anaplastic carcinoma), narrow surgical margin, or evidence of multicentricity. Complete thyroidectomy should be carried out within a few days of the initial procedure to avoid the increased degree of operative difficulty associated with longer delays.

GOALS OF TREATMENT

Prospects for cure of differentiated thyroid cancer are excellent, with anticipated 90% control rates. The goal of treatment is cure with minimum morbidity and fewest treatment interventions. Negative survival determinants for differentiated thyroid cancers include age (above 40 years), size of the primary tumor, evidence of extracapsular, extrathyroidal spread, and presence of systemic metastasis. While lymph node metastases are not negative survival determinants, regional recurrences result in more frequent therapeutic interventions.

ADJUVANT THERAPY (SEE ALSO APPENDIX 22)

Postoperative adjuvant therapy improves outcome in patients with more extensive disease. Tumors larger than 1.5 cm and those with evidence of cervical node metastasis or extracapsular or extrathyroid spread are all indications for adjuvant therapy. Fewer recurrences and improved survival are reported with adjunctive radioiodine therapy and thyroid hormone. When thyroid hormone suppression and thyroid remnant ablation are combined, results are significantly better than with any other form of adjuvant therapy. Complete postoperative ablation of the thyroid remnant with radioactive iodine leads to a lower death rate than when the patient is treated with surgery alone or when ablation is incomplete. Radioiodine therapy for systemic disease is most effective in treating miliary pulmonary metastases.

Adjunctive treatment with external radiation therapy has produced mixed results. Recent reports suggest improved local control for more advanced stages of all types of thyroid cancer after postoperative external irradiation. External irradiation may be employed to treat microscopic or minimal gross residual tumor in situations where surgical resection would result in sacrifice of important structures such as the recurrent laryngeal nerve or portions of the larynx or trachea. Improvement in survival has not been shown. Use of thyroglobulin levels in the surveillance for recurrent thyroid cancer remains unreliable because of difficulty in determining how levels should be measured, the significance of the various levels, and the inability to distinguish between recurrent disease and residual normal thyroid tissue. This lack of accuracy precludes the use of thyroglobulin as part of the routine follow-up for thyroid cancer patients.

TABLE 31-5 COMPONENTS OF ADEQUATE SURGICAL RESECTION FOR DIFFERENTIATED THYROID CANCER

The extent of thyroidectomy depends on the extent of disease present within the gland and experience of the surgeon. In selected circumstances, small tumors (< 1.5 cm) may be adequately treated with thyroid lobectomy. For larger tumors (extending to the capsule of the gland or evidence of multicentricity), subtotal or total thyroidectomy is recommended.

One or more parathyroid glands should be preserved with adequate blood supply to avoid permanent hypoparathyroidism. Central compartment neck dissection should be carried out in all thyroid cancer resections. Depending on extent of thyroidectomy, this may involve excision of lymph nodes in the paratracheal groove, superior mediastinum, and anterior neck between jugular veins.

Clinical or microscopic evidence of metastases into the lateral neck is an indication for modified neck dissection. This lymphadenectomy involves resection of the jugular lymph chain and posterior triangle nodes with preservation of sternomastoid muscle, jugular vein, and accessory nerve.

Rarely, tumor extending through capsule or invading neighboring structures may require extended resection of adjacent structures, such as strap muscles, trachea, or larynx.

MEDULLARY CARCINOMA

Meticulous excision of all thyroid tissue at the initial operation is critically important to avoid recurrence in the thyroid remnant. C-cell hyperplasia or microscopic carcinoma is common in the contralateral thyroid lobe in familial medullary carcinoma. Failure to remove the contralateral lobe completely may leave residual cancer or C cells, with a high probability of malignant transformation. Eighty-nine percent of patients with MEN syndromes, and 20% of sporadic cases have bilateral thyroid involvement.

In patients with palpable thyroid tumors, lymph node metastases occur in 90%. Central compartment neck dissection is essential at initial surgery, when the anatomy of the neck is most clearly defined. Selective removal of clinically enlarged nodes is inadequate. All fatty and lymphatic tissue must be excised in an operative field extending from the hyoid to the innominate vessels and laterally to the jugular veins. Midjugular nodes should also be sampled, and if they are positive for malignancy or if obvious metastatic tumor is evident on either side of the neck, modified neck dissection should be performed. Prognosis is best when all tumor can be removed at operation. Presence of nodal metastases indicates a poor prognosis, and the more advanced the tumor at initial surgery the less favorable the outcome. Both death and recurrence rates are significantly higher when disease has spread beyond the thyroid gland.

In selected patients with extensive disease, postoperative external radiation therapy has been associated with tumor regression, decreased local recurrence, and prolonged survival in some cases. Radioactive iodine is not useful in medullary carcinoma of the thyroid because these cells are unable to concentrate iodine.

If the diagnosis of medullary thyroid carcinoma is known before operation, the patient should be screened for pheochromocytoma and hyperparathyroidism. If pheochromocytoma is found, it should be excised first to avoid the possible effects of excessive catecholamine release during neck dissection. Aggressive screening should be undertaken in families with hereditary medullary thyroid carcinoma. This allows diagnosis to be made at an early stage and improves survival rates.

ANAPLASTIC CARCINOMA

Anaplastic carcinoma of the thyroid is one of the most lethal cancers in man. Studies of early therapy report a median survival of four months. Survival is much better for patients with intrathyroid containment of disease as opposed to those with extraglandular spread and is unaffected by lymph node metastases. Historically, local tumor invasion has been responsible for 38% to 60% of the deaths from anaplastic thyroid cancer. Every attempt should be made to excise all macroscopic tumor because 5-year survival is quadrupled when all gross disease can be removed. Multimodal treatment results in better survival rates than surgery, radiation therapy, or chemotherapy used independently. A combination of surgery and preoperative and postoperative radiation therapy with concomitant chemotherapy will markedly improve local control, decrease death from local tumor growth, and reduce the need for tracheostomy. In a similar study of combination radiation therapy and Adriamycin, patients died of systemic disease without evidence of local recurrence. Systemic toxicity was eliminated by using low-dose Adriamycin. Patients with large tumor masses at the time of irradiation did not show any significant response to combined treatment, and survival longer than one year was associated with radical surgery and minimal residual disease at the time of irradiation. Mean survival has improved to 12 months and long-term survivorship has been achieved in rare individuals.

POST-TREATMENT SURVEILLANCE

Sixty percent of recurrences for all histologic types appear within the first 12 months. This represents the majority of recurrences for medullary and anaplastic cancers. The pattern of recurrence for well-differentiated cancer reveals a cluster of recurrences in the first 12 months and then sporadic recurrences over more than 21 years. For all thyroid cancers we recommend follow-up every 3 months for the first 24 months, then every 6 months for three years, and yearly thereafter. Surveillance evaluation consists of detailed interview and physical examination. Further work-up should be guided by symptomatic complaints. Medullary carcinoma is a unique malignancy because of its synthesis and secretion of the hormone calcitonin. High basal or post-stimulation concentrations serve as a tumor marker capable of detecting occult or recurrent medullary thyroid carcinoma. Levels should be followed regularly with each interview and physical examination. Individuals with anaplastic carcinoma often fail to achieve a disease-free interval, and follow-up may be more individualized in these cases.

SUGGESTED READINGS

Ashcraft MW: Analysis of techniques to evaluate thyroid nodules

Benker G, Olbricht T, Reinwein D et al: Survival rates in patients with differentiated thyroid carcinoma. Influence of postoperative external radiotherapy. Cancer 65:1517–1520, 1990

Beierwaltes WH, Rabbani R, Dmuchowski C et al: An analysis of ablation of thyroid remnants with I-131 in 511 patients from 1947–1984: experience at University of Michigan. J Nucl Med 25:1287–1293, 1984

Brunt LM, Wells JA: Advances in the diagnosis and treatment of medullary thyroid carcinoma. Surg Clin North Am 67:263–279, 1987

Buhr HJ, Kallinowski F, Herfarth C: Therapeutic procedure in medullary thyroid carcinoma: surgical strategies and methods for the treatment of metastasizing medullary thyroid carcinoma. Recent Results Cancer Res 125:147–165, 1992

Cady B, Sedgwick CE, Meissmer WA et al: Changing clinical, pathologic, therapeutic, and survival patterns in differentiated thyroid carcinoma. Ann Surg 184:541–553, 1976

Cameron JL: Current surgical therapy. p. 572. In: Mosby Yearbook. 4th Ed. CV Mosby, St Louis, 1992

Caruso D, Mazzaferri EL: Fine needle aspiration biopsy in the management of thyroid nodules. Endocrinology 1:194–202, 1991

Cheung PSY, Lee JMH, Boey JH. Thyroxine suppressive therapy of benign solitary thyroid nodules: a prospective randomized study. World J Surg 13:818–822, 1989

delos Santos ET, Keyhani-Rofagha S, Cunningham JJ et al: Cystic thyroid nodules: the dilemma of malignant lesions. Arch Intern Med 150:1422–1427, 1990

Farrar WB, Cooperman M, James AG: Surgical management of papillary and follicular carcinoma of the thyroid. Ann Surg 192:701–704, 1980

Flynn MB, Tarter J, Lyons K et al: Frequency and experience with carcinoma of the thyroid at a private, a veterans administration, and a university hospital. J Surg Oncol 48:164–170, 1991

Gagel RF, Robinson MF, Donovan DT et al: Medullary thyroid carcinoma: recent progress. J Clin Endocrinol Metab 76:809–814, 1993

Gharib H, James EM, Charbonneau JW et al: Suppressive therapy with levothyroxine for solitary thyroid nodules: a double blind controlled clinical study. N Engl J Med 317:70–75, 1987

Grant CS, Hay ID, Gough IR et al: Long term follow-up of patients with benign thyroid fine needle aspiration cytologic diagnoses. Surgery 106:980–986, 1989

Hall TL, Layfield LJ, Philippe A et al: Sources of diagnostic error in fine needle aspiration of the thyroid. Cancer 63:718–725, 1989

Hamberger B, Gharib H, Melton LJ et al: Fine needle aspiration biopsy of thyroid nodules: impact on thyroid practice and cost of care. Am J Med 73:381–384, 1982

Hamming JF, Goslings BM, Van Steenis GJ et al: The value of fine needle aspiration biopsy in patients with nodular thyroid disease divided into groups of suspicion of malignant neoplasms on clinical grounds. Arch Intern Med 150:113–116, 1990

Harness JK, Fung L, Thompson NW et al: Total thyroidectomy: complications and technique. World J Surg 10:781–186, 1986

Hay ID, Grant CS, Taylor WF, McConahey WM: Ipsilateral lobectomy versus bilateral lobar resection in papillary thyroid carcinoma: a retrospective analysis of surgical outcome using a novel prognostic scoring system. Surgery 102:1088–1094, 1987

Hubert JP, Kiernan PD, Beahrs OH et al: Occult papillary carcinoma of the thyroid. Arch Surg 115:394–398, 1980

Jereb B, Stjernsward J, Lowhagen T: Anaplastic giant cell carcinoma of the thyroid: a study of treatment and prognosis. Cancer 35:1293–1295, 1975

Jossart GH, Clark OH: Well-differentiated thyroid cancer. Curr Probl Surg 31:935–1012, 1994

Kim JH, Leeper RD: Treatment of locally advanced thyroid carcinoma with combination doxorubicin and radiation therapy. Cancer 60:2372–2375, 1987

Lowhagen T, Granberg PO, Lundell G et al: Aspiration biopsy cytology (abc) in nodules of the thyroid gland suspected to be malignant. Surg Clin North Am 59:3–18, 1979

Mazzaferri EL: Management of a solitary thyroid nodule. N Engl J Med 328:553–559, 1993

Mazzaferri EL, delos Santos ET, Rofagha-Keyhani S: Solitary thyroid nodule: diagnosis and management. Med Clin North Am 12:1177–1211, 1988

Mazzaferri EL, Young RL, Oertel JE et al: Papillary thyroid carcinoma: the impact of therapy in 576 patients. Medicine 56:171–196, 1977

Mazzaferri EL, Young RL: Papillary thyroid carcinoma: a 10 year follow-up report of the impact of therapy in 576 patients. Am J Med 70:511–518, 1981

Nel CJC, vanHeerden JA, Goellner JR et al: Anaplastic carcinoma of the thyroid: a clinicopathologic study of 82 cases. Mayo Clin Proc 60:51–58, 1985

O'Connell ME, A'Hern RP, Harmer CL: Results of external beam radiotherapy in differentiated thyroid carcinoma: a retrospective study from the Royal Marsden Hospital. Eur J Cancer 30A:733–739, 1994

Ozata M, Suzuki S, Miyamoto T et al: Serum thyroglobulin in the follow-up of patients with treated differentiated thyroid cancer. J Clin Endocrinol Metab 79:98–105, 1994

Philips P, Hanzen C, Andry G et al: Postoperative irradiation for thyroid cancer. Eur J Surg Oncol 19:399–404, 1993

Rojeski MT, Gharib H: Nodular thyroid disease: evaluation and management. N Engl J Med 313:428–436, 1985

Rossi RL, Nieroda C, Cady B et al: Malignancies of the thyroid gland: the Lahey Clinic experience. Surg Clin North Am 65:211–230, 1985

Russel CF, van Heerden JA, Sizemore GW et al: The surgical management of medullary thyroid carcinoma. Ann Surg 197:42–48, 1983

Samaan NA, Schultz PN, Hickey RC et al: The results of various modalities of treatment of well differentiated thyroid carcinoma: a retrospective review of 1599 patients. J Clin Endocrinol Metab 75:714–720, 1992

Silverberg S, Hutter R, Foote F: Fatal carcinoma of the thyroid: histology, metastases, and causes of death. Cancer 25:2792–2802, 1970

Silverberg L: CA Cancer J Clin 36:9, 1986

Simpson WJ: Radioiodine and radiotherapy in the management of thyroid cancers. Otolaryngol Clin North Am 23:509–521, 1990

Starnes HF, Brooks DC, Pinkus GS, Brooks JR: Surgery for thyroid carcinoma. Cancer 55:1376, 1985

Tallroth E, Wallin G, Lundell G et al: Multimodality treatment in anaplastic giant cell thyroid carcinoma. Cancer 60:1428–1431, 1987

Thompson NW, Nishiyama RH, Harness JK: Thyroid carcinoma: current controversies. Curr Probl Surg 15:1–67, 1978

Tisell LE, Mansson G, Jansson S: Surgical treatment of medullary carcinoma of the thyroid. Horm Metab Res Suppl 21:29–31, 1989

Tubiana M: External radiotherapy and radioiodine in the treatment of thyroid cancer. World J Surg 5:75–84, 1981

Werner B, Abele J, Alveryd A et al: Multimodal therapy in anaplastic giant cell thyroid carcinoma. World J Surg 8:64–70, 1984

Witt TR, Meng RL, Economov SG, Southwick WW: The approach to the irradiated thyroid. Surg Clin North Am 59:45–63, 1979

32 Adrenal Cancer

Renato V. La Rocca

Adrenocortical Carcinoma

Incidence: 0.2 per 100,000/year

Prevalence: Mostly sporadic; in children and adolescents may be part of Li-Fraumeni syndrome

Goal of treatment: Curative for stages 1–2; largely palliative for stages 3–4

Primary modalities of treatment: Surgery for stages 1–3 or isolated metastases

Phase 1–2 drug studies, mitotane, chemotherapy, palliative surgery for stage 4

Prognosis: 5-year survival

Overall: 20%–35%

Stage 1   80%

Stage 2   50%

Stage 3   25%

Stage 4   <5%

Pheochromocytoma

Incidence: 0.005 to 0.1% of individuals (autopsy series)

Prevalence: 48% or more sporadic; up to 34% as von Hipple-Lindau syndrome; up to 18% as MEN-2 syndrome

Goal of treatment: Curative for localized disease (even if bilateral adrenal invovement); palliative for advanced disseminated disease

Primary modalities of treatment: α-Adrenergic blockade followed by surgery for localized disease or isolated metastases Medical treatment of hypertension, chemotherapy, [^{131}I]MIBG for advanced disseminated disease

Prognosis

	5-year survival
Localized benign	>90%
Malignant	36–60%

Cancers of the adrenal gland, although rare, may manifest a broad spectrum of clinical symptoms as a result of diverse unregulated hormone secretion. Adrenocortical carcinomas arise from cells of the adrenal cortex and are the most prevalent of these tumors, though comprising only a mere 0.05% to 0.2% of all cancers. This translates into an incidence of no more than 75 to 115 new cases each year in the United States. Retrospective studies have identified a slight female preponderance (female/male ratio of approximately 1.6/1) with a bimodal age distribution, initially in childhood and then in the fifth decade of life. Approximately 60% of these tumors present with symptoms referable to excessive steroid production. Pheochromocytomas on the other hand, arise from chromaffin cells in the adrenal medulla and secrete catecholamines that can result in intermittent or sustained hypertension. Most tumors of this histologic subtype, however, have a benign natural history. A management algorithm for a unilateral adrenal neoplasm is shown in Figure 32-1.

ADRENOCORTICAL NEOPLASMS

Adrenocortical carcinomas present either as a functioning tumor or as an intra-abdominal mass with associated symptoms referable to local pressure or hemorrhage. Functioning tumors of the adrenal cortex may produce a classic Cushing syndrome in which patients present with truncal obesity, striae of the skin, hypertension, and hyperglycemia. In females, some virilization is common as a result of the peripheral conversion of adrenally secreted androstendione and dihydroepiandrosterone. Distinguishing hypercortisolism secondary to functioning primary adrenal neoplasms from that resulting from ectopic adrenocorticotropic hormone (ACTH) production or pituitary-dependent hypercortisolism (Cushing's disease) often requires a formal endocrine evaluation. However, functioning adrenal cancers will typically have elevated levels of urinary ketosteroids and a very low or undetectable plasma ACTH level. Virilization in association with hypercortisolism almost always suggests a primary adrenal neoplasm. Feminization in adults with adrenocortical carcinoma is decidedly rare, as is a clinical presentation of primary hyperaldosteronism (Conn syndrome). The latter most often results from idiopathic hyperaldosteronism or an aldosterone-producing adenoma. An association of adrenocortical carcinoma, primarily in children, with kindreds having a high prevalence of breast cancer, sarcomas, leukemias, and primary brain tumors has been identified (Li-Fraumeni syndrome) and is attributed to inactivating germline mutations of the p53 gene.

The diagnosis of primary adrenocortical neoplasms relies upon clinical suspicion, endocrine evaluation and the use of diagnostic imaging studies, especially computed tomography (CT) scanning, and magnetic resonance imaging (MRI) of the abdomen. The differential diagnosis of a solitary adrenal mass includes a benign adenoma, an aldosteroma, a pheochromocytoma, a metatasis from another primary site as well as early adrenocortical carcinoma. Of these, adenomas and metastases from another primary site (especially lung and breast) are the most common. Adrenal gland metastases, adrenocortical carcinoma, and pheochromocytoma cannot, however, be readily differentiated by CT scan morphology alone. Distinguishing a primary adrenal cancer from an adenoma can also be difficult. The size of an adrenal mass is of importance because if greater than 6 cm in diameter, the incidence of cancer ranges from 35% to 98%, whereas if it is less than 3 cm, it is less likely to be a primary adrenocortical carcinoma. If an adrenal adenoma is documented radiographically and it is hormone-producing, resection of the involved adrenal gland is curative. This is usually done via a posterior approach, unless the mass is greater than 6 cm, in which case the probability of frank carcinoma is much higher and either an anterior or flank approach is preferred. In either instance, subsequent to resection of a functional adrenocortical mass, corticosteroid replacement is required during the surgical procedure and often for many months thereafter.

Preoperative staging workup for a suspected primary adrenocortical carcinoma includes a chest

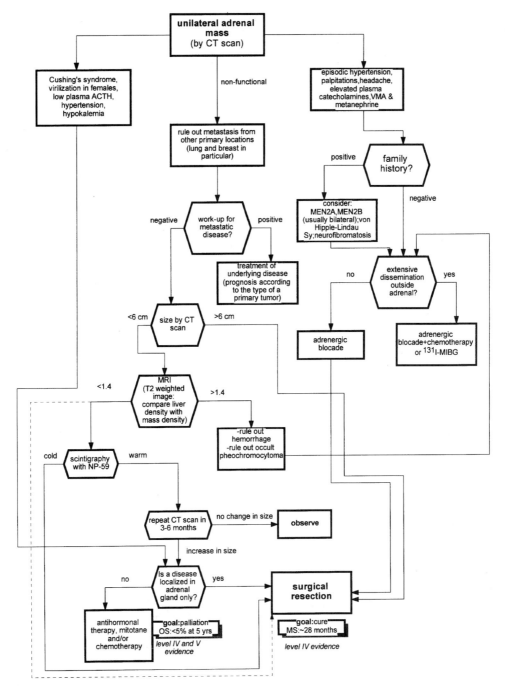

FIGURE 32-1 *Diagnostic and treatment management of adrenal carcinoma and pheochromocytoma. The key diagnostic principle is to distinguish between a benign and malignant mass. For noninvasive techniques, the size of the tumor on computed tomography (CT) scan, and density of T2-weighted image on magnetic resonance imaging (MRI) scan are two parameters with perhaps the best predictive values to help differentiate between malignant and benign lesions. However, in cases of high clinical suspicion invasive diagnostic techniques may be required to confirm the nature of the lesion. Determination of resectability represents the key reasoning principle in the management of a malignant adrenal mass. Goal in these patients is cure. In those unfortunate patients who are not deemed to have resectable mass, the goal is improvement in their quality of life. Because of the rarity of this tumor, there are no randomized trials evaluating the effectiveness of the various treatment options listed. Therefore, the recommended strategy is based on level III, IV, and V medical evidence. (See also Appendix 23.) OS, overall survival; MS, median survival; broken lines indicate alternative strategy.*

x-ray or CT scan and bone scan, in addition to the CT/MRI of the abdomen/pelvis. If a unilateral nephrectomy will be necessary as part of the surgical procedure, evaluation of the contralateral kidney function is necessary. If the cancer has not disseminated, complete surgical resection is indicated. This may also require resection of involved contiguous structures. If complete resection is not possible, surgical debulking may still be beneficial in reducing local complications and in decreasing the amount of unregulated steroid hormone production. The median survival for patients with unresectable adrenocortical carcinoma is only in the range of nine months, whereas for those patients having undergone complete resection it approaches 28 months. The presence of metastases at the time of diagnosis, age greater than 40 and the number of mitoses within the primary tumor specimen (i.e., greater than 20 mitoses per 50 high-power field) are predictive of a poorer prognosis. In the resection of a nonfunctioning malignancy, differentiation from renal cell carcinoma can be diffi-

cult. Adrenocortical carcinomas however, appear to reliably stain positive for vimentin whereas renal cell carcinomas do not. A surgical staging system is shown in Table 32-1. Approximately 66% to 72% of patients with adrenocortical carcinoma will have either stage 3 (locally advanced or with periadrenal lymph node involvement) or stage 4 (overtly disseminated) disease. Contiguous spread to adjacent organs (liver, kidney, diaphragm, and pancreas) is common, and distant metastases are most often found in the lungs, bone and within the mesentery. Surgery is also indicated in those select patients with isolated metastases. In the setting of surgically unresectable or recurrent disseminated disease, the drug o,p-DDD (mitotane) is often considered, though its true efficacy is of some debate (see Appendix 23). It exerts a direct effect on steroid metabolism in addition to a cytotoxic effect, resulting in reduction of abnormal 17 hydroxycorticosteroid secretion in up to 70% of patients. However, it induces an objective tumor regression in only 24% to 34% of treated patients with a median dura-

---

TABLE 32-1   STAGING SYSTEM FOR ADRENOCORTICAL CARCINOMA CRITERIA

Stage 1	T1N0M0	Primary tumor <5 cm, absent lymph node involvement; no local invasion
Stage 2	T2N0M0	Primary tumor >5 cm, absent lymph node involvement; no local invasion
Stage 3	T3N0M0	Primary tumor invades surrounding tissues
	T1–3N1M0	Periadrenal lymph node involvement
Stage 4	T4NXM0	Primary tumor invades adjacent organs
	TXNXM0	Distant metastases

TABLE 32-2   BENEFIT/RISK SHEET OF TREATMENT AGENTS USED IN ADVANCED ADRENOCORTICAL CARCINOMA

Drug	Dose	Response Rate
o,p-DDD (mitotane)	1–12 g/day	24–34% PR; control of hormone symptoms in 70% of pts
Cisplatin	40 mg/m²/day	2/2 pts achieved PR
VP-16	100 mg/m²/day for 3 days	
cisplatin &	75–100 mg/m² q 3 weeks	30% (1 CR, 10 PR)
o,p-DDD	1 g po qid	
5-Fluorouracil &	500 mg/m² days 1–3	25% (4 pts)
doxorubicin	60 mg/m² day 2 (q 4 weeks)	
Experimental drugs		
Suramin	850–1400 mg IV q week	17 pts (2 PR, 2 MR)
Gossypal	30–70 mg/day	21 pts (3 PR, 1 MR)
Chemotherapy for disseminated malignant pheochromocytoma		
Cyclophosphamide &	750 mg/m² day 1	14 pts (57% objective
Vincristine &	1.4 mg/m² day 1	79% biochemical)
Dacarbazine	600 mg/m² days 1 & 2 (q 3 weeks)	

Abbreviations: MR, minor response; PR, partial response; CR, complete response; GI, gastrointestinal; BM, bone marrow;

tion of response only in the range of 7–12 months. Its role in an adjuvant setting remains to be defined though some nonrandomized studies are suggestive of a possible benefit when compared to historical controls. In addition to mitotane, both aminoglutethimide and ketoconazole have both been used in patients with advanced functional cancers and symptoms of hormonal excess, in view of their ability to suppress steroid synthesis. Neither results, however, in reproducible significant regression in tumor size. The results with traditional chemotherapeutic agents in the setting of advanced disease have only been of modest and often transient benefit (Table 32-2). Suramin and gossypal are two experimental compounds that have been tried in patients with advanced disease, again with only modest results. Effective palliation of painful bone metastases can on occasion be obtained with radiation therapy. In view of its relative rarity, those patients with either completely resected adrenocortical carcinoma or those with advanced disseminated disease and good performance status should be considered for formal entry into adjuvant or phase 2 treatment studies.

ADRENAL MEDULLARY NEOPLASMS

Pheochromocytomas arise most commonly from the chromaffin cells of the adrenal medulla (90% of cases), as well as from the organ of Zuckerkandel, sympathetic and parasympathetic nerves (paragliomas), and, rarely, from within the heart or urinary bladder. They are estimated to cause 0.1% of cases of hypertension in which urinary catecholamines are measured, and occult pheochromocytomas have been found in autopsy series with an overall incidence of 0.005% to 0.1%. Approximately 10% to 50% of pheochromocytomas are familial and in such instances are usually histologically benign and often bilateral. Among the distinct syndromes in which there is an increased incidence of pheochromocytoma are the multiple endocrine neoplasia (MEN-IIa and MEN-IIb), neurofibromatosis (von Recklinghausen disease), von Hippel-Lindau disease, and Sturge-Weber syndrome. The frequency of this neoplasm appears to be particularly high in those patients with MEN syndrome and von Hippel-Lindau disease, where its penetrance approaches 25%.

Pheochromocytomas can cause a spectrum of symptoms, from labile hypertension to a hypertensive crisis, myocardial infarction or stroke, as a result of unregulated catecholamine release. Paroxysmal spells of headache, palpitations, diaphoresis, and hypertension are typical, although some patients present with sustained hypertension. The diagnosis is established with the demonstration of elevated 24-hour urine catecholamines and their metabolites vanilmandelic acid (VMA) and metanephrine. The urinary metanephrine level is considered the most specific single test. The clonidine suppression test is also helpful in those patients with borderline levels of plasma or urinary catecholamines. Serum neuron-specific enolase and neuropeptide levels are also often elevated in these patients, especially in those with metastatic dis-

Side Effects	Evidence Level	Comments	Author
GI, neuromuscular, abn LFts, rash	III	Measure level of drug	Icard et al. (1992), Van Slooten et al. (1994)
NV, BM suppression, peripheral neuropathy	V		Johnson et al. (1986)
GI, BM suppression peripheral neuropathy	III		Bukowski et al. (1993)
NV, BM suppression	IV		Schluberger et al. (1998)
malaise, rash keratopathy, neuropathy	III		La Rocca et al. (1990)
Ileus	III		Flack et al. (1993)
NV, peripheral neuropathy	III		Auerbach et al. (1988)

pts, patients; LFTS, liver function tests; abn, abnormality; NV, nausea and vomiting.

ease. Plasma chromogranin A levels may also be abnormal. CT scans and especially MRI can be used in the localization of clinically suspected pheochromocytomas. The latter is of particular benefit because on T2-weighted images pheochromocytomas, unlike other adrenal masses, have very high signal intensity. This is otherwise only seen in cases of adrenal hemorrhage. Another useful study available at some institutions is a radioisotope scan using [131I]MIBG. This is a catecholamine precursor which gives a "functional" image and is particularly useful in identifying small tumors in extra-adrenal sites.

The treatment of choice for localized pheochromocytomas is surgical resection following preoperative α-adrenergic blockade. Traditionally, phenoxybenzamine, an oral long-acting α blocker has been used. Subsequent β blockade may be added if supraventricular arrhythmias or angina are present. β blockade must never be used without prior α blockade for this can precipate a paradoxic rise in blood pressure. Phenoxybenzamine in conjunction with nifedipine or nicardapine alone have also been used. Medications such as atropine, droperidol, and fentanyl should be avoided.

The majority of pheochromocytomas are histologically benign (50% to 90%) and even after the resection of malignant lesions the disease-free interval can be prolonged. Follow-up subsequent to definitive resection should include use of some of the same modalities successfully used to detect the primary tumor (i.e., urinary and serum catecholamines, CT, MRI, clonidine suppression test, CT, MRI, or [131I]MIBG scan). In those patients with metastatic disease the clinical course may also be relatively indolent with 5-year survivals over 35%. Isolated metastases should be resected whenever possible. Otherwise, treatment with therapeutic doses of [131I]MIBG or combination chemotherapy may be warranted. Results with the former have yield an objective response of 17% in one study. The use of cyclophosphamide, vincristine, and dacarbazine has been reported to induce a 57% objective response rate and an improvement in catecholamine secretion in 79% (see Table 32-2). Both soft tissue and bone metastases on occasion respond well to external beam radiation therapy.

SUGGESTED READINGS

Averbuch SD, Steakley CS, Young RC et al: Malignant pheochromocytoma: effective treatment with a combination of cyclophosphamide, vincristine and dacarbazine. Ann Intern Med 109:267–273, 1988

Brennan MF: Adrenocortical carcinoma. Ca 37:348–364, 1987

Bukowski RM, Wolfe M, Levine HS et al: Phase II trial of mitotane and cisplatin in patients with adrenal carcinoma: a Southwest Oncology Group study. J Clin Oncol 11:161–165, 1993

Copeland PM: The incidentally discovered adrenal mass, diagnosis and treatment. Ann Intern Med 98:940–945, 1983

Flack MR, Pyle RG, Mullen NM et al: Oral gossypol in the treatment of metastatic adrenal cancer. J Clin Endocrinol Metab 76:1019–1024, 1993

Hutter AM, Kayhoe DE: Adrenal cortical carcinoma: results of treatment with o,p-DDD in 138 patients. Am J Med 41:581–592, 1966

Icard P, Chapuis Y, Andreassian B et al: Adrenocortical carcinoma in surgically treated patients: a retrospective study on 156 cases by the French Association of Endocrine Surgery. Surgery 112:972–980, 1992

Johnson DH, Greco FA: Treatment of metastatic adrenal cortical carcinoma with cisplatin and etoposide (VP-16). Cancer 58:2198–2202, 1986

Kasperlik-Zaluska AA, Migdalska BM, Zgliczynski S et al. Adrenocortical carcinoma: a clincial study and treatment results in 52 patients. Cancer 75:2587–2591, 1995

Krempf M, Lumbroso J, Mornex R et al: Use of 131 Im Iodobenzylguanidine in the treatment of malignant pheochromocytoma. J Clin Endocrinol Metab 72:455, 1991

La Rocca RV, Stein CA, Danesi R et al: Suramin in adrenal cancer: modulation of steroid hormone production, cytotoxicity in vitro and clinical antitumor effect. J Clin Endocrinol Metab 71:497–504, 1990

Li FP, Fraumeni JF, Mulvihill JJ et al: A cancer family syndrome in twenty-four kindreds. Cancer Res 48:5358, 1988

Loughlin KR, Gittes RF: Urological management of patients with von Hippel-Lindau disease. J Urol 136:789–791, 1986

Luton JP et al: Clinical features of adrenocortical carcinoma, prognostic factors and effect of mitotane therapy. N Engl J Med 322:1195–1201, 1990

McClennan BL: Oncology imaging: staging and followup of renal and adrenal carcinoma. Cancer 67:1199–1208, 1991

Neumann HP, Berger DP, Sigmund G et al: Pheochromocytomas, multiple endocrine neoplasia type 2 and von Hippel-Lindau disease. N Engl J Med 329:1531–1538, 1993

Pommier RF, Brennan MF: An eleven year experience with adrenocortical carcinoma. Surgery 112:963–971, 1992

Schluberger M, Ostronoff M, Bellaiche M et al: 5-Fluorouracil doxorubicin, and cisplatin in adrenal cortical carcinoma. Cancer 61:1492–1494, 1988

Schlumberger M, Gicquel C, Lumbroso J et al: Malignant pheochromocytoma: clinical, biologic, histologic and therapeutic data in 20 patients with distant metastases. J Endocrinol Invest 15:631–642, 1992

Sutton MG, Sheps SG, Lie JT: Prevalence of clinically unsuspected pheochromocytoma: review of 50-year autopsy series. Mayo Clin Proc 56:354–360, 1981

van Heerden JA, Sheps SG, Hamberger B et al: Pheochromocytoma: current status and changing trends. Surgery 91:367–373, 1982

Van Slooten H, Moolenaar AJ, Van Seters AP et al: The treatment of adrenocortical carcinoma with o,p-DDD: prognostic implications of serum level monitoring. Eur J Cancer 20:47–53, 1984

Weiss LM, Medeiros LJ, Vickery AL: Pathologic features of prognostic significance in adrenocortical carcinoma. Am J Surg Pathol 13:202–206, 1989

Wick MR, Cherwitz DL, McGlennan RC, Dehner LP: Adrenocortical carcinoma: an immunohistochemical comparison with renal cell carcinoma. Am J Pathol 122:343–352, 1986

33 Carcinoid Tumor

Ivana Pavlić-Renar
Aaron I. Vinik
Biljana Baškot

Incidence: 1.0–1.5/100,000 (around 2500 new cases in the United States yearly)
   (1 in 200–300 appendectomies; 1 in 2500 proctoscopies in middle-aged patients)

Localization: 95% in appendix, rectum, and small intestine (>60% of primary tumors in small intestine are clinically unrecognized; ectopic tumors may derive virtually at any location)

Treatment: Surgery is the only treatment for noninvasive tumors smaller than 1 cm in the largest diameter; debulking surgery may help for advanced disease
Medical: Ocleotide is the treatment of choice for carcinoid syndrome, but there is no strict evidence of tumor growth retardation
Interferon: Some evidence of growth retardation
Chemotherapy: Generally poor response

Prognosis: 5-year survival: 94% for localized tumor, 64% with lymph node involvement, 18% with distant metastases

Carcinoid tumors derive from enterochromaffin and argentaffin cells of the digestive tract, but the term "carcinoid tumor" can be expanded to cover "gut" tumors of paracrine and endocrine-like cells deriving from a stem cell that may differentiate into any of a variety of adult endocrine secreting cells.

The annual incidence and major sites are shown in Table 33-1. Carcinoids account for 56% of all neuroendocrine tumors of gastroenteropancre-atic axis, 13% to 34% of all tumors of the small bowel, and 17% to 46% of all malignant tumors in that location.

Appendiceal carcinoids have a good prognosis if smaller than 2 cm. Rectal carcinoids less than 1 cm in the largest diameter rarely metastasize, whereas those greater than 2 cm nearly always do. The median survival rates are shown in Table 33-2. Overall, the prognosis is good for a malignant disease.

TABLE 33-1 INCIDENCE AND SITES OF PRIMARY CARCINOIDS

Incidence: around 1.5/100 000 general population
Sites: 95% in appendix, rectum, and small intestine
   (1 in 200–300 appendectomies, incidence declining with age)
   (1 in 2,500 proctoscopies in middle-aged patients)
   (small intestine: 75% of all carcinoids found at autopsy, 25%
of carcinoids in clinical series)
1.5% bronchus and ovary
0.2% all other sites
3.3% primary site unknown

(Adapted from Vinik AI, Thompson NV, Averbuch AD: Neoplasms of the gastroenteropancreatic endocrine system. In Holland JF [ed]: Cancer Medicine. Lea & Febiger, Philadelphia, 1992, and Moertel CG, Dockerty MD, Judd ES: Carcinoid tumors of the vermiform appendix. Cancer 21:270–278, 1968, with permission.)

TABLE 33-2 SURVIVAL RATES FOR CARCINOIDS

Median 5-year overall survival	*(%)*
Localized tumor	94
Lymph node involvement	64
Distant metastases	18

Median survival after first flushing episode
   No lymph node involvement: 36 months (25% at 6 years)
   With regional lymph nodes: 14 months
   With 5-hydroxyindoleacetic acid > 150 mg/24 hours: 11 months

(Adapted from Godwin JD: Carcinoid tumors. An analysis of 2,837 cases. Cancer 36:560–569, 1975, and Moertel CG: Karnofsky memorial lecture. An odyssey in the land of tumors. J Clin Oncol 5:1502–1522, 1987, with permission.)

DIAGNOSIS

CLINICAL

The most prominent symptoms that might be related to carcinoid tumor are chronic abdominal pain, diarrhea or bowel hypermotility, and flushing. By the time of the diagnosis there generally has been a history of symptoms for an average duration of 2 to 9 years. The spectrum of symptoms is extremely broad because these tumors, especially those in the foregut, have the potential to produce a variety of hormones and bioactive amines. A carcinoid tumor's cosecretion of adrenocorticotropic hormone (ACTH) or gastrin is generally a sign of a poor prognosis.

A symptom complex, *carcinoid syndrome,* occurs in less than 10% of patients. The principle features of the syndrome include flushing (in 84% of patients), sweating, wheezing, diarrhea (usually secretory, in 70%), abdominal pain (in around 33%), bronchospasm (in 6%), and myopathy (in 7%). Dyspnea is found in 33%, some of which is due to cardiac fibrosis with development of valvular disease, predominantly right.

BIOCHEMICAL

Tryptophan metabolites, especially serotonin, are the key products in the biochemical diagnosis of carcinoids. A single measurement of 5-hydroxyindoleacetic acid (5-HIAA) in the urine seems to be the best for screening of midgut tumors, with *specificity approaching* 95%, although no single test is sufficient to identify all cases. Patients should be warned to avoid tryptophan-containing foods (such as avocados, bananas, eggplants, pineapples, walnuts, tomatoes) three days before testing. In patients with foregut carcinoids, the urine contains relatively little 5-HIAA but large amounts of 5-hydroxytryptophan (5-HTP). High-performance liquid chromatography, with ultraviolet, fluorometric, or electrochemical detection, is the method of choice for detection of tryptophan and its metabolites.

Serum chromogranin A and B levels and neuron-specific enolase are additional biochemical markers.

LOCALIZATION

Primary carcinoids in several sites are relatively easy to detect e.g., bronchial carcinoid by chest x-ray or computerized tomography and carcinoids of cecum, right colon, and rectum by barium enema and endoscopy. The greatest problem emerges in localizing common small bowel carcinoids. Barium examinations may demonstrate fixation, separation, thickening, and angulation of the bowel loops, but are rarely diagnostic. Uncommon tumors in extraintestinal sites are usually an incidental finding. Primary tumors of the small intestine are usually below the resolution capacity of CT or ultrasonography. However, CT is helpful in tumor staging and evaluation of treatment.

Scintigraphy with labeled somatostatin analogue seems to be the most accurate imaging method. Positron emission tomography (PET) using 5-HTP as ligand is still investigatory.

The role of angiography has decreased with time with the development of noninvasive methods of investigation. It is employed when the results of noninvasive techniques are equivocal, and surgery is being considered. In unclear cases in which the tumor has not been identified by any of the techniques mentioned, total body venous sampling may be considered, if there is production of a known and measurable peptide substance.

TREATMENT

The goals of treatment are

Relief of symptoms, at least to a bearable level.

Reduction of tumor mass to less than 50% as assessed by serial CT or other localization studies.

Reduction of the blood or urine levels of biochemical marker(s) to less than 50%. It is important to note, however, that no direct correlation between tumor mass and levels of any marker is uniformly present.

SURGERY

Local excision is recomended for incidental noninvasive tumors smaller than 2 cm in the largest diameter (Fig. 33-1). Palliative radical surgery should be performed to reduce symptoms and tumor bulk. It can also render further treatment more effective. Different centers have different approaches to timing and extent of surgery in metastatic carcinoids. An aggressive surgical approach adopted by Ahlman et al. for 41 patients seemed to give encouraging results. However, it is difficult to compare the effects of treatment without data on comparable surgical treatment and tumor staging.

Because of the slow growth of these tumors, patients with terminal liver disease caused by metastases might even be candidates for liver transplantation.

Gastric carcinoids can be associated with chronic atrophic gastritis type A (CGA-A). For small multiple tumors of this type, endoscopic removal may be the first step. Antrectomy combined with excision is performed for recurrent tumors or as a first treatment for larger and more numerous lesions, especially solitary tumors and those not associated with CGA-A and serum gastrin greater than 1,000 pg/L.

MEDIATORS OF BIOLOGIC RESPONSE

Somatostatin and its analogues inhibit secretion of a variety of peptides. *Octreotide* in doses of 1 to 2 µg/kg/day has been shown to suppress symptoms in at least 50% of patients with carcinoid syndrome

TABLE 33-3 SYSTEMIC ANTICANCER THERAPY FOR MALIGNANT CARCINOID

Drug	Number of Patients	Biochemical or Tumor Response (%)
Single agents		
5 Fluorouracil	19	26
Doxorubicin	33	21
	81	21
Streptozocin	23	30
Dacarbazine	15	13
	56	16
Dactinomycin	17	6
Etoposide	17	0
Cisplatin	15	6
Carboplatin	20	0
Interferon	99	50
	27	39
	22	58
Octreotide	85	71
	14	31
	55	37
Combinations		
Streptozocin + fluorouracil	154	33
Streptozocin + doxorubicin	10	40
Streptozocin + fluorouraci + doxorubicin	20	35
Streptozocin + cyclophosphamide	47	26
Etoposide + cisplatinum	13	0
Streptozocin + doxorubicin + interferon	11	0
Octreotide + interferon	19	71

(Figure 33-1). It has also been proven to reverse cardinoid crisis. There are reports of reduction of tumor mass with octreotide treatment. The starting dose of 100 to 300 µg/day could be further increased if there is no response after three months. A threefold increase in life expectancy after octreotide has been reported, with an even greater effect by increasing the dose to 1,500 µg/day. There is not a clear relationship between the effects on tumor growth and peptide production. In up to one third of patients, escalating doses of octreotide seems to stop or reverse the growth. A total response to recombinant *interferon* is reported to be 30% to 39%. One of the recommended schemes is 5 to 10 MU intramuscularly daily for three weeks, followed by the same dose three times weekly. Dosage differs for 2a and 2b interferon (Fig. 33-1). Side effects are fatigue, flu-like syndrome, and development of autoimmune disease. *Combined*

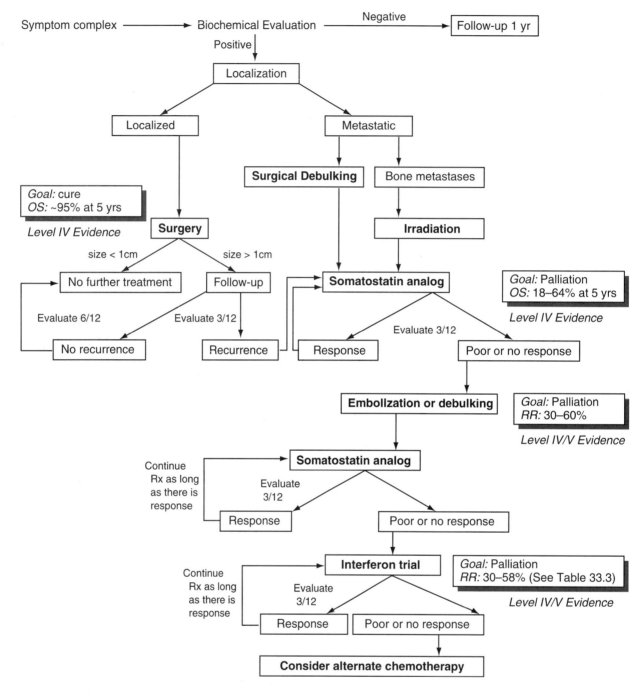

FIGURE 33-1 *Management of carcinoid tumor. Tumor size and its resectability dominates reasoning principles in the management of carcinoids. Small (< 1 cm) noninvasive tumors are surgically curable. In patients with such tumors, the goal of treatment is cure. However, carcinoids are slow growing, and overall survival is relatively long for a malignant disease. A long-term team (surgical, oncologic, medical) follow-up is thus necessary for patients with advanced disease with an active approach to treatment. The goals of the treatment are relief of symptoms and reduction of tumor mass. Strategy outlined is based mostly on level IV and V evidence. (See also Appendix 24 for practical details on the management of carcinoid tumors.) MO, months; RR, response rate; OS, overall survival; 6/12, q 6 months; 3/12, q 3 months; Rx, treatment. (From Vinik AI, Pavlic-Renar I: Neuroendocrine tumors of carcinoid variety. pp. 2803–2814. In De Groot LJ, Besser M, Burger HG et al. (eds): Endocrinology. WB Saunders, Philadelphia, 1995, with permission.)*

interferon-somatostatin analogue treatment seems to be beneficial in longterm management of disease, but long-term follow-up data are not yet available.

CHEMOTHERAPEUTIC AGENTS

Early nonrandomized studies of combinations of various chemotherapeutic regimens reported responses sometimes exceeding 50%. However, rigid criteria for measurement of responses were not always employed nor was a complete response ever seen. Multicentric studies by the Eastern and Southwest Cooperative Oncology Group of various regimens and agents, such as 5-fluorouracil, streptozotocin, cyclophosphamide, and doxorubicin, showed response rates not exceeding 33%. Combined etoposide and cisplatin is reported to be effective in anaplastic variants of neuroendocrine carcinomas.

HEPATIC ARTERY EMBOLIZATION

Hepatic arterial embolization is a relatively safe procedure for inducing regression of hepatic metastases (in 30%–60% of patients and even up to 80% with subsequent chemotherapy). Application of chemotherapy into the tumor vessel before arterial occlusion by gelatin sponge particles seems to improve the results further (regression or stabilization of liver tumor mass in 80% of patients). Complications of the procedure include abscess formation, gas formation without infection at the site of embolization, severe pain in virtually all patients, and pyrexia in one half. Renal failure may be prevented by vigorous hydration and allopurinol.

RADIOTHERAPY

Radiation can achieve symptomatic palliation for unresectable malignant tumors, especially in painful syndromes caused by bone metastases. However, there is no strict evidence that radiation decreases tumor mass.

SUGGESTED READINGS

Ahlman H, Kolby L, Lundell L et al: Clinical management of gastric carcinoid tumors. Digestion 55(suppl 3):77–85, 1994

Ahlman H, Wangberg B, Jansson S et al: Management of disseminated midgut carcinoid tumors. Digestion 49:78–96, 1991

Bajetta E, Zilembo N, DiBartelomeo M et al: Treatment of metastatic carcinoids and other neuroendocrine tumors with recombinant interferon- alpha- 2a. A study by the Italian Trial in Medical Oncology Group. Cancer 72:3099–3105, 1993

Chakravathy A, Abrams RA: Radiation therapy in the management of patients with malignant carcinoid tumors. Cancer 1386–1390, 1995

Clouse ME, Perry L, Stuart K, Stokes KR: Hepatic arterial chemoembolization for metastatic neuroendocrine tumors. Digestion 55(suppl 3):92–97, 1994

Hanssen LE, Schrumpf E, Kolbenstvedt AN, Tausjo J, Dolva LO: Treatment of malignant metastatic midgut carcinoid tumors with recombinant α-2b interferon with or without hepatic artery embolization. Scand J Gastroenterol 24:787–795, 1989

Krenning EP, Kwekkeboom DJ, Oei HY et al: Somatostatiu receptor scintigraphy in gastroenteropoucreatic tumors. An overview of European results. Amm NY Acad Sci 733:416–424, 1994

Loftus JP, van Heerden JA: Surgical management of gastrointestinal carcinoid tumors. Advances Surgery 28:317–336, 1995

Moertel CG: Karnofsky memorial lecture. An odyssey in the land of small tumors. J Clin Oncol 5:1502–1522, 1987

Moertel CG, Dockerty MB, Judd ES: Carcinoid tumors of the vermiform appendix. Cancer 21:270–278, 1968

Moertel CG, Johnson CM, McKusick MA et al: The management of patients with advanced carcinoid tumors and islet cell carcinomas. Ann Intern Med 120:302–309, 1994

Ruszniewski P, Rougier P, Roche A et al: Hepatic arterial chemoembolization in patients with liver metastases of neuroendocrine tumors. A prospective phase II study in 24 patients. Cancer 71:2624–2630, 1993

Schweitzer RT, Alsina AE, Rosson R, Bartus SA: Liver transplantation for metastatic neuroendocrine tumors. Transpl Proc 25:1973, 1993

Tiensuu J E, Oberg K: Long term management of the carcinoid syndrome. Treatment with octreotide alone and in combination with alpha interferon. Acta Oncol 32:225–229, 1993

Vinik Al, Moattari AR: Neuroendocrine tumors, secretory diarrhea, and responses to somatostatin. In Lebenthal E, Duffey M (Eds): Textbook of Secretory Diarrhea. pp. 309–324. Lippincott-Raven, Philadelphia, 1990

Vinik Al, Pavlic-Renar I: Neuroendocrine tumors of carcinoid variety. pp. 2803–2814. In De Groot LJ, Besser M, Burger HG et al (eds): Endocrinology. WB Saunders, Philadelphia, 1995

Vinik AI, Thompson NV, Averbuch AD: Neoplasms of the gastroenteropancreatic endocrine system. In Holland JF (ed): Cancer Medicine. Lea & Febiger, Philadelphia, 1992

34 Insulinoma

Ivana Pavlić-Renar
Aaron I. Vinik
Biljana Baškot

Incidence: 4/1,000,000

Localization: Of all causes of organic hyperinsulinemias, <90% are solitary tumors in pancreas (5%–6% malignant), and around 10% are multiple, or islet hyperplasia. Ectopic tumors are extremely rare.

Note: In 10% of patients, organic hyperinsulinemia is a feature of multiple endocrine neoplasias (MEA 1).

Diagnosis: Biochemical (prolonged fast with glucose and insulin sampling), angiography, and percutaneous transhepatic portal sampling for insulin.

Note: Extensive preoperative localization is seldom indicated in sporadic cases.

Treatment: *Surgery:* The only treatment for sporadic benign tumors

Medical:

Diazoxide for hypoglycemia

Chemotherapy for malignant tumors: combinations with streptozotocin or chlorozotocin

Prognosis: Benign sporadic tumors have no impact on life expectancy

Poor for sporadic metastatic tumors

The most common cause of organic hypoglycemia is a pancreatic β-cell tumor (insulinoma). These tumors are probably less rare than previously suspected, with an incidence of 4/1,000,000. In about 90% of the cases they are single, benign, and confined to the pancreas. Multiple adenomatosis (multiple microadenomas, several macroadenomas with or without microadenomas, and insular hyperplasia) occurs in 5% to 15% of the patients. In less than 10% of the patients, insulinoma is a feature of multiple endocrine neoplasia type 1 (MEN 1). Five to six percent of insulinomas are malignant.

Repeated prolonged hypoglycemia may be unrecognized for years, even decades, and may cause serious neurologic problems. Solitary insulinomas may appear at any age, with an even gender distribution. They are usually less than 1 cm in diameter, encapsulated, highly vascular, firmer than normal pancreatic tissue, and localized in any region of the pancreas. Ectopic tumors are extremely rare.

DIAGNOSIS

CLINICAL

Patients usually present with symptoms that can be attributed to neuroglycopenia (visual disturbances, confusion, clouding and loss of consciousness, weakness, transient motor deficits ranging from discrete deficits to hemiplegia, dizziness, fatigue, inappropriate behavior, speech difficulties—ranging from minor difficulties to aphasia, and headache). Unlike reactive hypoglycemia, symptoms attributable to adrenergic activation (sweating, shaking, trembling, anxiety, hunger, nausea, palpitations, tachycardia) are less frequent. Organic hyperinsulinemia presents as fasting hypoglycemia. Symptoms occurring during daytime can be the consequence of a prolonged interval between food consumption (5–6 hours). Some 40% of patients have a weight gain. Exacerbation of symptoms during or soon after exercise also suggests organic hyperinsulinism. In patients with reactive hypoglycemia, blood glucose tends to rise with exercise. There is progression of symptoms with time, unlike the symptoms of reactive hypoglycemia.

BIOCHEMICAL

Occasionally, biochemical hypoglycemia can be found in the work-up of patients not suspected of having hypoglycemia (this is particularly frequent in patients with MEA 1). If biochemical hypoglycemia occurs on fasting, or is severe, it must be pursued. Neither single insulin nor glucose level alone is diagnostic of insulinoma. The standard test is a prolonged fast (up to 72 hours). The prolongation of an overnight fast increases the yield of diagnostically relevant levels of insulin. In healthy individuals, plasma insulin declines with fasting, as does plasma glucose, to reach levels between 3 and 7 mU/mL in 63 to 72 hours. In patients with pancreatic cell disease, it may remain constant, fluctuate, or even rise. To improve the yield of positive tests, a variety of ratios of insulin to glucose have been developed. The "amended" *insulin/glucose ratio*, which is the plasma insulin (in mU/mL) multiplied by 100, divided by plasma glucose (in mg/dL),

minus 30 is one such iteration. The rationale for subtraction of 30 from plasma glucose level of 30 mg/dL derives from the observation that insulin secretion ceases at a plasma glucose level of 30 mg/dl in healthy subjects. This ratio does not exceed 50 in healthy subjects. In occasional insulin-requiring diabetics who developed organic hyperinsulinism, high levels of C-peptide are diagnostic. To rule out insulin abuse, plasma concentrations of C-peptide and insulin antibodies are essential. Patients abusing sulphonylureas do not have raised insulin and C-peptide levels. C-peptide also helps in diagnosis of a rare autoimmune form of hypoglycemia with formation of antibodies to insulin receptors in which insulin levels may be normal or high, whereas C-peptide is always low. In autoimmune hypoglycemia with anti-insulin antibodies, there is oversecretion of insulin. A careful assessment of insulin binding is necessary.

Various provocative tests are much less reliable in the identification of insulin-producing tumors than the ratio of insulin to glucose and hence are no longer used in practice. Specific tests may be employed to rule out hypoglycemia caused by endocrine, hepatic, or renal disease.

LOCALIZATION

An experienced surgeon has a 75% to 90% chance of identifying a solitary insulinoma during surgery (which is better than most localization studies, with the exception of transhepatic portal venous sampling). Intraoperative ultrasonography may improve the accuracy to 100%, making extensive preoperative localization studies less indicated for sporadic insulinomas. However, preoperative localization of the region of insulin oversecretion in cases of multiple lesions, such as adenomatosis, nesidioblastosis, or hyperplasia, may guide the decision as to which part, to what extent, and which region of the pancreas should be resected.

Several techniques have been employed to localize insulinomas preparatively. Computed tomography (CT) is accurate in the range of 35% to 66% in several published series. Magnetic resonance imaging (MRI) seems to be a little more reliable (around 75%). External ultrasonography is below the range of CT. Endoscopic ultrasonography seems to be a very powerful tool in localizing small tumors in the head of the pancreas and duodenum. Celiac arteriography has been reported as successful in localization of 60% to 70% of the insulinomas in a majority of more recent reports. It has a generally higher yield in comparison with CT and ultrasound. The most reliable technique for preoperative localization of insulin-producing tissue seems to be transhepatic portal venous sampling (THPVS) for insulin. Since its introduction in 1975 the reported success rates range from 25% to 100%. Simultaneous sampling from the celiac axis and hepatic vein provides basal reference insulin levels.

TREATMENT

SURGERY

Treatment is predominantly surgical. The overall prognosis is good, with no impaired long-term survival in benign sporadic tumors. In diffuse hyperinsulinism, if the results of transhepatic portal venous sampling THPVS suggest diffuse or multiple sources of hyperinsulinemia, an effort toward medical treatment of hypoglycemia is indicated. Successful preoperative treatment allows a more conservative approach in surgery. If, however, the patient does not respond to medical treatment, a resection of 85% of the pancreas is indicated. Frozen sections of the pancreas should be analyzed during surgical exploration, although proof of hyperplasia or nesidioblastosis is unlikely to emerge before the permanent sections. Patients with MEN 1 should be followed for life because of the high risk of developing another islet cell tumor in the remaining pancreas. For malignant insulinomas, a Whipple procedure (for potentially curable

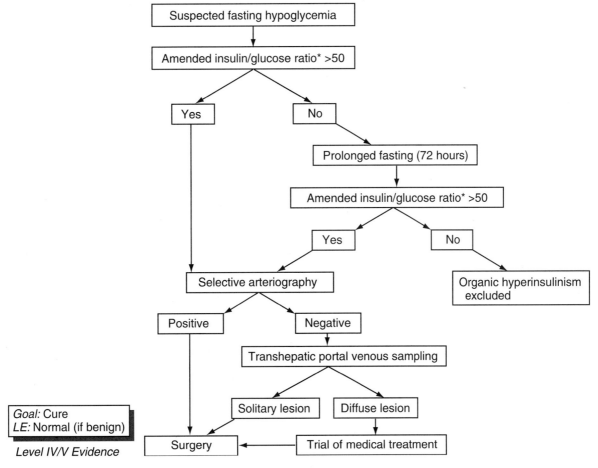

FIGURE 34-1 *Management of insulinoma. Tumor resectability dominates reasoning principles in the management of insulinoma. Sporadic noninvasive tumors are surgically curable. In patients with such tumors, the goal of treatment is cure. The strategy outlined is based on level IV and V evidence. Note that malignant insulinomas respond to combinations with streptozocin or chlorozotocin, which has been confirmed in randomized studies (not shown in the figure). LE, life expectancy. (From Vinik AI, Pavlić-Renar I: Insulin producing tumors. Adv Endocrinol Metabol 4:1–27, 1993, with permission.)*

tumors in the head of the pancreas) or distal pancreatectomy (for tumors in the neck and the tail) is necessary. In cases with metastatic disease, surgical debulking may mitigate the hypoglycemia and improve the response to chemotherapy.

MEDICAL

Diet is the first step in the treatment of insulin-producing tumors, similar to the other forms of hypoglycemia. More frequent meals and slowly absorbable forms of carbohydrates should be recommended. Hypoglycemic episodes are reversed by rapidly absorbable carbohydrates.

The most commonly used medication is diazoxide. It acts upon hypoglycemia through two mechanisms: (1) stimulation of adrenergic receptors that inhibit insulin secretion, and (2) inhibition of cyclic adenosine monophosphate (cAMP) phosphodiesterase, resulting in a higher tissue level of cAMP, which inhibits tissue glucose utilization and increases resistance to insulin. The side effect is sodium retention. Benzothiadiazine is thus added. Potassium supplement is often needed, especially with higher doses of benzothiadiazine. Patients with insulinoma are prone to hypokalemia because of hyperinsulinemia; the addition of diuretics easily induces overt hypokalemia. Other side effects of diazoxide treatment are nausea and hirsutism. The maintenance dose range is usually 150 to 600 mg diazoxide daily with an additional 2 to 8 mg trichlormethiazide.

Calcium channel blockers, propranolol, phenytoin, chlorpromazine, glucocorticoids, and glucagon have been occasionally used.

CHEMOTHERAPY

For advanced malignant disease, chemotherapy with streptozocin combined with fluorouracil and doxorubicin, as well as, more recently, chlorozotocin is used for insulinomas and for other malignant pancreatic islet tumors. The details of treatment are described in Chapter 35.

In summary, insulin-producing tumors are a rare cause of hypoglycemia. Their management is shown in Figure 34-1. Patients present with fasting hypoglycemia, evoked by prolonged fasting or exercise. The major test for establishing the diagnosis is a prolonged fast with repeated measurement of insulin and glucose. An amended insulin/glucose ratio of more than 50 at any time point is diagnostic of hyperinsulinemia.

Surgery is the treatment of choice for most patients. The majority of solitary tumors are below the discriminatory threshold of most imaging techniques. Arteriography and THPVS have an important place in localization of these tumors. THPVS for measurement of insulin levels permits proper localization of regions of diffuse lesions (nesidioblastosis and hyperplasia). Besides surgery, treatment of hyperinsulinism includes diet and hyperglycemic agents. In most patients medical treatment should only be regarded as supportive before surgery. Malignant insulinomas respond to streptozocin in combination with fluorouracil, doxorubicin, and chlorozotocin. However, the treatment is highly toxic and results are at best moderate.

SUGGESTED READINGS

Howard TJ, Stabile BE, Zinner MJ et al: Anatomic distribution of pancreatic endocrine tumors. Am J Surg 159:258–264, 1990

Miyazaki KA, Funakoshi S, Nishihara T et al: Aberrant insulinoma in the duodenum. Gastroenterology 90:1280–1285, 1986

Rosch TCJ, Lightdale JF, Botet GA et al: Localization of pancreatic endocrine tumors by endoscopic ultrasonography. N Engl J Med 326:1721–1726, 1992

Service FJ, McMahon MM, O'Brien PC, Ballard DJ: Functioning insulinoma—incidence, recurrence, and long-term survival of patients: a 60-year study. Mayo Clinic Proc 66:711–719, 1991

Stefanini P, Carboni M, Patrassi N, Basoli A: Beta-islet cell tumors of the pancreas: results of a study on 1,067 cases. Surgery 75:597–609, 1974

Thompson NW, Eckhauser FE: Malignant islet-cell tumors of the pancreas. World J Surg 8:940–951, 1984

van Heerden JA, Grant CS, Czako PF, Service FJ, Charboneau JW: Occult functioning insulinomas: which localizing studies are indicated? Surgery 112:1010–1014, 1992

Vinik AI, Pavlić RI: Insulin producing tumors. Adv Endocrinol Metabol 4:1–27, 1993

35 Zollinger-Ellison Syndrome

Ivana Pavlić-Renar
Aaron I. Vinik
Biljana Baškot

Incidence: Around 1/1,000,000

Localization: 90% in Passaro's triangle: junction of common bile and cystic duct junction of second and third portion of duodenum junction of pancreatic body and neck; *Note*: >40% in duodenum; >60% sporadic, solitary; 60% to 85% malignant, 30% with multiple endocrine neoplasia (MEA 1)

Treatment: After achieving control of gastric hypersecretion (by H2 blockers and/or proton pump inhibitors) and performing localization studies, surgery should be performed in patients with sporadic disease; in patients with MEA 1, surgical treatment is still controversial; chemotherapy: combinations with streptozotocin or chlorozotocin

Prognosis: Long-term cure is possible in 30% of operated patients with sporadic tumors (around 40% of patients); ten-year survival in patients with metastatic tumor: around 25%

Gastrinomas are the most frequent (excluding carcinoid and insulinomas, which can be classified in this category) among rare neuroendocrine tumors of gastroenteropancreatic origin. The incidence is about 1/1,000,000. They produce gastrin, a potent stimulator of acid release from the gastric parietal cells. Gastrin is a stimulator of the release of numerous biogenic amines and peptides but also acts as a growth factor. The clinical syndrome associated with gastrinoma has been described by Zollinger and Ellison in 1955. It consists of recurrent severe peptic ulcer disease in up to 95% of patients, with diarrhea in about 40% (in up to 15% of patients with Zollinger-Ellison syndrome [ZES] diarrhea is the sole manifestation of the disease)

and a gastrin-producing tumor. Radiologic features are hypertrophic mucosal folds in the stomach, sometimes in the duodenum and rarely in the jejunum. Major biochemical features are hypergastrinemia and elevated basal acid output (BAO) with high basal/maximal acid output (MAO). The original description of ZES included islet cell tumor of the pancreas. Indeed, the majority of reported primary tumors derive from pancreatic islets, mostly in the head of the pancreas. However, according to more recent reports, more than 40% gastrinomas are of duodenal origin. Around 90% of gastrinomas are found in anatomic triangle (Passaro's "gastrinoma triangle"): junction of common bile and cystic duct junction of the second and third portion of duodenum junction of pancreatic body and neck. Ectopic tumors may be found in lymph nodes, splenic hilum, mesenterial root, omentum, liver, gallbladder, and ovaries. More than 60% of tumors are sporadic, usually solitary *60% to 85% of them being malignant.* Ectopic tumors seem to be less likely to be malignant. Some 30% of gastrinomas are part of the multiple endocrine neoplasia syndrome I (MEN I). They tend to appear at an earlier age, are usually multiple and derive from the pancreas. Although earlier reports suggested malignancy in 7% to 12% of them, it may be more frequent.

DIAGNOSIS

Diagnosis of gastrinoma is based on elevated gastrin levels in patients with intractable peptic ulcers and diarrhea. In about 70% of patients the presenting symptom is peptic ulcer disease, in the remaining 30% it is diarrhea. A level of gastrin of 40 pmol/L or more strongly supports the diagnosis. Additional tests are acid output measurement (with pentagastrin stimulation) measurement: BAO exceeding 15 mmol/h and BAO/MAO exceeding 0.6 are characteristic of gastrinoma (parietal cells are already maximally stimulated by a tumor source of gastrin). If still in doubt, the secretin test (less cumbersome and more informative than calcium gluconate stimulation) can be performed. Patients with gastrinoma have a rise in gastrin level to more than 40 mmol/L or at least 50% above the basal level within 30 minutes after a bolus of 2 U/kg of secretin.

DIFFERENTIAL DIAGNOSIS

The differential diagnosis of hypergastrinemia with peptic ulcers is as follows:

1. *Peptic disease* with moderately elevated gastrin levels: There is no further gastrin elevation by a secretin provocative test.

2. *Isolated retained antrum* after partial gastrectomy with gastroduodenostomy, that is, Billroth II procedure. In this rare condition elevated gastrinemia decreases after secretin stimulation.

3. *Gastric outlet obstruction:* Monitoring of gastrin levels during and after mechanical or pharmacologic gastric emptying is required. In case of gastrinoma these procedures do not lead to a fall in gastrin levels.

4. *Renal failure:* This may be accompanied by a moderate hypergastrinemia with peptic ulcers.

5. Rare conditions of *antral cell hyperplasia and hyperfunction:* There is no rise in gastrin level on stimulation tests, localization studies are seldom necessary.

The differential diagnosis of hypergastrinemia without ulcer disease includes pernicious anemia, other forms of atrophic gastritis and gastric cancer. For unknown reasons some patients with rheumatoid arthritis and hyperthyroidism have hypergastrinemia.

LOCALIZATION

Ultrasound imaging and computed tomography (CT) scans are of limited value. Selective angiography visualizes the tumor in a minority of patients. When combined with secretin intra-arterial injection and catheter in portal circulation for sampling gastrin levels it seems to yield more accurate results than percutaneous transhepatic venous sampling alone. The most sensitive method is somatostatin receptor scintigraphy

TREATMENT

Since gastrinomas are most often malignant, the current strategy of treatment recommended by most authorities is to achieve control of acid hypersecretion while making every effort to localize the tumor and then removing it surgically.

MEDICAL

Acid secretion is manageable by H2 blockers (ranitidine, famotidine, nizatidine) or parietal cell H^+K^+-ATPase inhibitors (omeprazole, lansoprazole). The doses of H2 inhibitors necessary to control acid output are usually higher when compared with those used for the common duodenal ulcer. Once instituted, the treatment has to be maintained indefinitely. The dose required for maintenance may be assessed by measuring BAO in the hour before the next anticipated dose of the drug, the goal being BAO of less than 10 mmol/h at that time.

It is of critical importance to have good control of acid output preoperatively and perioperatively. The parenteral perioperative dose of H2 blockers can be predicted by the prior oral dose. Following successful curative gastrinoma resection, 40% of patients still require antisecretory therapy. Attempts to predict the need for continued antisecretory therapy by acid output criteria and other biochemical or clinical characteristic failed. Symptom evaluation and upper gastroscopy should be used as a guide in the attempt to withdraw the drug.

SURGERY

For the patients with Zollinger-Ellison syndrome without evidence of metastatic disease, surgical exploration with an attempt of curative tumor resection may alter the natural history of the syndrome, that is, it results in significant decrease of the incidence of hepatic metastases. Exploration should include mobilization of the pancreas along its entire length, allowing careful bimanual palpation and, according to some authors, intraoperative ultrasound. The most accurate method of detecting duodenal wall tumors seems to be duodenotomy with careful palpation. Such as aggressive approach allows resection of gastrinomas in most (78%) patients with sporadic localized ZES with 30% of them cured in terms of long-term disease-free survival. Duodenal tumors may be more malignant, since an improvement in detecting and resecting them did not result in an improvement in immediate disease-free period. For the diagnosis of recurrent disease-fasting gastrin determination and secretin test are methods of choice.

Surgical treatment of gastrinoma in patients with MEN I remains controversial. Most gastrinomas in these patients are multifocal, so preoperatively localized tumors might not be the sources of gastrin responsible for the clinical syndrome. Moreover, since a minority of these patients undergo the surgical exploration the true incidence of duodenal tumors in them remains unclear.

CHEMOTHERAPY

Patients with advanced unresectable or metastatic tumor are candidates for chemotherapy. A standard chemotherapy for islet cell carcinomas is a combi-

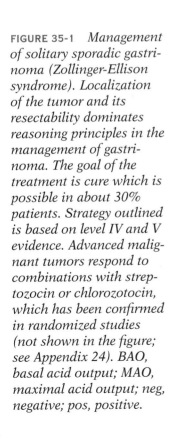

FIGURE 35-1 *Management of solitary sporadic gastrinoma (Zollinger-Ellison syndrome). Localization of the tumor and its resectability dominates reasoning principles in the management of gastrinoma. The goal of the treatment is cure which is possible in about 30% patients. Strategy outlined is based on level IV and V evidence. Advanced malignant tumors respond to combinations with streptozocin or chlorozotocin, which has been confirmed in randomized studies (not shown in the figure; see Appendix 24). BAO, basal acid output; MAO, maximal acid output; neg, negative; pos, positive.*

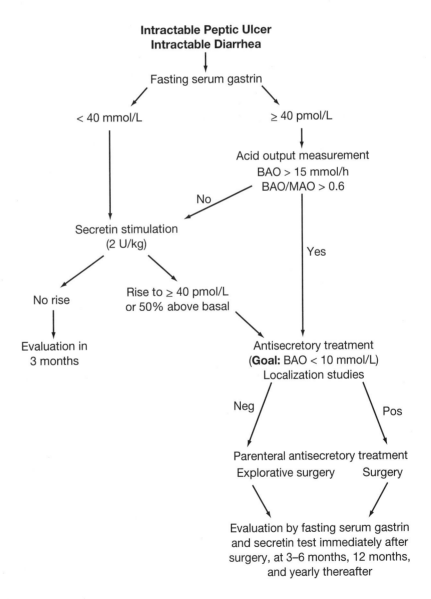

nation of streptozocin (500 mg/m² IV daily) and fluorouracil (400 mg/m² IV daily) for 5 consecutive days in 6-week intervals. It leads to 45% regression, with less than 5% complete regression. Combination of streptozocin and doxorubicin (50 mg/m² IV on days 1 and 22 of each six-week treatment cycle, maximal total dose of 500 mg/m²) was superior in a randomized study, with a 69% regression rate, 14% complete, whereas chlorozotocin (150 mg/m² IV in 7-week intervals) was comparable to the standard treatment (30% regression rate, 6% complete). Overall, although tumors do respond to chemotherapy the chance of long-term survival is still small.

In summary, in solitary sporadic gastrinoma the goal of the initial treatment is to control symptoms (by means of H2 blockers and parietal cell H+K+-ATPase inhibitors) along with localization studies to prepare patient for surgery (Fig. 35-1). The long-term goal is cure, which is now possible in 30% of patients.

Treatment of gastrinoma in MEA 1 syndrome is still controversial. In any case, the source of gastrin overproduction needs to be clearly documented before attempted surgery in those patients.

For unresectable advanced tumors there is no evidence of successful long-term cure. For the time being, the goal of the treatment is to increase the quality of life by symptom control. Effective chemotherapy is still the matter of clinical research studies (due to the rareness of these tumors a multicentric approach is mandatory).

SUGGESTED READING

Arnold WS, Fraker DL, Alexander HR et al: Apparent lymph node primary gastrinoma. Surgery 116:1123–1129, 1994

Fishbeyn VA, Norton JA, Benya RV et al: Assessment and prediction of long-term cure in patients with the Zollinger-Ellison syndrome: the best approach. Ann Intern Med 119:199–206, 1993

Fraker DL, Norton JA, Alexander HR et al: Surgery in Zollinger-Ellison syndrome alters the natural history of gastrinoma. Ann Surg 220:320–328, 1994

Gibril F, Reynolds JC, Doppman JL et al: Somatastatin receptor scintigraphy: its sensitivity compared with that of other imaging methods in detecting primary aud metastaic gastrinomas. A prospective study. Ann Int Med 125:26–34, 1996

Maton PN: Review artcle: the management of Zollinger-Ellison syndrome. Aliment Pharmacol Therap 7:467–475, 1993

Mc Guigan JE, Wolfe MM: Secretin injection test in the diagnosis of gastrinoma. Gastroenterology 79:1324–1331, 1980

Metz DC, Benya RV, Fishbeyn VA et al: Prospective study of the need for long-term antisecretory therapy in patients with Zollinger-Ellison syndrome following successful curative gastrinoma resection. Aliment Pharmacol Therap 7:247–257, 1993

Modlin IM, Lawton GP: Duodenal gastrinoma: the solution to the pancreatic paradox. J Clin Gastroenterol 193:184–188, 1994

Moertel CG, Lefkopoulo M, Lipsitz S et al: Streptozocin-doxorubicin, streptozocin-fluorouracil or chlorozotocin in the treatment of advanced islet cell carcinoma. N Engl J Med 326:519–523, 1992

Norton JA, Doppman JL, Jensen RT: Curative resection in Zollinger-Ellison syndrome: results of a 10-year prospective study. Ann Surg 215:8–18, 1992

Perry RR, Vinik AI: Diagnosis and management of functioning islet cell tumors. J Clin Endocrinol Metabol 80:2273–2278, 1995

Pipeleers-Marichal M, Somers G, Willems G et al: Gastrinomas in thc duodenums of patients with multiple endocrine neoplasia type I and Zollinger Ellison syndrome. N Engl J Med 322:723–727, 1990

Sugg SL, Norton JA, Fraker DL et al: A prospective study of intraoperative methods to diagnose and resect duodenal gastrinomas. Ann Surg 218:138–144, 1993

Thompson NW: Surgical treatment of the endocrine pancreas and Zollinger Ellison syndrome in the MEN 1 syndrome. Henry Ford Hosp Med J 40:195–198, 1992

Vinayek R, Hahne WF, Euler AR et al: Parenteral control of gastric acid hypersecretion in patients with Zollinger-Ellison syndrome. Digest Dis Sci 38:1857–1865, 1993

Zollinger RM, Ellison EH: Primary peptide ulcerations of the jejunum associated with islet cell tumors of the pancreas. Ann Surg 142:709–723, 1955

36 Breast Cancer

Karen K. Fields
Steven C. Goldstein
Robert A. Clark
Daniel M. Sullivan

Stage	0	I	II	III	IV
Presentation[a]	12.4%	41.8%	33.1%	8.0%	4.7%
Treatment[b]	S (R)	S (C, R)	S, C (R)	C, S, R	C, R
Goal	Cure	Cure	Cure	Cure	Palliation
Survival[c]	98%	90%	70%	50%	15%

[a]The incidence of breast cancer in women in the United States is 108.4/100,000. Listed under "presentation" is the percent of women with a given disease stage at the time of diagnosis.
[b]The main modality of treatment is listed first.
[c]Overall survival at 5 years.
Abbreviations: S, surgery; C, chemotherapy; R, radiation therapy.

INCIDENCE

The incidence of breast cancer has been increasing since the 1960s in the United States and worldwide, but the number of deaths resulting from breast cancer has remained relatively stable. This is likely due to earlier detection of the disease at a more curable stage as well as more effective treatment of later-stage disease. In the United States breast cancer accounts for 32% of all cancers in females and 18% of cancer deaths. In females 15 to 54 years of age, breast cancer is the most common cause of cancer-related death, and in the 40 to 55 years age group it is the leading cause of death. In the United States in 1995 there were 182,000 new cases of breast cancer diagnosed and 46,000 deaths from this disease. The lifetime risk of an American female developing breast cancer is about 11%, but more than one-half of this risk occurs after age 65. The lifetime risk of dying from this disease is 3% to 4%.

RISK FACTORS

Several risk factors are associated with the development of breast cancer, but at least 70% of females diagnosed with this cancer have no identifiable risk factors. An increased risk of breast cancer is associated with an increased total duration of menstrual life, which can result from earlier menarche (relative risk 1.1–1.9 for <14 years old) or later menopause (relative risk 1.5–2.0 for >55 years old). Nulliparous women have an increased risk of breast cancer (relative risk 3.0), as do females older than 30 years when they have their first term pregnancy (relative risk 1.9). The postmenopausal use of estrogens is associated with a decreased risk of osteoporosis and coronary artery disease, but also with an increased risk of breast cancer (relative risk 1.5–2.0). The risk of breast cancer from long-term use of oral contraceptives has probably been obviated by the much lower concentration of estrogens in present-day oral contraceptives. There is no conclusive evidence that increased dietary fat intake is associated with an increased risk of breast cancer; however, a relative risk of 1.4 is associated with a two-drink per day alcohol intake (the greatest effect here is seen in females <30 years old). A benign breast biopsy interpreted as nonproliferative disease is not associated with an increased risk of breast cancer, whereas a proliferative biopsy has a 1.9 relative risk; the subcategory of atypical hyperplasia has an even greater risk (relative risk 4.4).

The family pedigree is also very important in determining the risk of breast cancer in an individual. In this regard a distinction must be made between genetically inherited breast cancer and a family history of breast cancer. Approximately 5% to 10% of patients are thought to have hereditary breast cancer. This may be part of a cancer family syndrome (e.g., the Li-Fraumeni syndrome, in which p53 mutations have been demonstrated or associated with the recently described *BRCA1* gene on human chromosome 17q21 or *BRCA2* gene on chromosome 13q12–13). *BRCA1* gene mutations are highly heritable, and a female with this mutated gene has a 50% risk of breast cancer before the age of 50 years. An individual has a 1.5 to 3.0 relative risk of breast cancer if the mother or sister has had breast cancer. If in addition to a breast cancer diagnosis in a first-degree relative, the individual has an atypical hyperplasia biopsy, then the person has a 20% risk of developing breast cancer within 15 years; this risk is 8% in the presence of atypical hyperplasia alone.

Breast cancer may be classified as either infiltrating or in situ. In ductal carcinoma in situ (DCIS) and lobular carcinoma in situ (LCIS) the malignant cells are confined to the mammary ducts or lobules and have not invaded through the basement membrane. The majority of infiltrating carcinomas are ductal (78.1%). Infiltrating lobular carcinoma, which presents more often with multicentric tumors and spreads to meningeal and serosal surfaces, is the next most common (8.7%), followed by comedo (4.6%), medullary (4.3%), colloid (2.6%), and papillary (1.2%). Paget's disease and inflammatory breast cancer are seen in about 1% and 2%, respectively, of all those diagnosed with breast cancer. The primary site of breast cancer, which is not related to survival, is most often the upper outer quadrant (48%), followed by a central location within 1 cm of the areola (17%), the upper inner quadrant (15%), lower outer quadrant (11%), lower inner quadrant (6%), and a diffuse presentation (3%). The regional lymph nodes most commonly involved are the axillary nodes, which are involved in about 40% of those diagnosed with breast cancer. The internal mammary lymph nodes are the next most frequently site of regional spread, followed by the supraclavicular lymph nodes. The physical examination of the axillae is only moderately reliable in detecting regional spread, as palpable axillary nodes are pathologically negative 25% of the time and nonpalpable axillary nodes are involved with tumor in 30% of patients. While several prognostic factors for breast cancer have been described (see Table 36-5), the single most important prognostic factor is the presence and extent of axillary node involvement with tumor. The 2 year survival of patients treated with a radical mastectomy was found to be 73% in axillary node negative patients, 51% when one to three lymph nodes were involved, and 23% when more than four nodes were involved. In addition to lymph node involvement, survival has been correlated with primary tumor size. If the primary tumor is greater than 2 cm, the 10 year survival is 82% and 68% in node-negative and node-positive patients, respectively. For tumors 2 to 5 cm, the corresponding numbers are 65% and 51%, and for primary tumors greater than 5 cm, the survival is 44% and 37%.

STAGING

Guidelines for staging breast cancer at the time of initial diagnosis depend on whether the patient is a candidate for any form of systemic treatment, whether the patient is eligible for an investigational protocol, and on the presence or absence of symptoms suggestive of metastatic disease. In all cases a detailed history and physical examination should be performed, as well as a chest radiograph, complete blood count, and chemistry panel (which includes liver chemistries). If the patient is to be enrolled in a protocol, then further evaluation will be dictated by the investigational study and will likely include a bilateral mammogram, bone scan, computed tomography scan of the abdomen and pelvis, magnetic resonance imaging of the brain, and CEA and CA15-3 levels. For patients who are ineligible for protocols but are candidates for systemic treatment, further initial evaluation depends on the stage of their breast cancer and the presence of symptoms. Patients should be evaluated with the appropriate test at any stage for bone pain, change in mental status, abnormal liver chemistries, hepatomegaly, or significant weight loss. Asymptomatic stage I and "low risk" stage II patients need no further evaluation than that initially outlined above (increased risk is defined here as younger patients, larger primary tumors, ≥ four lymph nodes involved, increased S phase, aneuploid tumors, and estrogen and progesterone receptor-negative tumors). Higher risk stage II, as well as stage III and IV patients, should be evaluated for the presence of metastatic disease, which is found most often (in decreasing order of incidence) in lung, liver, bone, pleura, and adrenal glands. Less than 5% of asymptomatic stage I and II patients will have positive bone scans, whereas 20% to 25% of asymptomatic stage III patients will have bone metastases demonstrated by a bone scan. Tables 36–1 to 36-7 and Figures 36-1 to 36-5 cover the

TABLE 36-1 GUIDELINES FOR BREAST CANCER SCREENING[a]

	Organization		
	ACS	*ACP*	*USPSTF*
Breast self-examination	> age 20, monthly	Not recommended	Not recommended
Breast clinical physical examination	ages 20–40, every 3 years > age 40, annually	> age 40, annually	> age 40, annually
Screening mammography	ages 40–49, every 1 or 2 years[d] > age 50, annually[b]	> age 50,[c] annually[d]	ages 50–75,[c] every 1 or 2 years[d]

[a]*As endorsed by the American Cancer Society (ACS), American College of Physicians (ACP), and United States Preventive Services Task Force (USPSTF). These guidelines are based on evidence from several randomized, controlled, clinical trials (level 1, grade A evidence). The expected benefit of screening is reduction of breast cancer mortality by one third in screened women.*

[b]*Also endorsed by the American Medical Association, American College of Radiology, American Association of Family Practice, American College of Obstetrics and Gynecology, College of American Pathologists, National Medical Association, American Association of Women in Medicine.*

[c]*High-risk women, i.e., history of first degree family member with breast cancer, may begin screening at an earlier age.*

[d]*Similar to the recommendations of the National Cancer Institute (annual screening ages 50 to 74 years).*

TABLE 36-2 STANDARDIZED MAMMOGRAPHY REPORTING CATEGORIES DEVELOPED BY THE AMERICAN COLLEGE OF RADIOLOGY

0. **Incomplete. Needs further radiographic assessment (A)**
   This is a temporary category to be used in screening examinations and in more definitively examining a detected abnormality. Further assessment may include additional mammographic images (e.g., localization views, magnification, or spot compression or sonography). Following the additional assessment, the case is then reported in one of the following five completed categories.
1. **Negative (N). Routine subsequent screening is recommended.**
   This category is to be used for reporting a negative, or normal, examination.
2. **Negative, with benign findings (B). Routine subsequent screening is recommended.**
   This category is to be used for reporting a negative examination with additional comments on benign findings (e.g., intramammary lymph nodes, benign calcifications).
3. **Abnormal, probably benign (P). Short-term interval follow-up is recommended.**
   This category is to be used for abnormal findings that have a very low likelihood, or probability, of representing cancer (e.g., asymmetric parenchymal density, sharply circumscribed mass, smooth or punctate clustered calcifications). The short-term follow-up is usually done 4 to 6 months later and may continue at 6-month intervals for a period of 1 to 2 years, confirming benignity by a lack of progression of the findings. The follow-up procedures may include diagnostic mammography, ultrasound, clinical breast examination, or a combination. Biopsy of findings in this category may be done occasionally, if the woman or her physician so desires.
4. **Abnormal, suspicious for malignancy (S). Biopsy should be considered.**
   This category is to be used for findings that carry a higher likelihood, or probability, of representing cancer (e.g., irregularly marginated mass, indeterminate clustered calcifications, architectural distortion). Biopsy may be done with image-guided needle techniques or open surgical excision.
5. **Abnormal, highly suggestive of malignancy (M). Biopsy is recommended.**
   This category is to be used for findings that are characteristic for cancer (e.g., branching or pleomorphic microcalcifications, spiculated mass). Biopsy may be done with image-guided needle techniques or open surgical excision.

The expected benefits of standardized results reporting are improved communication among women and physicians and reduced variability in radiologists' interpretations of mammography.

TABLE 36-3 **BENCHMARKS FOR OUTCOME MEASURES OF BREAST CANCER SCREENING**

Benign biopsies: < 75% of total biopsies
Malignant biopsies: >25% of total biopsies
Noninvasive cancers: > 20% detected cancers
Invasive cancers: < 80% detected cancers
Stage distribution of detected cancers (TNM staging of cancers at diagnosis (i.e., size, invasiveness,
    nodal status):   Tis + T1a + T1b = > 40% cancers; Stages 0 + 1 = > 70% cancers
Sensitivity of mammography: > 0.85
Specificity of mammography: > 0.95

*These outcome measures are derived from intermediate endpoints of several randomized, controlled,
clinical trials (Level 1, grade A evidence). The expected benefit of screening is reduction of breast cancer
mortality by one-third in screened women.*

TABLE 36-4 **BREAST CANCER STAGING**

Stage 0	Carcinoma in situ (DCIS, LCIS, or Paget's disease of the nipple without tumor)
Stage I	Primary tumor ≤2 cm
Stage IIA	No primary tumor with metastasis to movable ipsilateral axillary lymph nodes, or tumor ≤2 cm with metastasis to movable ipsilateral axillary lymph nodes, or tumor >2 cm and ≤5 cm without regional lymph node metastasis
Stage IIB	Tumor >2 cm and ≤5 cm with metastasis to movable ipsilateral axillary nodes or tumor >5 cm and no regional lymph node metastasis
Stage IIIA	Tumor ≤ 5 cm with metastasis to ipsilateral axillary lymph node(s) fixed to one another or to other structures, or tumor >5 cm with metastasis to ipsilateral axillary lymph nodes that are either movable or fixed to one another or to other structures
Stage IIIB	Tumor of any size that directly extends to chest wall or skin associated with any nodal status (includes inflammatory cancer), or tumor of any size with metastasis to ipsilateral internal mammary node(s)
Stage IV	Any tumor size and any nodal status with distant metastasis including metastasis to ipsilateral supraclavicular lymph node(s)

*(From Beahrs OH, Henson DE, Hutter RVP, Kennedy BJ [eds]: American Joint Committee on Cancer:
Manual for Staging of Cancer. JB Lippincott, Philadelphia, 1992, pp. 149–154, with permission.)*

TABLE 36-5 COMMONLY MEASURED PROGNOSTIC INDICATORS

Indicator	Favorable
Tumor size	≤ 1 cm
Histologic grade	Grade 1
Histologic type	Tubular, medullary
Nuclear grade	Grade 1
Estrogen receptor	Positive
Progesterone receptor	Positive
Ploidy	Diploid
Percent S phase	≤ 7%
Cathepsin D	<30
p53 gene product	None
P-glycoprotein	None

Prognostic indicators are used to determine the risk of developing systemic disease in patients with newly diagnosed breast cancer. Although several prognostic factors are commonly evaluated at the time of initial surgical intervention, their role in guiding therapy is currently limited. The presence or absence of lymph node involvement remains the most important prognostic indicator, with the majority of node-negative women disease-free (65% to >80%) over a lifetime following local therapy alone. It is this group of patients for whom the assessment of prognostic factors is clinically useful, since a minority of these women actually need or benefit from adjuvant systemic therapy. Other prognostic indicators, such as estrogen receptor status, play a role in determining optimal adjuvant or systemic therapy (i.e., antihormonal therapy and/or chemotherapy). For example, if both estrogen and progesterone receptors are positive, the clinical response rate to antihormonal therapy is >75%, while estrogen and progesterone-negative tumors exhibit only about a 10% response rate to antihormonal therapy. A myriad of new prognostic factors are currently being evaluated, but their role remains investigational. Percent S phase reflects the number of cells entering the synthesis phase of the cell cycle, reflecting cell proliferation; this indicator is strongly associated with prognosis in several studies. Ploidy refers to the DNA content, with diploid tumors associated with less aggressive tumors and improved survival. p53 gene product, a nuclear phosphoprotein, regulates cell proliferation, and excessive amounts of this protein result in inactivation of tumor-suppressor function. P-glycoprotein expression is associated with resistance to several chemotherapeutic agents, including paclitaxel, doxorubicin, etoposide, and mitoxantrone. The evidence to support the use of these indicators is generally level II and III. The key reasoning principle is that using these indicators to assess the risk of developing systemic disease in early stage breast cancer provides further support for the use of adjuvant therapy in high-risk patients, especially node-negative patients.

TABLE 36-6 CONTRAINDICATIONS TO BREAST CONSERVATION

Absolute

Tumor size ≥ 5 cm

Two or more gross malignancies in separate quadrants of the breast

Diffuse malignant or indeterminate-appearing microcalcifications on mammogram

Inability to achieve negative surgical margins

Extensive intraductal component

Prior breast irradiation prohibiting adequate radiation dosing

First- or second- trimester pregnancy

Large tumor in small breast prohibiting adequate cosmesis

Relative

History of collagen vascular disease (interference with healing)

Tumor location that prohibits adequate cosmesis

Large breast size may prohibit adequate dose homogeneity

Multiple large, prospective, randomized clinical trials comparing breast conservation therapy (lumpectomy with axillary node dissection and breast irradiation) to mastectomy for the treatment of early-stage breast cancer have demonstrated that, in appropriate circumstances, overall survival does not differ significantly for patients who receive lumpectomy compared with patients who receive mastectomy. The addition of radiation therapy following lumpectomy decreases the risk of local recurrence following lumpectomy by approximately one third. Although the risk of local recurrence following lumpectomy and irradiation ranged from 4% to 19% in several large, prospective trials, this did not affect overall survival when compared with mastectomy. The pattern of relapses varies in these patients, however, with local relapses seen more commonly in lumpectomy patients as the first site of recurrence and distal relapses seen more commonly as the first site of recurrence in patients undergoing more extensive primary surgery. Ipsilateral breast tumor recurrence within 4 years of lumpectomy and radiation is associated with a 50% incidence of developing distal metastases and a 50% 5-year overall survival. However, in patients with ipsilateral breast tumor recurrence greater than 4 years following lumpectomy and radiation, only 17% of patients develop distal metastases and 78% are alive at 5 years. Therefore, early breast relapse should be treated aggressively with consideration of adjuvant therapy (seeAppendix 25). This table defines which patients are candidates for breast conservation. The evidence to support these decisions is level I. The key reasoning principle is based on the premise that local therapy does not influence long-term survival in patients with breast cancer; rather, breast cancer is a systemic disease at diagnosis, and initial therapy should address this possibility. The goal of therapy in all cases is local control and cure.

TABLE 36-7 RECOMMENDATIONS FOR POST-TREATMENT SURVEILLANCE

	Years 1 and 2	Years 3–5	>5 Years
History/Physical Exam	Every 3–4 months	Every 6 months	Every 12 months
Mammography[b]			
S/P Mastectomy	Every 12 months	Every 12 months	Every 12 months
S/P Lumpectomy	Every 6 months	Every 12 months	Every 12 months
Serology			
Tumor markers[c]	Every 6 months	Every 6 months	Every 6 months
Liver function studies (sensitivity[d] 1%–12%)	Every 6 months	Every 6 months	Every 12 months
Radiology			
Chest x-ray (sensitivity[d] 0%–5%)	Every 12 months	Every 12 months	Every 12 months
Bone scan (sensitivity[d] 0%–8%)	As indicated	As indicated	As indicated
CT scan abdomen	As indicated	As indicated	As indicated

The use of serial physical examinations/history, serologic, and radiographic studies as a means for following patients who have undergone therapy for breast cancer would be medically appropriate and cost effective only if early asymptomatic detection of relapse could be demonstrated to have a clear beneficial effect on long-term survival. Because treatment for local regional recurrence can still be considered curative for a significant number of patients, serial physical examinations/history and mammograms are warranted. Whether systemic relapse is curable in enough patients (e.g., with high-dose chemotherapy) to warrant the costs of early asymptomatic detection via more invasive and expensive studies remains controversial, as is the survival benefit of early institution of salvage therapy. Therefore, it is important to enroll patients in clinical trials to define the role and optimal timing of salvage therapy, including high-dose chemotherapy, in the treatment of stage IV disease. It is from these analyses that the benefits, if any, of post-treatment surveillance and institution of early salvage therapy will be defined.

[b]See section on screening. Patients undergoing lumpectomy should be studied every 6 months unilaterally for local recurrence for 1 to 2 years, then bilaterally every 12 months.

[c]Primary utility is as part of an IRB-approved protocol. Isolated elevation should not be interpreted as definitive evidence for metastatic disease.

[d]Clinical utility and cost effectiveness of surveillance beyond history/physical examination and serial mammography remains controversial because of low sensitivity.

(From Loprinzi C: J Clin Oncol 12:881–883, 1994, with permission.)

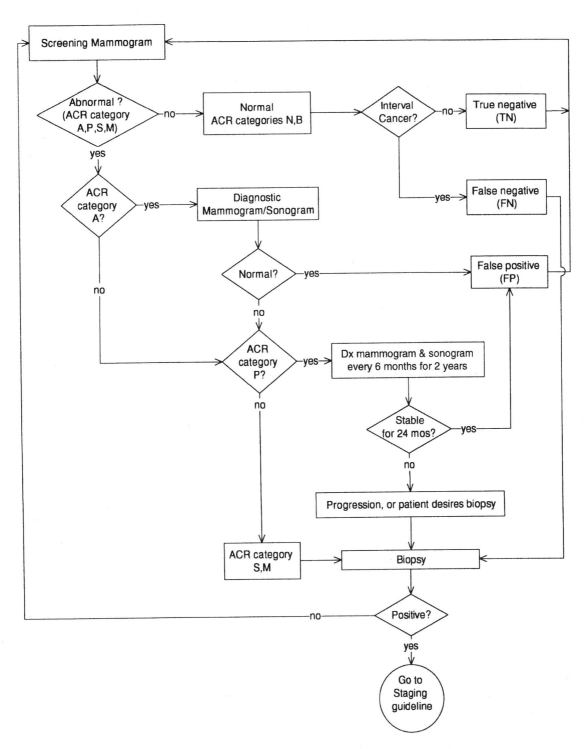

FIGURE 36-1 *Algorithm for the interpretation of screening mammography and management of detected abnormalities. This approach is based on evidence from several randomized, controlled clinical trials (level 1, grade A evidence). The expected benefit of screening is reduction of breast cancer mortality by one third in screened women. ACR, American College of Radiology; see Table 36-2 for other abbreviations.*

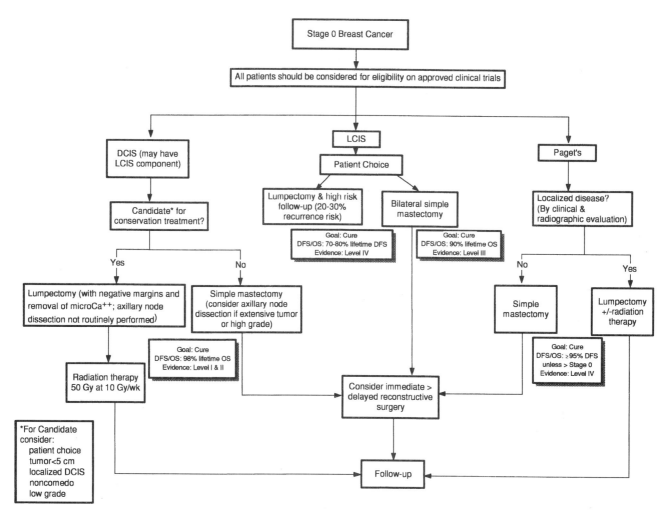

FIGURE 36-2 *Treatment of ductal carcinoma in situ (DCIS), lobular carcinoma in situ (LCIS), and Paget's disease. The key reasoning principle is the malignant (invasive) potential of these stage 0 breast cancers, which determines the aggressiveness of the treatment approach. The goal of treatment in all cases is cure. The evidence used to support these recommendations is level I and II for DCIS and level IV for LCIS and Paget's. The addition of radiation therapy to lumpectomy for localized DCIS tumors decreases the 5-year cumulative incidence of ipsilateral noninvasive cancers from 10.4% to 7.5%, and of ipsilateral invasive cancers from 10.5% to 2.9% (p < 0.001). The recurrence rate after lumpectomy and radiation therapy at 10 years is 10% to 15%. One half of these are invasive cancers (5% to 7%) and one half of these will be curable. Therefore, the mortality risk using this treatment approach in localized DCIS is 2% to 3%. LCIS is considered a premalignant diffuse (bilateral) disease found in 0.8% to 8% of breast biopsies. There is no good evidence in favor of lumpectomy versus bilateral mastectomy. However, the patient may not be willing to accept a 20% to 30% risk of recurrence after conservation treatment. The risk of invasive cancer after biopsy alone in LCIS is 16% in the ipsilateral breast and 9% in the contralateral breast. About 50% of those with Paget's disease have a breast mass at presentation and should be staged according to the size of the tumor.*

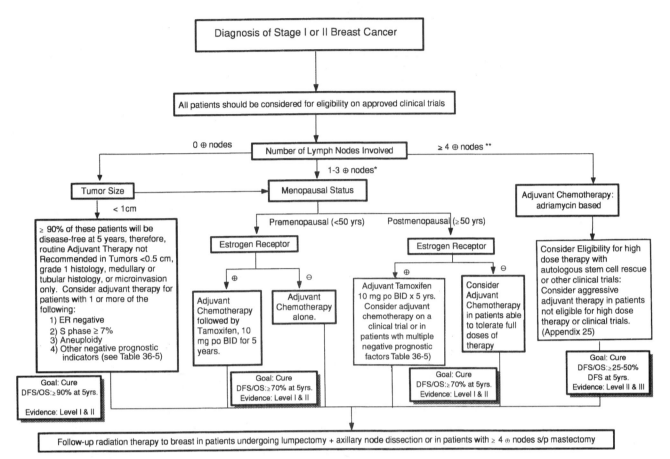

FIGURE 36-3 *Strategies for adjuvant therapy for patients with stage I and II breast cancer are outlined. In node-negative patients with small tumors (< 1 cm), the decision to give adjuvant therapy is based on the assessment of other prognostic indicators. For patients with larger tumors with or without nodal metastases, adjuvant therapy is based on menopausal status, estrogen receptor status, as well as other prognostic factors. The goal of therapy in all instances is cure. Key reasoning principles are based on the assessment of risk of systemic disease at the time of initial therapy, with the presence and number of nodal metastases remaining the most important determinants of long-term prognosis. Recent data suggest that adjuvant hormonal therapy is associated with an overall reduction in the risk of mortality at 15 years of 27%; adjuvant chemotherapy is associated with an overall reduction in mortality of 18% at 15 years. The greatest reduction following adjuvant chemotherapy is seen in patients with node-negative disease (27% compared with a 14% decrease in patients with nodal involvement). Adjuvant chemotherapy with or without antihormonal therapy has been associated with up to 80% progression-free at 5 years in patients with 1 to 3 positive nodes (*) in some series. However, for women with four or more positive nodes (**), the benefits of adjuvant therapy are limited, and 50% or fewer of these women would be expected to remain disease free with long-term follow-up, the risks increasing with increasing numbers of positive nodes. For this reason, all women with four or more positive nodes should be considered for investigational protocols with aggressive or novel treatment regimens. The evidence to support treatment decisions in these patients is based on the analysis of multiple large prospective, randomized clinical trials including several meta-analyses and is therefore considered level I.*

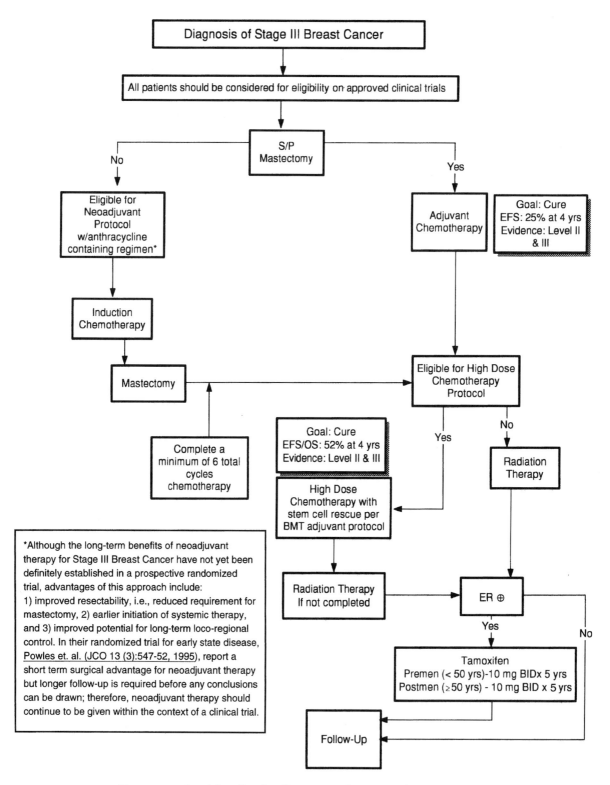

FIGURE 36-4 *Treatment algorithm for the diagnosis of stage III breast cancer. Treatment strategies should be pursued with curative intent, although relapse rates approximate 60% to 80% with standard therapy. In the Autologous Blood and Marrow Transplant Registry (ABMTR) data base, the probability of progression-free survival at 3 years for patients with stage III disease undergoing high-dose chemotherapy and stem cell rescue is 52%. The evidence to support this algorithm is considered level III.*

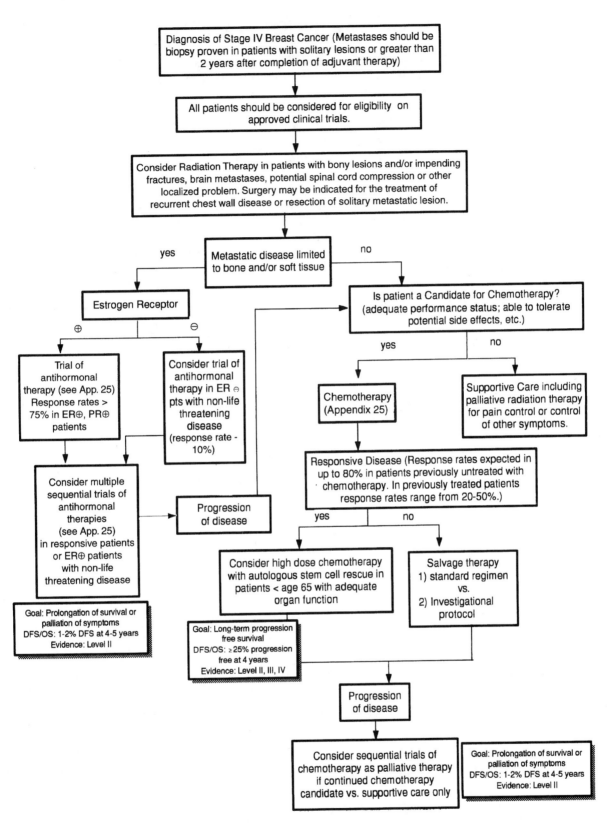

FIGURE 36-5 *Strategies for the treatment of patients with metastatic breast cancer are outlined. Long-term survival is limited in these patients, with approximately 1% to 2% of patients alive and disease free at 5 years after a diagnosis of metastatic breast cancer. The key reasoning principle is, therefore, that metastatic breast cancer is generally an incurable disease. However, breast cancer can be very chemo- or hormonal-sensitive, especially in previously untreated patients, and treatment of metastases frequently results in improvement of symptoms early in the course of disease. The goals of this*

therapy are generally palliative, although high-dose therapy has resulted in prolonged progression-free survival in a group of patients with chemoresponsive, metastatic breast cancer. As noted, diagnosis and treatment should be based on biopsy-proven disease whenever possible. Initial treatment should be based on the extent and location of disease and the estrogen receptor status of the patient. Women with limited, nonlife-threatening disease should be considered for antihormonal therapy as primary management. However, this approach is palliative in nature. Guidelines for this type of therapy are described in Appendix 25. Patients considered for chemotherapy should be approached with a goal of palliation of symptoms while limiting side effects, except in younger patients and chemoresponsive patients who may be candidates for high-dose therapy or other aggressive novel treatments. In patients with good performance status who fail initial therapy for metastatic disease, salvage therapy with different single agents or combinations of chemotherapy is appropriate. Selection of patients for multiple trials of salvage therapy should be individualized based on the performance status and the extent and location of disease, since the strategy is palliative in nature, not curative. Responses to second-line therapy are generally in the 20% to 25% range, with decreasing response rates after each subsequent therapeutic trial. Therefore, more than two to three trials of different chemotherapy regimens would not be expected to yield meaningful responses. Evidence for this approach is level II and III, with few large randomized trials comparing standard therapy to no therapy and one randomized trial comparing high-dose therapy to standard therapy.

following topics: breast cancer screening by mammography, the staging of breast cancer, commonly measured prognostic indicators, contraindications for breast conservation, treatment of DCIS and LCIS, treatment of clinically stage I and II disease, treatment of clinically stage III disease, management of stage IV disease, and guidelines for post-treatment follow-up. Examples of commonly used antihormonal agents, standard adjuvant chemotherapy regimens, high-dose chemotherapy protocols, salvage regimens, and antiemetic regimens can be found in Appendix 25.

SUGGESTED READINGS

Antman K, Corringham R, DeVries E et al: Dose intensive therapy in breast cancer. Bone Marrow Transplantation 10(suppl):67–73, 1992

Antman K et al: High dose chemotherapy with autologous hematopoietic stem cell support for breast cancer in North America (in press)

Bezwoda WR, Seymour L, Dansey RD: High-dose chemotherapy with hematopoietic rescue as primary treatment for metastatic breast cancer: A randomized trial. J Clin Oncol 13:2483–2489, 1995

Bilimoria MM, Morrow M: The woman at increased risk for breast cancer: evaluation and management strategies. CA: Cancer J Clin 45:263–278, 1995

Bondy ML, Lustbader ED, Halabi S, Ross E, Vogel VG: Validation of a breast cancer risk assessment model in women with a positive family history. JNCI 86:620–625, 1994

Early Breast Cancer Trialist's Collaborative Group: Systemic treatment of early breast cancer by hormonal, cytotoxic, or immune therapy. 133 randomised trials involving 31,000 recurrences and 24,000 deaths among 75,000 women. Lancet 339: 1–15, 71–85, 1992

Early Breast Cancer Trialist's Collaborative Group: Effects of radiotherapy and surgery in early breast cancer. N Engl J Med 333:1444–1455, 1995

Eddy DM: Common Screening Tests. American College of Physicians, Philadelphia, 1991, Ch. 9, pp. 229–254

Fletcher SW, Black W, Harris R, Rimer BK, Shapira S: Report of the International Workshop on Screening for Breast Cancer. J Natl Cancer Inst 85:1644–1656, 1993

Fisher B, Anderson S, Redmond CK et al: Reanalysis and results after 12 years of follow-up in a randomized clinical trial comparing total mastectomy with lumpectomy with or without irradiation in the treatment of breast cancer. N Engl J Med 333:1456–1461, 1995

Gail MH, Brinton LA, Byar DP et al: Projecting individualized probabilities of developing breast cancer for white females who are being examined annually. NCI 81:1879–1886, 1989

Haffty BG, Reiss M, Beinfield M et al: Ipsilateral breast tumor recurrence as a predictor of distant disease: implication for systemic therapy at the time of local relapse. J Clin Oncol 14:52–57, 1996

Harris JR, Morrow M, Bonadonna G: Cancer of the breast. In DeVita V.T Jr Hellman S, Rosenberg SA (eds): Cancer: Principles and Practice of Oncology. Lippincott-Raven, Philadelphia, 1993

Henderson IC: Chemotherapy for metastatic disease. pp. 604–665. In Harris JR, Hellman S, Henderson IC, Kinne DW (eds): Breast Diseases. 2nd Ed. Lippincott-Raven, Philadelphia, 1991

Hortobagyi GN, Buzdar AU: Current status of adjuvant systemic therapy for primary breast cancer: progress and controversy. CA: Cancer Clin 45:199–226, 1995

Horton J: Special report: 1995 Oxford Breast Cancer Overview-preliminary outcomes. Cancer Control 3:80–81, 1996

Kerlikowske D, Grady D, Rubin SM, Sandrock C, Ernster VL: Efficacy of screening mammography: a meta-analysis. JAMA 273:149–154, 1994

Loprinzi C: It is now the age to define the appropriate follow-up of primary breast cancer patients. JCO 12:881–883, 1994

McGuire WL, Clark GM: Prognostic factors for recurrence and survival in ancillary factors for recurrence and survival in axillary node-negative breast cancer. J Steroid Biol 34:145–148, 1989

McGuire WL, Clark GM: Prognostic factors and treatment decisions in axillary-node-negative breast cancer. N Engl J Med 326:1756–1761, 1992

Muss HB, Case LD, Richards F et al: Interrupted versus continuous chemotherapy in patients with metastatic breast cancer. N Engl J Med 325:1342–1348, 1991

Mettlin C, Smart CR: Breast cancer detection guidelines for women aged 40–49 years: rationale for the American Cancer Society reaffirmation of recommendations. CA Cancer J Clin 44:248–255, 1994

Olivotto IV, Bajdik CD, Math M et al: Adjuvant systemic therapy and survival after breast cancer. N Engl J Med 330:805–810, 1994

Pandya K et al: A retrospective study of earliest indicators of recurrence in patients on ECOG adjuvant chemotherapy trials for breast cancer. Cancer 55:202–205, 1985

Powles T et al: Randomized trial of chemoendocrine therapy started before or after surgery for treatment of primary breast cancer. J Clin Oncol 13:547–552, 1995

Sigurdsson H, Baledtorp B, Borg A et al: Indicators of prognosis in node-negative breast cancer. N Engl J Med 322:1045–1053, 1990

United States Preventive Services Task Force. Guide to clinical preventive services. Williams & Wilkins, Baltimore, 1989, Ch. 6, pp. 39–46

Winchester DP, Cox JD: Standards for Breast Conservation Treatment. CA Cancer J Clin 42:134–162, 1992

Wingo PA, Tong T, Bolden S: Cancer statistics. CA Cancer J Clin 45:8–30, 1995

Wood WC, Budman DR, Korzun AH et al: Dose and dose intensity of adjuvant chemotherapy for stage II, node-positive breast carcinoma. N Engl J Med 330:1253–1259, 1994

37 Ovarian Cancer

James R. Bosscher
David L. Doering

EPITHELIAL OVARIAN CANCER

Epidemiology: Fourth most common cause of death from cancer in women in the United States. Mean age at diagnosis is 59 years; 80% found in postmenopausal women. Lifetime incidence 1/70 and 1/100 will die from it. Accounts for 90% of ovarian cancers

Goal of treatment: Cure except for recurrent/persistent disease

Main modality of treatment: Surgery with adjuvant chemotherapy (except for stage Ia grade 1 tumors)

Prognosis:

Stage	5-Year Survival (%)
Stage Ia	70–100
Stage Ib	70–100
Stage Ic	60–90
Stage IIa	75
Stage IIb	50
Stage IIc	40
Stage IIIa	30–40
Stage IIIb	20
Stage IIIc	5–10
Stage IV	5

GERM CELL TUMORS

Epidemiology: Represent less than 5% of ovarian tumors. In first two decades of life, 70% of ovarian tumors are of germ-cell origin. Median age of diagnosis between 16 to 20 years. Majority are unilateral

Goal of treatment: Cure

Main modality of treatment: Surgery (conservative unilateral oophorectomy with staging laparotomy and removal of readily resectable metastasis) and chemotherapy (except for stage Ia dysgerminoma and stage Ia grade 1 immature teratoma, which need no adjuvant chemotherapy)

Prognosis: *Stage*   *5-year survival (%)*

Stage I   95

Stage II–IV   30–70

SEX CORD STROMAL TUMORS

Epidemiology: Account for 5% to 8% of all ovarian malignancies. Adult-type granulosa cell tumors (95%) occur in the perimenopausal years, with a mean age of 50 to 53 years. Juvenile granulosa cell tumors (5%) occur in the first two decades of life. Sertoli-Leydig tumors are low-grade malignancies that are usually diagnosed in the third and fourth decades. Majority are unilateral

Goal of treatment: Cure

Main modality of Treatment: Surgery (unilateral oophorectomy in young patient). The optimal treatment for metastatic disease has not been defined but chemotherapy (BEP, VAC, PAC) has been used.

Prognosis: Granulosa cell tumors: 10-year survival, 90%

20-year survival, 75%

Sertoli-Leydig cell tumor: 5-year survival, 70%–90%

Ovarian cancer is the fourth most common cause of death from cancer in American women. The prevalence is 30 to 50/100,000 and the lifetime incidence is about 1 in 70. The most frequent ovarian neoplasms, termed epithelial carcinomas, account for 85% to 90% of all cases. Seventy-five percent of epithelial tumors are of the serous histologic type. Less common types are mucinous (20%), endometrial (2%), clear cell, Brenner, and undifferentiated carcinomas, each of the latter three representing less than 1% of the epithelial tumors. Sex cord-stromal tumors as well as germ cell ovarian neoplasms are much less common.

The majority of women with ovarian cancer have no symptoms. When they do develop, they are often nonspecific. This is why 75% of epithelial tumors are first diagnosed at an advanced stage. Advanced ovarian cancer symptoms include abdominal distension, bloating, constipation, nausea, anorexia, and early satiety. Premenopausal women may complain of irregular or heavy menses and postmenopausal women may have vaginal bleeding.

Although the cause is unknown, some women are at a higher risk of developing ovarian cancer. Advanced age, nulliparity, North American or Northern European descent, a personal history of endometrial, colon, and breast cancer, or a family history of ovarian cancer are some of the risk factors. The lifetime risk for ovarian cancer with no affected relatives is 1.4%. With one first-degree relative, the risk approaches 5%, and with two or more first-degree relatives the lifetime risk rises to 7%. Three to five percent of the latter group will have one of the hereditary ovarian cancer syndromes. They include the site-specific familial cancer syndrome, the breast/ovary familial cancer syndrome, and the Lynch II syndrome. For patients with a hereditary ovarian cancer syndrome, the lifetime risk is approximately 40%, assuming an autosomal dominant inheritance with 80% penetrance.

Certain factors have been established as protective and include more than one full-term pregnancy, oral contraception, and breast feeding, all of which reduce the total number of ovulatory cycles. Tubal ligation has also been described as protective. Oral contraception use for more than five years reduced the lifetime risk by 35% in one study.

The most common finding of ovarian cancer is an adnexal or pelvic mass. It is estimated that 5% to 10% of women in the United States will undergo a surgical procedure for a suspected ovarian neoplasm during their lifetime and of these, 10% to 20% will be found to have an ovarian malignancy. Since the majority of masses found are benign, it is important to determine preoperatively whether the patient is at high risk for ovarian cancer to ensure proper management. A complete history and physical examination including a bimanual and rectovaginal examination should be performed. Transvaginal ultrasound (TVS) can further help to evaluate a pelvic mass. CA-125 levels in postmenopausal women are also helpful. Management depends on a combination of many predictive factors. They include age, menopausal status, size of the mass, TVS features, CA-125 level, presence or absence of symptoms, and whether the mass is unilateral or bilateral. In premenopausal women, a cystic mass greater than 8 cm has a higher probability of being neoplastic. In postmenopausal women, most adnexal masses will require surgical exploration with the exception of a unilocular, less than 5-cm cyst with a normal CA-125. Before surgical exploration, a chest x-ray, on electrocardiogram, a complete blood count, and liver and renal function tests, should be evaluated.

Routine screening of women with current screening modalities is not recommended. It is only encouraged in the context of clinical trials, to determine the efficacy of the available modalities and their potential impact upon ovarian morbidity and mortality.

STAGING

Proper surgical staging is imperative to assess the extent of disease accurately before selecting the most appropriate treatment (Table 37-1). An attempt should be made to remove all macroscopic disease if possible or remove the bulk to smaller than a predetermined size or diameter (0.5–2 cm). It has been shown that patients whose largest residual lesions were less than or equal to 5 mm had a superior survival. In one study by Van Linden et al, the survival was 40 months, compared with 18 months for patients whose lesions were less than 1.5 cm, and 6 months for patients with nodules less than 1.5 cm. When only microscopic or pelvic tumor is found, surgical staging should be completed. The staging procedure usually will include a unilateral oophorectomy, when a conservative procedure is required; otherwise, a total abdominal hysterectomy with bilateral oophorectomy is done. Staging also includes collecting any free ascitic fluid; if none is present, peritoneal washings should

TABLE 37-1 FIGO STAGING FOR OVARIAN CANCER

Stage I	Growth limited to the ovaries
Ia	Growth limited to one ovary; no ascites; no tumor on the external surface; capsule intact
Ib	Growth limited to both ovaries; no ascites; no tumor on the external surface; capsule intact
Ic	Tumor either stage la or lb, but with tumor on the surface of one or both ovaries; or with capsule ruptured; or with ascites present containing malignant cells, or with positive peritoneal washings
Stage II	Growth involving one or both ovaries with pelvic extension
IIa	Extension and/or metastasis to the uterus and/or tubes
IIb	Extension to other pelvic tissues
IIc	Tumor either stage IIa or IIb, but with tumor on the surface of one or both ovaries; or with capsule(s) ruptured; or with ascites present containing malignant cells, or with positive peritoneal washings
Stage III	Tumor involving one or both ovaries with peritoneal implants outside the pelvis and/or positive retroperitoneal or inguinal nodes; superficial liver metastasis equals stage III; tumor limited to the true pelvis, but with histologically verified malignant extension to the small bowel or omentum
IIIa	Tumor grossly limited to the true pelvis with negative nodes, but with histologically confirmed microscopic seeding of the abdominal peritoneal surfaces
IIIb	Tumor of one or both ovaries with histologically confirmed implants of 2 cm in diameter; nodes negative
IIIc	Abdominal implants exceeding 2 cm in diameter and/or positive retroperitoneal or inguinal nodes
Stage IV	Growth involving one or both ovaries with distant metastasis; if pleural effusion is present, cytologic test results must be positive to allot a case to stage IV; parenchymal liver metastasis equals stage IV

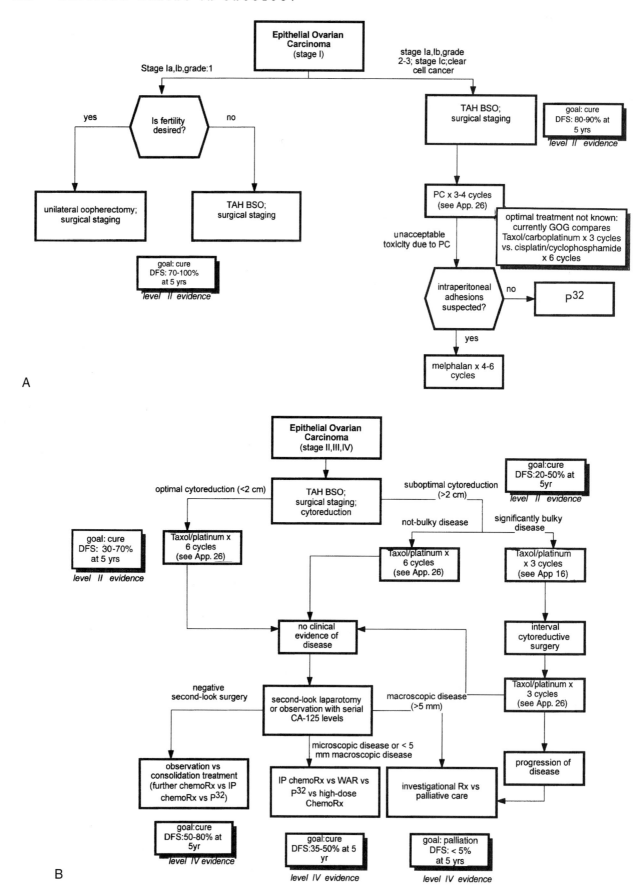

FIGURE 37-1 *(A & B) Management of ovarian cancer.*
Determining the stage and assessing prognostic category represent key management principles in the treatment of ovarian cancer. The goal of the treatment is cure for all patients except those with recurrent/persistent disease. Recommended strategy is based on solid data for initial treatment options (level II evidence); data are of lower quality for recommendations on persistent/recurrent disease (level IV/V). DFS, disease-free survival; TAH, total abdominal hysterectomy; BSO, bilateral salpingo-oophoritis; WAR, whole abdominal irradiation. (See also Appendix 26.)

be obtained. Washings from the cul-de-sac, both paracolic gutters, and the diaphragms are necessary. A systematic exploration of the intra-abdominal surfaces and viscera should be done, and biopsies from any suspicious lesion as well as the pelvic cul-de-sac, bladder serosa, pelvic sidewalls, both paracolic gutters, and diaphragms are recommended. An infracolic omentectomy and exploration of the retroperitoneal spaces with a pelvic and paraaortic lymph node sampling should also be included. All this is usually performed through a midline vertical incision.

Early stage epithelial ovarian carcinoma can be divided into favorable and unfavorable prognosis categories. The favorable prognosis category includes all stage IA and IB well-differentiated tumors. After a proper staging procedure is completed, no further therapy is needed. The unfavorable category includes all stage IA and IB, moderate to poorly differentiated carcinomas, stage IC tumors, and all clear-cell ovarian carcinomas. After the staging laparotomy has been completed, further adjuvant therapy is recommended. As shown in the flow diagram, a combination platinum-based chemotherapy for four cycles is the standard of care. For those patients unable to tolerate platinum combination intravenous chemotherapy, four to six cycles of melphalan or intraperitoneal ^{32}P can be substituted. The GOG is currently investigating whether the combination of paclitaxel and cisplatin is superior to the standard cisplatin and Cytoxan combination currently being used.

Patients with an *advanced ovarian epithelial adenocarcinoma should initially* undergo cytoreductive surgery to debulk as much tumor as possible (Fig. 37-1). Postoperative patients can be divided into those cytoreduced to residual tumor implants less than or equal to 2 cm and those with residual tumor greater than 2 cm. Approximately 50% of stage IIIC patients can be optimally cytoreduced. The GOG has recently shown a significant survival advantage in advanced ovarian cancer with the use of cisplatin and paclitaxel. Therefore, the optimally debulked group should be offered combination chemotherapy with a platinum compound (cisplatin or carboplatin) and paclitaxel given every 21 days for a total of six cycles. In the suboptimally debulked group, a similar regimen of chemotherapy can be used. In addition, if a significant amount of residual tumor is remaining after the initial cytoreductive surgery, an initial three courses of chemotherapy can be given, followed by an interval cytoreductive surgery. Three additional courses of chemotherapy should follow.

In patients with no clinical evidence of disease after the initial therapy, there are several treatment options. Routinely a physical examination, abdominal-pelvic computed tomograpy (CT) scan, and CA-125 level are reviewed. If the patient has evidence of persistent disease, further chemotherapy, investigational therapy, or palliative care is indicated. Although second-look laparotomies have not been shown to influence patient survival, they may be an option if the results have an impact on further treatment or are required in a research setting. Patients with a negative second look have up to a 50% recurrence rate. Besides observation, these patients may benefit from some form of consolidation of therapy by continued conventional, high-dose, or intraperitoneal chemotherapy, or possibly intraperitoneal^{32}P. Microscopic residual disease could be treated similarly or with whole abdominal radiation (WAR). Greater than 5-mm residual disease should be treated as persistent disease and after further cytoreductive surgery is attempted the patient can be offered further chemotherapy, investigational treatment or palliative care. Follow-up surveillance requires regular physical examinations with serial CA-125 levels every 3 months for 2 years, every 6 months for 3 years, and yearly thereafter. Radiographic studies should be ordered, as deemed necessary, by the clinician to include yearly chest x-rays and mammograms.

Patients with recurrent disease within 6 months of therapy have a poor prognosis. They are considered platinum-refractory and if they have not received paclitaxel as part of the initial regimen, paclitaxel should be administered. Patients who have received paclitaxel may receive other regimens, including Hexalin or topotecan. Patients who have recurred more than 6 months after therapy can receive a platinum-based therapy. They

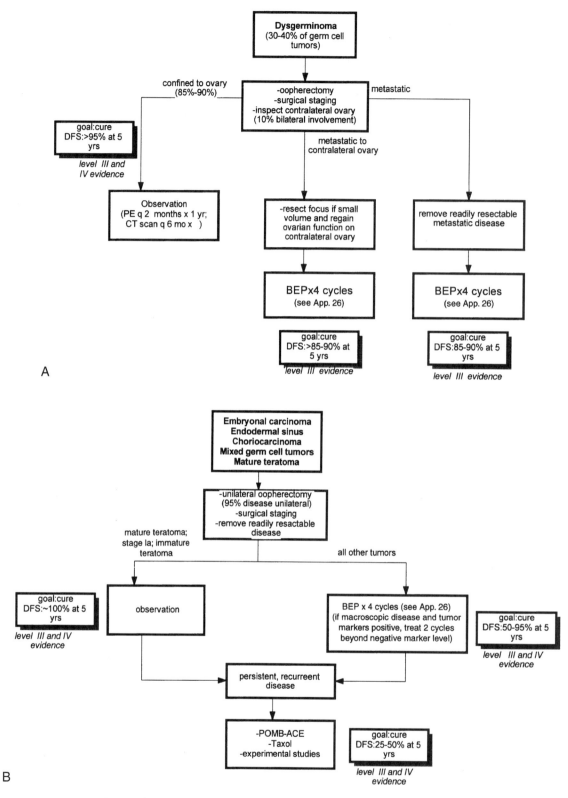

FIGURE 37-2 *(A & B) Management of ovarian germ cell tumors (GCT). Key management principle resides on identification of dysgerminoma versus "all other GCT." Further principle involves determination of the extent of the disease (metastatic versus localized disease). The goal of the treatment is cure. Recommended strategy is mainly based on single-arm and retrospective studies (level III and IV). DFS, disease-free survival; PE, physical examination.*

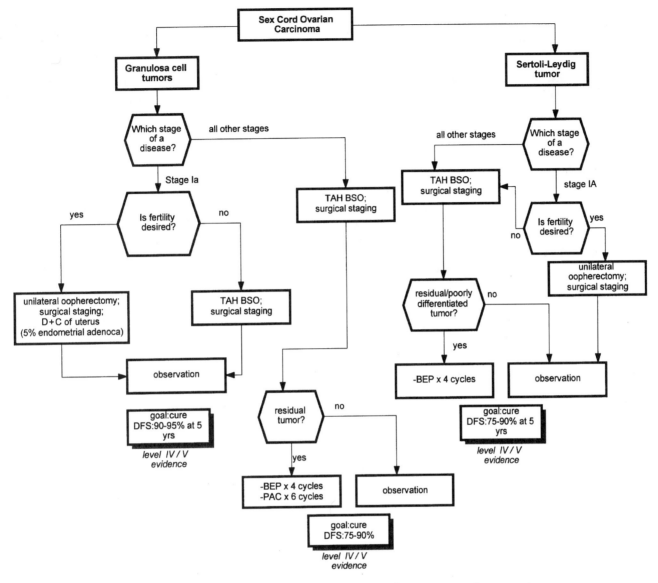

FIGURE 37-3 *Management of sex cord ovarian cancer. This is a rare, slow growing tumor with late recurrences, management of which is stage dependent. The goal of the treatment is cure. Recommended strategy is mainly supported by level IV and V data. DFS, disease-free survival; TAH, total abdominal hysterectomy; BSO, bilateral salpingo-oophrectomy; D+C, dilation and curettage.*

can expect a 30%-60% response rate and a 5%–20% complete response to retreatment with a platinum-based therapy depending on the disease-free interval. Patients subsequently progressing after the above therapy should be referred for protocol salvage chemotherapy.

Patients with epithelial ovarian tumors of low malignant potential should undergo a similar surgical procedure. A TAH/BSO, staging laparotomy and optimal debulking procedure should be performed. Stage IA tumors can be treated conservatively by a unilateral oophorectomy. There is no evidence that

adjuvant therapy of any kind improves the disease-free interval or overall survival.

Germ cell tumors account for less than 5% of all ovarian malignancies. They typically occur in the first two decades of life and are more frequent among Asians and blacks. Most germ cell cancers are unilateral, with the exception of dysgerminomas. Any persistent 2-cm adnexal mass in a pre-menarchal girl or 8-cm adnexal mass in a postmenarchal woman requires further evaluation. Tumor markers include human chorionic gonadtrophin (hCG) alpha fetoprotein (AFP), placental alkaline phosphatase (PLAP), and LDH. A complete blood count (CBC) and liver function tests are also often evaluated. A chest radiograph is important because germ cell tumors can metastasize to the lungs or mediastinum. A karyotype should be obtained preoperatively on all premenarchal girls because of the propensity of these tumors to arise in dysgenetic gonads.

Germ cell tumors can be divided into two groups for treatment, dysgerminomas and all others. Germ cell tumors commonly arise in young women in whom future fertility is a priority. Since most tumors are unilateral, conservative surgery can be performed. Therefore, when a germ cell tumor is suspected, an exploratory laparotomy, unilateral oophorectomy, and staging procedure are done. In most circumstances, TAH-BSO does not alter outcome and should not be routinely done. When a dysgerminoma is confined to one ovary, an oophorectomy is all that is necessary. When metastatic disease is found, the readily resectable implants should be removed to include a small metastatic focus on the contralateral ovary, if present before the patient receive four cycles of adjuvant chemotherapy. The most active combination chemotherapy for germ cell tumors is bleomycin, etoposide, and cisplatin (BEP). All germ cell tumors with the exception of a stage IA grade I immature teratoma should undergo an oophorectomy and staging laparotomy followed by four cycles of BEP chemotherapy. The stage IA, grade I immature teratoma requires no further treatment. A rule of thumb when positive markers are found is to treat two cycles beyond a negative marker. Follow-up is

TABLE 37-2 **SUMMARY OF STUDIES SUPPORTING CURRENT MANAGEMENT PROTOCOLS**

	No. of Patients	Survival (5 year)	Evidence Level	Reference
Stage I				
Epithelial ovarian cancer				
Scully (1980)	Favorable 81	98%	I	N Engl J Med
	Unfavorable 141	81%	I	322:1021, 1990
	86	83%	II	Am J Obstet Gynecol 138:139, 1980
	104	^{32}P, 61%	II	Multimodal Treatment of
		Cisplatin, 84%		Ovarian Cancer
	47	Observation, 70%	II	Multimodal Treatment
		Cisplatin, 71%	II	of Ovarian Cancer
Stage II, III, IV				
	386	Median survival (PC),	I	N Engl J Med 334:1–6, 1996
		24 months (PT),	II	N Engl J Med 332:629–634, 1995
		38 months		
			III	Semin Oncol 18:213–221, 1991
			I	Am J Obstet Gynecol 166:504–511, 1992
Germ cell tumors				
	93 (BEP)	96%	III	J Clin Oncol 12:701–706, 1994
	89 (PVB)	53%	III	Proc Am Soc Clin Oncol 8:150, 1989
	20 (BEP) completely resected	100%	III	J Clin Oncol 8:715–720, 1990
	6 (BEP) advanced disease	83%	III	
Sex cord-stromal tumors				
	11 (PVB)	6, CR	IV	Obstet Gynecol 67:265–268, 198
	6 (VAC)	2, CR	IV	Am J Obstet Gynecol 125:402–409, 1976
	VAC		IV	Semin Oncol 11:299, 1984

GOG currently looking at PEB for advanced/recurrent disease.

Abbreviations: CR, complete remission; PC, cisplatin cytoxan; PR, partial remission; PT, cisplatin paclitaxel; PVB, cisplatin, vincristine, bleomycin; VAC, vincristine, actinomycin, cytoxan.

similar to the epithelial cancers, using tumor markers when appropriate.

Sex cord-stromal tumors are rare and are characterized by a somewhat unpredictable biologic behavior. Most are unilateral and can be treated with an adnexectomy and staging in young women. In women who have completed their childbearing, surgical staging and TAH/BSO are appropriate. *Granulosa cell tumors* often produce estrogen and in 75% of cases are associated with pseudoprecocity puberty in the premenarchal female. In the older age group 25–50% of the cases are associated with endometrial hyperplasia and in 5% of cases, endometrial adenocarcinoma. *Sertoli-Leydig tumors* typically produce androgens and can be associated with clinical virilization in 70% to 85% of patients. Optimal adjuvant therapy has not been determined. Only when these low-grade malignancies metastasize and residual tumor is present is chemotherapy indicated. Four to six cycles of BEP, VAC (vincristine, actinomycin-D, and Cytoxan) or PAC (cisplatin, Adriamycin and Cytoxan) can be used. In addition, poorly differentiated or stage II or greater Sertoli-Leydig tumors need adjuvant chemotherapy, since they are more likely to reoccur. Since the majority of these tumors are a low-grade malignancy, late recurrences after primary therapy is a hallmark in this group, especially with the adult granulosa cell tumors.

The management of ovarian cancer is detailed in Figures 37-1 to 37-3. Supporting data on the recommended treatment protocols are provided in Table 37-2. Appendix 26 describes practical details of the management of ovarian cancer.

SUGGESTED READINGS

Berek JS: Epithelial ovarian cancer, pp. 327–375. In Berek JS, Hacker NF (eds). Practical Gynecologic Oncology. 2nd Ed. Williams & Wilkins, Baltimore, 1994

Berek JS, Hacker NF, Lagasse LD et al: Survival of patients following secondary cytoreductive surgery in ovarian cancer. Obstet Gynecol 61:189, 1983

Boring CC, Squires TS, Tong T et al: Cancer Statistics, 1994. CA 44:7–26, 1994

Colombo N, Sessa C, Landoni F et al: Cisplatin, vinblastine and bleomycin combination chemotherapy in metastatic granulosa cell tumor of the ovary. Obstet Gynecol 67:265–268, 1986

Copeland LJ, Gershenson DM, Wharton JT et al: Microscopic disease at second-look laparotomy in advanced ovarian cancer. Cancer 55:472, 1985

Gershenson DM, Morris M, Cangir A et al: Treatment of malignant germ cell tumors of the ovary with bleomycin, etoposide and cisplatin. J Clin Oncol 8:715, 1990

Hoskins WJ, Rubin SC: Surgery in the treatment of patients with advanced ovarian cancer. Semin Oncology 18:213–221, 1991

Hoskins WJ, Rubin SC, Dulaney E et al: Influence of secondary cytoreduction at time of second-look laparotomy on the survival of patient with epithelial ovarian carcinoma. Gynecol Oncol 34:365, 1989

McGuire WP, Hoskins WJ, Brady MF et al: Cyclophosphamide and cisplatin compared with paclitaxel and cisplatin in patients with stage III and stage IV ovarian cancer. N Engl J Med 334:1–6, 1996

National Institutes of Health Consensus Development Conference Statement: Ovarian Cancer: Screening, Treatment and Follow-up: April 5–7, 1994, pp. 1–25

Ozols RF: Ovarian cancer, part II: treatment. Curr Prob Cancer March/April:67–126, 1992

Ozols RF, Rubin SC, Dembo AS et al: Epithelial cancer. pp. 731–781. In Hoskins WJ, Perez CA, Young RC (eds): Principles and Practice of Gynecologic Oncology. 3rd Ed. Lippincott-Raven, Philadelphia, 1992

Ponder BAJ, Easton DF, Peto J: Risk of ovarian cancer associated with a family history: preliminary report or the OPCS study. p. 3. In Sharp F, Mason WP, Leake RE (eds): Ovarian Cancer: Biological and Therapeutic Challenges. Chapman and Hall Medical, Cambridge, 1990

Rubin SC, Hoskins WJ, Hakes TBC et al: Recurrence after negative second-look laparotomy for ovarian cancer; analysis of risk factors. Am J Obstet Gynecol 159:1094, 1988

Slayton RE: Management of germ cell and stromal tumors of the ovary. Semin Oncol 11:299, 1984

Van der Berg MEL, Van Lent M, Kobierska A et al: The effect of debulking surgery after induction chemotherapy in the prognosis in advanced ovarian cancer. N Engl J Med 332:629–634, 1993

Williams SD, Blessing SA, Hatch K, Homesly HD: Chemotherapy of advanced ovarian dysgerminoma: trial of the GOG. J Clin Oncol 9:1950, 1991

Williams SD, Blessing JA, Liao SC et al: Adjuvant therapy of ovarian germ cell tumors: chemotherapy with cisplatin, etoposide and bleomycin: a trial of the GOG. J Clin Oncol 12:701–706, 1994

Williams SD, Blessing JA, Slayton RC et al: Ovarian germ cell tumors: adjuvant trials of the GOG. Proc Am Soc Clin Oncol 8:150, 1989

The WHO collaborative study of neoplasia and steroid contraceptives: epithelial ovarian cancer and combined oral contraceptives. Int J Epidemiol 18:538–545, 1989

Young RE, Scully RE: Ovarian sex cord—stromal tumors: recent progress. Int J Gynecol Pathol 1:153, 1980

Young RE, Scully RE: Ovarian Sertoli-Leydig cell tumors. Am J Surg Pathol 9:543–569, 1985

Young RC, Waltin LA, Ellenberg SS et al. Adjuvant therapy in stage I and stage II epithelial ovarian cancer. N Engl J Med 322:1021–1027, 1990

38 Endometrial Cancer

Ward Katsanis
Randall Gibb
Nermina Obralić
David L. Doering

Incidence: 22.7/100,000

Mortality: 3.4/100,000

Goal of treatment: Cure, except in patients with extrapelvic disease other than periaortic nodal metastases (Stage 4B)

Main modality of treatment: Surgery with or without adjuvant radiotherapy

Prognosis: 85% five-year overall survival

INCIDENCE AND RISK FACTORS

Endometrial carcinoma is the *most common female genital tract cancer* in the United States, with 34,000 new cases expected in 1996. It is also the gynecologic tumor with the most favorable prognosis (85% five-year relative survival for all stages). Endometrial carcinoma is a hormone-related cancer, often associated with the use of unopposed estrogen. The incidence is increased in women using postmenopausal estrogen replacement without progestins, as well as in patients with polycystic ovarian disease or estrogen-secreting tumors of the ovary. Other risk factors include nulliparity, late onset of menopause, diabetes, hypertension, and obesity.

DIAGNOSIS

Abnormal uterine bleeding (menorrhagia, metrorrhagia, postmenopausal bleeding) occurs early and is the most common presenting symptom. When postmenopausal uterine bleeding occurs, it must be considered to be due to endometrial cancer until proven otherwise. Persistent or heavy bleeding in the perimenopausal woman mandates evaluation for endometrial cancer as well. Fractional dilatation and curettage (D&C) has been the standard diagnostic method for confirming this diagnosis. However, office endometrial biopsy has a sensitivity up to 90% for detecting endometrial carcinoma and can often eliminate the need for D&C. Other techniques useful in making the diagnosis include vaginal ultrasonography to assess endometrial thickness and hysteroscopy with D&C and directed biopsies.

Adenocarcinoma is the most common histology of endometrial carcinoma, accounting for 60% of all tumors encountered. Less common subtypes include adenosquamous, clear cell, papillary serous, and secretory carcinomas. These tumors are further categorized according to FIGO grading criteria: Grade 1, well differentiated; Grade 2, moderately differentiated; Grade 3, poorly differentiated. Endometrial cancers may appear as a localized nodule or polyp or as a mass that fills the uterine cavity. Tumor can penetrate the myometrium and may locally infiltrate the vagina, parametria, ovaries, and adjacent pelvic structures.

Pretreatment evaluation of the patient, coupled with the pathologic diagnosis, allows the physician to individualize therapy. Important prognostic variables include histologic type, depth of myometrial invasion, tumor grade, stage of disease, and lymph node metastases. Therefore, accurate and complete surgical staging is essential for proper clinical management of these patients. Tables 38-1 and 38-2 show the current FIGO staging system and survival data according to stage, depth of myometrial invasion, and histology. The overall five-year survival rate for patients treated for endometrial carcinoma is 85%, with surgical stage being the strongest predictor of survival. Cell type, regardless of histologic grade, also influences prognosis. Papillary serous carcinoma, clear cell carcinoma, and adenosquamous carcinoma all imply a worse prognosis. Myometrial invasion irrespective of the grade of the tumor is also an important prognostic factor. Deep myometrial invasion is more often associated with high-grade lesions: 42% in grade 3 vs. 10% in grade 1. Patients without lymph node metastases have a better prognosis; however, the likelihood of lymphatic spread is related to tumor grade (3% pelvic and 2% aortic in grade 1 vs. 18% pelvic and 11% aortic in grade 3) and depth of myometrial invasion (1% pelvic and 1% aortic when tumor is confined to the endometrium vs. 25% pelvic and 24% aortic when deep myometrial invasion is present). Other prognostic factors commonly recognized are vascular space invasion, presence or absence of hormonal receptors, and the age of the patient. On the basis of these prognostic factors it is possible to identify those patients with a low risk of recurrence who may be spared from the morbidity of extended surgical staging or postoperative adjuvant therapy. The low-risk group includes patients with grade 1 or grade 2 endometrial adenocarcinoma, myometrial invasion less than 50%, no cervical extension, and negative lymph-vascular space involvement. All other patients are considered high risk and should receive adjuvant therapy.

TABLE 38-1 SURGICAL STAGING OF ENDOMETRIAL CARCINOMA (FIGO 1988)

Stage	
1A	Tumor confined to the endometrium
1B	Invasion to less than one half myometrium
1C	Invasion to greater than one half myometrium
2A	Endocervical glandular involvement
2B	Endocervical stromal invasion
3A	Tumor invades serosa, and/or adnexa, and/or positive peritoneal cytology
3B	Vaginal metastases
3C	Metastases to pelvic and/or aortic lymph nodes
4A	Tumor invasion to bladder and/or rectal mucosa
4B	Distant metastases including intra-abdominal and/or inguinal lymph nodes

TABLE 38-2 FIVE-YEAR SURVIVAL ACCORDING TO PROGNOSTIC INDICATORS

Stage	Survival Rate
1	72%
2	56%
3	32%
4	11%

Myometrial Invasion	Survival Rate
< 1/3	82%
1/3–1/2	78%
>1/2	67%

Grade	Survival Rate
1	80%
2	73%
3	58%

(From Peterson F [ed]: Annual report on the results of treatment in gynecological cancer, Vol. 20, Stockholm, 1988, International Federation of Gynecology and Obstetrics, with permission.)

TREATMENT

SURGERY

Surgery is the mainstay of treatment in early endometrial carcinoma, and in many cases surgery itself may be the definitive therapy. Appropriate steps include extrafascial hysterectomy, bilateral salpingo-oophorectomy, peritoneal cytology, selective pelvic and aortic lymphadenectomy, omental biopsy, and resection of intra-abdominal disease if present. Further treatment is defined by the results of surgical staging obtained at initial laparotomy.

RADIATION THERAPY

Radiation therapy alone can be used in medically inoperable patients with stage 1 or stage 2 disease, but the results are inferior to operative intervention. Patients with clinical stage 3 or 4A have also been treated with primary radiation therapy. Post-

TABLE 38-3 SUMMARY OF STUDIES SUPPORTING MANAGEMENT AS OUTLINED IN FIGURE 38-1

	Number of Patients	5-Year Survival (%)	Evidence Level	References	Comments
Stage 1					
Stokes et al.	304	87	III	Int J Radiat Oncol Biol Phys 12:339, 1986	Preoperative or postoperative radiation therapy beneficial especially for myometrial invasion >1/2, decreased local failure and pelvic recurrence
Underwood et al.	220	91	III	Am J Obstet Gynecol 128:86, 1977	
Grigsby et al.	858	84	III	Int J Radiat Oncol Biol Phys 21:379, 1991	
Aalders	540	85	II	Obstet Gynecol 56:419, 1980	
Stage 2	*RT and Surgery*				
Onsrud et al.		85	III	Gynecol Oncol 13:76, 1982	Same decrease observed as in stage 1 above
Gagnon et al.	20	45 (5-year only)	III	Cancer 44:1247, 1979	
	RT Alone				
Landgren et al.	38	65 (Act. 5 yrs.)	III	AJR 126:148, 1976	Radiation and surgery superior
Stage 3					
Danoff et al.	17	12	III	Int J Radiat Oncol Biol Phys 6:1491, 1980	Dismal survival but increased disease-free interval with surgery and radiation
Homesley et al.	49	18	III	Obstet Gynecol 49:604, 1977	
Chemotherapy					
Cohen et al.	*Single Agent* Cisplatin Doxorubicin		IV	Clin Obstet Gynecol 13:811, 1986	Single agent chemotherapy recurrence rate is 15%–30%
Hancock et al.	*Combination* Cisplatin 50 mg/m^2 Doxorubicin 50 mg/m^2 Cyclophosphamide 500 mg/m^2		III	Cancer Treat Rep 70:789, 1986	28% complete remission 28% partial remission with significant toxicity; no benefit over single agent therapy
Hoton et al.	Cyclophosphamide 400 mg/m^2 Doxorubicin 40 mg/m^2 5-FU 300 mg/m^2 × 3 days		IV	Cancer 49:2441, 1982	Same as above

operative adjuvant radiation therapy is employed for patients assigned to the high-risk category to reduce the risk of local recurrence. Available data evaluating postoperative radiation therapy are mostly retrospective and based on small numbers (level IV). Prospective comparative data useful in the evaluation of these treatment modalities is lacking. Adjuvant irradiation of the upper vagina reduces the incidence of vaginal cuff failure, and external beam therapy reduces regional recurrence but may not affect overall survival. Extending the radiation field to cover the aortic region is indicated if positive aortic lymph nodes are encountered, while whole abdominal radiation may be recommended for control of microscopic or small abdominal metastases. Radiation therapy is indicated for palliation in patients with metastatic disease. Late sequelae of whole pelvis radiation therapy include chronic cystitis and proctitis, which are seen in 5%–10% of patients.

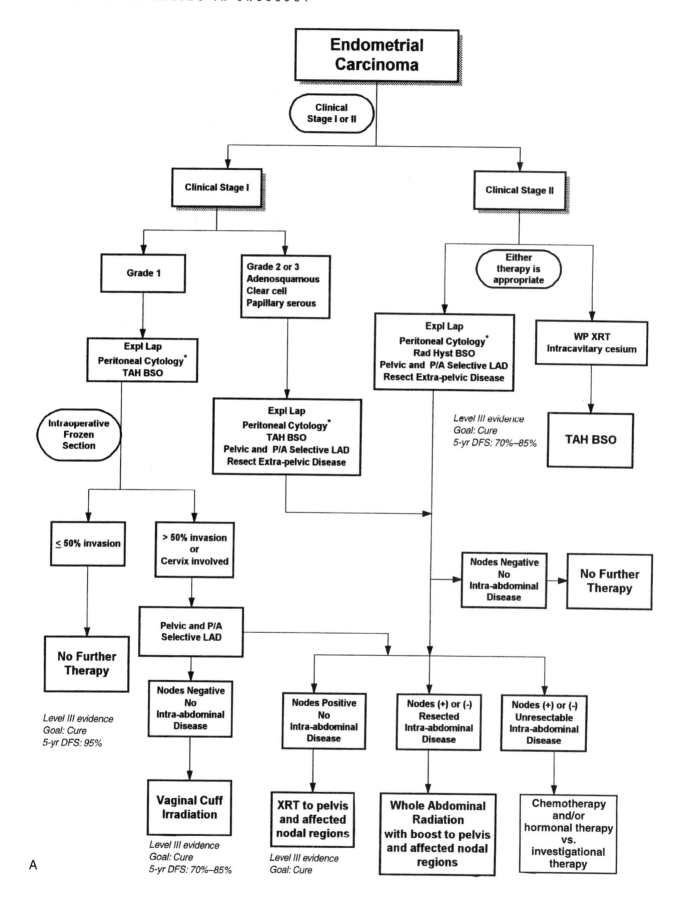

A

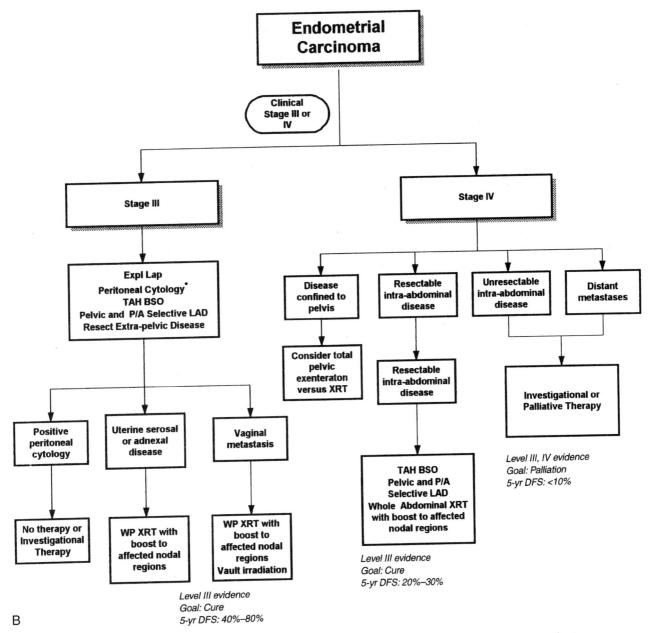

FIGURE 38-1. *(A & B) An algorithm for the management of endometrial carcinoma clinically confined to the corpus and cervix. Management strategies are based on suspected extent of pelvic disease and depth of myometrial invasion. Treatment is intended to be curative except for unresectable extrapelvic disease. Expl Lap, exploratory laparotomy; TAH BSO, total abdominal hysterectomy, bilateral salpingo-oophorectomy; Rad Hyst, radical hysterectomy; P/A, periaortic; LAD, lymphadenectomy; WP, whole pelvis; XRT, radiation therapy. The algorithm is based on level III and IV studies. *If peritoneal cytology is positive but other risk factors are negative, consider investigational protocol versus no further therapy. †Consider vaginal cuff irradiaton if myometrial invasion is present. ††Consider whole pelvis irradiation for high grade or deeply invasive tumors if surgery did not include radical hysterectomy.*

CHEMOTHERAPY

Endometrial carcinoma is considered a tumor that does not respond well to chemotherapy. The most extensively used single agents are doxorubicin (60 mg/m² every 3 weeks) and cisplatin (100 mg/m² every 3 weeks). Objective responses are 37% and 46% respectively. The most frequently used combinations of chemotherapy are doxorubicin and cisplatin; doxorubicin, cisplatin, and cyclophosphamide; or doxorubicin, cyclophosphamide, and 5-fluorouracil 5FU. Reported response rates range from 15% to 58%. The duration of the response to chemotherapeutic agents is short in most patients, and significant toxic effects are reported in many patients. Chemotherapy is currently used in the treatment of advanced or recurrent endometrial tumors and is considered palliative.

The sensitivity of endometrial carcinomas to progestational agents is well known. The most commonly used progestins, depo-provera (400 mg intramuscularly weekly) and megesterol acetate (160 mg/day) produce similar results. The response rate to both agents is similar and ranges from 15% to 29%. At least three months are necessary to determine the maximum response, with duration of the response averaging 30 months. Other hormonal therapies include tamoxifen and Danazol. Hormonal therapy is used in the treatment of patients with metastatic or recurrent disease. The treatment should be maintained as long as a response is observed. Based on these findings the algorithm was constructed in Figure 38-1. Supporting studies used to create the algorithms are summarized in Table 38-3.

SUGGESTED READINGS

Boronow RC, Morrow CP, Creasman WT et al: Surgical staging in endometrial cancer: clinical-pathologic findings of a prospective study. Obstet Gynecol 63:825, 1984

Cowles TA, Magrina JF, Masterson BJ, Capen CV: Comparison of clinical and surgical staging in patients with endometrial carcinoma. Obstet Gynecol 66:413,1985

Deppe G, Malviva VK, Malone JN: Treatment of recurrent and metastatic endometrial carcinoma with cisplatin and doxorubicin. Eur J Gynecol Oncol 15:263, 1994

Eifel PJ, Ross J, Hendrickson M et al: Adenocarcinoma of the endometrium: analysis of 256 cases with disease limited to the uterine corpus: treatment comparisons. Cancer 52:1026, 1983

Grigsby PW, Perez CA, Kuten A: Clinical stage 1 endometrial cancer: prognostic factors for local control and distant metastases and implications of the new FIGO surgical staging system. Int J Radiat Oncol Biol Phys 22:905, 1992

Lewis GS, Slack NH, Mortel R: Adjuvant progesterone therapy in the primary definitive treatment of endometrial carcinoma. Gynecol Oncol 2:368, 1974

Reisinger SA, Staros EB, Mohiudden M: Survival and failure analysis in stage 2 endometrial cancer using the revised 1988 FIGO staging system. Int J Radiat Oncol Biol Phys 21:1027,1991

Wolfson AH, Sightler SE, Markoe AM: The prognostic significance of surgical staging for carcinoma of the endometrium. Gynecol Oncol 45:142, 1992

39 Cervical Cancer

Nermina Obralić
Ward Katsanis
Randall Gibb
David L. Doering

Incidence: 7.8/100,000

Mortality: 2.7/100,000

Goal of treatment: Cure, except in patients with extra pelvic dissemination of disease (stage 4B)

Main modality of treatment: Surgery and radiation therapy

Prognosis: 55% 5-year survival (all stages combined)

Stage I	85%
Stage II	60%
Stage III	30%
Stage IV	10%

INCIDENCE AND PATHOLOGY

After cancer of the endometrium and ovary, carcinoma of the cervix is *the third most common gynecologic neoplasm*. About 15,700 cases of invasive carcinoma and nearly 4,900 deaths are expected in the United States for 1996. The peak age of incidence is 52 years for invasive cervical cancer. Cervical carcinoma is more frequent in black women, in low socioeconomic classes, in women who have had intercourse at an early age, multiparas, women with sexual promiscuity, and in women with certain types of human papilloma virus (HPV) infection. Other cofactors such as smoking and oral contraceptives have been included in theories of the carcinogenesis of cervical carcinoma.

Eighty-five to 90% of invasive cervical tumors are squamous cell carcinomas, while approximately 5% to 15% are classified as adenocarcinomas. Other epithelial tumors of the cervix include adenosquamous, glassy cell, small cell, undifferentiated, and carcinoid tumors. By definition, invasive cervical carcinoma has broken the basement membrane of the epithelium and has invaded the underlying cervical stroma. As the lesion becomes visible, it may appear as a surface ulceration with an exophytic component or endophytic infiltration of the stroma. When tumor expands and extends into the endocervix the term "barrel-shaped" cervix is used. Cervical carcinoma may spread by direct extension to the vaginal fornices, the paracervical and parametrial tissues, or the lower uterine segment and endometrium. The bladder or rectum may also be directly invaded. Lymphatic spread occurs to the parametrial lymph nodes, then to the obturator, iliac, and aortic lymph nodes. Distant metastases are less frequent; the most common sites are the lungs, mediastinal and supraclavicular nodes, bones, and the liver.

MANAGEMENT

Vaginal discharge, postcoital spotting, and metrorrhagia are symptoms of early invasive tumors, while pelvic pain and urinary or rectal pressure are manifestations of advanced disease. Preinvasive and early invasive carcinomas are usually detected by exfoliative cytology (*Pap smear*) on routine periodic evaluation. Successful screening and early detection of cervical carcinoma has resulted in a decrease in the overall mortality from the disease. Diagnosis of cervical carcinoma should always be confirmed by biopsy. The recommended procedures in detection, diagnosis, and evaluation of cervical carcinoma are presented in Table 39-1 and Figure 39-1. This disease is clinically staged according to the revised International Federation of Gynecology and Obstetrics (FIGO) staging scheme presented in Table 39-2.

The five-year survival for treated patients with all stages of cervical cancer is 55%. Extent of disease as defined by FIGO staging is the single most important predictive factor for survival in carcinoma of the cervix. Approximate cure rates include 80% for stage 1, 60% for stage 2, 30% for stage 3, and 7% for stage 4. Other significant prognostic

TABLE 39-1   PROCEDURES USED FOR THE EVALUATION AND STAGING OF CERVICAL CARCINOMA

Complete physical examination (including under anesthesia if indicated)
Colposcopically directed biopsy with endocervical curettage
Conization (if indicated)
Radiologic studies
    Chest x-ray
    Intravenous pyelogram
    Barium enema (if indicated clinically)
    Skeletal x-ray (if indicated clinically)
Cystoscopy and proctoscopy as needed

TABLE 39-2   FIGO STAGING SYSTEM FOR CERVICAL CARCINOMA

Stage 0	Carcinoma in situ	
Stage I	Tumor confined to the cervix	
	IA1	Measured invasion of stroma no greater than 3.0 mm in depth and no wider than 7.0
	IA2	Measured invasion os stroma greater than 3 mm and no greater than 5 mm and no wider than 7 mm
	IB	Clinical lesions confined to the cervix or preclinical lesions greater than stage IA
		IB1 Clinical lesions no greater than 4.0 cm in size
		IB2 Clinical lesions greater than 4 cm in size
Stage II	Extends beyond cervix but not to pelvic wall or involves vagina but not lower one-third	
	IIA	No obvious parametrial involvement
	IIB	Obvious parametrial involvement
Stage III	Extends to pelvic sidewall or lower third of vagina or hydronephrosis/nonfunctioning kidney	
	IIIA	Extension to lower third of vagina
	IIIB	Extension to pelvic sidewall and/or hydronephrosis or nonfunctioning kidney
Stage IV	Extends beyond true pelvis or involves bladder or rectal mucosa	
	IVA	Spread to adjacent organs
	IVB	Distant spread

indicators as they relate to survival are outlined in Table 39-3.

Surgery, radiation therapy, and chemotherapy have been used in the management of patients with carcinoma of the cervix. The major surgical procedures are cervical conization, extrafascial abdominal hysterectomy, radical hysterectomy with bilateral pelvic lymphadenectomy (PLND), and pelvic exenteration. *Extrafascial hysterectomy* consists of removal of the uterus and cervix, adjacent tissues, and upper vagina with minimal disturbance to the bladder or ureters and is typically performed for microinvasive carcinoma. *Cervical conization* includes a conical removal of a large

TABLE 39-3   PROGNOSTIC INDICATORS FOR CERVICAL CARCINOMA

Presence and number of nodal metastases
Tumor size (i.e., barrel-shaped cervix >4 cm)
Depth of stromal invasion
Lymph-vascular space involvement
Positive surgical margins and/or parametrial involvement
Histologic type of cancer

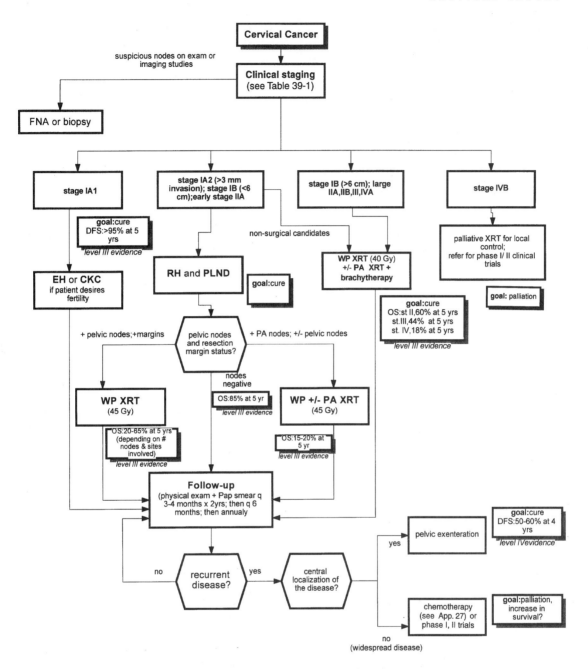

FIGURE 39-1 *Management of cervical carcinoma. Assessing the extent of disease as defined by the International Federation of Gynecology and Obstetrics (FIGO) (Table 39-2) represents a key reasoning principle in the management of cervical cancer. Radical surgery with or without adjuvant radiation therapy is the treatment of choice for stage IB and early stage IIA cancers. Radiation therapy may also be used for patients who are not candidates for radical surgery. More advanced disease is managed with radiation therapy. The goal of treatment is cure, except for stage IVB. Strategies for primary curative surgery or radiation are based on level II and III evidence. Palliation and treatment of recurrent disease is based on level III and IV evidence. FNA, fine needle aspiration; EH, extrafascial hysterectomy; CKC, cold knife conization; RH, radical hysterectomy; PLND, pelvic lymph node dissection; WP, whole pelvis; PA, periaortic; XRT, external radiation therapy; T&O, tandem and ovoid brachytherapy; OS, overall survival (See Table 39-1 for additional information.)*

portion of the ectocervix and endocervix and is reserved for those women who desire fertility and who have microinvasive disease. *Radical hysterectomy with PLND* consists of a wider resection of the pericervical tissues with dissection of the ureters, mobilization of the bladder neck as well as removal of the medial portion or all of the surrounding parametrial tissue. Radical hysterectomy with PLND is indicated in stages 1A, 1B, and 2A cervical carcinomas. The most common complication of the procedure is neurogenic bladder dysfunction which occurs acutely in one-third of the patients. Long-term bladder dystonia affects only 3%. Other complications include fistulas, hemorrhage, bowel obstruction, and pulmonary embolism. *Pelvic exenteration* is reserved for central pelvic tumor recurrence and includes an *en bloc* resection of the cervix and uterus (if present) with removal of the vagina as well as the bladder and/or rectum. Significant morbidity is associated with the procedure, including perioperative infections, hemorrhage, thromboembolic events, and bowel or urinary obstruction or fistula. Operative mortality from this procedure is 9%.

Radiation therapy is also effective treatment of carcinoma of the cervix. Treatment plans are designed individually based on the stage of disease with most patients receiving a combination of external beam radiation therapy and brachytherapy. External beam therapy using high-energy sources provides a tumoricidal dose to the parametria, pelvic lymph nodes, and other pelvic structures. Extended field irradiation includes the aortic lymph nodes and may be used when aortic nodal metastases are present or suspected. Brachytherapy is used to irradiate the cervix and the medial one-half of the parametria, while sparing the bladder and rectum. Most commonly, the combination of vaginal colpostats and a uterine tandem is used; however, vaginal cylinders or interstitial needles are also employed. High dose rate and low dose rate brachytherapy are equally effective treatments with similar complication rates. Approximate cure rates with radiation therapy are 85% for stage 1, 60% for stage 2, 30% for stage 3, and 10% for stage 4. Cure rates for early stage disease (stage 1 and 2A) are similar for surgery and radiation. Radiation therapy may also be used in combination with surgery as preoperative or postoperative irradiation. The most frequent complications of radiation therapy are vaginal stenosis, radiation enteritis, thrombophlebitis, and rectovaginal or vesicovaginal fistulas. In order to improve the results of treatment, radiosensitizers such as hydroxyurea, cisplatin, and 5-fluorouracil are often combined with radiation therapy.

TABLE 39-4   SUPPORTING DATA FOR MANAGEMENT SCHEME PRESENTED IN FIGURE 39-1

		Radical Hysterectomy and PLND in Stage I	
Patients	*Evidence Level*	*Comments*	*Reference*
Stage IB, 139	III	86% 5-year survival	Underwood et al: Am J Obstet Gynecol 134:889, 1979
Stage IB, 56	III	84% 5-year survival	Hoskins et al: Gynecol Oncol 4:278, 1976
		Primary Radiation Therapy in Stage I and II	
IB, 312		IB 85% 5-year survival	Perez et al: Int J Radiat Oncol Biol Phys 12:339, 1986
IIA, 90	III	IIA 70% 5-year survival	
		Radical Hysterectomy And Adjuvant RT for Stage I and II	
95	III	67% 5-year disease-free survival	Monk et al: Gynecol Oncol 54:4, 1994
30 surgery only	II	41% 10-year survival (surgery alone)	Stock et al: Int J Radiat Oncol Bio Phys 31:31, 1995
29 surgery + RT		65% 10-year survival (surgery + RT)	

		Chemotherapy for Advanced and Recurrent Carcinoma		
Patients	*Chemo*	*Evidence Level*	*Comments*	*Reference*
24	Cisplatin 100 mg/m² d1			Rotmensch et al: Gynecol Oncol 29:76, 1988
	5 FU 1000 mg/m² d1-5	III	17% CR	
			33% PR	
30	Cisplatin 90 mg/m²			
	5 FU 1500 mg/m²	III	17% CR	Fanning et al: Gynecol Oncol 56:235, 1995
	Ifosfamide 3 gm/m² Q 28 d		36% PR	

Abbreviations: PLND, pelvic lymph node dissection; RT, radiation therapy; CR, complete response; PR, partial response.

Chemotherapy of cervical carcinoma may play a role in the treatment of patients with metastatic or recurrent disease or as an adjuvant treatment to surgery or radiation therapy in locally advanced disease or aortic metastases. Among the various single agents tested in advanced cervical carcinoma, three have demonstrated significant activity: platinum-based compounds, doxorubicin, and ifosfamide. Platinum compounds are the most extensively studied with an overall response rate of 23%, while doxorubicin has 17% and ifosfamide has 14%. Compared to single-agent therapy, none of the combination regimens has yet been shown to offer a significant survival advantage. The responses to chemotherapy are brief and are associated with significant toxicity. Responses usually last 6 months, with median survival ranging from 6 to 9 months. Chemotherapy as a radiosensitizer to reduce tumor size and eradicate micrometastases is currently under investigation in prospective randomized trials. However, there does appear to be a subset of patients that can benefit from currently available drugs (see Table 39-4).

SUGGESTED READINGS

Creasman W, Soper J, Clarke-Pearson D: Radical hysterectomy as therapy for early carcinoma of the cervix. Am J Obstet Gynecol 155:964, 1986

Delgado G, Bundy BN, Fowler WC et al: A prospective surgical pathological study of stage I squamous carcinoma of the cervix: a Gynecologic Oncology Group study. Gynecol Oncol 35:314, 1989

Perez CA: Uterine Cervix in Principles and Practice of Radiation Oncology, pp. 1143–1202, JB Lippincott Company, Philadelphia, 1993

Stehman F, Thomas GM: Prognostic factors in locally advanced carcinoma of the cervix treated with radiation therapy. Semin Oncol 21:25–29, 1994

Vermorken JB: The role of chemotherapy in squamous cell carcinoma of the uterine cervix; a review. Int J Gynecol Cancer 3:129, 1993

40 Gestational Trophoblastic Disease

David L. Doering
James R. Bosscher

Incidence: 1/1,000 pregnancies (United States)

Goal of treatment: Cure

Main modality of treatment: Chemotherapy

Prognosis

Nonmetastatic gestational trophoblastic disease (GTD)	>98% (cure)
Metastatic GTD (low risk)	>98% (cure)
Metastatic GTD (high risk)	85% (cure)

Gestational trophoblastic disease (GTD) comprises a spectrum of neoplastic disorders of trophoblast, including hydatidiform mole, invasive mole, placental-site trophoblastic tumor, and gestational choriocarcinoma. Hydatidiform mole is a benign lesion that is usually cured by removal, while persistent GTD ranks among the most curable of human malignancies, largely because of its sensitivity to chemotherapy and the ability to monitor the course of the disease with a sensitive tumor marker. Malignant GTD is unique among malignancies in that it is typically diagnosed without tissue for histologic examination, usually when a woman has a rising or plateauing human chorionic gonadotropin (HCG) level or develops metastatic disease after evacuation of a molar pregnancy. Persistent GTD most often follows a molar pregnancy, but it may occur after any gestational event, including normal pregnancy.

MOLAR PREGNANCY

Molar pregnancies may be classified as *complete* or *partial*. Complete moles have no fetal tissue and exhibit diffuse villous swelling and trophoblastic proliferation. Most have a 46XX karyotype, with all the molar chromosomes of paternal origin. Approximately 10% have a 46XY karyotype, also all paternal in origin. Partial moles have identifiable fetal tissue and have only focal villous swelling and trophoblastic proliferation. Characteristic scalloping of the villi is often present. Partial moles generally have a triploid karyotype.

SYMPTOMS

The most common symptom of molar pregnancy is vaginal bleeding. Other symptoms may include excessive uterine size, toxemia, hyperemesis gravidarum, theca lutein ovarian cysts, trophoblastic embolization, and hyperthyroidism. Diagnosis is usually made at the time of ultrasonic evaluation of the uterus for vaginal bleeding or absent fetal heart tones. Complete moles produce a characteristic vesicular ultrasonic appearance often referred to as a "snowstorm" pattern. Partial moles may demonstrate focal cystic areas in the placenta as well as an identifiable fetus. Eighty per cent of molar pregnancies regress after removal, but approximately 20% of patients will develop persistent GTD; 15% as locally invasive disease within the uterus, and 5% as distant metastases.

THERAPY

Therapy for molar pregnancy consists of surgical removal of the molar tissue. Once the diagnosis is made, the patient should be carefully evaluated for associated medical complications such as anemia, preeclampsia, or hyperthyroidism. If future fertility is not desired, hysterectomy may be performed with the molar pregnancy in situ. Oophorectomy is not necessary, even if large theca lutein cysts are present. Hysterectomy eliminates the risk of persistent locally invasive disease, but does not affect the risk of metastatic disease.

Suction curettage is the treatment of choice for patients who desire to preserve fertility. The patient is begun on an oxytocin infusion in order to facilitate uterine contraction. The cervix is then dilated, and suction curettage is performed. Following completion of the suction curettage, sharp curettage is often recommended in order to remove any residual molar tissue. Prophylactic single-agent chemotherapy at the time of uterine evacuation has been demonstrated to reduce the risk of subsequent persistent GTD. Either methotrexate or actinomycin D may be utilized. However, since 80% of patients will not develop persistent disease, prophylactic chemotherapy is often reserved for high-risk patients only. An algorithm for the management of hydatid mole is depicted in Figure 40-1.

FOLLOW-UP

Close follow-up is essential in the management of molar pregnancy. All patients require weekly monitoring of β-HCG levels until normal values are obtained for 3 consecutive weeks. Levels are then followed monthly until normal for 6 consecutive months. Effective contraception is critical during the follow-up period, so that another pregnancy does not occur. Patients who have had one molar pregnancy are at increased risk for subsequent GTD. Therefore, prompt ultrasonic evaluation is indicated with future pregnancies.

MALIGNANT GESTATIONAL TROPHOBLASTIC DISEASE

Malignant GTD most commonly occurs following molar pregnancy. Clinical presentation may include irregular vaginal bleeding, theca lutein cysts, persistent uterine enlargement, and persistently elevated serum HCG levels. Diagnosis is usually made when serum HCG levels plateau or rise after evacuation of a molar pregnancy. When malignant GTD occurs following a nonmolar pregnancy, diagnosis may be delayed until the patient presents with symptoms due to metastatic disease. After diagnosis, evaluation focuses on establishing the extent of disease and identifying risk factors for treatment failure. Malignant GTD is classified as nonmetastatic versus metastatic; metastatic GTD is further subclassified as low risk versus high risk. Table 40-1 outlines the International Federation of Gynecology and Obstetrics (FIGO) anatomic staging system. Table 40-2 lists the factors which have traditionally been used to classify patients with metastatic GTD into the high-risk category. The World Health Organization scoring system for assessment of risk is depicted in Table 40-3. Once the diagnosis of persistent GTD is established, evaluation should include a careful history and physical examination, serum β-HCG level, complete blood count, and hepatic, renal, and thyroid function tests. Assessment for metastatic disease should include a chest x-ray as well as computed tomography (CT) of the head, abdomen, and pelvis. Selective angiography may be useful, particularly for identifying disease in the pelvis. Determination of cerebrospinal fluid (CSF) hCG levels can identify occult cerebral metastases when the head CT is normal. The plasma/CSF HCG ratio is generally less than 60 when cerebral metastases are present.

THERAPY

Stage I. Therapy is determined by the *stage of disease and presence of other risk factors*. Patients with stage I disease who do not desire fertility may be treated with hysterectomy and single-agent chemotherapy. If future fertility is desired, these patients are treated with single-agent chemotherapy. Various regimens have been employed, all with excellent results. Single-agent chemotherapy regimens are summarized in Appendix 27. No direct comparisons have been performed, but the success rates are similar and morbidity is comparable. Selection of a regimen should take into consideration such factors as cost and systemic toxicity. Many centers use the methotrexate-folinic acid regimen because of excellent results and minimal toxicity. Disease resistance to one agent can often be overcome by switching to the alternate agent. If disease resistance persists despite use of another agent, combination chemotherapy is indicated. Cure rates for

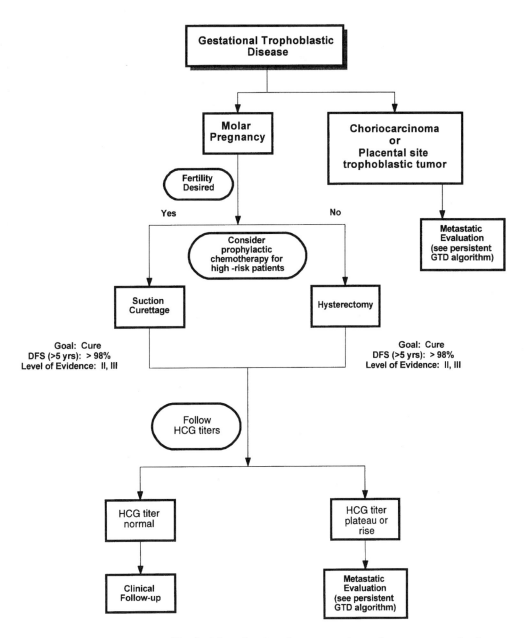

FIGURE 40-1 *Management of hydatid mole. Suction curettage or hysterectomy is the mainstay of therapy for this benign disease with a propensity to develop into malignant gestational trophoblastic disease (GTD). If human chorionic gonadotropin (HCG) titer plateaus or rises, or if histology reveals choricarcinoma or placental site throphoblastic disease, proceed to persistent GTD algorithm (Fig. 40-2). Goal of treatment is cure. Recommended strategy is based on levels II and III evidence. DFS, disease-free survival.*

nonmetastatic and good-prognosis metastatic GTD approach 100%.

Follow-up for nonmetastatic or low-risk metastatic GTD involves weekly hCG levels until normal for 3 consecutive weeks, then monthly for 12 consecutive months. Effective contraception should be employed during the follow-up period.

Stages II and III. Patients with high-risk (World Health Organization [WHO] score ≥ 8) stage II or

TABLE 40-1   THE INTERNATIONAL FEDERATION OF GYNECOLOGY AND OBSTETRICS (FIGO) STAGING OF GESTATIONAL TROPHOBLASTIC DISEASE

Stage I	Confined to uterine corpus
Stage II	Metastases to pelvis and/or vagina
Stage III	Metastases to lung
Stage IV	Distant metastases

TABLE 40-2   HIGH-RISK METASTATIC GESTATIONAL TROPHOBLASTIC DISEASE

Urinary hCG > 100,000 IU/24 hours
Interval since antecedent pregnancy > 4 months
Brain or liver metastasis
Following term pregnancy
Serum β-HCG > 40,000 mIU/mL
Failed prior chemotherapy
WHO score > 8

Abbreviations: HCG, human chorionic gonadotropin; WHO, World Health Organization.

III disease, and all patients with stage IV disease will require combination chemotherapy. Numerous regimens have been utilized, with varying results. MAC (methotrexate, actinomycin D, and cyclophosphamide) was formerly used, but recent data indicate a remission rate of only approximately 50% in high-risk metastatic GTD. The combination of etoposide, methotrexate, actinomycin D, cyclophosphamide, and vincristine (EMA-CO), first reported by Bagshawe in 1984, results in a remission rate of about 85% in these high-risk patients. This regimen is depicted in Appendix 27. Whole head irradiation (3,000 cGy) is added for cerebral metastases, and surgical resection is employed selectively for resistant disease or to manage complications such as hemorrhage. Treatment should be continued until the patient achieves 3 consecutive normal HCG levels. Two courses of therapy are administered after attainment of a normal HCG level. Figure 40-2 outlines the management of malignant GTD.

PLACENTAL-SITE TROPHOBLASTIC DISEASE

Placental-site trophoblastic disease (PSTT) is an unusual variant of malignant GTD, which arises from the intermediate trophoblast. Human placental lactogen as well as HCG may be secreted, but HCG levels are usually only modestly elevated. Response to chemotherapy has been poor; therefore hysterectomy should be the mainstay of therapy for this condition, after careful evaluation for metastatic disease.

Resistant disease requires a multidisciplinary approach with careful attention to the patient's cardiovascular, renal, hepatic, and hematopoietic function. Therapeutic options may be limited by accumulated toxicity; however, even heavily pretreated patients are often salvaged. Cisplatin is active against GTD, and regimens combining this agent with other active drugs have been successful in some patients. Substitution of cisplatin and

TABLE 40-3   WHO SCORING SYSTEM[a]

Prognostic Factor	Prognostic Score			
	0	1	2	4
Age (years)	<39	>39		
Antecedent pregnancy	Hydatid mole	Abortion	Term	
Interval between antecedent pregnancy and start of chemotherapy (months)	<4	4–6	7–12	>12
HCG (mIU/mL)	<10^3	10^3–10^4	10^4–10^5	>10^5
ABO blood groups (female x male)		O × A	B	
		A × O	AB	
Largest tumor, including uterine (cm)		3–5	>5	
Site of metastases	Lung, vagina, pelvis	Spleen, kidney	Gastrointestinal tract, liver	Brain
Number of metastases identified		1–4	4–8	>8
Prior chemotherapy		Single drug	Two or more drugs	

Abbreviations:HCG, human chorionic gonadotropin; WHO, world health organization.

[a] Total score ≤ 4 = low risk, 5–7 = intermediate risk, ≥ 8 = high risk.

(From Bagshawe KD: Treatment of high-risk choriocarcinoma. J Reprod Med 29:813, 1984, with permission.)

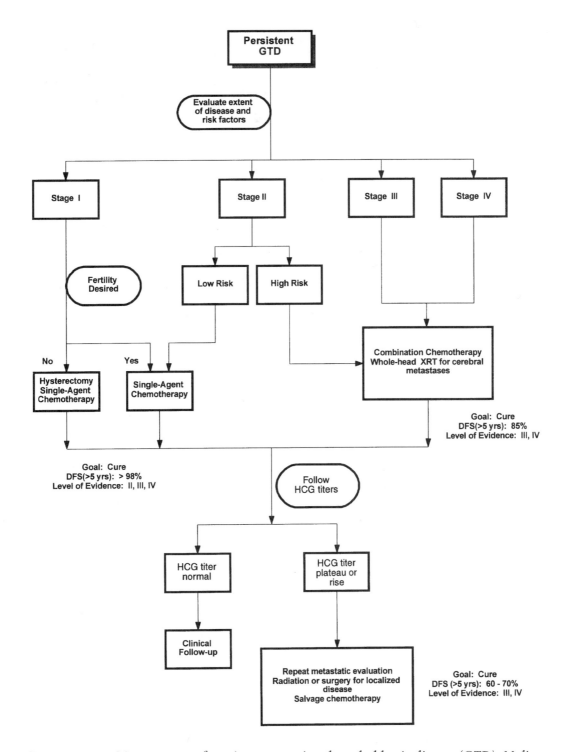

FIGURES 40-2 *Management of persistent gestational trophoblastic disease (GTD). Malignant GTD is unique among malignancies in that it is typically diagnosed without tissue for histologic examination, usually when a woman has a rising or plateauing human chorionic gonadotropin (HCG) level or develops metastatic disease after evacuation of a molar pregnancy. Persistent GTD ranks among the most curable of human malignancies, largely because of its sensitivity to chemotherapy and the ability to monitor the course of the disease with a sensitive tumor marker. Recommended strategy is based on levels II, III, and IV evidence. DFS, disease-free survival. (See also Appendix 27.)*

etoposide for the cyclophosphamide and vincristine on day 7 of the EMA-CO regimen has resulted in cures of patients who had failed EMA-CO. The combination of ifosfamide, cisplatin, and etoposide has also been used.

After successful treatment for high-risk disease, HCG levels should be followed weekly until normal for 3 consecutive weeks, and then monthly for 24 consecutive months. Effective contraception should be utilized during the follow-up period.

SUGGESTED READINGS

Bagshawe KD, Harland S: Immunodiagnosis and monitoring of gonadotropin-producing metastases in the central nervous system. Cancer 38:112, 1976

Bagshawe KD: Treatment of high-risk choriocarcinoma. J Reprod Med 29:813, 1984

Berkowitz RS, Goldstein DP: Gestational trophoblastic neoplasia. pp. 457–480. In Berek JS, Hacker NF (eds): Practical Gynecologic Oncology. 2nd Ed. Williams & Wilkins, Baltimore, 1994

Berkowitz RS, Goldstein DP, Bernstein MR: Ten years' experience with methotrexate and folinic acid as primary therapy for gestational trophoblastic disease. Gynecol Oncol 23:111, 1986

Bolis G, Bonazzi C, Landoni F et al: EMA-CO regimen in high-risk gestational trophoblastic tumor (GTT). Gynecol Oncol 31:439, 1988

Curry SL, Blessing JA, DiSaia PL et al: A prospective randomized comparison of methotrexate, dactinomycin and chlorambucil versus methotrexate, dactinomycin, cyclophosphamide, doxorubicin, melphalan, hydroxyurea and vincristine in "poor prognosis" metastatic gestational trophoblastic disease: a Gynecologic Oncology Group study. Obstet Gynecol 73:357, 1989

DeBaz BP, Lewis TJ: Imaging of gestational trophoblastic disease. Semin Oncol 22:130, 1995

DuBeshter B, Berkowitz RS, Goldstein DP et al: Metastatic gestational trophoblastic disease: experience at the New England Trophoblastic Disease Center, 1965–1985. Obstet Gynecol 69:390, 1987

Feldman S, Goldstein DP, Berkowitz RS: Low-risk metastatic gestational trophoblastic tumors. Semin Oncol 22:166, 1995

Finkler NJ: Placental site trophoblastic tumor diagnosis, clinical behavior and treatment. J Reprod Med 36:27, 1991

Finkler NJ, Berkowitz RS, Driscoll SD et al: Clinical experience with placental site trophoblastic tumors at the New England Trophoblastic Disease Center. Obstet Gynecol 71:854, 1988

Goldstein DP: Prevention of gestational trophoblastic disease by use of actinomycin-D in molar pregnancies. Obstet Gynecol 43:475, 1974

Goldstein DP, Berkowitz RS: Prophylactic chemotherapy of complete molar pregnancy. Semin Oncol 22:157, 1995

Gordon AN, Gershenson DM, Copeland LJ et al: High-risk metastatic gestational trophoblastic disease: further stratification into clinical entities. Gynecol Oncol 34:54, 1989

Greenfield AW: Gestational trophoblastic disease: prognostic variables and staging. Semin Oncol 22:142, 1995

Kim DS, Moon H, Kim KT et al: Effects of prophylactic chemotherapy for persistent trophoblastic disease in patients with complete hydatidiform mole. Obstet Gynecol 67:690, 1986

Kennedy AW: Persistent nonmetastatic gestational trophoblastic disease. Semin Oncol 22:161, 1995

Lurain JR, Elfstrand EP: Single-agent methotrexate chemotherapy for the treatment of nonmetastatic gestational trophoblastic tumors. Am J Obstet Gynecol 172:574, 1995

Rose PG: Hydatidiform mole: diagnosis and management. Semin Oncol 22:149, 1995

Rustin GJS, Newland ES, Begent RHJ et al: Weekly alternating etoposide, methotrexate, actinomycin D/vincristine and cyclophosphamide chemotherapy for the treatment of CNS metastases of choriocarcinoma. J Clin Oncol 7:900, 1989

Semer DA, Macfee MS: Gestational trophoblastic disease: epidemiology. Semin Oncol 22:109, 1995

Soper JT, Clarke-Pearson DL, Berchuck AB et al: 5-day methotrexate for women with metastatic gestational trophoblastic disease. Gynecol Oncol 54:76, 1994

Soper JT, Evans AC, Clarke-Pearson DL et al: Alternating weekly chemotherapy with etoposide-methotrexate-dactinomycin/cyclophosphamide-vincristine for high-risk gestational trophoblastic disease. Obstet Gynecol 83:113, 1994

Soper JT: Identification and management of high-risk gestational trophoblastic disease. Semin Oncol 22:172, 1995

Wong LC, Choo YC, Ma HK: Primary oral etoposide therapy in gestational trophoblastic disease: an update. Cancer 58:14, 1986

Yordan EL Jr, Schlaerth J, Gaddis O, Morrow CP: Radiation therapy in the management of gestational choriocarcinoma metastatic to the central nervous system. Obstet Gynecol 69:627, 1987

41 Vaginal Cancer

David L. Doering
James R. Bosscher
Nermina Obralić

Epidemiology: 1% of gynecologic cancers; second most rare gynecologic malignancy after fallopian tube cancer

Goal of treatment: Cure, except when disease has spread beyond the pelvis

Main modality of treatment: Radiation therapy; surgery for selected cases of early stage disease confined to the upper vagina

Prognosis: Overall 5-year survival 43%

Primary cancer of the vagina is a rare disease, comprising only about 1% of all gynecologic malignancies. Squamous cell carcinomas account for 95% of vaginal cancers, although other histologic types are also encountered. Additional vaginal malignancies include adenocarcinomas, sarcomas, melanomas, and germ cell tumors. *Most cancers found in the vagina are metastatic lesions from other sites*, usually the cervix or vulva. The International Federation of Gynecology and Obstetrics (FIGO) classification and staging system requires that tumors which involve both the vagina and cervix be classified as cervical cancers, while those that involve both the vulva and vagina are considered to represent vulvar cancers. Endometrial carcinomas and choriocarcinomas also frequently metastasize to the vagina.

INCIDENCE

The incidence of the various histologic types of vaginal cancer varies with the age of the patient population. Embryonal rhabdomyosarcoma (sarcoma botryoides) and endodermal sinus tumors occur in infancy and early childhood. Clear cell adenocarcinomas are found in adolescents and young adults, often associated with *in utero* exposure to diethylstilbestrol (DES). Squamous cell carcinoma and melanoma are generally diseases of postmenopausal women. The mean age of diagnosis is 60 years for squamous cell carcinoma and 58 years for melanoma.

SYMPTOMS

Vaginal bleeding and discharge are the most common symptoms of vaginal cancer. The bleeding is usually painless and may be postcoital. Urinary frequency may indicate bladder wall involvement, or tenesmus may occur with posterior wall tumors involving the rectum. Pelvic pain is generally a sign of disease extension beyond the vagina. The disease is usually detected on routine pelvic examination and cervicovaginal cytology in 5% to 10% of patients who have no symptoms.

DIAGNOSIS AND STAGING

Diagnosis is accomplished by biopsy of any gross lesions noted on physical examination. When no obvious lesion is present, colposcopic evaluation with application of 3% acetic acid is indicated. Examination under anesthesia may be necessary for diagnosis and staging.

Vaginal cancer is staged clinically. The FIGO staging system is depicted in Table 41-1. Staging is based on clinical findings, including physical examination, cystoscopy, proctoscopy, and chest x-ray. Imaging studies such as computed tomography (CT) or magnetic resonance imaging (MRI) may be useful for pretreatment evaluation of the primary tumor, the peritoneal contents, and the retroperitoneal lymph nodes; however, these studies are not utilized in the formal FIGO staging process.

THERAPY

Most vaginal cancers are best treated with radiation therapy. Surgery has only a limited role, because of the inability to achieve adequate surgical margins due to the proximity of the bladder and rectum. Small lesions involving the upper posterior vaginal wall can be treated by radical hysterectomy, partial vaginectomy, and pelvic lymphadenectomy. If the patient has previously had a hysterectomy, radical upper vaginectomy and pelvic lymphadenectomy may be appropriate. In patients with locally advanced disease (stage IVa), primary pelvic exenteration is a therapeutic option, especially if a vesicovaginal or rectovaginal fistula is present. When vaginal cancer occurs in a patient who has received prior pelvic radiation therapy, pelvic exenteration may be the only treatment option.

Vaginal cancers that do not meet the specific criteria for surgical intervention outlined above will be treated with radiation therapy. Whole pelvis external beam radiation therapy is administered to a dose of approximately 5,000 cGy, followed by intracavitary or interstitial therapy. Small superficial lesions may be treated with intracavitary therapy alone. Better dose distribution is often achieved in larger lesions by the use of interstitial radiation. If the lower one-third of the vagina is involved, it is important to include the inguinal nodes in the treatment field or to perform inguinal lymph node dissection.

Survival for vaginal cancer patients is not as high as survival for patients with similar stage cervical cancer. Even patients with stage I disease have only approximately 70% 5-year survival. Improved outcome awaits further refinements in radiation therapy.

Figure 41-1 shows the recommended approach to the management of vaginal cancer. Due to the rare incidence of this tumor no randomized trial evaluating different treatment options has been performed; all recommendations are, therefore, based on indirect evidence (mostly levels IV and V).

SUGGESTED READINGS

Al-Kurdi M, Monaghan JM: Thirty-two years experience in management of primary tumors of the vagina. Br J Obstet Gynaecol 88:1145, 1981

Andrassy RJ, Hays DM, Raney RB et al: Conservative surgical management of vaginal and vulvar pediatric rhabdomyosarcoma: a report from the Intergroup Rhabdomyosarcoma Study III. J Pediatr Surg 30:1034–1036, 1995

Choo YC, Anderson DG: Neoplasms of the vagina following cervical carcinoma. Gynecol Oncol 14:125, 1982

Chung AF, Casey MJ, Flannery JT et al: Malignant melanoma of the vagina: report of 19 cases. Obstet Gynecol 55:720, 1980

Herbst AL, Ulfelder H, Poskanzer DC: Adenocarcinoma of the vagina: association of maternal stilbestrol therapy with tumor appearance in young women. N Engl J Med 284:878, 1971

Hilgers RD, Malkasian GD, Soule EH: Embryonal rhabdomyosarcoma (botryoid type) of the vagina: a clinicopathologic review. Am J Obstet Gynecol 107:484, 1970

Kirkbridge P, Fyles A, Rawlings GA et al: Carcinoma of the vagina — experience at the Pricess Margaret Hospital (1974–1989). Gynecol Oncol 56:435–443, 1995

Kucera H, Langer M, Smekal G et al: Radiotherapy of primary carcinoma of the vagina: management and results of different therapy schemes. Gynecol Oncol 21:87, 1985

Kumer APM, Wrenn EL, Fleming ID et al: Combined therapy to prevent complete pelvic exenteration for rhabdomyosarcoma of the vagina or uterus. Cancer 37:118, 1976

Nanavati PJ, Fanning J, Hilgers RD et al: High-dose-rate brachytherapy in primary stage I and II vaginal cancer. Gynecol Oncol 51:61–71, 1993

Perez CA, Arneson AN, Dehner LP et al: Radiation therapy in carcinoma of the vagina. Obstet Gynecol 44:862, 1974

TABLE 41-1 FIGO STAGING FOR CARCINOMA OF THE VAGINA

Stage 0	Carcinoma in situ, intraepithelial neoplasia
Stage I	Limited to the vaginal wall
Stage II	Subvaginal tissue is involved but not extended to the pelvic wall
Stage III	Extended to the pelvic wall
Stage IV	Extended beyond the true pelvis or has clinically involved the mucosa of the bladder or rectum
Stage IVa	Spread to adjacent organs and/or direct extension beyond the true pelvis
Stage IVb	Spread to distant organs

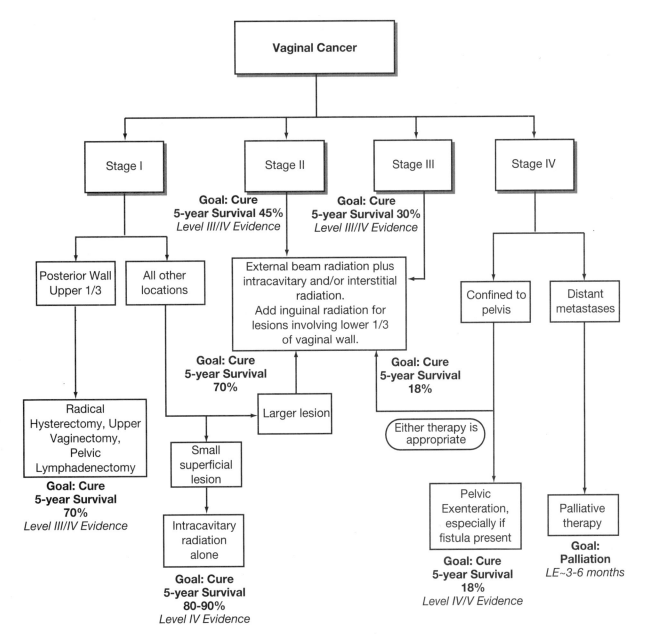

FIGURE 41-1 *Management of vaginal cancer. Determination of the stage (see Table 41-1.) and resectability, which is possible only in rare cases, represent the key reasoning principle in the management of vaginal cancer. The goal of treatment is curative in all stages except in metastatic disease beyond pelvis. The recommended strategy is based mainly on indirect (levels IV and V evidence) and on some level III evidence (single-arm prospective studies).*

Stock RG, Chen AS, Seski J: A 30-year experience in the management of primary carcinoma of the vagina: analysis of prognostic factors and treatment modalities. Gynecol Oncol 56:45–52, 1995

Sulak P, Barnhill D, Heller P et al: Nonsquamous cancer of the vagina. Gynecol Oncol 165:282, 1991

Weinstock MA. Malignant melanoma of the vulva and vagina in the United States: patterns of incidence and population-based estimates of survival. Am J Obstet Gynecol 171:1225–1230, 1994

42 Vulvar Cancer

Ward Katsanis
Randall Gibb
Nermina Obralić
David L. Doering

Incidence: 0.6/100,000

Mortality: 0.3/100,000

Goal of treatment: In disease limited to the pelvis (stages I, II, III, IVA) treatment is with curative intent. Palliation is the only option for disseminated disease (IVB)

Main modality of treatment: Surgery with or without adjuvant radiation therapy, preoperative radiation ± chemotherapy indicated for advanced disease

Prognosis: Overall five-year survival 70%; status of groin lymph nodes most important prognostic factor:

(–) groin nodes	90%
(+) groin nodes	50%
(+) pelvic lymph nodes	10%

INCIDENCE

Carcinoma of the vulva is a relatively rare tumor, accounting for only 3% to 5% of gynecologic malignancies and 1% to 2% of all malignant tumors in women. Vulvar cancer is primarily a disease of the elderly, with a median age at diagnosis of 61 years. It is often associated with a history of venereal disease, vulvar and vaginal inflammatory conditions, chronic vulvar irritation, diabetes, hypertension, obesity, and smoking. Emerging data also suggests a role for human papilloma virus in the development of some vulvar carcinomas.

HISTOLOGY AND PATHOPHYSIOLOGY

These tumors are exophytic in two-thirds of cases, with the remainder being endophytic and ulcerated. Invasive lesions arise in the labia majora or minora in over 70% of patients, 10% to 15% originate near the clitoris, and 4% to 5% on the perineum. *Squamous cell cancers are the predominant histologic type, comprising nearly 90% of cases.* Other less common histologies include malignant melanomas, adenocarcinomas, basal cell cancers, adenoid cystic carcinomas, verrucous carcinomas, and sarcomas.

Typically, vulvar carcinomas are slow growing and spread to adjacent tissues by direct extension. Lymphatic dissemination occurs first to the superficial inguinal femoral nodes, next to the deep femoral nodes and, in the presence of positive deep nodes, possibly to the pelvic lymph nodes. Risk of lymph node involvement depends on tumor size, depth of invasion, and lymphvascular space invasion (Table 42-1). Incidence of regional lymph node involvement also correlates well with the International Federation of Gynecology and Obstetrics

(FIGO) clinical staging system and is found in 8.9% of patients with stage I, 25.3% with stage II, 31.5% with stage III, and 62.5% with stage IV disease.

MANAGEMENT

The most common presenting *symptoms* of vulvar carcinoma are pruritis, bleeding, pain, and dysuria; however many patients are either asymptomatic or simply complain of a vulvar mass. Delay in diagnosis is common with this disease. Because of this, it is important that the clinician *perform a biopsy whenever suspicious lesions are noted on the vulva.* In addition, complete evaluation includes a Pap smear, careful colposcopic inspection of the cervix, vagina, and vulva, as well as a bimanual examination and palpation of the inguinal and femoral lymph nodes. Routine laboratory studies (CBC, SMA-18) and chest x-ray are also performed. Additional studies including cystoscopy, proctoscopy, barium enema, or abdominal and pelvic computed tomography (CT) scanning are indicated when more advanced disease is suspected.

Previously, vulvar carcinoma was clinically staged according to FIGO guidelines. Clinical staging is inaccurate in 18% to 45% of cases, thus leading to the adoption of FIGO surgical staging system

TABLE 42-1 PROGNOSTIC FACTORS RELATING TO REGIONAL LYMPH NODE METASTASES

	Regional nodes (% +)
Lesion size (cm)	
≤ 1	5
1–2	15
2–4	33
>4	50
Depth of invasion (mm)	
<1	0
1–2	7
2–3	8
3–5	27

TABLE 42-2 FIGO AND TNM CLASSIFICATION OF VULVAR CARCINOMA (1988)

	TNM			FIGO
T	Primary tumor		Stage 0	Carcinoma in situ
	Tis	Carcinoma in situ	Stage I	Confined to the vulva and or perineum, <2 cm; negative nodes
	T1	Tumor confined to vulva and/or perineum, < 2 cm		
	T2	Tumor confined to vulva and/or perineum, >2 cm	Stage II	Confined to the vulva and or perineum, > 2 cm; negative nodes
	T3	Tumor of any size with spread to urethra, vagina, anus or all of these	Stage III	Tumor of any size with spread to lower urethra, lower vagina anus and/or unilateral positive nodes
	T4	Tumor of any size infiltrating the bladder, rectum, upper urethra, or fixed to bone	Stage IVA	Tumor invades upper urethra, bladder, rectum, pelvic bone and/or bilateral positive nodes
N	Regional lymph nodes		Stage IVB	Distant metastases, including pelvic nodes
	N0	No palpable nodes		
	N1	Unilateral regional metastases		
	N2	Bilateral regional metastases		
M	Distant metastases			
	M0	No clinical metastases		
	M1	Distant metastases (including pelvic nodes)		

Abbreviations: FIGO, International Federation of Gynecology and Obstetrics; TNM, tumor, node, metastasis.

in 1988, as outlined in Table 42-2. Five-year survival rates based on stage of disease have been examined by the Gynecologic Oncology Group and reported as stage I, 98%; stage II, 85%; stage III, 74%; and stage IV, 31%. Overall, prognosis is related to lymph node involvement regardless of clinical stage (80% to 85% five-year survival for patients with negative nodes vs 40% to 50% with positive nodes). *The depth of tumor invasion is critical in determining the risk of nodal metastases and in this way strongly influences prognosis and treatment recommendations.*

En bloc radical vulvectomy and bilateral inguinofemoral lymphadenectomy with or without pelvic lymphadenectomy was the traditional treatment for operable vulvar carcinoma. Based on level II, III, and IV evidence, management has become more conservative. Management decisions are now individualized to achieve the best control of disease, to reduce acute and long-term therapy-related morbidity (Table 42-3), and to maintain sexual function when possible. Unilateral lesions less than 2 cm in diameter can be effectively treated with radical local excision and unilateral inguinofemoral lymph node dissection. This is supported by level II data. One randomized study comparing groin dissection to groin irradiation was stopped prematurely due to excess recurrences and deaths in the groin radiation therapy arm. Pelvic radiation therapy has been shown to be superior to pelvic lymph node dissection for patients with positive groin nodes. Primary curative radiation therapy is possible, but is generally reserved for periclitoral lesions or patients who are not operative candidates. Larger lesions or bilateral tumors are treated with radical vulvectomy and bilateral inguinofemoral lymphadenectomy. When patients present with very large, unrespectable lesions, preoperative radiation therapy (with or without radiation-sensitizing chemotherapy) is used to shrink the tumor, followed by resection of any residual tumor (Table 42-4). The emergence of less radical surgery, more specific guidelines for nodal dissections, and the use of preoperative chemoradiation with advanced tumors have been incorporated into contemporary treatment schemes as presented in Figure 42-1.

TABLE 42-3 ACUTE AND LATE COMPLICATIONS FROM SURGICAL MANAGEMENT OF VULVAR CANCER

Acute	Late
Wound breakdown (50%)	Chronic leg edema
Urinary tract infection	Recurrent lymphangitis
Wound seromas	Introital stenosis
Deep venous thrombosis	Femoral hernia (rare)
Pulmonary embolus	Fistulas (rare)
Myocardial infarction	Pubic osteomyelitis (rare)
Hemorrhage	
Osteitis pubis (rare)	

TABLE 42-4 COMBINED CHEMORADIATION IN ADVANCED VULVAR CARCINOMA

Patients	Treatment	Evidence Level	Outcomes (Comments)	Reference
33	5-FU 1000 mg/m²; ± MC 6 mg/m²; XRT individualized	III	Effective therapy for advanced disease	Thomas et al: Gynecol Oncol 34:263, 1989
12	DDP 50 mg/m²; 5-FU 1000 mg/m²; XRT 44–54 Gy	III	67% CR; 25% PR	Berek et al: Gynecol Oncol 42:197, 1991
20	5-FU 750–1000 mg/m² × 3–d; ± cisplatin 50–100 mg/m² × 1 day; XRT 40–54 Gy	III	50% CR; 40% PR	Koh et al: Int J Radiat Oncol Biol Phys 26:809, 1993
19	5-FU 1000 mg/m²; MC 10 mg/m²; XRT 45–50 Gy to pelvis and groin	III	74% local control	Wahlen et al; Cancer 75:2289, 1995

Abbreviations: 5-FU, 5-fluorouracil; MC, mitomycin C; XRT, radiation therapy; DDP, cisplatin; CT, chemotherapy; Gy, gray; CR, complete response; PR, partial response.

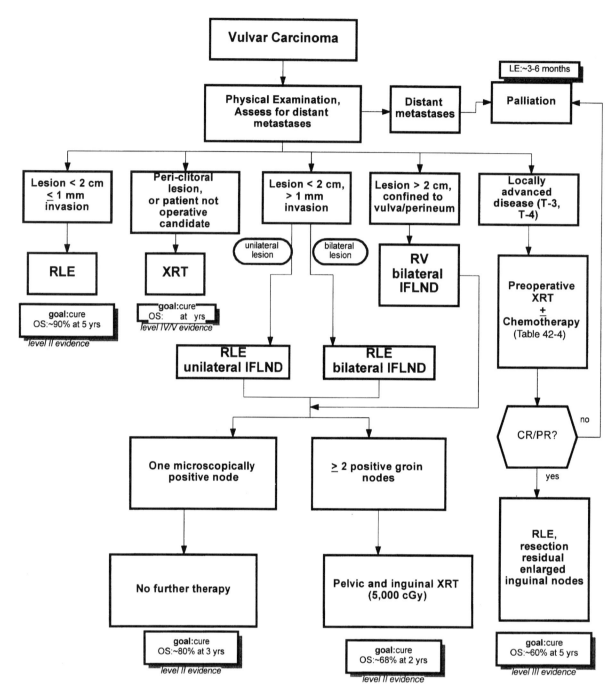

FIGURE 42-1   *An algorithm for the treatment of vulvar carcinoma. Management strategies are based on size and location of primary lesion, depth of invasion, and stage of disease. Treatment is given with curative intent in most cases. Recommended strategies are mainly based on level IV and some level III evidence. Note that IFLND compared to elective groin radiation is based on level II evidence. Pelvic radiation therapy for patients with 2 or more positive groin nodes is also supported by level II evidence. RLE, radical local excision; IFLND, inguinal femoral lymph node dissection; RV, radical vulvectomy; XRT, radiation therapy; CR, complete response; PR, partial response; OS, overall survival; LE, life expectancy (see also Tables 42-3 and 42-4 for details regarding management).*

SUGGESTED READINGS

Berek JS, Hacker NF: Practical Gynecologic Oncology. 2nd Ed. pp. 403–439. Williams & Wilkins, Baltimore, Maryland, 1994

Burger MF, Hollema H, Emanuels AG: The importance of the groin node status for the survival of T1 and T2 vulvar cancer patients. Gynecol Oncol 57:327–334, 1995

Giles GG, Kneale BL: Vulvar cancer: the Cinderella of gynecological oncology. Aust NZJ Obstet Gynecol 35:71–75, 1995

Hacker NF, Berek JS, Juillard GJF, Lagasse LD: Preoperative radiation therapy for locally advanced tumor. Cancer 54:2059–2063, 1984

Homesley HD, Bundy BN, Sedlis A, Adcock L: Radiation therapy versus pelvic node resection for carcinoma of the vulva with positive groin nodes. Obstet Gynecol 68:733, 1986

Hopkins MP, Reid GC, Morley GW: Radical vulvectomy: the decision for the incision. Cancer 72:799–803, 1993

Keys H: Gynecologic Oncology Group randomized trials of combined technique therapy for vulvar cancer. Cancer 71:1691–1696, 1986

Stehman FB: Groin dissection versus groin radiation in carcinoma of the vulva: a Gynecologic Oncology Group study Int J Rad Oncol Biol Physics 24:389–396, 1992

Stehman FB, Bundy BN, Dvoretsky PM, Creasman WT: Early stage I carcinoma of the vulva treated with ipsilateral superficial inguinal lymphadenectomy and modified radical hemivulvectomy: a prospective study of the Gynecologic Oncology Group. Obstet Gynecol 79:490–497, 1992

43 Renal Adenocarcinoma

James I. Harty

Synonyms: Renal cell carcinoma, hypernephroma, Grawitz tumor.

Incidence/prevalence: Incidence is approximately 9.6/100,000; 10th most common cancer in United States; 3% of all malignancies; 30,000 new cases diagnosed in 1996; 11,700 deaths in 1996.

Goal of treatment: Curative nephrectomy in patients with localized disease. Palliative nephrectomy in symptomatic patients with metastatic disease (e.g., hematuria/flank pain).

Main modality of treatment: Surgery, radical nephrectomy.

Prognosis: Dependent on stage of disease. Actuarial 10-year survival is 50%.

INCIDENCE

Renal adenocarcinoma arises from the cells of the proximal tubule and accounts for 3% of all neoplasms. It accounts for 85% of renal malignancies; the remaining 15% are made up of transitional cell neoplasms (12%), Wilms' tumors, and various types of sarcomas (3%). In the United States, there were approximately 30,000 new cases of renal adenocarcinoma and almost 12,000 deaths secondary to it in 1996. The incidence appears to be rising, which may be due to the fact that more incidental tumors are being found on abdominal ultrasound, computerized tomography (CT) scans, and magnetic resonance imaging (MRI) studies. The male-to-female ratio is 2:1, with a median age at diagnosis of 55 years. There is no known etiology.

DIAGNOSIS

Renal adenocarcinoma may present in several ways. The classic presentation is hematuria (40%), flank pain (35%–40%), or a palpable flank mass

(30%). This classic triad of symptoms only appear together in 10% of cases, and these patients usually have a poor prognosis because the disease is likely to be advanced. As many as 40% of renal adenocarcinomas are detected incidentally during abdominal imaging studies. These tend to be smaller tumors at a lower stage of disease and, therefore, have a better prognosis. A significant number of patients (10%–40%) may have symptoms of a paraneoplastic syndrome. This syndrome and its symptoms are due to the production of hormones specifically produced by the kidney, such as renin (causing hypertension, 38%) and erythropoietin (causing erythrocytosis, 35%), as well as true atopic hormones such as parathyroid-like hormone (causing hypercalcemia, 5%), ACTH-like hormone (causing Cushing syndrome), and human chorionic gonadotrophin (causing gynecomastia). Some patients present with nonspecific findings— anemia (37%), weight loss (35%), pyrexia (17%). Hepatic dysfunction that may reverse after nephrectomy, *Stauffer's syndrome*, is seen in approximately 15% of cases. Finally, approximately 10% of the patients present with symptoms of metastatic disease alone, and a renal primary is found only on further investigation.

Making the initial choice to use radiologic imaging to evaluate a patient suspected of having a renal adenocarcinoma depends largely upon the presenting symptoms. Patients who present with hematuria or flank pain should have an intravenous pyelogram as their initial study. An intravenous pyelogram, performed on a well-prepared patient, has a sensitivity rate of 85% and a specificity rate of greater than 90% for a kidney mass larger than 3 cm. In addition, an intravenous pyelogram will give useful information about the urinary collecting and drainage system, which might help in detecting the source of hematuria and flank pain. The finding of a renal mass on intravenous pyelogram should be further investigated with a renal ultrasound, which can further determine whether the mass is a cyst (benign) or a solid mass (malignant), with an 84% to 98% sensitivity rate. The sonographic characteristics of a benign simple renal cyst are sonolucency, good through transmission without internal echoes, far-wall enhancement, and smooth, regular walls. A solid mass is not sonolucent and has many internal echoes. Occasionally, a mass found on ultrasound may be equivocal, in that it shows some but not all of the ultrasound characteristics of a simple cyst. For example, it may be sonolucent but has thick walls or internal echoes secondary to septae. In these cases, as well as in those showing an obvious solid mass, the next study should be an abdominal CT scan performed with and without intravenous and oral contrast material. A CT scan can distinguish between a cystic and a solid mass with 95% rate of sensitivity and specificity. The remaining 5% of cases will be equivocal on CT scan and require further investigation—either a percutaneous puncture of the cystic mass or an arteriogram. The aim of the percutaneous puncture is to obtain fluid, which can be evaluated cytologically for malignant cells, and also to examine the internal characteristics of the cyst by injecting contrast material into it. Renal arteriography may be used instead of a cyst puncture. Since renal adenocarcinomas are highly vascular tumors in approximately 85% of cases, the presence of a vascular mass on renal arteriography is diagnostic of a renal adenocarcinoma. Renal arteriography has the added advantage of providing a detailed picture of the renal vasculature, which may assist with planning any surgical procedure, and, indeed, is mandatory in those patients in whom partial nephrectomy is contemplated because there is a solitary kidney or a poorly functioning contralateral kidney.

Renal adenocarcinoma has the unusual ability to form a tumor thrombus that may grow enough to extend into small intrarenal veins (70%), the main renal vein (15%), the vena cava (5%–10%), and even as far as the right atrium (1%–2%). This occurs more commonly from the right kidney because of the shorter right renal vein. The presence of a thrombus may be suggested clinically by delayed function of the kidney, shown on intravenous pyelogram or CT scan, lower extremity swelling, the presence of collateral circulation on the anterior abdominal wall, or a right-sided varicocele that fails to empty on lying down. While a thrombus may be seen on CT scan, MRI is superior in defining the extent of the tumor within the venous system. It is important to determine the extent of the tumor within the vena cava before any surgical procedure. MRI is 100% accurate in diagnosing vena cava thrombus, 88% accurate in diagnosing renal vein thrombus, and 80% accurate in diagnosing an atrial thrombus. MRI cannot distinguish those tumor thrombi that actually invade the vein as opposed to laying within it. Besides determining the presence and extent of a venous tumor thrombus, MRI is indicated in patients with a serious contrast allergy and in those with a significant degree of renal insufficiency.

STAGING

The TNM staging system proposed by the American Joint Committee on Cancer provides the most information concerning the stage of the disease (Table 43-1 and Fig. 43-1). Previously Robson's modification of Flocks and Kadesky's was utilized. It is important to try to stage the local disease accurately within the kidney. Intravenous pyelography and ultrasound have limited abilities in this regard. However, CT scan has a sensitivity rate of 46% for perinephric invasion, 78% for venous invasion into the renal vein or vena cava, 83% sensitivity for detecting regional lymphadenopathy, and 60% for adjacent organ invasion. In one study using CT scanning, 91% of patients were correctly diagnosed, and if patients with stage I and stage II disease were omitted, the overall accuracy rate was 96%.

Approximately 50% of patients with renal adenocarcinoma will have demonstrable metastatic disease at the time of diagnosis. An additional 25% of the patients who do not have metastases at the time of diagnosis will subsequently develop them, occasionally many years later. It is important to establish or rule out metastatic disease before surgical therapy since surgical removal of the kidney, in the presence of gross metastatic disease, is

TABLE 43-1 PROGNOSIS FOR SURVIVAL BASED ON STAGE OF RENAL DISEASE

	Modified Robson Stage	AJC TNM	5-Year(%)	10-Year(%)
Confined to renal capsule	I	T1T2N0M0	85	82
Confined to Gerota's fascia	II	T3aN0M0	78	64
Renal vein involvement	IIIA	T3bN0M0	57	50
Lymphatic involvement	IIIB	T1T3bN1–4M0	46	34
Vein and nodal involvement	IIIC	T3bN1–4M0	22	16[a]
Antigen organ involvement	IVA	T1–T4N0–4M0	14	10
Metastatic spread	IVB	T1–T4N0–4M1	5	3[b]

Unique features: Paraneoplastic syndromes; delayed metastases; unusual metastatic sites; spontaneous regression; some responses to immunotherapy.

[a], 9 years

[b], 8 years

Patient identification
Name _____
Address _____
Hospital or clinic number _____
Age _____ Sex _____ Race _____

Institution identification
Hospital or clinic _____
Address _____

Oncology Record

Anatomic site of cancer _____
Histologic type _____
Grade (G) _____
Date of classification _____

Chronology of classification
[ ] Clinical (use all data prior to first treatment)
[ ] Pathologic (if definitively resected specimen available)

DEFINITIONS

Primary Tumor (T)

Clin	Path		
[ ]	[ ]	TX	Primary tumor cannot be assessed
[ ]	[ ]	T0	No evidence of primary tumor
[ ]	[ ]	T1	Tumor 2.5 cm or less in greatest dimension limited to the kidney
[ ]	[ ]	T2	Tumor more than 2.5 cm in greatest dimension limited to the kidney
[ ]	[ ]	T3	Tumor extends into major veins or invades adrenal gland or perinephric tissues but not beyond Gerota's fascia
[ ]	[ ]	T3a	Tumor invades adrenal gland or perinephric tissues but not beyond Gerota's fascia
[ ]	[ ]	T3b	Tumor grossly extends into renal vein(s) or vena cava below diaphragm
[ ]	[ ]	T3c	Tumor grossly extends into vena cava above diaphragm
[ ]	[ ]	T4	Tumor invades beyond Gerota's fascia

Lymph Node (N)

Clin	Path		
[ ]	[ ]	NX	Regional lymph nodes cannot be assessed
[ ]	[ ]	N0	No regional lymph node metastasis
[ ]	[ ]	N1	Metastasis in a single lymph node, 2 cm or less in greatest dimension
[ ]	[ ]	N2	Metastasis in a single lymph node, more than 2 cm but not more than 5 cm in greatest dimension, or multiple lymph nodes, none more than 5 cm in greatest dimension
[ ]	[ ]	N3	Metastasis in a lymph node more than 5 cm in greatest dimension

Distant Metastasis (M)

Clin	Path		
[ ]	[ ]	MX	Presence of distant metastasis cannot be assessed
[ ]	[ ]	M0	No distant metastasis
[ ]	[ ]	M1	Distant metastasis

FIGURE 43-1 *Data form for staging renal adenocarcinoma. (From American Joint Committee on Cancer: Staging of Cancer Forms (Renal Adenocarcinoma). 3rd Ed. Lippincott-Raven, Philadelphia, 1988, with permission.)*

unlikely to prolong survival. Much has been written about the spontaneous regression of renal adenocarcinoma following removal of the primary tumor. The true incidence of this appears to be less than 1%, with the vast majority (90%) being cases involving pulmonary metastases. Only 8% to 11% of patients have a solitary resectable metastasis. However, these patients have a 30% to 45% 5-year survival rate following surgical removal of the primary tumor and the solitary metastasis.

The most common sites of metastatic disease are the lungs (76%), regional lymph nodes (64%), bone (43%), and liver (41%). Also, renal cell carcinoma has the ability to metastasize to unusual sites, including skin, vagina, and penis.

Much of the information required to stage renal cell carcinoma in terms of distant metastases is obtained from the same studies used to detect its local extent. The adrenal gland can be assessed on CT scan, and if it appears normal, it is almost always not involved pathologically. The liver can be evaluated by CT scan and also by liver function tests. Anteroposterior and lateral chest x-rays are usually sufficient to detect parenchymal lung metastases. However, if the retroperitoneal lymph nodes are enlarged, it is advisable to do a CT scan of the chest to look for mediastinal lymphadenopathy. The value of bone scans in the metastatic work-up is controversial. In general, if the serum calcium and alkaline phosphatase are normal, and the patient does not have symptoms of bone pain, there is no necessity to perform a bone scan. Fifty-two percent of the patients with hypercalcemia have bone metastasis, but only 6% of asymptomatic patients have positive bone scans.

TREATMENT

Surgery for renal cell carcinoma is unique because it is performed without prior biopsy and without tissue confirmation of a neoplasm. Percutaneous renal biopsy before surgery is not routinely used because of the high accuracy of radiologic procedures in diagnosing renal carcinoma, the risk of bleeding from the highly vascular tumors, the risk of seeding the needle tract with tumor cells, and, finally, a negative biopsy may not actually prove that the mass is not a malignancy, and surgical exploration would be recommended anyway.

Renal adenocarcinoma is one of the most resistant tumors to both chemotherapy and radiation therapy. The primary form of therapy is a radical nephrectomy as described by Robson. When a tumor thrombus is present in the vena cava, an extended surgical procedure will be required, even to the point of placing the patient on cardiac bypass with hypothermic cardiac arrest, to remove thrombi extending as far as the right atrium. In the absence of any distant metastases, these patients have a 5-year survival rate of 72%, and a 10-year survival rate of 62%.

When renal adenocarcinoma occurs bilaterally (1%–2%), or in a solitary kidney where the contralateral kidney has significantly diminished renal function, partial nephrectomy is indicated. Partial nephrectomy is not usually performed when the contralateral kidney is normal, because there is a 7% to 10% risk of local recurrence, and concomitant satellite tumors occur in 5% to 10% of renal cell carcinomas. Most partial nephrectomies can be performed in situ with hypothermia, and only rarely must the tumor be removed from the kidney *ex vivo*, followed by autotransplantation of the residual kidney.

Once the kidney has been removed and examined by the pathologist, the carcinoma can be staged more accurately and the need to refer for further therapy determined.

Renal cell carcinoma responds poorly to both chemotherapy and radiation therapy. The complete response rate to combination chemotherapy is only 4% to 6%. Therefore, adjunctive therapy is not used in cases of T1, T2, or T3 disease. These patients are followed up for evidence of metastatic disease and are only considered for additional therapy should metastasis develop. Radiation therapy is used for palliation of painful metastases, with palliation achieved in 67% to 77% of patients.

The frequency and extent of follow-up is controversial since the treatment options are limited. However, a yearly physical examination, chest x-ray, and serum chemistry studies should be performed in patients with stage T1-T2 disease, while those with T3 and T3a disease should also have an abdominal CT scan. Patients with T3b or T3c disease should have similar studies in addition to a yearly CT chest scan.

METASTATIC DISEASE

For patients who present with metastatic disease (50%) or who develop metastatic disease after nephrectomy (25%), treatment options are limited. They have a very poor prognosis, with a median survival time ranging from 6 to 12 months. As mentioned previously, renal cell carcinoma is not very responsive to chemotherapy because of the phenomenon of multi-drug resistance. The 4% to 6%

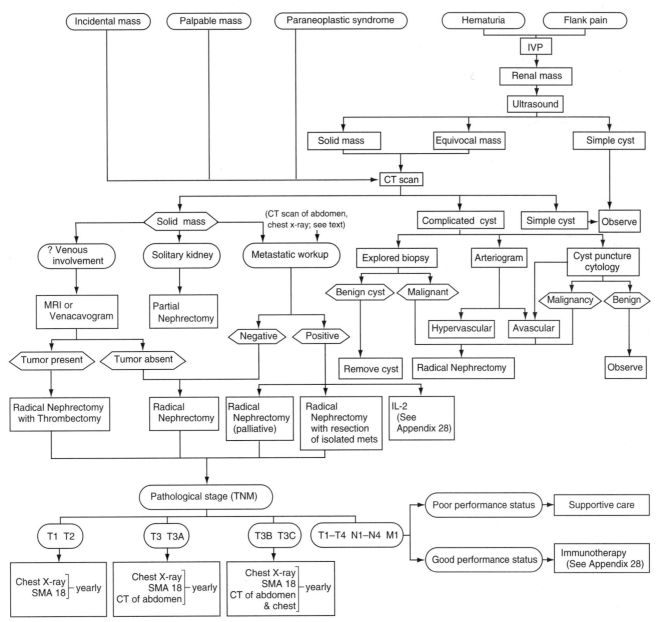

FIGURE 43-2 *Management of renal adenocarcinoma. Determination of extent of disease and resectability represents the key reasoning element in the management of renal cancer. Goal of treatment is curative surgery in patients with localized disease. Note that (curative) surgery can be undertaken for a solid mass without resorting to the biopsy first. This is an example of the probabilistic reasoning technique, which is based on estimate of the likelihood of renal cancer after imaging studies are performed (see Ch. 1). This is a rare deviation from the usual reasoning in oncology in which treatment is almost always based on the results of a biopsy. Recommended strategy is based on solid nonexperimental evidence about the role of surgery in the management of renal cancer (level II evidence) and level III and IV evidence on the role of biologic response modifiers in the treatment of metastatic disease (see also Appendix 28 for details on treatment protocols).*

success rate is not much higher than in the untreated population. Attention therefore has shifted to immunotherapy using biologic response modifiers, such as the interferons and interleukins. Interleukin-2 (IL-2) has been used alone and together with lymphokine-activated killer cells (LAK cells) or with tumor infiltrating lymphocytes (TIL cells).

Most attention is now directed at IL-2 used alone (see Appendix 28) or combined with one of the other biologic response modifiers, with a 10% to 30% partial response rate and a 5% to 10% complete response rate reported. In addition, these responses appear more durable than those that are occasionally seen with standard cytotoxic chemotherapy. The major limiting factors with high-dose IL-2 have been its toxicity and a mortality rate of 4%. This has led to the use of low-dose regimens of IL-2, but large enough series are not available today. The results of therapy are shown in Figure 43-2.

SUGGESTED READINGS

Licht MR, Novick AC: Nephron-sparing surgery for renal cell carcinoma. J Urol 149:1–7, 1993
McDougal WS, Garnick MB: Clinical signs and symptoms of the renal cell carcinoma. p. 154. In: Comprehensive Textbook of Genitourinary Oncology. Williams & Wilkins, 1996
Rosenberg SA, Yang JC, Topahan SL et al: Treatment of 283 consecutive patients with metastatic melanoma or renal cell cancer using high dose bolus interleukin-2. JAMA 271:907–913, 1994
Warshaver DM, McCarthy SM, Street L et al: Detection of renal masses: sensitivities and specificities of excretory urography/linear tomography, ultrasound and CT. Radiology 169:363–365, 1988
Zagoria RJ, Bechtold RE, Dyer RB: Staging of renal adenocarcinoma: role of various imaging procedures. Am J Roentgenol 184:363–370, 1995

44 Bladder Cancer

Terence Hadley

Incidence/prevalence: 17/100,000 population per year; 2% of all cancers in the United States.

Goal of treatment: Cure (stages O, A, Cis, B, C, and small minority of patients with D1 disease); prolongation of survival (for rest of patients with D1 disease and those with D2 stage) or *palliation* depending on co-morbid conditions.

Main modality of treatment: *Superficial disease (stages 0 and A):* Surgical resection plus BCG vaccine.

Local and regional disease (stages B, C, and D1): Cystectomy (segmental or radical) plus adjuvant chemotherapy or radiation therapy.

Distant disease (D2): Chemotherapy

Prognosis (5-year survival): Localized: ~90%

Regional: ~45%

Distant: ~10%

Bladder cancer accounts for about 2% of cancers in the United States. Approximately 50,000 new cases are diagnosed each year. The male to female ratio is about 3:1. Cigarette smoking is a significant risk factor as is industrial exposure to aromatic carcinogens, such as aryl amines.

Most bladder cancers (90%–95%) are transitional cell carcinomas. Less common histologic variants are squamous cell carcinoma (3%–8%), adenocarcinoma (2%), and undifferentiated carcinoma (< 1%). Although the less common types of bladder cancer are often managed in a fashion similar to muscle-invasive transitional cell carcinoma, more data are required to verify the usefulness of this approach. Most studies on bladder cancer have focused on transitional cell carcinoma, and therefore conclusions are relevant primarily to tumors of this histology.

DIAGNOSIS

The diagnosis of transitional cell carcinoma of the bladder depends upon cystoscopy and biopsy. Prognostic features include stage, histologic grade, and the presence or absence of a mutated p53 tumor suppressor gene. The staging system is summarized in Table 44-1, in which the Marshall-Jewett classification is correlated with the system of the American Joint Committee on Cancer (AJCC) and the International Union against Cancer (UICC). Clinical staging (which includes the results of biopsy) is important because it divides patients into three categories: superficial disease, muscle invasive disease without distant metastases, and metastatic disease. Each of these categories requires a different approach. For example, cystectomy is usually not required initially for patients with superficial disease. Also, cystec-

TABLE 44-1 BLADDER CANCER: STAGING SYSTEMS

Marshall (1952)	AJC-UICC (1972)	Description
Superficial		
0	To	No tumor in specimen
0	Tis	Carcinoma in situ
0	Ta	Noninvasive papillary tumor
A	T1	Lamina propria invasion
Invasive		
B1	T2	Superficial muscle invasion
B2	T3a	Deep muscle invasion
C	T3b	Perivesical fat invasion
D1	T4	Invasion of contiguous viscera
D1	N1-3	Pelvic node metastases
D2	N4	Juxtaregional node metastases
D2	M1	Distant metastases

tomy is usually not appropriate for patients with distant metastases, unless they have had a complete response to systemic chemotherapy with the bladder being the sole site of residual disease. Accurate clinical staging is hampered by the fact that computed tomography (CT) and magnetic resonance imaging (MRI) are less than optimal for detecting metastatic disease in the pelvic lymph nodes. Therefore, clinical stage (denoted T1-T4) does not always correspond with pathologic stage (P1-P4), especially in muscle-invasive disease. Pathologic stage, determined at the time of surgery, is a better correlate of overall prognosis than clinical stage.

GRADING SYSTEM

There are several grading systems for transitional cell carcinoma, including the World Health Organization System, which classifies transitional cell carcinomas into three grades. Grade 1 denotes the most differentiated tumors; grade 3 denotes the least differentiated tumors; grade 2 denotes tumors of intermediate differentiation. There is some correlation between the grade of tumor determined at the time of biopsy and the pathologic stage of tumor determined at the time of surgery. Recently, mutations in the p53 tumor-suppressor gene were shown to confer a poor prognosis. There is some evidence that mutational status of p53 may be more significant than either stage or grade in determining ultimate prognosis.

TREATMENT

The therapeutic approach to transitional cell carcinoma of the bladder depends primarily on stage and grade, as methods to identify mutations in p53 are not yet generally available. The goals of treatment of bladder cancer are cure (stages O, A, Cis, B, C, and small minority of patients with D1 disease); prolongation of survival (for rest of patients with D1 stage and those with D2 disease), or palliation, depending on co-morbid conditions. The key reasoning principle in the management of bladder cancer is to distinguish between superficial tumors and muscle-invasive tumors, as determined by examination of carefully obtained biopsies and clinical staging (Fig. 44-1). *Superficial tumors* include those that are confined to the mucosa (Ta) or invade only the lamina propria (T1). These stages can be treated by transurethral resection, often followed by topical intravesicular therapy (e.g., BCG). *Muscle-invasive tumors* (T2, T3a) and tumors that extend into perivesicular fat (T3b) or contiguous viscera (T4) require more extensive intervention (e.g., radical cystectomy with pelvic lymphadenectomy) to achieve local and regional control and the possibility of long-term survival.

There is the expected inverse correlation between the stage of bladder cancer and prognosis. Estimates of 5-year survivals according to stage are as follows: Ta, 80% to 90%; Tis and P1, 70% to 85%; P2, 62% to 88%; P3a, 57% to 74%; P3b, 29% to 57%, P4 or N+, 10% to 15%. The goal of therapy in each of these stages is long-term survival or cure, although the probability of achieving this goal in more advanced disease is low.

The use of intravesicular therapy after surgery in selected superficial tumors has been shown to be beneficial, and a meta-analysis of randomized prospective trials demonstrated the superiority of BCG over other agents (level I evidence, large randomized trial). *Radical cystectomy* is the standard therapy for muscle-invasive disease for patients able to tolerate the surgery (Fig. 44-1). Single-arm surgical series indicate that long-term survival with radical cystectomy is superior to that obtained with radiation therapy alone or conservative bladder-sparing surgery. The operative mortality of radical cystectomy is around 1%. Prospective randomized trials between radiation followed by surgery and surgery alone for muscle-invasive disease indicate that neoadjuvant radiation therapy does not provide a benefit.

As many patients eventually succumb to distant metastases, interest has emerged in adjuvant and neoadjuvant chemotherapy. One nonrandomized trial (level 3 evidence) compared survival in patients treated with CISCA (cisplatin, cytoxan, and Adriamycin) with patients who did not receive adjuvant chemotherapy for high-risk disease (positive nodes, invasion of perivesicular fat, lymphatic or blood vessel invasion). Patients who received adjuvant chemotherapy had a significantly longer survival than those who did not (level 3 evidence, nonrandomized comparison). A small randomized single-institution trial (level 2 evidence) suggested that adjuvant chemotherapy prolongs disease-free survival in patients with P3, P4, +/–N disease although patients with two or more positive nodes did not appear to benefit. Based on these studies, many oncologists recommend adjuvant chemotherapy for high-risk patients with the above pathologic stages. However, further studies are required to define the risks and benefits of adjuvant chemotherapy more clearly and to test new chemotherapeutic combinations.

The use of neoadjuvant chemotherapy (i.e., the administration of chemotherapy before surgery) is currently being investigated in the treatment of muscle-invasive bladder cancer. This approach has the advantage of allowing the clinician to determine whether the tumor is indeed sensitive to the combination of drugs being administered. Another potential advantage of neoadjuvant therapy is that it can "down-size" large tumors, thereby facilitating surgical resection (Fig. 44-1).

Another important line of investigation in the treatment of muscle-invasive bladder cancer involves the use of chemotherapy and radiation therapy with a view toward avoiding radical cystectomy and sparing the bladder. This approach is based on the following considerations: (1) radical cystectomy cures only 40% to 50% of patients with muscle-invasive disease, and most of the remaining 50% to 60% of patients die from distant metastases (systemic disease); therefore, systemic therapy should theoretically play a major role in the treatment of bladder cancer; (2) preliminary studies indicated that concomitant radiation and chemotherapy can be given safely with good results in terms of tumor response and maintenance of bladder function, and (3) in patients who do not have a complete response to chemotherapy plus radiation therapy, salvage radical cystectomy can be safely performed.

TABLE 44-2   FOLLOW-UP OF THE PATIENT WITH BLADDER CANCER

	1st Year (Months)				2nd–5th Year (Months)		Thereafter (Months)
	3	6	9	12	6	12	12
History							
Complete				×		×	×
Hematuria	×	×	×		×		
Dysuria	×	×	×		×		
Frequency	×	×	×		×		
Bone pain	×	×	×		×		
Physical							
Complete				×		×	×
Abdomen	×	×	×		×		
Rectal	×	×	×		×		
Stoma (if any)	×	×	×		×		
Lymph nodes	×	×	×		×		
Cystoscopy[a]	×	×		×	×	×	×
Ureteroscopy		×	×		As indicated		
Pelvic (female)		×	×		×	×	×
Tests							
Chest x-ray				×		×	×
Complete blood count		×	×			×	×
Urine	×	×	×	×	×	×	×
BUN alkaline phosphatase		×		×		×	×
IVP[b]				×		×	
Urine cytology		×		×		×	

[a]This should revert to the inital follow-up (i.e., every 3 months for the first 6 months after each occurrence).

[b]IVP should be performed at 3 months following a urinary diversion and at 6-month intervals in the first year for upper-tract tumors.

(Modified from Lytton , Esrig D: Bladder Cancer. p. 62. In Fischer (ed): Follow-up of Cancer: A Handbook for Physicians. 4th Ed. Lippincott-Raven, Philadelphia, 1996, with permission.)

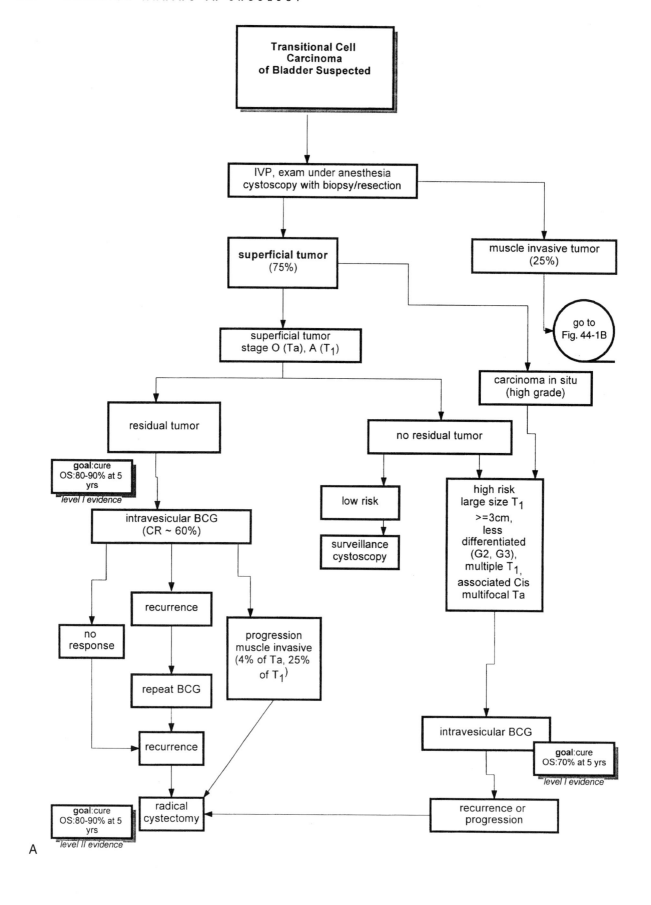

A

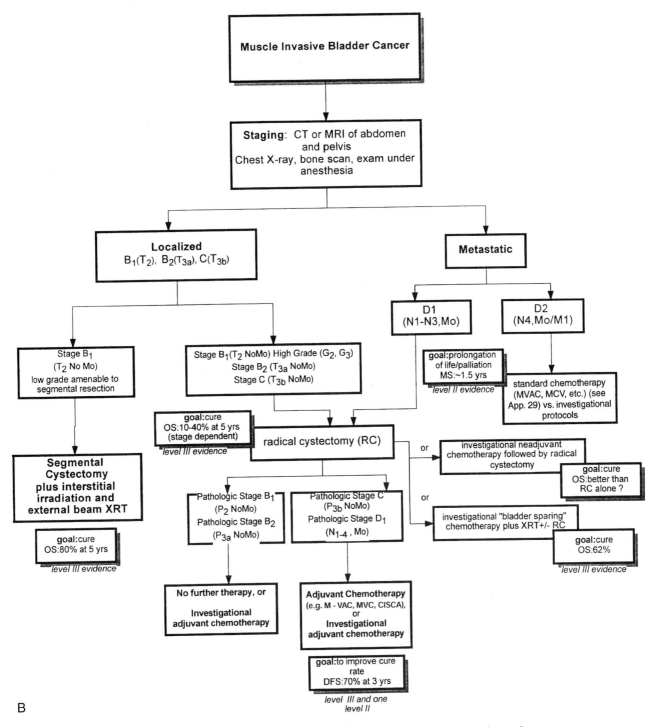

B

FIGURE 44-1 *Management of bladder cancer. The key reasoning principle in the management of bladder cancer is to distinguish between superficial tumors and muscle-invasive tumors as determined by examination of carefully obtained biopsies and clinical
staging. The goals of treatment of bladder cancer are cure (stages O, A, Cis, B, C, and
minority of patients with D1 stage); prolongation of survival (for the rest of patients
with D1 stage and those with D2 stage) or palliation, depending on co-morbid conditions. Recommended management strategies in early stages of disease are based upon
high quality data on the role of BCG following surgery (level I evidence); level II evidence exists for the role of chemotherapy in advanced stages of disease; data for management of localized advanced stages are more of indirect type (most of level III
evidence). For details on chemotherapy regimen, see Appendix 29.*

The Radiation Therapy Oncology Group reported results of a phase II trial using neoadjuvant combined radiation and chemotherapy after local resection. Patients were treated initially with two cycles of methotrexate, vinblastine, and cisplatin (MCV) followed by radiation with two additional cycles of single-dose cisplatin. Patients were then reevaluated with cystoscopy. If a complete response was achieved, the patient was treated with radiation and another cycle of single-dose cisplatin. If residual tumor was identified after induction, patients were treated with radical cystectomy. In this study, 37 of 91 patients (40%) required cystectomy. The 4-year actuarial survival rate of the entire group was 62%, which is similar to survival rates obtained with radical cystectomy alone. The 4-year actuarial survival with the bladder intact was 44%. Thus, it appears that a bladder sparing protocol combining chemotherapy and radiation therapy may be a reasonable option in the management of muscle-invasive bladder cancer.

Patients with distant metastases from bladder cancer are considered incurable with current therapeutic modalities; however, there is evidence (level 1) that systemic chemotherapy can prolong survival. The two most commonly used chemotherapeutic regimens are M-VAC (methotrexate, vinblastine, Adriamycin, and cisplatin) and MVC (methotrexate, vinblastine, and cisplatin). M-VAC was shown to be more effective than single-agent cisplatin and CISCA (cisplatin, cyclophosphamide, and Adriamycin) in the treatment of metastatic disease. In a large intergroup trial comparing M-VAC to single-agent cisplatin, M-VAC was superior to cisplatin in terms of response (33% vs. 5%), complete response (13% vs. 3%) and median survival (12.6 vs. 8.7 months). In a trial comparing M-VAC to CISCA, M-VAC produced a higher response rate (65% vs. 46%) and a longer median survival (82 vs. 40 weeks) than CISCA. Studies using MVC have yielded results similar to M-VAC, although MVC has not been directly compared with M-VAC. There is evidence that surgical removal of residual disease in patients who have had a complete response to chemotherapy may be of benefit. Guidelines for follow-up of patients with bladder cancer following treatment are given in Table 44-2.

SUGGESTED READINGS

Amendola MA, Glazer GM, Grossman HB et al: Staging of bladder carcinoma: MRI-CT-surgical correlation. AJR 146:1179, 1986

Brodsky GL: Pathology of bladder cancer. Hematol Oncol Clin North Am 6:59, 1992

Denis LJ: Clinical staging: its importance in therapeutic decisions and clinical trials. Hematol Oncol Clin North Am 6:41, 1992

Esrig D, Elmajian D, Groshen S et al: Accumulation of nuclear p53 and tumor progression in bladder cancer. N Engl J Med 331:1259, 1994

Gilbert HA, Logan JL, Kagan AR et al: The natural history of papillary transitional cell carcinoma of the bladder and its treatment in an unselected population on the basis of histological grading. J Urol 119:488, 1978

Herr HW: Intravesical therapy. Hematol Oncol Clin North Am 6:117, 1992

Herr HW, Laudone VP, Badalament RA et al: BCG therapy alters the progression of superficial bladder cancer. J Clin Oncol 6:1450, 1988

Igawa M, Ohkuchi T, Ueki T et al: Usefulness and limitations of methotrexate, vinblastine, doxorubicin and cisplatin for the treatment of advanced urothelial cancer. J Urol 144:662, 1990

Kantoff PW: Bladder cancer. Curr Probl Cancer 14:233, 1990

Kantoff PW, Scher HI: Chemotherapy for metastatic bladder cancer. Hematol Oncol Clin North Am 6:195, 1992

Laudone VP, Rogatko A, Herr HW: Intravesical therapy: a meta-analysis.

Loehrer PJ, Elson KP, Kuebler JP et al: Advanced bladder cancer: a prospective intergroup trial comparing single agent cisplatin versus M-VAC combination chemotherapy. Proc Am Soc Clin Oncol 9:132, 1990

Logothetis CJ, Dexeus FH, Finn L et al: A prospective randomized trial comparing M-VAC and CISCA chemotherapy for patients with metastatic urothelial tumors. J Clin Oncol 8:1050, 1990

Logothetis CJ, Johnson DE, Chong C: Adjuvant cyclophosphamide, doxorubicin, and cisplatin chemotherapy for bladder cancer: an update. J Clin Oncol 6:1590, 1988

Lytton B, Esrig D: Bladder cancer. P.LL. In Fischer DS (ed): Follow-up of Cancer: A Handbook for Physicians, 4th Eed. Lippincott-Raven, Philadelphia, 1996

Martinez-Piniero JA, Martin MG, Arocenta F et al: Neoadjuvant cisplatin chemotherapy before radical cystectomy in invasive transitional cell carcinoma of the bladder: a prospective randomized phase III study. J Urol 153:964, 1995

Rintala E, Hannisdahl E, Fossa SD et al: Neo-adjuvant chemotherapy in bladder cancer: a randomized study. Nordic Cystectomy Trial I. Scand J Urol Nephrol 27:355, 1993

Silverberg E, Boring CC, Squires TS: Cancer statistics. CA 40:9, 1990

Silverman DT, Hartge P, Morrison AS, Devesa SS: Epidemiology of bladder cancer. Hematol Oncol Clin North Am 66:1, 1992

Skinner DG, Daniels JR, Russell CA et al: The role of adjuvant chemotherapy following cystectomy for invasive bladder cancer: a prospective comparative trial. J Urol 145:459, 1991

Skinner DG, Lieskovsky G: Contemporary cystectomy with pelvic node dissection compared to preoperative radiation therapy plus cystectomy in the management of invasive bladder cancer. J Urol 131:1069, 1984

Sternberg CN, Yagoda A, Scher HI et al: Methotrexate, vinblastine, doxorubicin and cisplatin for advanced transitional cell carcinoma of the urothelium. Efficacy and patterns of response and relapse. Cancer 64:2448, 1989

Tester W, Caplan R, Heaney J et al: Neoadjuvant combined modality program with selective organ preservation for invasive bladder cancer: results of Radiation Therapy Oncology Group phase II trial 8802. J Clin Oncol 14:119, 1996

Thrasher JB, Crawford ED: Current management of invasive and metastatic transitional cell carcinoma of the bladder. J Urol 149:957, 1993

45 | Prostate Cancer

Renato V. La Rocca

Prevalence: Most common form of cancer diagnosed in men (except for skin cancer)

Incidence: 317,000 new cases of prostate cancer diagnosed in the United States in 1996. Probability of developing prostate cancer (birth to death): 1 in 6

Mortality: 44,000 deaths per year in the United States

Goals of treatment: Potentially curative if cancer discovered early, palliative if in advanced stage

Treatment modalities:

Early stage disease: Surgery, radiation, or watchful waiting

Advanced stage disease: Hormonal therapy

Relapsed advanced stage disease: second hormone manipulation, androgen withdrawal, chemohormonal therapy, external beam radiation to sites of painful bone metastases, entry into phase 2 drug studies, systemic radioactive isotopes

Prognosis	5-Year Disease-Free Survival (%)	5-Year Overall Survival (%)
Stage A	82–92	84–87
Stage B	63–71	73–78
Stage C	48–70	61–65
Stage D	—	29

Prostate cancer is commonly, although not exclusively diagnosed in men older than 60 years. An estimated 317,000 men in the United States will be diagnosed with prostate cancer in 1996, making it the *most commonly diagnosed neoplasm other than carcinomas of the skin*. It is also the *second-leading cause of cancer-related deaths* (after lung cancer) in men. The increase in incidence that has occurred in the United States over the last decade is in part the result of mass screening of asymptomatic individuals who are discovered to have localized disease. Most often, it is found after patients develop signs and symptoms caused by pressure on nearby structures from cancerous mass within the prostate. The use of the serum PSA (prostate specific antigen) measurement has emerged as an important method primarily for the detection of early stage prostate cancer, although its role as a screening tool remains controversial. The mainstay of diagnosis of this cancer is the transperineal or transrectal core biopsy, most often of a suspicious lesion detected by digital rectal examination. Histologically, *adenocarcinomas compose over 85% of the tumor types*. Ten per cent of tumors manifest extensive neuroendocrine cell differentiation and are histologically similar to small cell tumors. The biology of this subtype of prostate cancer appears to be somewhat different, with perhaps an increased propensity for soft tissue involvement rather than predominantly bone, which is typical for adenocarcinoma; this subtype also appears to have a higher susceptibility to conventional systemic chemotherapeutic agents.

STAGING

Once the diagnosis of prostate cancer is established histologically, clinical staging is undertaken to determine treatment options. This includes a bone scan and chest x-ray to assess dissemination and transrectal ultrasound and pelvic computed tomography (CT) to evaluate for possible tumor extension beyond the prostate or within pelvic lymph nodes. Indeed, up to 24% of all prostate cancers initially present with radiographic evidence of dissemination.

THERAPY

The *management* of patients with prostate cancer is stage dependent. A staging system for prostate cancer is shown in Table 45-1. When therapeutic intervention is undertaken for *early stage (i.e. localized) disease*, it is with *curative intent*. Indeed, the 5-year survival rate for patients presenting with localized disease is over 90%. Determining, however, the optimal treatment modality in this setting (*watchful waiting, prostatectomy, or radiation*) remains under study. The Prostate Cancer Clinical Guidelines Panel recently reviewed all published articles from 1966 to 1993 on stage T2 (B) prostate cancer and systematically analyzed outcomes data for the three management options noted above. The panel concluded that each of the three options are acceptable treatment alternatives, and patients should be counseled regarding each. The patient most likely to benefit from either radical prostatectomy or radiation should have a relatively long life expectancy and no significant surgical or radiation toxicity risk factors, whereas those most likely to benefit from surveillance are those with a shorter life expectancy and/or

TABLE 45-1 STAGING SYSTEMS FOR PROSTATE CANCER

Modified Jewett Classification		TNM Classification	
Clinically nonpalpable tumor			
A1	Nonpalpable, involving <5% of gland by volume	T1a	≤3 Foci
A2	Diffuse, both sides of gland, >5% of gland, nonpalpable	T1b	>3 Foci
Clinically confined to the prostate			
BO/B1	Palpable, <1.5 cm circumscribed nodule to palpation	No comparable stage	
B1	Palpable, not circumscribed, occupying one lobe <1.5 cm	T2	Palpable
B2	Palpable, occupies two lobes >1.5 cm	T2	Palpable
Clinically extends through the prostatic capsule			
C1	Extracapsular extension to periprostatic fat	T3	Not fixed
C2	Extracapsular extension producing bladder, outlet or ureteral obstruction		
	Invasion of the bladder neck, rectum and/or fixed to the pelvic wall	T4	
Metastatic disease			
D1	Regional pelvic lymph node involvement	TXN1–3	
	Single lymph node, ≤2 cm	N1	
	Multiple lymph nodes, none >5 cm	N2	
	Lymph node, >5 cm	N3	
D2	Metastases outside the true pelvis or bone	TXNXM1	
D3	Prostate cancer that has relapsed after adequate endocrine therapy		

a low-grade tumor histology. The potential complications associated with radical prostatectomy and radiation therapy are shown in Table 45-2.

TABLE 45-2 POTENTIAL COMPLICATIONS OF RADICAL PROSTATECTOMY AND EXTERNAL BEAM RADIATION THERAPY

Radical Prostatectomy	Radiation Therapy
Incontinence	Diarrhea
Impotence	Proctitis
Urethral stricture	Cystitis
Fistula	Rectal bleeding
Rectal injury	Rectal stricture
Surgical/anesthetic risk	Bowel obstruction
(e.g., myocardial infarction,	Urethral stricture
pulmonary embolism)	Impotence

In the setting of *advanced disease*, primary *hormonal manipulation* remains the mainstay of initial therapeutic intervention, although the choice and precise form of treatment remains variable (Table 45-3). The five-year survival rate for patients presenting with radiographic evidences of tumor dissemination approaches only 30%. African-Americans, however, appear to fare significantly worse, perhaps in part as a result of socioeconomic issues and less readily available access to health care, although some investigators have now also postulated a more aggressive tumor biology in this population. Additional prognostic indicators in patients presenting with newly diagnosed advanced prostate cancer are shown in Table 45-4.

When addressing the types of hormonal manipulation with the patient, the physician should

TABLE 45-3 PRIMARY HORMONAL THERAPY IN PROSTATE CANCER—TREATMENT ORDERS

Primary Hormonal Manipulation	Median TTP (months)	Type of Evidence	Side Effects	Reference
Bilateral orchiectomy	11.5	II	Impotence, psychological	Denis et al. (1993)
Leuprolide 1 mg SQ qd (no longer used) 7.5 mg IM q 28d 22.5 mg IM q 3 mos	13.9	II	Hot flashes, impotence, bone pain (early flare)	Crawford et al. (1989)
Zoladex 3.6 mg depot SQ q28d 10.8 mg depot SQ q 3 mos	14.5	II	Hot flashes, impotence, bone pain (early flare)	Waymont et al. (1992)
Leuprolide 7.5 mg IM q 28d 22.5 mg IM q 3 mos 1 mg SQ qd (no longer routinely used) plus *Flutamide 250 mg po tid*	16.5	II		Crawford et al. (1989)
Diethylstilbestrol 3 mg po qd (1mg po qd now routinely used)	11.4	II	Diarrhea (ameliorates leuprolide flare), cardiovascular and thromboembolic events, impotence, gynecomastia	Waymont et al. (1992)

Abbreviation: TTP, time to progression.

TABLE 45-4 PROGNOSTIC INDICATORS IN NEWLY DIAGNOSED METASTATIC PROSTATE CANCER

Prognostic Factor	Favorable	Unfavorable
Gleason Score	2–4	8–10
Number of bone metastases	≤3	>3
Liver/lung/pleural metastases	Absent	Present
Pretreatment testosterone levels	>200 mg%	<200 mg%
Pretreatment PSA level	10–100 ng/mL	<10 or >500 ng/mL
PSA nadir	<10 ng/mL	>10 ng/mL
Performance status	<2 (ECOG)	>2(ECOG)

Abbreviations: ECOG, Easter Cooperative Oncology Group; PSA, prostate specific antigen.

take into consideration the following information: *Orchiectomy* avoids the issue of compliance with medical regimens but is not accepted by all patients. Gonadotropin-releasing hormone agonists (LHRH agonists) are as effective as orchiectomy and offer the psychological advantage of avoiding castration. Significant disadvantages include the need for repeated monthly injections and its cost. Either orchiectomy or LHRH agonists can be used alone, or in conjunction with an antiandrogen (such as flutamide), which blocks the binding of androgens to their intracellular receptors. The combination regimens are known as maximum androgen blockade (MAB). Two North American studies initially demonstrated as much as a 6-month improvement in overall survival as compared with monotherapy (i.e., orchiectomy or use of a LHRH agonist alone). However, the Prostate Cancer Trialists' Collaborative Group has published a meta-analysis of 22 trials comparing conventional castration (medical or surgical) with MAB. They found only a 2.1% reduction in absolute risk of death in those patients treated with MAB, which corresponded to a nonsignificant reduction of only 6.4% ± 3.9% in the annual odds of death. Thus, a formal recommendation regarding the optimal form of primary hormonal therapy (monotherapy vs. MAB) cannot be made at this time. Factors to be considered with the patient as part of the decision making process are shown in Table 45-5.

Although retrospective studies do reveal an apparent survival advantage with some form of hormonal manipulation versus no treatment of approximately 12 months in patients with advanced prostate cancer, the timing of therapeutic intervention (immediate vs. expectant) remains unresolved. Investigators at the Mayo Clinic did, however, report on a subset of patients with pathologic stage D1 disease (i.e., underwent surgery for apparent early stage disease, but were found at that time to have pelvic lymph node involvement) who fared better after immediate hormonal manipulation. These investigators found that the time interval to evidence of first progression was prolonged in those patients who received immediate endocrine therapy (in this case, bilateral orchiectomy) versus those who did not undergo immediate therapy. In general, the decision regarding early versus expectant primary hormonal therapy in the newly diagnosed patient with stage D disease remains an individual choice, with careful consideration of both quality-of-life issues and eventual cost.

In those patients who eventually progress through primary hormonal manipulation, no treatment modality has yet emerged that has been shown to impact significantly on survival, which is usually less than one year. Evaluating treatment regimens in advanced prostate cancer is particularly difficult given the inability to assess response of bone metastases objectively. Many early studies included subjective responses and considered stable disease in the category of objective response, making comparisons among different trials quite difficult (Table 45-6). Finally, the role of a declining serum PSA in documenting response is not entirely resolved.

Traditionally, a second hormonal manipulation has been the most commonly employed treatment in patients who progress through primary hormonal manipulation (Table 45-7). This is perhaps most beneficial in those patients whose serum testosterone level is not at castrate level as a result of the primary hormonal manipulation. In those patients taking an antiandrogen at the time of relapse, its discontinuation can result in a transient decline in PSA levels and reduction in pain symptoms, but this is usually of brief duration (3–4 months). Over the last 5 years some potentially promising chemohormonal combinations and a number of novel compounds have emerged that may prove to have a significant impact on survival in those patients with prostate cancer refractory to primary hormonal manipulation. A list of these is shown in Table 45-8. A thorough knowledge of pain management (see Ch. 55) is also critical in care of this patient population. In addition to oral and par-

TABLE 45-5 FACTORS TO CONSIDER IN SELECTING PRIMARY HORMONAL MODALITY

LHRH Agonist
Administration not convenient
Cost
Hot flashes

Bilateral Orchiectomy
Psychological impact
Hot flashes

Estrogen
Gynecomastia
Cardiovascular risk, edema, skin changes

Abbreviation: LHRH agonist, leutinizing hormone-releasing agonist; PSA, prostate specific antigen.

TABLE 45-6 TYPES OF RESPONSES IN PROSTATE CANCER

Objective response (OR)
  Complete response (CR)
  Partial response (PR)
PSA response (decline by 50%)
Subjective response (SR)

TABLE 45-7 TREATMENT OPTIONS IN PATIENTS REFRACTORY TO PRIMARY HORMONAL MANIPULATION (SEE ALSO APPENDIX 30)

Secondary Hormonal	No. of Patients	Response (type)	Type of Evidence	Reference	Median Duration of Response (months)
1) Antiandrogen withdrawal	41	28% (PSA)	III	Herrada et al., (1996)	3.3
2) Prednisone 10 mg po qd	37	38% (SR)	III	Tannock et al., (1989)	4
3) Ketoconazole 200–400 mg po tid	38	14% (PR)	III	Trump et al., (1989)	3
4) Stilphosterol 1 g IV qd for 7–10 d	151[a]	61% (SR)	III	Dawson, (1993)	
5) Megestrol acetate 40 mg po qid	118[a]	5% (PR)	III	Dawson, (1993)	
6) Aminoglutethimide 250 mg po qid with replacement hydrocortisone	58	19% (PR)	III	Murray and Pitt, 1985	10

Abbreviations: PR, partial response; SR, subjective response; PSA, prostate specific antigen.

[a] *Aggregate number of patients from multiple studies.*

TABLE 45-8 CHEMOTHERAPEUTIC REGIMENS FOR PROSTRATE CANCER REFRACTORY TO PRIMARY HORMONAL MANIPULATION

Regimen	No. of Patients	Evidence Level	Response (type)	Reference
Mitoxantrone 12 mg/m^2 IV q 3 weeks with prednisome 5 mg po twice daily	80	II	29% (palliative)	Tannocks et al., (1996)
Estramustine 280–420 mg po bid	217	III	2% (OR)	Murphy et al., (1983)
Estramustine 10–15 mg/kg po daily with vinblastine 3–4 mg/m^2 IV q week	24	III	40% (OR), 54% (PSA)	Seidmon et al., (1992)
Estramustine 15 mg/kg/day and VP-16 50 mg/m^2/day in divided doses for 21 days, off seven days, then repeat	42	III	22.5% (OR), 57% (PSA)	Pienta et al., (1994)
Doxorubicin 20 mg/m^2 IV q week (to a total dose of 400 mg/m^2)	25	III	16% (OR)	Torti et al., (1983)
Ketoconazole 400 mg po tid daily with doxorubicin 20 mg/m^2 q week IV for 6 weeks, then off 2 weeks		III	58% (OR), 55% (PSA)	Sella et al., (1994)

Experimental Therapies

Regimen	No. of Patients	Response	Reference
Suramin	26	58% (OR)	Tkaczak et al., (1992)
Liarozole	17	53% (OR)	Denis et al., (1992)

Abbreviations: IV, intravenous; OR, objective response; PSA, prostate specific antigen.

TABLE 45-9 RECOMMENDED FOLLOW-UP IF ENROLLED IN A CLINICAL STUDY

Stages A, B and C
History and physical examination (incl DRE) every 3-4 months for 4 visits, every 6 months for 5 years, then every year
Prostate biopsy, physical examination 18–24 months after radiation therapy, then as clinically indicated
PSA, every 3–4 months × 4, every 6 months for 5 years, then every year
Baseline bone scan, every year, then more frequently as dictated by symptoms
Other tests, as dictated by symptoms and physical examination
Stage D
History and physical examination, every 3–4 months for 4 visits, then every 6 months as symptoms dictate
PSA, every month until no change, then every 3 months
Bone scan, every 3 months × 2, then every 6 months
Other tests, as dictated by symptoms and physical examination

Abbreviations: DRE, digital rectal examination; PSA, prostate specific antigen.

enteral analgesics, localized palliative radiation can alleviate otherwise excruciating bone pain. Radioactive isotopes such as strontium 89 can also have a role in the palliation of symptomatic bone metastases. Figure 45-1 summarizes the management recommendations for prostate cancer. Data used

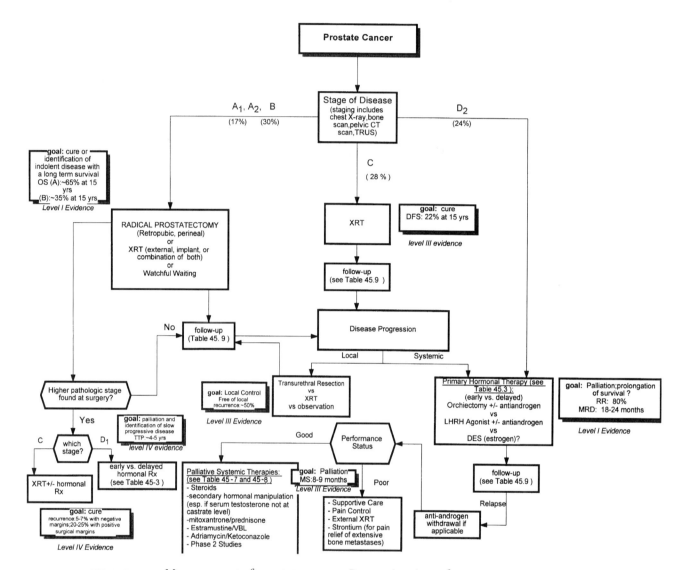

FIGURE 45-1. *Management of prostate cancer. Determination of tumor stage represents a key reasoning principle in the management of patients with prostate cancer. Goal of treatment is cure and/or identification of indolent disease in early (A & B) stages of disease; cure in stage C, and palliation in advanced disease (stage D). Note that many alternative equally efficacious treatment options exist and that the patient's preference is one the most critical variables in decision making (see also Tables 45-2, 45-3, and 45-5 on benefit/risk of various treatment alternatives). Recommended strategies for treatment of early stages are based on level I and III evidences and for the treatment of advanced stages on the results of large meta-analysis (level I evidence); data for management of recurrent disease are mainly of level IV quality. For practical details on the management of hormone retractory prostate cancer see Appendix 30. MS, median survival; MRD, median response duration; DFS: disease-free survival; OS, overall survival; XRT, radiation therapy; TRUS, transrectal ultrasound; TTP, time to progression; For practical details on the management of hormone refractory prostate cancer see Appendix 30. VBL, vinblastine.*

for its construction are of level I for the management of early and advanced stages, but of level III and IV for the management of stage C and of recurrent disease.

SUGGESTED READINGS

Amato RJ, Logothetis CJ, Hallihan R et al: Chemotherapy for small cell carcinoma of prostatic origin. J Urol 147:935–937, 1992

Beland G, Elhilai M, Fradet Y et al: Total androgen ablation: Canadian experience. Urol Clin North Am 18:75–82, 1991

Crawford ED, Eisenberger MA, McLeod DG et al: a controlled trial of leuprolide with and without flutamide in prostatic carcinoma. N Engl J Med 321:419–424, 1989

Dawson NA: Treatment of progressive metastatic prostate cancer. Oncology 7:17–25, 1993

Denis L, Mahler C, De Smedt E et al: R 75251: a new cytotoxic agent for relapsed prostate cancer (abstract 702), Eur J Cancer 28A (suppl 2):S119, 1992

Denis LJ, Whalen P, De Moura JL et al: Goserelin acetate and flutamide versus bilateral orchiectomy, a phase II EORTC trial (30853). Urology 42:119–130, 1993

Herrada J, Dieringer P, Logothetic CJ: Characterization of patients with androgen-independent prostatic carcinoma whose serum prostate specific antigen decreased following flutamide withdrawal. J Urol 155:620–623, 1996

Johansson JE, Adami MD, Anderssonp SO et al: Natural history of localized prostate cancer, a population-based study in 223 untreated patients. Lancet 1:799, 1989

Logothetis CJ: Chemotherapeutic approaches in advanced prostate cancer. Oncology (suppl 8):15–24, 1994

Middleton RG, Thompson IM, Austenfeld MS et al: Prostate cancer clinical guidelines panel summary report on the management of clinically localized prostate cancer. J Urol 154:2144–2148, 1995

Murphy GP, Slack NH, Mittelman H: Experiences with Estramustine phosphate (Estracyt, Emcyt) in prostate cancer. Semin Oncol (suppl 3) 10:34, 1983

Murray R, Pitt P: Treatment of advanced prostate cancer. Eur J Cancer Clin Oncol 21:453–458, 1985

Nesbit RM, Baum WC: Endocrine control of prostatic carcinoma. JAMA 143:1317–1320, 1950

Parker SL, Tong T, Bolden S, Wingo PA: Cancer Statistics 1996. CA J 46:5–27, 1996

Pienta KJ, Eman B, Hussein M et al: Phase II evaluation of oral estramustine and oral etoposide in hormone-refractory adenocarcinoma of the prostate. J Clin Oncol 12:2005–2012, 1994

Prostate Cancer Trialists' Collaborative Group: Maximum androgen blockade in advanced prostate cancer: an overview of 22 randomized trials with 3283 deaths in 5710 patients. Lancet 346:265–269, 1995

Seidman AD, Scher HI, Petrylak D et al: Estramustine and vinblastine: use of prostate specific antigen as a clinical trial endpoint for hormone refractory prostatic cancer. J Urol 147:931–934, 1992

Sella A, Kilbourn R, Amata R et al: Phase II study of ketoconazole combined with weekly doxorubicin in patients with androgen-independent prostate cancer. J Clin Oncol 12:683–688, 1994

Tannock I, Gospodarowicz M, Meakin W et al: Treatment of metastatic prostatic cancer with low-dose prednisone: evaluation of pain and quality of life as pragmatic indices of response. J Clin Oncol 7:590–597, 1989

Tannock I, Osoba D, Stockler MR et al: Chemotherapy with mitoxantrone plus prednisone or prednisone alone for symptomatic hormone-resistant prostate cancer: a Canadian randomized trial with palliative end points. J Clin Oncol 14:1756–1764, 1996

Tkaczak K, Eisenberger M, Sinibaldi V et al: Activity of suramin in prostate cancer observed in a phase 1 trial (abstract). Proc Am Soc Clin Oncol 11:201, 1992

Torti ErM, Aston D, Lum B et al: Weekly doxorubicin in endocrine-refractory carcinoma of the prostate. J Clin Oncol 1:477–482, 1983

Trump DL, Havlin KH, Messing EM et al: High dose ketoconazole in advanced hormone refractory prostate cancer: endocrinologic and clinical effects. J Clin Oncol 7:1093–1098, 1989

Waymont B, Lynch TH, Dunn JA et al: Phase III randomized study of Zoladex versus stilboestrol in the treatment of advanced prostate cancer. Br J Urol 69:614–620, 1992

Zincke H, Bergstralh EJ, Larsen-Keller JL et al: Stage Dl prostate cancer treated by radical prostatectomy and adjuvant hormonal therapy. Cancer 70:311–322, 1992

46 | Carcinoma of the Female Urethra

James I. Harty

Incidence/prevalence: Very rare—only 1200 cases reported in the literature.

Goal of treatment: Cure with surgery and radiation for localized disease and some patients with inguinal node metastasis.

Palliation with radiation and chemotherapy for patients with unresectable lymph node metastasis.

Main modality of treatment: Surgery alone or combined with radiation.

Prognosis: 75% 5-year survival with surgery and radiation for anterior urethral cancer.

40% 5-year survival with surgery and radiation for posterior urethral cancer.

Unique features: More common than male urethral carcinoma.

INCIDENCE

Carcinoma of the female urethra is a rare tumor. Approximately 1,200 cases have been reported in the world literature, which is twice the number reported in men. It usually occurs in patients over the age of 60 years. Although there is no known etiology, human papilloma virus is a possible cause in some cases.

The majority of urethral tumors are squamous cell carcinomas (55%), but adenocarcinomas (18%), transitional cell carcinomas (16%), and miscellaneous tumors (11%) may also occur.

SIGNS AND SYMPTOMS

The symptoms include hemorrhagic spotting, dyspareunia, or a palpable urethral mass. Most tumors arise in the distal third of the urethra, which is designated the anterior urethra, while the remainder occur in the proximal two thirds, called the posterior urethra. Besides being more common, anterior urethral tumors are usually of a lower stage and grade and, therefore, carry a better prognosis than posterior urethral tumors. Urethral tumors progress locally at the primary site and spread by lymphatic embolization to the regional lymph nodes. They only metastasize to distant sites when they are locally and regionally extensive. Lymphatics of the posterior urethra drain into the pelvic lymph nodes while those of the anterior urethra drain into the superficial and deep inguinal lymph nodes. Approximately 20% of patients have palpably enlarged inguinal nodes at the time of diagnosis, and this usually represents metastatic spread rather than inflammatory changes. The TNM system is the most commonly used staging system for female urethral cancers (Fig. 46-1).

Patient identification
Name _____
Address _____
Hospital or clinic number _____
Age _____ Sex _____ Race _____

Institution identification
Hospital or clinic _____
Address _____

Oncology Record

Anatomic site of cancer _____
Histologic type _____
Grade (G) _____
Date of classification _____

Chronology of classification
[ ]   Clinical (use all data prior to first treatment)
[ ]   Pathologic (if definitively resected specimen available)

Clin	Path		

DEFINITIONS

Primary Tumor (T)

Clin	Path		
[ ]	[ ]	TX	Primary tumor cannot be assessed
[ ]	[ ]	T0	No evidence of primary tumor
[ ]	[ ]	Ta	Noninvasive papillary, polypoid, or verrucous carcinoma
[ ]	[ ]	Tis	Carcinoma *in situ*
[ ]	[ ]	T1	Tumor invades subepithelial connective tissue
[ ]	[ ]	T2	Tumor invades corpus spongiosum or prostate or periurethral muscle
[ ]	[ ]	T3	Tumor invades corpus cavernosum or beyond prostatic capsule or the anterior vagina or bladder neck
[ ]	[ ]	T4	Tumor invades other adjacent organs

Lymph Node (N)

Clin	Path		
[ ]	[ ]	NX	Regional lymph nodes cannot be assessed
[ ]	[ ]	N0	No regional lymph node metastasis
[ ]	[ ]	N1	Metastasis in a single lymph node, 2 cm or less in greatest dimension
[ ]	[ ]	N2	Metastasis in a single lymph node, more than 2 cm but not more than 5 cm in greatest dimension, or multiple lymph nodes, none more than 5 cm in greatest dimension
[ ]	[ ]	N3	Metastasis in a lymph node more than 5 cm in greatest dimension

Distant Metastasis (M)

Clin	Path		
[ ]	[ ]	MX	Presence of distant metastasis cannot be assessed
[ ]	[ ]	M0	No distant metastasis
[ ]	[ ]	M1	Distant metastasis

Histopathologic Type

Cell types can be divided into transitional, squamous, and glandular.

Histopathologic Grade (G)

[ ] GX   Grade cannot be assessed
[ ] G1   Well differentiated
[ ] G2   Moderately differentiated
[ ] G3-4   Poorly differentiated or undifferentiated

FIGURE 46-1 *Data form for staging cancer of the urethra. (From American Joint Committee on Cancer: Staging of Cancer Forms (Carcinoma of the Urethra). 3rd Ed. Lippincott-Raven, Philadelphia, 1988, with permission.)*

MANAGEMENT

The diagnosis is usually made on cystourethroscopy and biopsy (Fig. 46-2). The inguinal nodes are assessed by palpation, and the pelvic nodes by CT scan.

Treatment of urethral carcinoma in the female depends largely on the portion of the urethra (anterior or posterior) in which the carcinoma occurs, the depth of invasion of the primary tumor, and the presence or absence of palpably enlarged inguinal lymph nodes. Low-grade, low-stage (Tis, T1) tumors of the anterior urethra can usually be cured with local destruction by means of laser (neodymium YAG), diathermy, or surgical excision (Fig. 46-2). Interstitial radiation with irridium 192 has been reported to be equally successful for these superficial lesions (Fig. 46-2). More invasive lesions are

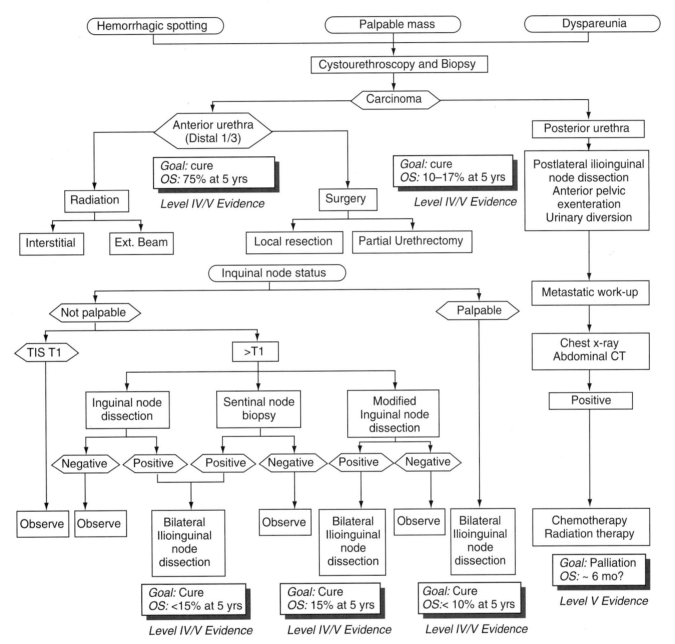

FIGURE 46-2 *Management of carcinoma of the female urethra. Anatomical presentation of the tumor (an anterior urethra vs. posterior urethra) determines the approach to the management of patients with female urethral cancer. Goal of treatment is cure for patients with localized disease and some patients with inguinal node metastasis. Recommended strategy is based on nonexperimental evidence about the role of surgery in the management of early stages of female urethral cancer (level II and III evidence) and level IV and V evidences on the role of surgery and chemotherapy in the treatment of advanced disease (see also Appendix 31 for details on treatment protocols). OS, overall survival; LE, life expectancy.*

best treated with an anterior urethrectomy, which can be performed with preservation of urinary continence. Carcinomas of the posterior urethra tend to be at a higher stage at the time of diagnosis. Patients with high-stage posterior urethral carcinomas require an anterior pelvic exenteration and bilateral iliac node dissection. Results, even with this extensive procedure, are poor, with 10% to 17% survival rates at 5 years, and recurrences in 66% to 100% of the patients.

All patients with palpably enlarged inguinal lymph nodes should have a bilateral ilioinguinal node dissection (Fig. 46-2). Bulky, fixed, unresectable nodes have been treated with combination radiation and chemotherapy for palliation. Finally, for patients who develop distant metastatic disease, a combination of methotrexate, bleomycin, and cisplatin (see Appendix 31) has been used in a small number of patients to palliate pain and to prolong survival.

SUGGESTED READINGS

Ali MM, Klein FA, Hazra TA: Primary female urethral carcinoma: a retrospective comparison of different treatment techniques. Cancer 62:54–57, 1988

Johnson DE, O'Connell JR: Primary carcinoma of the female urethra. Urology 21:42–45, 1983

Johnson DW, Keseler JF, Ferrigni RG et al: Low dose combined chemotherapy/radiotherapy in the management of locally advanced urethral squamous cell carcinoma. J Urol 141:615–616, 1989

Klein FA, Whitmore WF Jr, Herr HW et al: Inferior pubic rami resection with en bloc radical excision for invasive proximal urethral carcinoma. Cancer 51:1238–1242, 1983

47 Carcinoma of the Male Urethra

James I. Harty

Incidence/prevalence: Very rare neoplasm; less than 600 cases reported in literature

0.01% of all urologic neoplasms

Goal of treatment: Cure with surgery for localized disease and some patients with inguinal node metastasis

Palliation with radiation and chemotherapy for patients with unresectable lymph node metastasis

Main modality of treatment: Surgery

Prognosis: 22% 5-year survival for penile urethra

10% 5-year survival for bulbomembranous urethra

Unique features: Associated with chronic urethritis and urethral stricture disease

INCIDENCE

Primary carcinoma of the male urethra is a very rare tumor. Only approximately 600 cases have been reported in the world literature. Urethral carcinoma usually occurs in men over the age of 50 years. Chronic inflammation secondary to urethritis is the major etiologic factor, and as many as 35% of patients have been treated for venereal disease or a urethral stricture before diagnosis.

SIGNS AND SYMPTOMS

Presenting symptoms include difficulty voiding, bloody urethral discharge, dysuria, and initial hematuria (Fig. 47-1). When the lesion is in the penile portion of the urethra, a mass may be palpable. Eighty percent of urethral cancers in the male are squamous cell carcinomas. Transitional cell carcinomas occur in 15% of the patients (most of these are associated with transitional cell carcinoma of the bladder and are addressed in Ch. 44); the remaining 5% are adenocarcinomas. Sixty percent of urethral cancers in the male arise in the bulbomembranous urethra, 30% in the penile urethra, and 10% in the prostatic urethra. They tend to progress silently at the primary site and spread by lymphatic embolization to the regional lymph nodes. They only metastasize to distant sites when they are locally and regionally extensive. The lymphatics of the bulbomembranous urethra drain into the pelvic lymph nodes, while those of the penile urethra drain into the superficial and deep inguinal nodes. Approximately 20% of the patients have palpable nodes at presentation, and unlike penile cancer, this finding almost always represents metastatic disease. Several different staging systems have been described, but the tumor, node, metastasis (TNM) system is the most useful (see Fig. 46-1).

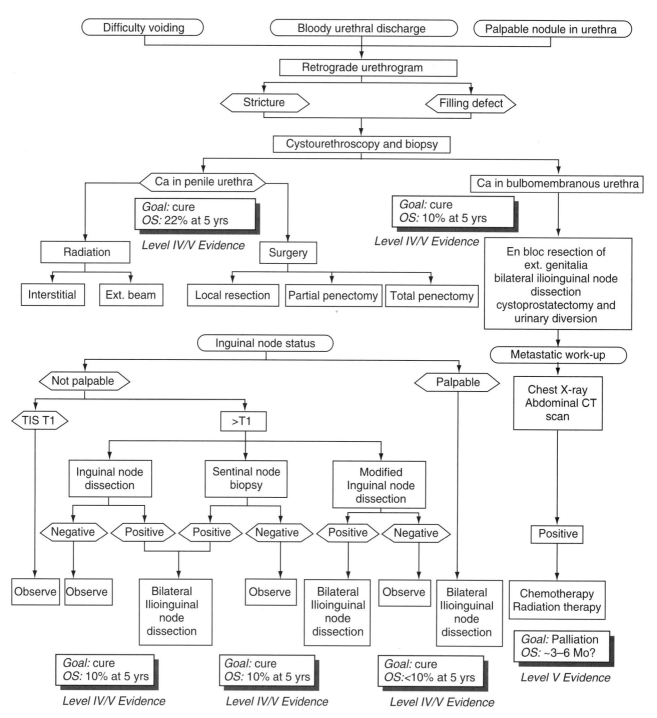

FIGURE 47-1 *Management of carcinoma of the male urethra. Anatomical presentation of the tumor (cancer in penile urethra vs. bulbomembranous urethra) determines the approach to the management of the patients with male urethral cancer. Goal of treatment is cure for patients with localized disease and some patients with inguinal node metastasis. Recommended strategy is based on nonexperimental evidence about the role of surgery in the management of early stages of male urethral cancer (level III) and level IV and V evidences on the role of surgery and chemotherapy in the treatment of advanced disease (see also Appendix 31 for details on treatment protocols). OS, overall survival.*

MANAGEMENT

While the diagnosis may be suspected with the presenting symptoms, and retrograde urethrography will usually locate the site of the lesion in the urethra, urethroscopy with biopsy is necessary to make the diagnosis. A pelvic computed tomography (CT) scan is used to determine the status of the pelvic lymph nodes.

The treatment of urethral carcinoma depends largely on the portion of the urethra (bulbomembranous or penile) in which the carcinoma occurs, the depth of invasion of the primary tumor, and the presence of palpably enlarged inguinal lymph nodes. Tumors in the penile urethra have a more favorable prognosis than those in the bulbomembranous urethra, because the latter may be more locally extensive at the time of diagnosis and spread to the pelvic lymph nodes rather than the inguinal lymph nodes, where they are less likely to be detected.

Carcinomas of the penile urethra, which are superficial (T1), may be managed either by radiation therapy, or local destruction by laser (neodymium YAG), or surgical excision (Fig. 47-1). These patients must be carefully selected or local recurrence rates will be high. Larger or more invasive tumors of the penile urethra usually require either a partial penectomy or total penectomy with perineal urethrostomy. The decision to perform a partial or total penectomy depends on the length of penis remaining after amputation, with a 2-cm tumor-free margin proximal to the tumor. Despite performing a total penectomy, 20% of the patients will die of their disease because of local recurrences from subsequent metastases. This probably represents poor patient selection or failure to recognize the extent of the local disease at the time of penectomy. Patients with penile carcinoma in the bulbomembranous urethra should be treated with an en bloc resection of the penis, urethra, scrotum, and then to pubic ramus, with a cystoprostatectomy and bilateral ileoinguinal lymph node dissection (Fig. 47-1).

Thirty-eight percent of patients treated with en bloc radical incision for bulbomembranous carcinoma remain free of disease for variable periods.

All patients with palpably positive inguinal nodes should have a bilateral inguinal node dissection. Patients with nonpalpable nodes and invasive tumors should have at least a modified inguinal node dissection as described by Catalona (see Ch. 48). Several small series have shown that prophylactic lymphadenectomy for male urethral cancer provides a survival benefit over observation.

Chemotherapy has been used neoadjuvantly for large tumors of the bulbous urethra in an attempt to improve disease-free survival rates. Vincristine, bleomycin, and methotrexate have produced partial responses, which were converted to complete responses with surgery. There are no large series of patients treated with chemotherapy, and most chemical agents have been chosen based on their success in patients with squamous cell carcinoma of the penis. The most promising combination is cisplatin, bleomycin, and methotrexate, administered either intra-arteriorly or intravenously (see Appendix 31). Local recurrences in the groin after lymphadenectomy may be treated with a combination of radiation and chemotherapy, but the prognosis is usually very poor. There are no large series reported.

SUGGESTED READINGS

Hopkins SC, Nag SK, Soloway MS: Primary carcinoma of the male urethra. Urology 23:128–133, 1984

Hussein A, Benefetto P, Sridhar KS: Chemotherapy with cisplatin and 5-fluorouracil for penile and urethral squamous cell carcinomas. Cancer 65:433–438, 1990

Kaplan GW, Bulkley GJ, Grayback JT: Carcinoma of the male urethra. J Urol 98:365–371, 1967

Raghavaich NV: Radiotherapy in the treatment of carcinoma of the male urethra. Cancer 41:1313–1316, 1978

48 | Penile Carcinoma

James I. Harty

Incidence/prevalence: Incidence is aproximately 0.5–1/100,000 in the United States

20% of male carcinomas in South America; 0.4% of male carcinomas in the United States

Goal of treatment: Cure is possible with early detection

Early lymphadenectomy for high-grade disease may be curative

Main modality of treatment: Surgery

Prognosis: 66% 5-year survival if nodes are negative

27% 5-year survival if nodes are positive

50% overall 5-year survival rate

Unique features: Slow growing cancer

Diagnosis delayed because of patient embarassment

Only 20% die from distant metastasis

Most die from local and regional complications

Lymphadenectomy can be *curative* rather than prognostic

Could be avoided with better hygiene and neonatal circumcision

INCIDENCE

Penile cancer accounts for 0.4% of all male malignancies in the United States. It is estimated that the relative risk of a male in the United States developing penile cancer is 0.5 to 1 per 100,000. However, penile cancer represents a greater health risk in other areas of the world where personal hygiene is poor and circumcision is not widely practiced.

Squamous cell carcinoma accounts for 95% of all penile cancers; the remainder are soft tissue sarcomas (2.6%), melanomas (1.7%), basal cell carcinomas (0.5%), lymphomas (0.2%), and metastatic tumor (0.1%). Squamous cell carcinoma is most commonly seen in men over 60 years of age who are uncircumcised and have phimosis. Other suggested etiologic factors include smegma acting as a carcinogen and human papilloma virus. However, there are conflicting reports concerning their role in the development of penile cancer.

DIAGNOSIS

Unfortunately, because penile cancer is rare and because it may be confused with benign or premalignant conditions, the diagnosis and treatment may be delayed. Any suspicious penile lesion should be biopsied before any topical or locally destructive treatment is performed (Fig. 48-1). The earliest form of penile cancer is carcinoma in situ (Tis). This

333

occurs in two forms—erythroplasia of Queyrat on the glans penis and Bowen's disease on the penile shaft. Both of these conditions are identical histologically. Approximately 10% of cases of erythroplasia of Queyrat will become invasive (i.e., break into the subepithelial tissue). Patients with invasive penile cancer usually present either with a palpable ulcer or nodule on the glans penis, the foreskin, or the penile shaft, commonly associated with phimosis and balanitis. Patients often delay seeking medical attention because of embarrassment.

As a first step, a biopsy should be performed to distinguish benign and premalignant conditions from carcinoma and to determine the depth of penetration of any carcinoma into the underlying tissue. Traditionally, the depth of invasion is determined by physical examination and biopsy results. Using these parameters, underestimation of the extent of the disease is very common. More recently, there have been reports of the use of ultrasound, cavernosography, computed tomography and magnetic resonance imaging (MRI) in the staging of the penile lesion. All these reports include only small numbers of patients, but MRI appears to be the most useful. Two established staging systems are in use: the Jackson system and the American Joint Committee on Cancer tumor, node, metastasis (AJCC TNM Fig. 48-2) system. McDougal has more recently proposed a new system, based on the TNM system combined with the grade of the tumor.

TREATMENT

Surgery is the principal form of therapy for the primary lesion on the penis. The type of surgical procedure is determined by the depth of penetration and the location (Fig. 48-1). Penile cancers occur most frequently on the glans penis (48%), prepuce (21%), glans and prepuce (9%), coronal sulcus (6%), and the penile shaft (2%). Several forms of therapy that permit penile preservation can be used for carcinoma in situ and superficial noninvasive tumors (Tis, T1). These include Mohs micrographic surgery, laser destruction, cryotherapy, topical 5-fluorouracil cream, local surgical excision, and radiation therapy—either brachytherapy or external beam. Failure to eradicate the tumor with subsequent local recurrence is the biggest drawback to all these forms of conservative therapy, and they should be avoided in patients who are likely to be noncompliant. Tumors situated on the glans penis that have invaded through the basal layer of the dermis and involve the underlying corporal bodies (T2–T4) should be treated with a partial penectomy,

including a 2-cm, tumor-free margin proximally. Those invasive tumors situated on the penile shaft require either a partial penectomy, as described above, if it would allow residual penile length sufficient to enable the patient to stand to void and to engage in sexual intercourse, or a total penectomy and perineal urethrostomy when the lesion is more proximal, since a partial penectomy with a 2-cm tumor-free proximal margin would not preserve enough penile length to allow normal voiding and sexual intercourse.

METASTATIC DISEASE

Carcinoma of the penis metastasizes primarily through the lymphatic channels to the *regional lymph nodes*. Hematogenous spread is rare. The penile lymphatics drain primarily into the superficial inguinal nodes located around the junction of the saphenous and femoral vein. From there, the lymph passes through the deep inguinal nodes located in the femoral canal to the pelvic lymph nodes. In rare instances, the lymphatics of the glans penis and corporal bodies may bypass the superficial nodes and drain directly into the deep inguinal and pelvic nodes. Also, the lymphatics of the penis decussate at the base of the penis and pass to both inguinal groups of nodes. This accounts for bilateral inguinal node involvement and the necessity for bilateral lymph node dissection.

The status of the inguinal lymph nodes is the most important prognostic indicator in cases of penile cancer (Fig. 48-1). The 5-year survival rate for patients with cancer in the nodes is 25% compared to 66% in patients with negative nodes. The superficial inguinal lymph nodes are best evaluated by palpation, although lymphangiograms and fine-needle aspiration may also be used, while the deep inguinal and pelvic nodes may be imaged by either computed tomography (CT) or MRI.

Overall, approximately 50% of patients with penile cancer have palpably enlarged superficial inguinal lymph nodes at the time of presentation. Approximately 50% of these palpably enlarged nodes will actually contain cancer, while the other 50% are enlarged secondary to inflammation. In addition, it is also important to realize that up to 20% of patients with nonpalpable lymph nodes will have malignancy within those nodes. The treatment of this group of patients is one of the most controversial issues in penile cancer.

Patients with superficial (Tis, T1), low-grade primary tumors and no palpable lymph nodes should be observed because the instance of positive

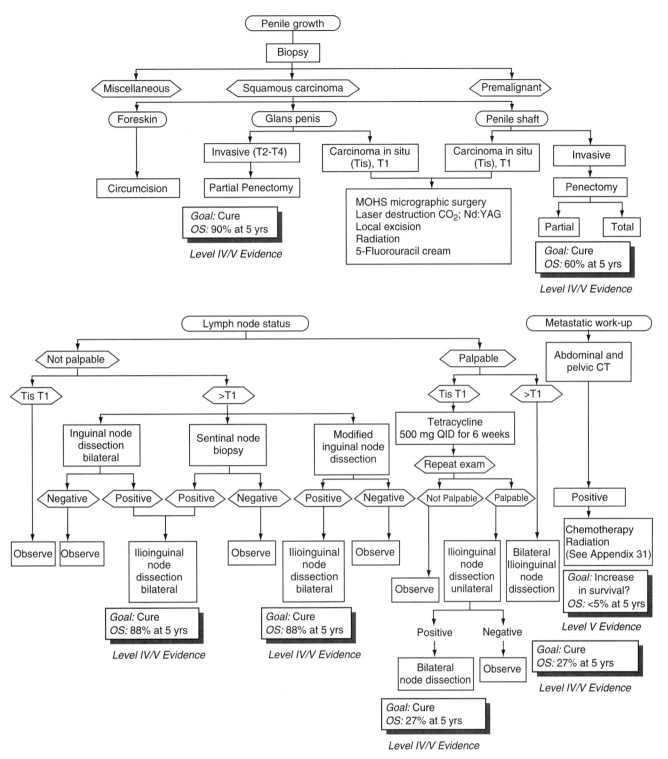

FIGURE 48-1 *Management of penile cancer. Determination of extent of disease and resectability and inguinal lymphadenectomy represent the key reasoning elements in management. Goal of treatment is curative surgery in patients with localized disease and prolongation of survival with lymphadenectomy in node-positive tumor. Metastatic disease may respond to chemotherapy, but it is not clear whether this translates into survival advantage. Recommended strategy is based on nonexperimental evidence about the role of surgery in the management of penile cancer (level II and III evidence) and level IV and V evidences on the role of chemotherapy in the treatment of metastatic disease (see also Appendix 31 for details on treatment protocols).*

nodes is extremely low (<5%). With observation only, one may avoid the 30% to 50% morbidity (lymphadema, poor wound healing, hemorrhage) and 3% mortality rates associated with inguinal lymphadenectomy.

Those with an invasive T2 to T4 primary tumor and impalpable nodes are the patients who provide the greatest challenge and the most controversy. Cabanas has suggested doing a biopsy of a sentinel node located at the junction of the superficial epigastric and saphenous veins to avoid a full superficial lymphadenectomy with its attendant complications. He showed, through the use of penile lymphangiograms and a clinical study, that this node is the first site of metastasis in patients with carcinoma of the penis; the 5-year survival rate among 31 patients with negative biopsies was 90%, with the remaining 10% being lost to follow-up. However, several others report cases in which the sentinel node biopsy was negative, and the patients subsequently developed extensive inguinal adenopathy secondary to metastatic disease. Catalona and others suggest a more extensive dissection of the inguinal nodes—removing all the nodes in the upper medial quadrant of the groin but sparing the saphenous vein and the nodes lateral to the

---

Patient identification
Name _____
Address _____
Hospital or clinic number _____
Age _____ Sex _____ Race _____

Institution identification
Hospital or clinic _____
Address _____

Oncology Record

Anatomic site of cancer _____
Histologic type _____
Grade (G) _____
Date of classification _____

Chronology of classification
[ ]   Clinical (use all data prior to first treatment)
[ ]   Pathologic (if definitively resected specimen available)

Clin	Path		
		DEFINITIONS	
		Primary Tumor (T)	
[ ]	[ ]	TX	Primary tumor cannot be assessed
[ ]	[ ]	T0	No evidence of primary tumor
[ ]	[ ]	Tis	Carcinoma *in situ*
		Ta	Noninvasive verrucous carcinoma
[ ]	[ ]	T1	Tumor invades subepithelial connective tissue
[ ]	[ ]	T2	Tumor invades corpus spongiosum or cavernosum
[ ]	[ ]	T3	Tumor invades urethra or prostate
[ ]	[ ]	T4	Tumor invades other adjacent structures
		Lymph Node (N)	
[ ]	[ ]	NX	Regional lymph nodes cannot be assessed
[ ]	[ ]	N0	No regional lymph node metastasis
[ ]	[ ]	N1	Metastasis in a single, superficial inguinal lymph node
[ ]	[ ]	N2	Metastasis in multiple or bilateral superficial inguinal lymph nodes
[ ]	[ ]	N3	Metastasis in deep inguinal or pelvic lymph node(s), unilateral or bilateral
		Distant Metastasis	
[ ]	[ ]	MX	Presence of distant metastasis cannot be assessed
[ ]	[ ]	M0	No distant metastasis
[ ]	[ ]	M1	Distant metastasis

Histopathologic Grade (G)

[ ] GX   Grade cannot be assessed
[ ] G1   Well differentiated
[ ] G2   Moderately differentiated
[ ] G3-4   Poorly differentiated or undifferentiated

Histopathologic Type

Cell types are limited to carcinomas.

FIGURE 48-2 *Data form for cancer staging. (From American Joint Committee on Cancer: Staging of Cancer Forms (Penile Carcinoma). 3rd Ed. Lippincott-Raven, 1988, with permission.)*

femoral vein. This results in fewer postoperative complications, but the risk of false-negative results is unknown. Therefore, in this group of patients, since the risk of positive nodes may be as high as 66%, an early (prophylactic) bilateral superficial inguinal lymphadenectomy should be performed. McDougal has shown that early lymphadenectomy has an 88% 5-year survival rate compared with a 27% survival rate in those whose lymphadenectomy was delayed until the nodes became palpable.

Those patients with superficial (Tis, T1) low-grade (grade I) primary tumors and palpable lymph nodes should be treated with 500 mg of tetracycline 4 times a day for 4 to 6 weeks, and then be reevaluated. Those patients whose nodes are no longer palpable on reevaluation should be followed very carefully with physical examination of the inguinal area every 2 to 3 months for at least 2 years. On the other hand, patients whose nodes remain palpable after antibiotic therapy should undergo a superficial inguinal node dissection with frozen section of the enlarged nodes. If these nodes have tumor, then a bilateral ileoinguinal lymphadenectomy should be performed. A bilateral node dissection is recommended, as there is a 50% chance of finding positive nodes on the contralateral groin, even if they are not palpable. Patients with invasive T2–4 lesions and palpable nodes require a bilateral ileoinguinal node dissection. If the nodes are large and fixed, it may be advisable to perform the pelvic node dissection first, and if this is positive, abort the inguinal node dissection since the prognosis is very poor. Thereby the complications of inguinal lymphadenectomy can be avoided.

The incidence of positive pelvic nodes in patients with penile cancer is 14% to 27%. Patients with extensive nodal involvement or recurrent inoperable disease may benefit from palliative radiation and chemotherapy.

Distant metastases are rare in patients with penile cancer. They are usually found only in the presence of extensive local regional disease. Such patients should be staged with chest x-ray, abdominal and pelvic CT, and a bone scan. If distant metastases are found, systemic chemotherapy with either intra-arterial or intravenous agents may be used. A combination of methotrexate, vinblastin, and cisplatin produced a 43% response rate in 14 patients, with squamous cell carcinoma of the penis, urethra, and scrotum at the MD Anderson Hospital in Houston, Texas (see Appendix 31). Because of the rarity of this disease, especially in its most advanced stage, no large series are reported.

SUGGESTED READINGS

Burgers JK, Badalament RA, Drago JR: Penile cancer: Clinical presentation, diagnosis and staging. Urol Clin North Am 19:247–256, 1992

Cabanas RM: An approach for treatment of penile carcinoma. Cancer 39:456–466, 1977

Catalona WJ: Modified inguinal lymphadenectomy for carcinoma of the penis with preservation of the saphenous veins: technique and preliminary results. J Urol 140:306–310, 1988

Dexeus FH, Logothetis CJ, Sella A et al: Combination chemotherapy with methotrexate, bleomycin, and cisplatin for advanced squamous cell carcinoma of the male genital tract. J Urol 146:1284–1287, 1991

McDougal WS: Carcinoma of the penis: improved survival by early regional lymphadenectomy based on the histological grade and depth of invasion of the primary lesion. J Urol 154:1364–1366, 1995

49 Transitional Cell Carcinoma of the Renal Pelvis and Ureter

James I. Harty

Incidence: <1% of all neoplasms

5–10% of all renal neoplasms (renal pelvis)

1–2% of all transitional cell neoplasms (ureter)

Goal of treatment: Cure with nephroureterectomy for localized disease

Palliative with nephroureterectomy in symptomatic patients with metastatic disease (e.g., hematuria)

Survival prolonged with chemotherapy

Main modality of treatment: Surgery (nephroureterectomy)

Prognosis: 95% 5-year survival with low-stage and low-grade disease

25% 5-year survival with high-stage and high-grade disease

Unique features: Prognosis depends mainly on grade

Multicentricity throughout urothelium

Cigarette smoking responsible for 50% of cases

INCIDENCE AND EPIDEMOLOGY

Transitional cell carcinoma of the renal pelvis and ureter is a very uncommon tumor constituting less than 1% of all neoplasms. Tumors of the renal pelvis account for approximately 12% of renal malignancies, and 85% of these are transitional cell carcinomas, with the remainder being either squamous carcinoma (9%), adenocarcinoma (1%), or a miscellaneous group (5%). Transitional cell carcinomas occur much more commonly in the bladder than in either the renal pelvis or the ureter—the ratio of bladder to renal pelvis to ureter being 80:4:1. Transitional cell carcinomas tend to be multifocal. Of patients who have transitional cell carcinoma of the bladder, 2% to 4% will have a transitional cell carcinoma of the renal pelvis or ureter, whereas 30% to 75% of patients who present with upper tract tumors will subsequently develop transitional cell carcinoma of the bladder.

There are some well recognized carcinogens for transitional cell carcinoma—cigarette smoking, industrial carcinogens, and phenacetin abuse. A genetically transmitted form of transitional cell carcinoma occurs in the Balkan countries and is associated with a nephropathy. Squamous cell carcinoma is often associated with chronic infection and renal stone disease.

DIAGNOSIS

The initial presenting symptom in patients with transitional cell carcinoma of the renal pelvis and ureter is usually hematuria (75%)—either gross or microscopic (Fig. 49-1). Flank pain occurs in 30% of patients and is due to ureteral colic secondary to passage of blood clots, or to hydronephrosis secondary to a ureteral obstruction from a ureteral tumor. In 10% to 15% of patients, there may be no symptoms. The initial study in a patient presenting with hematuria and flank pain should be an intravenous pyelogram with nephrotomograms to visualize the calyces and the renal pelvis. This study has a 50% to 75% sensitivity rate in detecting an abnormality. A transitional cell carcinoma may demonstrate calyceal distortion, a radiolucent filling defect, or, if very large, nonvisualization of the collecting system. There are several other causes of a radiolucent filling defect, such as a radiolucent stone (uric acid), a blood clot, a sloughed papilla secondary to papillary necrosis, or a fungus ball. A radiolucent stone will show up clearly on a computed tomography (CT) scan performed without intravenous contrast. A sloughed papilla will leave a defect that gives a characteristic clubbed appearance to the calyces, and a fungus ball will be associated with funguria. When the intravenous pyelogram is in any way suspicious or inconclusive, a cystoscopic examination with retrograde pyelography should be performed (Fig. 49-1). This test has a 75% accuracy rate in detecting an abnormality. In addition, washings and brushings of the renal pelvis or ureter for cytology can be carried out. Cytology may not be diagnostic, as it is associated with high false-positive (10%) and false-negative (10%) results. Cytology is more reliable in high-grade lesions, especially if it is obtained with brushing. Cytology results with high-grade lesions have rates of 91% sensitivity and 88% specificity.

The ureter is more difficult to visualize on an intravenous pyelogram, and any abnormality of the ureter should be studied with retrograde ureteropyelogram. A ureteral tumor will usually show either a meniscus-like appearance (Bergman's sign) when a polypoid tumor is present, or a ureteral stenosis, which may indicate a more sessile invasive tumor, since sessile tumors are more likely to invade the ureteral wall, producing obstruction. When the washings and brushings are negative, a CT scan performed without intravenous contrast may show a radiolucent uric acid stone. Such a stone can generally be treated with sodium bicarbonate and allopurinol without resorting to surgical therapy.

The absence of a stone on CT scan compels the investigator to perform ureteroscopy and biopsy. However, ureteroscopy may be associated with complications, which include ureteral perforation and potential tumor implantation.

It is difficult to determine the stage of local disease within the renal pelvis or ureter based on the radiologic studies alone. It is important to remember that high-grade tumors are more likely to be invasive than low-grade tumors. Therefore, grade does play a very important role in the management of these tumors.

Once the primary tumor has been diagnosed, staging for distant disease includes chest x-ray, liver function tests, and abdominal CT scan (Fig. 49-2). The role of bone scan is limited unless the patient has hypercalcemia, elevated alkaline phosphatase, bone pain, or a high-grade tumor.

TREATMENT

The treatment of transitional cell carcinoma of the renal pelvis and ureter is primarily surgical (Fig. 49-1). The type of surgical procedure depends largely on the location of the tumor within the renal pelvis or ureter, as well as on the status of the opposite kidney. As mentioned previously, another factor that must be considered is the grade of the tumor since high-grade tumors tend to be more invasive and therefore are at the higher stage. The standard treatment for all transitional cell tumors of the upper urinary tract, regardless of their precise location, is a nephroureterectomy, provided that the other kidney is normal and there is no evidence of metastatic disease. However, if the opposite kidney is absent or is functionally severely impaired, and the tumor is of low grade and stage, then nephron-sparing procedures are indicated. These include open surgical procedures, such as an open pyelotomy with excision and fulguration of the tumor, partial nephrectomy, or segmental or distal ureterectomy. Alternatively, endoscopic procedures, either percutaneous nephroscopy or ureteroscopy, can be performed. However, with any of these nephron-sparing procedures, there is a 43% rate of recurrence and a 5-year survival rate of 58% compared with a 94% 5-year survival rate associated with a nephroureterectomy.

Older patients, especially those who have nephron-sparing procedures, require careful follow-up with repeat intravenous pyelogram, cystoscopy, retrograde pyelography, urinary cytology, and even ureteroscopy, especially for the first 2 years.

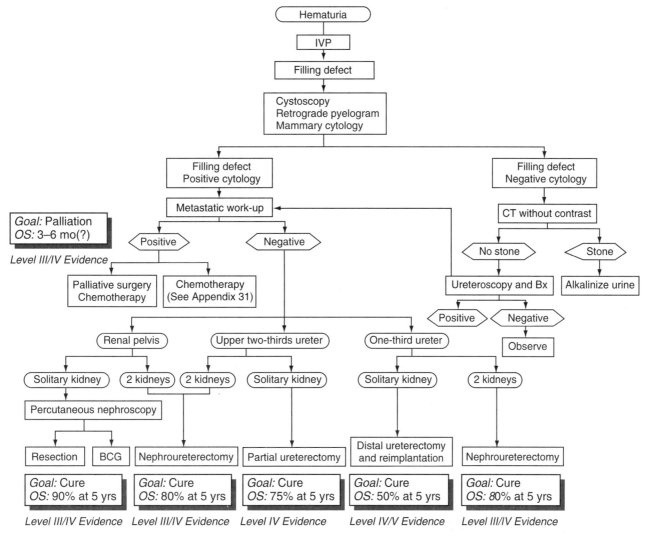

FIGURE 49-1 *Management of transitional cell carcinoma of the renal pelvis and ureter. Determination of extent of disease and resectability represents the key reasoning element in management. Note that determination of the grade of tumor may play a role in planning the extent of surgery. Goal of treatment is curative surgery in patients with localized disease and prolongation of survival with chemotherapy. Recommended strategy is based on solid nonexperimental evidence about the role of surgery in the management of this cancer (level II evidence) and level III and IV evidences on the role of chemotherapy in the treatment of metastatic disease (see also Appendix 31 for details on treatment protocols). OS, overall survival.*

METASTATIC DISEASE

Metastatic disease from transitional cell carcinomas of the renal pelvis and ureter may be found after the primary tumor has been diagnosed. Usual sites of metastases are the regional lymph nodes, liver, lung, and bone. Should metastatic disease occur, patients may be treated with the same chemotherapeutic agents used for patients with metastatic bladder cancer (see Ch. 44 and Appendix 31). Unfortunately, the results in these patients do not appear to be as good as in those with metastatic transitional cell carcinoma of the bladder.

Patient identification
Name _____
Address _____
Hospital or clinic number _____
Age _____ Sex _____ Race _____

Institution identification
Hospital or clinic _____
Address _____

Oncology Record

Anatomic site of cancer _____
Histologic type _____
Grade (G) _____
Date of classification _____

Chronology of classification
[ ]   Clinical (use all data prior to first treatment)
[ ]   Pathologic (if definitively resected specimen available)

Clin	Path		
		DEFINITIONS	
		Primary Tumor (T)	
[ ]	[ ]	TX	Primary tumor cannot be assessed
[ ]	[ ]	T0	No evidence of primary tumor
[ ]	[ ]	Ta	Papillary noninvasive carcinoma
[ ]	[ ]	Tis	Carcinoma *in situ*
[ ]	[ ]	T1	Tumor invades subepithelial connective tissue
[ ]	[ ]	T2	Tumor invades muscularis
[ ]	[ ]	T3	Tumor invades beyond muscularis into peripelvic fat or renal parenchyma (For renal pelvis only)
[ ]	[ ]	T3	Tumor invades beyond muscularis into periureteric fat (For ureter only)
[ ]	[ ]	T4	Tumor invades adjacent organs or through the kidney into perinephric fat
		Lymph Node (N)	
[ ]	[ ]	NX	Regional lymph nodes cannot be assessed
[ ]	[ ]	N0	No regional lymph node metastasis
[ ]	[ ]	N1	Metastasis in a single lymph node, 2 cm or less in greatest dimension
[ ]	[ ]	N2	Metastasis in a single lymph node, more than 2 cm but not more than 5 cm in greatest dimension, or multiple lymph nodes, none more than 5 cm in greatest dimension
[ ]	[ ]	N3	Metastasis in a lymph node more than 5 cm in greatest dimension
		Distant Metastasis (M)	
[ ]	[ ]	MX	Presence of distant metastasis cannot be assessed
[ ]	[ ]	M0	No distant metastasis
[ ]	[ ]	M1	Distant metastasis

Histopathologic Grade (G)

[ ] GX   Grade cannot be assessed
[ ] G1   Well differentiated
[ ] G2   Moderately differentiated
[ ] G3-4   Poorly differentiated or undifferentiated

Histopathologic Type

The histopathologic types are:

Transitional cell carcinoma
Papillary carcinoma
Squamous cell carcinoma
Epidermoid carcinoma
Adenocarcinoma
Urothelial carcinoma

FIGURE 49-2 *Data form for staging cancer of the renal pelvis and ureter. (From American Joint Committee on Cancer: Staging of Cancer Forms (Carcinoma of the Renal Pelvis and Urethra). 3rd Ed. Lippincott-Raven, Philadelphia, 1988, with permission.)*

SUGGESTED READINGS

Bagley DH, Huffman JL, Lyon ES: Flexible ureteropyeloscopy: diagnosis and treatment in the upper urinary tract. J Urol 138:280–285, 1987

Catalona WJ: Urothelial tumors of the urinary tract. pp. 1137–1158. In Walsh PC, Retik AB, Stamey TA, Vaughan ED, Jr, (eds): Campbell's Urology. WB Saunders, Philadelphia, 1992

Eastham J, Huffman JL: Topical therapy in the upper urinary tract. J Urol 150:324–325, 1993

Tasca A, ZaHoni F: The case for a percutaneous approach to transitional cell carcinoma of the renal pelvis. J Urol 143:902, 1990

Yagada A: Chemotherapy for advanced urothelial cancer. Semin Urol 1:60–74, 1983

50 | Testicular Cancer

Geetha Joseph

Incidence: 5.5/100,000 white men

0.5/100,000 African-American men

Goal of treatment: Cure in all stages

Main modality of treatment: Surgery for stage I and II nonseminoma

Radiation for stage I and II seminoma

Chemotherapy for all bulky stage II and stage III of either type

Prognosis (5-year survival): Stage I and II germ cell tumors: > 90%

Stage III germ cell tumors: 50%–70%

Cancer of the testis may be germ cell (> 95%) or nongerm cell in origin. Germ cell tumors (GCT) of the testis are the most common malignancy in males aged 15 to 35, with an incidence of 5.5 in 100,000. There are about 7000 new cases every year in the United States. The majority are nonseminomatous cancers (60%), while the remainder are pure seminomas. With the advent of cisplatin-based chemotherapy, GCT are now among the few solid tumors that are frequently cured by combination chemotherapy.

Risk factors for GCT include cryptorchidism (12% of GCT), testicular feminization, Klinefelter's syndrome, or testicular atrophy from any cause. Human immunodeficiency virus (HIV) positive men have also been reported to have an increased risk of GCT. Despite these risk factors, most patients (> 80%) have no identifiable risk factors.

The most common presenting symptom is painless enlargement of the testis. Pain, caused by torsion, infarction or bleeding, is seen in 20% of patients. Gynecomastia may be seen because of high β-HCG (human chorionic gonadotropin) levels.

DIAGNOSIS

The diagnosis is made by radical inguinal orchiectomy (RIO) with high ligation of the spermatic cord (Fig. 50-1). Trans-scrotal biopsy is contraindicated because of the risk of scrotal contamination and inguinal lymph node spread.

GCT are *classified histologically* into five categories (Table 50-1). For treatment purposes, pure *seminoma* (Fig. 50-2) is distinguished from the other types, which are classified as *nonseminoma* (Fig. 50-3). Laboratory tests, including β-HCG and

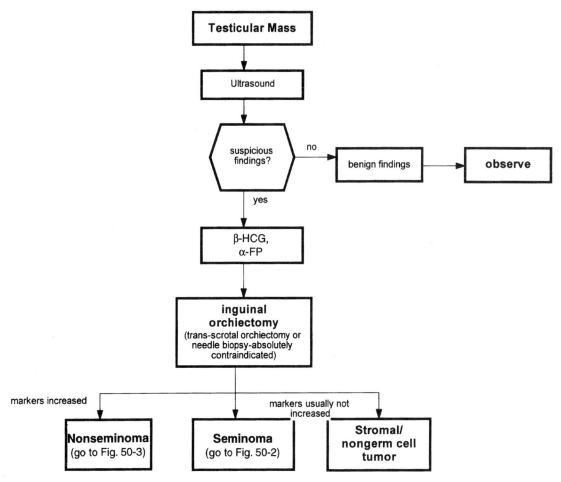

FIGURE 50-1 *Radical inguinal orchiectomy is ultimately the procedure of choice in the diagnosis of testicular cancer and can also be curative in early stages. It can only be avoided in those patients with extragonadal germ cell tumors with normal physical examination and ultrasound. Any elevation of AFP and/or HCG greater than 100u regardless of histologic type qualifies the tumor as a nonseminomatous GCT.*

TABLE 50-1 **HISTOLOGIC CLASSIFICATION OF GCT**

WHO classification (17)

A. Tumor showing single cell type
    1. Seminoma[a]
    2. EC
    3. Teratoma
    4. CC
    5. YST
B. Tumor showing more than one histologic pattern
    1. EC + teratoma with or without seminoma
    2. EC + YST with or without seminoma
    3. EC + seminoma
    4. YST + teratoma with or without seminoma
    5. CC + any other element

Abbreviations: GCT, germ cell tumors, EC, enbryonal carcinoma; CC, choriocarcinona; YST, yolk sac tumor.

[a]Classified as pure seminoma; all other types are classified as nonseminomatous GCT. Seminomas are subclassified as classic, anaplastic, and spermatocytic.

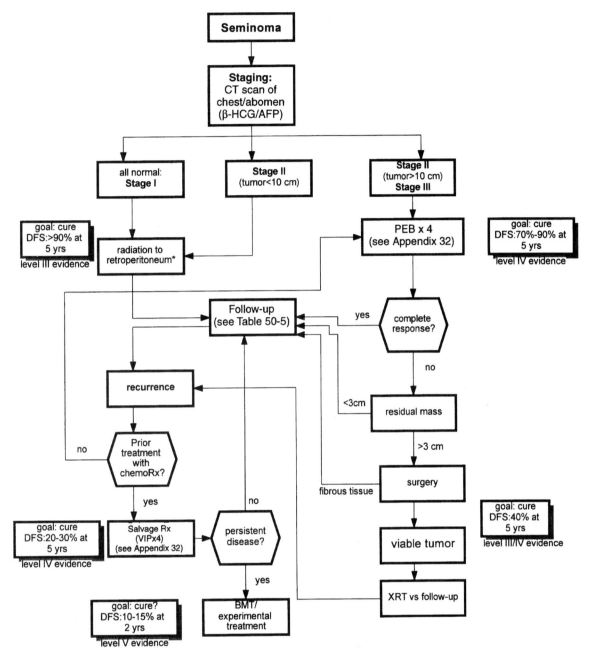

FIGURE 50-2 *Management of seminoma. Exclusion of nonseminomatous elements repre-sents the key decision-making strategy. The goal of treatment is cure in all stages of dis-ease. The recommended strategy is based on level II/III evidence. *(Preliminary data suggests a surveillance strategy is equally effective in clinical stage I; see text for details.)*

α-fetoprotein (AFP), are also used in this distinc-tion. Any elevation of AFP and/or HCG greater than 100u regardless of histologic type qualifies the tumor as a nonseminomatous GCT. Pure semino-mas may have HCG elevations of less than 100u. These tumor markers are useful in follow-up and as markers of response to treatment. The half-life of β-HCG is 24 hours and of AFP is 4 to 6 days. This should be taken into account when following treated patients. Primary nongerm cell tumors of the testes include gonadal stromal tumors (Leydig and Sertoli cell), sarcomas, melanomas, and lymphomas. In men over 60 years of age, 75% of testicular tumors are metastatic, usually from the lung and prostate.

Once the diagnosis of GCT is made, the patient is staged to determine the treatment modality. *Staging* includes physical examination, laboratory evaluation of liver functions, AFP, β-HCG, and computed tomography (CT) scans of the chest and abdomen. Different staging classifications are used in different parts of the country. Memorial Sloan-Kettering Cancer Center (MSKCC) and Walter Reed (WR) Hospital use one based on tumor volume to distinguish minimal, moderate, and advanced tumor load (Table 50-2). The American Joint Committee on Cancer (AJCC) and tumor, node, metastasis (TNM) systems are also commonly used (Table 50-3).

TREATMENT

Treatment of seminoma and nonseminoma differ because of the sensitivity of seminoma to radiation therapy. Below are detailed recommendations regarding GCT tumors.

NONSEMINOMATOUS TUMORS

The main modality of treatment for nonseminoma is surgery for early stages and chemotherapy with adjuvant surgery for late-stage disease. Determining the risk/benefit of retroperitoneal node dissection (RPND) versus surveillance is the key decision-making principle in early stage disease. The goal of treatment is cure in all stages. Depending on the stage and sensitivity to the treatment, the cure rate varies from more than 90% for early stage disease and 70% to 90% for sensitive advanced disease, but drops to 10% to 15% in primary refractory disease.

Clinical Stage I Nonseminoma In this situation the staging workup is negative, and AFP and HCG are not elevated after RIO. The risk of occult node involvement is about 25% and the cure rate is more than 95%. *Standard therapy is a RPND* followed by close follow-up for 2 years as most relapses (30%) occur in this period. A modification of RPND called a nerve-sparing RPND is recommended if preservation of fertility is an important consideration. This approach is associated with a greater than 95% cure rate. The main morbidity of RPND is infertility caused by ejaculatory dysfunction.

Although not standard therapy, an equally acceptable option to RPND is *close surveillance* after RIO, with abdominal scans every 2 months for 2 years along with monthly examination and measurement of tumor markers. RPND is done if there is evidence of tumor either with marker elevation or nodal enlargement. This approach also has cure rates of greater than 95% and avoids the morbidity of RPND in 75% of patients. The negative aspect of this approach is the risk that the patient will not comply with surveillance and not be cured when he relapses because of late detection. A subset of patients with vascular invasion identified in the orchiectomy specimen have a higher risk of relapse (19% in pathologic stage I [PSI] to 60%, PSII) and this group may be better managed with elective RPND.

Pathologic Stage II (After RPND) This situation can be managed in 2 ways: (1) cycles of PEB (cisplatin, etoposide, bleomycin) chemotherapy, or (2) close follow-up and salvage with PEB chemotherapy for relapse (usually in the chest). Both these options have high cure rates (>95%, but as the risk of relapse with microscopic disease is low (10%), option (2) may be better.

Clinical Stage II Nonseminoma This implies visible retroperitoneal nodal involvement on computed tomography (CT) scans and/or elevated tumor markers after RIO and is curable in more than 95% of patients. This stage is subclassified based on the volume of a disease in the retroperitoneum into bulky (> 5 cm mass) and low volume.

Patients with low-volume disease treated with RPND whose tumor markers normalize are managed by (1) close follow-up or (2) two cycles of adjuvant PEB chemotherapy. A randomized trial showed no difference in survival for either approach. The relapse rate is 49% without adjuvant chemotherapy, but the salvage rate with chemotherapy at the time of relapse is 96%, making this option equally effective. The presence of more than 6 positive nodes, tumor diameter more than 2 cm, and extracapsular extension is associated with a higher relapse rate. Persistent marker elevation after RPND requires chemotherapy.

Patients with masses greater than 5 cm have unresectable (bulky) disease and are best managed with 4 cycles of PEB chemotherapy. After chemotherapy, if CT scans and tumor markers are normal, follow-up is instituted. Persistent marker elevation is an indication for salvage chemotherapy, although 20% to 25% of patients may be rendered disease free by surgery (RPND) in this setting. Persistent masses greater than 3 cm without marker elevations should be surgically resected, especially if the initial RIO specimen had a component of teratoma.

TABLE 50-2 **STAGING OF GERM CELL TUMORS**

Memorial Sloan-Kettering Cancer Center	Walter Reed Hospital	Definition
A	I	Tumor confined to testis
B1	IIA	Minimal RP node spread (microscopic disease; <6 nodes involved)
B2	IIB	Moderate RP node spread (± gross; >6 nodes)
B3	IIC	Bulky RP nodes (palpable, > 5 cm)
C	III	Above diaphragm/extranodal sites

Abbreviation: RP, retroperitoneal. (From American Joint Committee on Cancer: Staging of Cancer. 4th Ed. Lippincott, Philadelphia, 1993, with permission.)

TABLE 50-3 **TNM STAGING SCHEME FOR ALL GERM CELL TUMORS**

Code	Definition
Primary tumor (T; the extent of primary tumor is classified after radial orchiectomy)	
pTX	Primary tumor cannot be assessed (if no radical orchi ectomy has been performed, TX is used)
pTO	No evidence of primary tumor (e.g., histologic scar in testis)
pTis	Intratubular tumor: preinvasive cancer
pT1	Tumor limited to the testis, including the rate testis
pT2	Tumor invades beyond the tunica albuginea or into the epididymis
pT3	Tumor invades the spermatic cord
pT4	Tumor invades the scrotum
Regional lymph nodes (N)	
NX	Regional lymph nodes cannot be assessed
NO	No regional lymph node metastasls
N1	Metastasis in a single lymph node, 2 cm or less in greatest dimension
N2	Metastasis in a single lymph node, more than 2 cm but not more than 5 cm in greatest dimension, or multiple lymph nodes, none more than 5 cm in greatest dimension
N3	Metastasis in a lymph node more than 5 cm in greatest dimension
Distant metastasis (M)	
MX	Presence of distant metastasis cannot be assessed
MO	No distant metastasis
M1	Distant metastasis

Stage	T	N	M
O	pTis	NO	MO
I	Any pT	NO	MO
II	Any pT	N1	MO
	Any pT	N2	MO
	Any pT	N3	MO
III	Any pT	Any N	Ml

(From American Joint Committee on Cancer: Manual for Staging of Cancer. 4th Ed. Lippincott-Raven, Philadelphia, 1993, with permission.)

The use of positron emission tomography (PET) is being tested in the evaluation of residual masses. The finding of viable nonseminomatous germ cell malignant elements in the specimen at surgery is an indication for further chemotherapy.

Failure of PEB chemotherapy to lower markers or shrink nodal masses or recurrent nodal masses or marker elevations after initial normalization is an indication for salvage chemotherapy (Appendix 32). Fifty percent to 60% of relapsing patients with nonseminoma and 70% with seminoma achieve a long-term survival, especially with late relapses. Patients with primary resistance to chemotherapy have a very poor outcome with standard chemotherapy two-year survival, 9%–15% and should be included in trials evaluating effectiveness of high-dose chemotherapy with or without stem-cell support.

Clinical Stage III Nonseminoma

Clinical Stage III Nonseminoma This stage has supradiaphragmatic involvement or visceral involvement and is cured 70% of the time. Standard therapy is 4 cycles of PEB, although 3 courses are equally effective in low-volume disease (minimal/moderate disease; see Tables 50-2 and 50-3). High-volume disease has a 30% to 40% cure rate. Residual disease/persistent marker elevation after PEB is managed as in bulky stage II. If residual disease is present above the diaphragm, thoracotomy is indicated.

Relapse after initial response is managed with salvage regimen (Appendix 32). *Primary resistant disease* should be treated on clinical trials. Radiation therapy is indicated for brain metastases.

SEMINOMA

The main treatment modality for early stage seminoma is radiation and chemotherapy for advanced disease. The key decision making principle is to exclude nonseminomatous elements that will not respond to radiation. The goal of treatment is cure, which depends on the stage of disease and sensitivity of the tumor to the treatment. The cure rates are greater than 90% in early-stage disease, 70% to 90% for advanced stage disease, and 20% to 30% for relapsed disease.

Stage I Seminoma This clinical stage is defined by a negative staging work-up after RIO. Standard therapy is radiation therapy (XRT) to the retroperitoneal and inguinal lymph nodes (15% relapse rate without XRT). The cure rate with this strategy is greater than 95%. Early data suggest a watch and wait approach is equally effective, but the risk of relapse continues beyond 2 years and requires longer surveillance than nonseminomatous GCT.

Stage II Seminoma Standard treatment is radiation therapy for nonbulky disease, with a cure rate of 80% to 90%. For bulky disease (> 10 cm), 4 cycles of PEB or etoposide/cisplatin is recommended (85% to 95% cure) as treatment with XRT alone has a relapse rate of 30% to 40%. Controversy exists regarding the management of residual masses after XRT or chemotherapy. Stable masses may be observed, but use of newer imaging techniques, such as PET, may delineate active disease that is best biopsied and treated with additional chemotherapy.

Stage III Seminoma This stage is managed like stage II bulky disease. Recurrent disease is managed with the same salvage chemotherapy used for nonseminoma GCT. Refractory disease should be treated in the setting of a clinical trial.

RESIDUAL MASS AFTER CHEMOTHERAPY IN GCT

Seminoma Patients with bulky seminoma undergoing chemotherapy may have residual masses after completion of therapy (60% to 85%). These are best followed radiologically unless they are greater than 3 cm in size, when surgical removal may be warranted. Only 20% to 25% of all masses have viable tumor, while 42% of masses greater than 3 cm do. Radiation or 2 additional cycles of chemotherapy may be given if viable tumor is found.

Nonseminoma In nonseminoma, residual masses are more likely to represent teratoma or viable tumor and should be surgically resected, especially if they are greater than 3 cm or the original tumor had a component of teratoma. The survival of patients with viable tumor is less than those with fibrosis or teratoma. Experimental approaches, including PET scanning, are being used to identify patients most likely to benefit from surgery. Residual masses in the lung should be resected; 10% to 20% contain malignancy; 20% to 60%, teratoma; 15% to 60%, fibrosis. Two additional cycles of PEB should be given if viable tumor is found.

PROGNOSTIC FACTORS

Various prognostic factors have been studied and schemas have been proposed to classify patients. The Indiana University classification defines patients into minimal, moderate, and extensive disease based on certain features (Table 50-4). Strategies to decrease toxicities of therapy and maintain high cure rates are being tested, primarily in "good risk" groups. "Poor risk" groups are being targeted for experimental approaches to improve cure rates. MSKCC has shown that cisplatin plus etoposide (EP) is equivalent to their VAB-6 regimen (Table 50-5) in response and survival in their good risk subgroup. To date no widely accepted risk assessment schema has been developed, and individual institutional schema vary widely. The lack of a uni-

TABLE 50-4 INDIANA UNIVERSITY PROGNOSTIC CLASSIFICATION SCHEMA

Minimal Disease	*Response Rates*
Elevated HCG ± AFP levels only	
Cervical nodes, ± non PAM	88%–90%
Nonresectable but non-PAM LA nodes	
LM < 5/lung field and < 2 cm largest diameter	
Moderate Disease	
PAM as only anatomic site	
LM = 5-10/lung field and largest < 3 cm Or mediastinal mass	
< 50% of intrathoracic diameter or solitary LM > 2 cm diameter (± non-PAM)	
Advanced disease (poor risk)	
Mediastinal mass > 50% of intrathoracic diameter or > 10 LM/lung field	
or multiple > 3 cm diameter (± non-PAM)	38%–60%
PAM with any LM	
Liver, bone, or central nervous system metastases	

Abbreviations: AFP, alphafetoprotein; HCg, human chorionic gonadotropin; LA, lumboaortic; LM, lung metastases; PAM, palpable abdominal mass.

form prognostic classification underscores the dangers of altering therapy based on randomly chosen classifications.

LONG-TERM SEQUELAE OF TREATMENT

Because of the high cure rate of GCT and long-term survival of these patients, the sequelae of treatment may impact on survival/quality of life. Efforts are currently underway to decrease the toxicities of treatment without lowering cure rates. Sequelae include the following:

Fertility is often impaired before therapy because of oligospermia or abnormalities of the sperm themselves. RPND may impair fertility owing to ejaculatory dysfunction. Chemotherapy causes oligospermia in almost all patients, but this reverses in many patients who then can father children

Renal and hearing dysfunction caused by cisplatin is seen in a minority of patients

Pulmonary toxicity caused by bleomycin can be seen but is rarely fatal with cumulative doses below 400 units.

Secondary leukemias such as acute myeloid leukemia (AML) have been reported with cumulative etoposide doses of more than 2,000 mg (relative risk for AML > 15) with a typical 11q23 translocation. This is particularly frequent with primary mediastinal extragonadal GCT.

FOLLOW-UP CARE

After standard therapy most patients are followed intensively for 2 years and then less often for the next 3 years. Patients have a 5% risk of a contralateral GCT and should be taught testicular self-examination (Table 50-5).

SURVEILLANCE

This term refers to the follow-up strategy used after RIO when neither radiation nor RPND have been used and the patient is at risk for occult disease in the retroperitoneum. CT of the abdomen is done frequently during surveillance, unlike routine follow-up after RPND or abdominal radiation when chest x-rays are usually adequate.

Figures 50-1 to 50-3 summarize the clinical approach to the patient with a testicular cancer. Recommended strategies are based on solid level I

TABLE 50-5 FOLLOW-UP AND SURVEILLANCE STRATEGIES

Surveillance
Nonseminoma (after radical inguinal orchiectomy with no other treatment)
    Monthly examination with chest x-rays; markers (β-HCG and AFP) q month × 12, then q 2 months × 12
    Computed tomography of abdomen q 2 months × 1 year; q 3 month × 1 year; q 4 month × 1 year; q 6 month × 1 year; annually × 2 year
Seminoma (not standard therapy at this time; see Fig. 50-2)
Follow-up (after RPND or chemotherapy)
    Monthly physical examination with chest x-ray, AFP/HCG q month × 12, then q 2 months × 1 year, q 6 months × 3 years
    Computed tomography scan of abdomen as clinically indicated (residual disease)

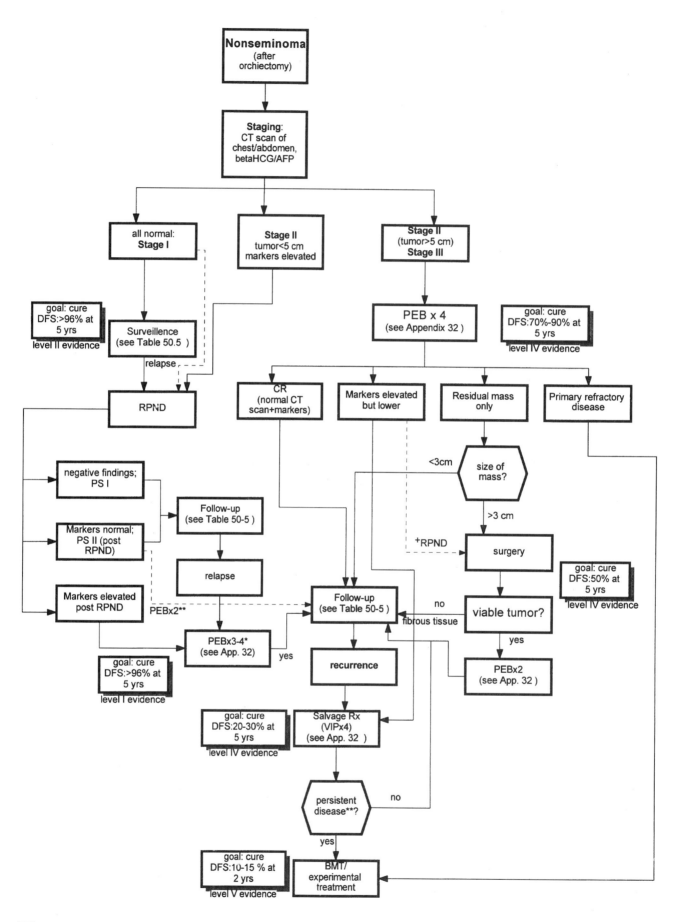

Nonseminoma
(after orchiectomy)

Staging:
CT scan of chest/abdomen, betaHCG/AFP

all normal:
Stage I

Stage II
tumor<5 cm
markers elevated

Stage II
(tumor>5 cm)
Stage III

goal: cure
DFS:>96% at 5 yrs
level II evidence

Surveillence
(see Table 50.5)

PEB x 4
(see Appendix 32)

goal: cure
DFS:70%-90% at 5 yrs
level IV evidence

relapse

RPND

CR
(normal CT scan+markers)

Markers elevated but lower

Residual mass only

Primary refractory disease

negative findings;
PS I

size of mass?

<3cm

Markers normal;
PS II (post RPND)

Follow-up
(see Table 50-5)

>3 cm

+RPND

surgery

goal: cure
DFS:50% at 5 yrs
level IV evidence

relapse

Follow-up
(see Table 50-5)

no

viable tumor?

fibrous tissue

Markers elevated post RPND

PEBx2**

goal: cure
DFS:>96% at 5 yrs
level I evidence

PEBx3-4*
(see App. 32)

yes

recurrence

yes

PEBx2
(see App. 32)

goal: cure
DFS:20-30% at 5 yrs
level IV evidence

Salvage Rx
(VIPx4)
(see App. 32)

persistent disease**?

no

goal: cure
DFS:10-15 % at 2 yrs
level V evidence

BMT/
experimental treatment

yes

350

FIGURE 50-3 *Management of nonseminoma. Evaluating the risk/benefit of retroperitoneal node dissection versus observation in early stages is the key decision-making principle. The goal of treatment is cure in all stages. The recommended strategy is based on level I evidence for early disease and level IV for advanced disease. *(Three cycles of PEB are adequate for small-volume disease. **Alternative strategy for close surveillance could be administration of two cycles of PEB. †Patients with elevated markers may benefit from surgery; see text for details.) RPND, Retroperitoneal node dissection.*

and II evidence of effectiveness of the various management options for the treatment of early stages of testicular cancer; less solid (level III/IV) but still convincing are data about curability with the management options for advanced stage disease. Appendix 32 shows practical methods of administering chemotherapy.

SUGGESTED READINGS

American Joint Committee on Cancer: Manual for Staging of Cancer. 4th Ed. Lippincott-Raven, Philadelphia, 1993

Bokemeyer C, Schmoll H. Treatment of testicular cancer and the development of secondary malignancies. J Clin Oncol 13:283, 1995

Einhorn EH, Williams SD, Loehrer PJ et al: Evaluation of optimal duration of chemotherapy in favorable-prognosis disseminated germ cell tumors: a Southeastern Cancer Study Group protocol. J Clin Oncol 7:387, 1989

Foster RS, Donohue JP: Surgical treatment of clinical stage A nonseminomatous testis cancer. Semin Oncol 19:166, 1992

Fox EP, Weathers TD, Williams SD et al: Outcome analysis for patients with persistent nonteratomatous germ cell tumor in postchemotherapy retroperitoneal lymph node dissections. J Clin Oncol 11:1294, 1993

Jansen RHL, Sylvester R, Sleyfer DT et al: Long term follow up of nonseminomatus testicular cancer patients with mature teratome or carcinoma at postchemotherapy surgery. Eur J Cancer 27:695, 1991

Kleep O, Olsson AM, Henrikson H et al: Prognostic factors in clinical stage I nonseminomatous germ cell tumors of the testis: multivariate analysis of a prospective multicenter study. J Clin Oncol 8:509, 1990

Loehrer PJ, Einhorn LH, Williams SD: VP-16 plus ifosfamide plus cisplatin as salvage therapy in refractory germ cell cancer. J Clin Oncol 4:528, 1986

Mostofi FK, Sesterhenn IA, Davis CJ: Developments in histopathology of testicular germ cell tumors. Semin Urol 6:171, 1988

Motzer RJ, Bosl GJ, Heelan R et al: Residual mass: an indication for further therapy in patients with advanced seminoma following systemic chemotherapy. J Clin Oncol 5:1064, 1987

Sesterhenn IA, Weiss RB, Mostofi SK, Stablein DM et al: Prognosis and other clinical correlates of pathologic review in stage I and stage II testicular carcinoma: a report from the Testicular Cancer Intergroup Study. J Clin Oncol 10:69–78, 1992

Stephens AW, Gonin R, Hutchins GD, Einhorn LH: Positron emission tomography evaluation of residual radiographic abnormalities in postchemotherapy germ cell tumor patients. J Clin Oncol 14:1637, 1996

Sturgeon JF, Jewett MA, Alison RE et al: Surveillance after orchidectomy for patients with clinical stage I nonseminomatous testis tumors. J Clin Oncol 10:564, 1992

Stutzman RE, McLeod DG: Radiation therapy: a primary treatment modality for seminoma. Urol Clin North Am 7:753, 1980

Sujka SK, Huben RP: Clinical stage I nonseminomatous germ cell tumors of testis: observation versus retroperitoneal lymph node dissection. Urology 38:29, 1991

Thomas G: Management of metastatic seminoma: role of radiotherapy. P. 211. In Horwich A (ed): Testicular Cancer—Clinical Investigation and Management. Chapman and Hal Medical, New York, 1991

Warde P, Gospadarowicz MK, Panzarella T et al: Stage I testicular seminoma: results of adjuvant irradiation and surveillance. J Clin Oncol 13:2255, 1995

Williams SD, Stablein DM, Einhorn LH et al: Immediate adjuvant chemotherapy versus observation with treatment at relapse in pathologic stage II testicular cancer. N Engl J Med 317:1433, 1987

51 Brain Tumors

Baby O. Jose

Prevalence: 1% of all cancers

Goal of treatment: Histology dependent; cure for meningioma
Prolongation of survival for glioma

Main modality of treatment: Surgery (plus adjuvant radiation
therapy plus chemotherapy for glioma)

Prognosis (median survival): 10–14 months (glioblastoma)

In the United States, approximately 18,000 primary brain tumors are diagnosed every year. *Astrocytoma* is the most common primary brain tumor (50%). There is an increased incidence of primary brain tumors, especially primary *non-Hodgkin's lymphoma* of the brain. The general symptoms are due to mass effect, increased intracranial pressure, and from destruction of adjacent brain tissue. The focal symptoms depend on the location of the tumor. The suggested guidelines for work-up, management, and follow-up are shown in Figure 51-1. The histopathologic types are depicted in Table 51-1.

GLIOMAS

The most important prognostic factors are age, Karnofsky score, histopathology, duration of symptoms, and extent of surgery. The staging used is mainly surgical, based on size, extent, and location of tumors (Table 51-2). Low-grade gliomas are primarily treated initially with surgical resection. If a total resection is possible, most of the patients will be followed or considered for clinical trials. If only partial resection is possible, patients should be advised to participate in clinical trials with radiation therapy. The timing of irradiation in these tumors is in question, as some of them can grow

very slowly. Untreated, thirty percent or more of patients with low grade gliomas will develop a higher grade tumor.

High-grade gliomas are treated with radiation therapy after surgery, with or without chemotherapy. Since the overall outcome is poor in these patients, they should be advised to participate in clinical trials with radiation and different chemotherapy regimens. In most centers, 60 Gy in 6 to 7 weeks to the involved site using custom blocks and computerized treatment planning is usually done. Attempts are being made to increase the dose using conforming methods, implants, or radiosurgery. Attempts to improve local control using radiosensitizers have not been very successful so far.

Chemotherapy with N, N-bis (2-chloroethyl)-N-nitrosourea (BCNU) shows a statistically significant improvement in survival based on Brain Tumor Study Group trials. The other drugs used in combination are procarbazine N-(2-chloroethyl)-N'-cyclohexyl-N-nitrosourea (CCNU), and vincristine (PCV). Intra-arterial BCNU showed poor results compared with intravenous BCNU. BTCG (Brain Tumor Study Cooperative Group) is investigating the use of iodine 125 seed implantation, in addition to the external beam, with intravenous BCNU in high-grade gliomas, in a phase III

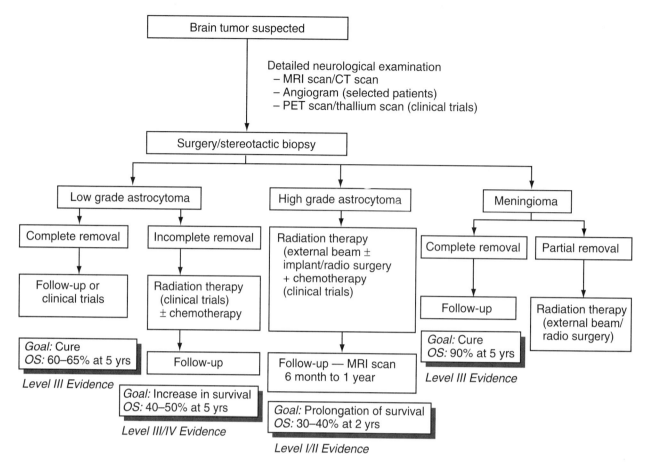

FIGURE 51-1 *Management of brain tumors. The approach is histology dependent. Goal of treatment varies from cure in meningioma and completely resected low-grade astrocytoma to increase in survival in high-grade astrocytoma. Recommended strategy is based on level I and II evidence. (See also Appendix 33 for details on treatment.) OS, overall survival.*

prospective randomized trial (BTCG-87-01). Other areas of investigation include gene therapy in selected brain tumors.

With the current treatment methods, the outcome in glioblastoma multiforme has improved to a median survival of 10 to 14 months and a 2-year survival of about 10% to 15%. The median survival of patients with anaplastic astrocytoma is about 18 to 20 months, with a 2-year survival of 30% to 40%. With the current use of modern computerized treatment plans, the amount of brain tissue to be irradiated will be less, thus minimizing the acute and long-term effects of radiation treatment.

TABLE 51-1 HISTOPATHOLOGIC TYPES OF BRAIN TUMORS

Astrocytomas
Oligodendrogliomas
Ependymal and choroid plexus tumors
Glioblastomas
Medulloblastomas
Meningiomas, malignant
Neurilemmomas (neurinomas, schwannomas), malignant
Hemangioblastomas
Neurosarcomas
Sarcomas

PRIMARY CENTRAL NEVOUS SYSTEM LYMPHOMA

The incidence of this disease is increasing, especially among patient with acquired immunodeficiency syndrome (AIDS). It can present as a focal or multiple lesions. Patients are treated with combination chemotherapy and irradiation. Studies are being done by the Radiation Therapy Oncology Group (RTOG) using combination chemotherapy

TABLE 51-2 STAGING OF BRAIN TUMORS

Primary tumor (T)

TX   Primary tumor cannot be assessed

T0   No evidence of primary tumor

Supratentorial Tumor

T1   Tumor 5 cm or less in greatest dimension; limited to one side

T2   Tumor more than 5 cm in greatest dimension; limited to one side

T3   Tumor invades or encroaches upon the ventricular system

T4   Tumor crosses the midline, invades the opposite hemisphere, or invades infratentorially

Infratentorial Tumor

T1   Tumor 3 cm or less in greatest dimension; limited to one side

T2   Tumor more than 3 cm in greatest dimension; limited to one side

T3   Tumor invades or encroaches upon the ventricular system

T4   Tumor crosses the midline, invades the opposite hemisphere, or invades supratentorially

Regional lymph nodes (N)

This category does not apply to this site.

Distant metastasis (M)

MX   Presence of distant metastasis cannot be assessed

M0   No distant metastasis

M1   Distant metastasis

Histopathologic grade (G)

GX   Grade cannot be assessed

G1   Well differentiated

G2   Moderately well differentiated

G3   Poorly differentiated

G4   Undifferentiated

Stage grouping

Stage	G	T	M
Stage IA	G1	T1	M0
Stage IB	G1	T2	M0
	G1	T3	M0
Stage IIA	G2	T1	M0
Stage IIB	G2	T2	M0
	G2	T3	M0
Stage IIIA	G3	T1	M0
Stage IIIB	G3	T2	M0
	G3	T3	M0
Stage IV	G1, 2, 3	T4	M0
	G4	Any T	M0
	Any G	Any T	M1

with irradiation to improve the outcome. The details of treatment and outcomes are described in Chapter 9.

MENINGIOMA

Meningiomas are benign tumors, and the primary treatment is surgery. If complete resection is possible, most patients are followed. Radiation reduces recurrence and also prolongs the time to recurrence based on retrospective studies. Radiosurgery and brachytherapy are also used in recurrent or residual disease.

PITUITARY ADENOMA

The symptoms and signs of pituitary adenomas are caused by the hormones they produce or by local effects on the optic chiasm and surrounding tissues. Most of the patients are treated with surgery followed by involved field radiation therapy with doses up to 45 to 50 Gy based on the type and size of the tumor. Fractionated radiosurgery is added in the management of pituitary tumors. In selected patients with prolactinomas, bromocriptine has been used successfully, before the initiation of radiation therapy.

Rare tumors, such as medulloblastomas in adults, are treated with craniospinal irradiation, with or without chemotherapy, because of the extent of the disease at the time of surgery.

COMPLICATIONS AND FOLLOW-UP

Patients with brain tumors should be closely followed at intervals of 2 to 3 months for the first 1 to 2 years, every 4 to 6 months for 2 to 5 years, and yearly afterwards. The acute reactions from surgery and radiation, which include edema in the brain, will improve in 4 to 6 months. The significant late effects, which include necrosis of brain tissues, changes in cognitive function, and vascular effects, can occur for many years. These effects depend on the extent of surgery, volume of brain tissue radiated, and total dose and duration of treatment. The patients with these effects should be reevaluated with magnetic resonance imaging or magnetic resonance spectroscopy or SPECT scans to distinguish between recurrence versus radionecrosis. The management of radionecrosis includes steroids and surgery if possible. Patients who receive radiation and chemotherapy should be followed for second malignancy, either solid or hematologic.

SUGGESTED READINGS

Abeloff MP, Armitage JO, Lichter AS, Niederhuber JE (eds): Clinical Oncology. Churchill Livingstone, New York, 1995

Barbaro, Gurtin PH, Wilson CB: Radiation therapy in the treatment of partially resected meningomas. Neurosurgery 20:525, 1987

Fine HA, Dear KBG, Loeffler JS et al: Meta-analysis of radiation therapy with and/without adjuvant chemotherapy for malignant gliomas in adults. Cancer 71:2585, 1993

Haskell: Cancer Treatment, 4th Ed. Saunders, Philadelphia, 1995

Kondgiolka, Lunsford LD: Radiosurgery for meningioma. Neurosurg Clin North Am 3:219, 1992

Shapiro, Green SB, Burger PC et al: Randomized trial of three chemotherapy regimens and two radiotherapy regimens in postoperative treatment of malignant gliomas. J Neurosurg 71:1, 1989

Walker MD, Alexander E, Hunt WE et al: Evaluation of BCNU and/or radiotherapy in the treatment of anaplastic gliomas. J Neurosurg 49:333, 1978

Walker MD, Strike TA, Shehine GE: An analysis of dose effect relationship in the radiotherapy of malignant gliomas. Int J Radiat Oncol Biol Phys 5:1725, 1979

Walker MD, Green SB, Byar DP et al: Randomized comparison of radiotherapy and nitrosureas for the treatment of malignant glioma. N Engl J Med 303:1323, 1980

52 | Osteosarcoma

Linda Garland

Incidence: 2.1 cases/1,000,000

Goal of treatment: Cure using preoperative chemotherapy to reduce significantly the tumor burden, followed by limb-sparing surgery (or amputation if unable to salvage a well-functioning limb) and adjuvant chemotherapy

Main modalities of treatment: Involve surgical resection by an expert in bone neoplasms with preoperative and postoperative chemotherapy

Prognosis: 5-year disease-free survival 60%–65% overall

Osteosarcomas (OS) are highly malignant tumors of bone that most commonly affect children and adolescents. Over the last twenty years, long-term survival with good functional status has greatly improved for OS patients. Before the advent of chemotherapy for OS, the 5-year survival rate for high-grade OS treated with amputation alone was 12% to 15%. The five-year survival has improved to 60% to 70% in similar patients treated with combined modality therapy in the mid-1970s to mid-1980s, reflecting improved understanding of the biology of OS coupled with improvements in diagnosis and treatment. These include multimodality imaging for accurate staging and presurgical planning, surgical advances in limb-sparing procedures, and the development of active chemotherapy regimens used in the neoadjuvant (preoperative) and adjuvant settings. Still, patients with metastatic disease at presentation have a poor prognosis, and there is significant disease recurrence despite intensive treatment of the primary tumor and micrometastatic disease. These outcomes can be related to the intrinsic resistance of some OS tumors to chemotherapeutic agents, superimposed on an aggressive histologic nature. Unique ways to overcome tumor resistance and improve disease-free and overall survival are being addressed by current multi-institutional clinical trials for OS.

EPIDEMIOLOGY

Osteosarcoma is a rare malignancy seen mainly during childhood and adolescence, a period characterized by the skeletal growth spurt. The overall incidence is 2.1 cases per million, with a peak incidence between ages 10 and 19. A small number of patients present after age 40, often with secondary OS arising in abnormal bone because of Paget's disease, bone infarcts, fibrous dysplasia, and irradiation. There is a slight male predominance, with a male to female ratio of 1:6 to 1. Familial cases of OS are extremely rare.

CLASSIFICATION AND GRADING

Bone tumors are classified according to the cell of origin and the material produced by the tumor stroma. Osteosarcomas are classified as osteogenic tumors in which malignant spindle cells and osteoblasts produce osteoid matrix or immature bone. Most OS are classic high-grade intramedullary tumors, which can be further divided by histologic subtype. More rare forms include low-grade intra-medullary and juxtacortical tumors (Table 52--1).

SKELETAL DISTRIBUTION

The long bones of the extremities are the most common sites of involvement (70%), especially the areas of growth around the knee. In a series of 1,095 patients, the knee region was involved in about half the patients, and the femur was involved in 44% of patients. Pelvic tumors represent 8% of cases, with spine tumors 1.5% and jaw bone tumors 6%.

PATTERNS OF TUMOR GROWTH AND METASTASIS

Ninety percent of osteosarcomas arise in the meta-physis of tubular long bones. Local growth often results in a large soft-tissue component. The tumor can involve the epiphysis and also the articular aspect of the involved bone, and tumor can embolize into the marrow sinusoids, causing skip metastases. Hematogenous spread commonly leads to pulmonary metastases, and secondarily to involvement of other osseous sites. It is assumed that the majority of patients with OS have micro-metastatic pulmonary disease at presentation. Lymph node involvement is rare and portends a poor prognosis.

PROGNOSTIC FACTORS

Important prognostic factors include metastatic disease at presentation (survival 15% overall), site of primary tumor (appendicular skeleton better than axial skeleton), histologic response to preoper-ative chemotherapy when limited drugs are given for a limited time, and the serum lactate dehydro-genase and alkaline phosphatase. Current studies are evaluating multiple drug resistance (mdr 1) gene expression by tumor as a predictor of out-come, as mdr expression relates to responsiveness of OS to important classes of chemotherapeutic agents.

TABLE 52-1 MAJOR HISTOLOGIC VARIETIES OF PRIMARY INTRAMEDULLARY AND JUXTACORTICAL OSTEOSARCOMA

Dominant Histologic Patterns	Incidence
Primary, solitary, high-grade intramedullary osteosarcoma (75% of entire set of osteosarcomas)	
Mixed patterns	73
Bone rich or "sclerosing"	9
Cartilage rich (chondrosarcoma-like)	5
Spindle cell rich (fibrosarcoma-like)	4
Malignant histiocyte rich (MFH-like)	3
Large vascular spaces or telangiectatic (ABC-like)	3
Small cell rich (Ewing's sarcoma-like)	1
Benign giant cell rich (giant cell tumor-like)	1
Epithelioid cell rich (metastatic carcinoma-like)	1
Chondroblastoma-like	0.2
	Total 100
Low-grade intramedullary osteosarcoma (4%–5% of entire set of osteosarcomas)	
Fibrous dysplasia-like	50
Nonossifying fibroma-like	25
Osteoblastoma-like	15
Chondromyxoid fibroma-like	10
	Total 100
Juxtacortical osteosarcoma (7%–10% of entire set of osteosarcomas)	
Parosteal osteosarcoma	65
Periosteal osteosarcoma	25
High-grade surface osteosarcoma	10
	Total 100

(From Mirra JM, Picci P, Gold RH: Bone Tumors: Clinical, Radiologic and Pathologic Correlations. Lea & Febiger, Philadelphia. 1989, p. 254, with permission.)

DIAGNOSIS

Patients with osteosarcomas report progressive pain related to an expanding mass, which on examination is fixed to underlying bone. Plain radiographs characteristically show a mass involving intramedullary bone, with radiodense areas of bone or cartilage in sclerotic lesions and nonossified lytic areas in lytic lesions. More typically, the radiograph shows a mixture of density and lucency. There may be signs of permeative bony destruction with periosteal elevation that appear in a "sunburst" or "hair-on-end" periosteal pattern, or Codman's triangle representing a wedge of new bone formation adjacent to tumor pushing through raised periosteum. Very frequently there is soft-tissue calcification, which represents extraosseous extension of tumor.

Patients who are suspected of having osteosarcoma should be referred to cancer centers with bone tumor expertise *before* biopsy is undertaken. The type of biopsy (fine needle aspiration, core needle, or open biopsy) and its location can impact on diagnostic accuracy and risk of contamination of compartments adjacent to the tumor. Biopsy should be performed by an orthopedic surgeon with a specialty in bone neoplasms. Review of biopsy tissue should be performed by a pathologist well-versed in bone tumor histology.

STAGING

Careful staging of osteosarcoma requires the combined use of imaging modalities. Bone radiographs are important initial imaging studies that show characteristic bone and soft-tissue abnormalities and direct attention to areas distant from the primary tumor that may be the site of osseous metastases. Computed tomography (CT) helps to distinguish between infection and neoplasm and further defines the extent of intramedullary tumor and extension into adjacent structures. Osseous and pulmonary metastases are imaged with CT. Magnetic resonance imagine (MRI) can accurately define the extent of tumor involvement in adjacent soft tissues, aiding the orthopedic surgeon in planning lines of resection.

TREATMENT

The treatment of OS involves a combined modality approach, which includes surgery, chemotherapy, rehabilitation, and psychological support for the patient. The treatment plan should be designed and implemented by a multispecialty team. All eligible patients should be enrolled into clinical research trials that are based on this approach and that address current questions regarding tumor biology and optimal treatment schemes.

Most OS tumors originate in the extremities, and a general treatment scheme is illustrated by the algorithm for OS of the extremity (Fig. 52-1). The primary goal of treatment is to achieve a state of minimal residual disease by administering preoperative chemotherapy, followed by resection of all gross local and metastatic disease. This is followed by adjuvant therapy administered to treat locoregional and distant microscopic disease.

Limb-sparing surgery involves resection of the primary tumor with adequate margins of resection, which is followed by reconstruction to yield a functional limb. With careful planning and selection of patients, it can be used in the majority of patients with extremity OS without jeopardizing long-term survival. When limb-sparing surgery is not possible or will result in an increased risk of local or distant disease recurrence, amputation is the procedure of choice. The complete tumor specimen is carefully evaluated for degree of necrosis after preoperative chemotherapy. Huvos has devised a frequently used grading system for preoperative tumor necrosis (Table 52-2) that has prognostic significance when used with limited preoperative chemotherapy (Fig. 52-1).

There is a well-defined role for both preoperative and adjuvant chemotherapy in the treatment of OS (Fig. 52-1). Active agents include doxorubicin, cisplatin, high-dose methotrexate, ifosfamide, bleomycin, and dactinomycin. In general, intensive combination chemotherapy is administered for several months before definitive surgery, and the same or a different combination of agents is administered postoperatively for a duration of 3 to 4 months. A chemotherapy scheme that shows typical dose-intensity of agents and timing of administration is presented in Figure 52-2.

OS of the axial skeleton (e.g., spinal and deep pelvic tumors) and tumors originating in the craniofacial bones may not be able to be completely resected; this applies to bulky pulmonary or hepatic metastases as well. Still, the treatment approach described above is used as possible with these tumor presentations. In general, radiation therapy plays a limited role in selected patients.

The lungs are the most common site of metastatic disease at initial presentation, as well as recurrent disease after definitive treatment of OS. The number of metastatic nodules per se is not a

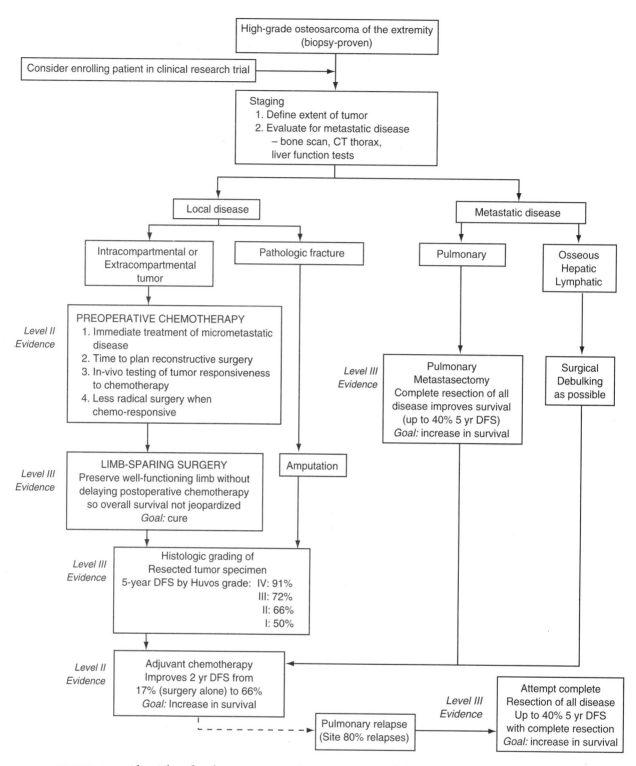

FIGURE 52-1 *Algorithm for the treatment of osteosarcoma of the extremity. The key reasoning principles for treating local disease are that preoperative chemotherapy will often allow limb-sparing surgery and provides early treatment of micrometastatic disease, while postoperative chemotherapy improves disease-free survival. For metastatic disease, basic principles are major surgical debulking followed by adjuvant chemotherapy to improve survival. The goal of an aggressive combined chemotherapy/surgical approach in local disease is cure. Prolongation of survival is the goal for aggressive treatment of metastatic disease. The levels of evidence supporting this algorithm are level II/III. Selected patients who present with pathologic fracture can have preoperative chemotherapy followed by limb-sparing surgery.*

TABLE 52-2 HUVOS SYSTEM FOR HISTOLOGIC GRADING OF EFFECT OF PREOPERATIVE CHEMOTHERAPY ON PRIMARY OSTEOSARCOMA

Grade	Effect
I	Little or no effect identified
II	Areas of acellular tumor osteoid, necrotic, and/or fibrotic material attributable to the effect of chemotherapy, with other areas of histologically viable tumor
III	Predominant areas of acellular tumor osteoid, necrotic, and/or fibrotic material attributable to the effect of chemotherapy, with only scattered foci of histologically viable tumor cells identified
IV	No histologic evidence of viable tumor identified within the entire specimen

(From Huvos AG et al: Arch Pathol Lab Med 101:14–18, 1977, with permission.)

contraindication to resection, and some patients have more than 30 nodules resected via bilateral thoracotomies. In some series, patients who are treated for pulmonary metastases have a 40% 5-year disease free survival when metastatic nodules can be completely resected.

PROGNOSIS

In large series of patients treated on multi-institutional protocols and some single institution protocols at cancer centers, the 5-year disease free survival for patients with **OS** is 60% to 65% (level of

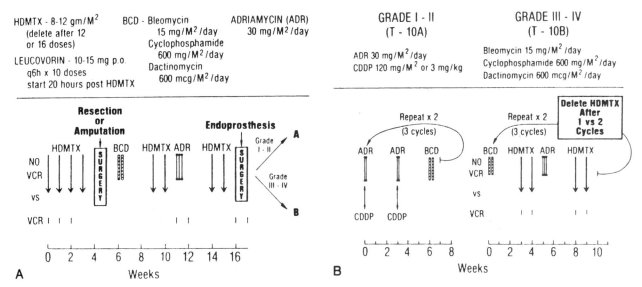

FIGURE 52-2 *The T-10 regimen from Memorial Sloan-Kettering Cancer Center. (A) All patients receive the initial 16-week regimen. The presurgical chemotherapy regimen features four weekly courses of high-dose methotrexate and leucovorin rescue followed by resection of amputation. Patients undergoing endoprosthetic replacement receive 16 weeks of presurgical chemotherapy. (B) Postoperative chemotherapy is determined by the histologic grade of response of the primary tumor to presurgical chemotherapy. Patients achieving an unfavorable response in the primary tumor (grades I and II) receive T-10A regimen postoperatively, featuring doxorubicin, cisplatin, and the bleomycin–cyclophopsphamide–dactinomycin (BCD) combination. Patients achieving a favorable response (grades III and IV) receive the T-10B regimen postoperatively and continue to receive high-dose methotrexate with doxorubicin and the BCD combination. (See Appendix 34 for detailed orders.) (From Malawer MM, Link MP, Donaldson SS: Sarcomas of bone 1528. Devita VT Jr, Hellmans, Rosenberg SA [eds]: Cancer: Principles and Practice of Oncology. JB Lippincott, Philadelphia, 1993 with permission.)*

evidence II and III). Improved 5-year disease free survival, in the range of 75%, is seen in younger patients who have extremity tumors. Patients who present with metastatic disease as a group have an extremely poor prognosis, with a 10% to 15% 5-year disease-free survival. Patients in this group do best when there is aggressive surgical resection of all macroscopic metastatic disease.

SUGGESTED READINGS

Goorin AM, Delorey MJ, Lack EE et al: Prognostic significance of complete surgical resection of pulmonary metastases in patients with osteogenic sarcoma: analysis of 32 patients. J Clin Oncol 2:425–431, 1984

Huvos AG: Bone Tumors: Diagnosis, Treatment and Prognosis. WB Saunders, Philadelphia, 1991

Huvos AG, Rosen G, Marcove RC: Primary osteogenic sarcoma. Pathologic aspects in 20 patients after treatment with chemotherapy, en bloc resection and prosthetic bone replacement. Arch Pathol Lab Med 101:14–18, 1977

Link MP, Goorin AM, Miser AW et al: The effect of adjuvant chemotherapy on relapse-free survival in osteosarcoma of the extremity. N Engl J Med 314:1600–1606, 1986

Meyers PA, Heller G, Healey JH et al: Chemotherapy for non-metastatic osteogenic sarcoma: the Memorial Sloan-Kettering Experience. J Clin Oncol 10:5–15, 1992

Meyers PA: Malignant bone tumors in children: osteosarcoma. Hem/Oncol Clin North 1:655–665, 1987

Meyers PA, Heller G, Healey JH et al: Osteogenic sarcoma with clinically detectable metastasis at initial presentation. J Clin Oncol 11:449–453, 1993

Mirra JM, Picci P, Gold RH: Bone Tumors: Clinical, Radiologic and Pathologic Correlations. Lea & Febiger, Philadelphia, 1989

Provisor A, Nachman J, Krailo M, Ettinger L, Hammond D: Treatment of non-metastatic osteosarcoma of the extremities with pre- and post-operative chemotherapy. Pro Am Soc Clin Oncol 6:217, 1987

Rosen G, Forscher CA, Eilber FR, Eckhardt JJ, Fu Y: Osteosarcomas. In Haskell CM, Berek JS (eds): Cancer Treatment. WB Saunders, Philadelphia, 1995

Stark A, Krieberg S, Nilsonne U, Silversward C: The age of osteosarcoma patients is increasing. An epidemiological study of osteosarcoma in Sweden 1971 to 1984. J Bone Joint Surg 72(B):89–93, 1990

53 Nutritional Support for the Cancer Patient

Ellen Gesser

Gerry Sheehan

Malnutrition is a common finding in oncology patients, with progressive weight loss and depletion of body tissues present in up to 87% of all patients. Many patients present with malnutrition at the time of diagnosis, however, extensive and progressive depletion of nutritional reserves is even more prevalent after multimodality therapy.

Despite the overwhelming evidence of nutritional deficiency, specific nutritional interventions are often ignored until severe malnutrition is evident, thus diminishing response to therapy, quality of life, and overall survival. Weight loss itself has been shown to be an important predictor of survival, independent of tumor type or stage of disease, and precludes the impact of therapy for some types of cancer. A weight loss of 6% or more from usual body weight is a significant negative prognostic factor for survival. In cooperative chemotherapy trials, the apparent effect of weight loss at initial diagnosis on median survival for certain common cancers was greater than the impact of chemotherapy. Malnutrition further complicates survival with concomitant muscle wasting, susceptibility to pulmonary complications, and decreased immunologic reactivity with susceptibility to infection. In cancer-related malnutrition, data suggests that metabolic abnormalities and responses interfere with the normal response to undernutrition and therefore accelerate the development of severe nutrition deficit. Cella et al. have shown that with appropriate nutrition therapy, it is possible to influence quality of life, provide a sense of well being, and control and improve functional status.

Improved clinical effect is demonstrable both in patients who are already malnourished and in those at high risk of malnutrition through prolonged anorexia and gastrointestinal (GI) dysfunction. Since malnutrition is certainly related to the underlying disease and disease progression, the appropriate intervention outcome should be defined as it relates to survival opportunity, quality of life, and tolerance to potentially beneficial medical therapies.

NUTRITIONAL ASSESSMENT AND EVALUATION

The effectiveness of nutrition interventions is contingent upon *early nutritional assessment and ongoing evaluation*. With weight loss as an important predictor of survival and treatment tolerance, assessment of nutritional status should be a routine part of the initial and ongoing oncology evaluation, particularly in cancers of the esophagus, pancreas, stomach, lung, non-Hodgkin's lymphoma, and colonic and prostate cancers in which the highest prevalence of weight loss has been documented.

Attention to early deficits related to depression, diagnostic tests, mild anorexia, and taste changes can be most easily addressed using calorie-dense foods and fluids in the context of the individual's usual eating plan. Thus, it is prudent to initiate assessment at the time of diagnosis and in conjunction with the overall treatment plan and follow-up.

Nutrition evaluation consists of a thorough nutritional history including present symptoms affecting oral intake, food records, and a gross calculation of calorie and nutrient needs based on weight, activity and stress factors, clinical treatment plan, prognosis, and therapeutic goals. It is essential to quantify oral intake *to compare assessed nutritional needs with the actual intake*. Table 53-1 lists the ideal body weights (IBW) for adults. Tables 53-2 and 53-3 show the composition for common foods. These tables can aid in assessing a patient's actual intake of nutrients and in

TABLE 53-1 IDEAL BODY WEIGHTS[a] **(IN POUNDS**[b]**)**

Females				Males			
Height (feet, inch)	Height[c] (inches)	Range	Mean	Height(feet, inch)	Height (inch)	Range	Mean
4'6"	54	76–94	85	5'0"	60	95–117	106
4'7"	55	79–97	88	5'1"	61	101–123	112
4'8"	56	81–99	90	5'2"	62	106–130	118
4'9"	57	84–102	93	5'3"	63	112–136	124
4'10"	58	85–105	95	5'4"	64	117–143	130
4'11"	59	88–108	98	5'5"	65	122–150	136
5'0"	60	90–110	100	5'6"	66	128–156	142
5'1"	61	94–116	105	5'7"	67	133–163	148
5'2"	62	99–121	110	5'8"	68	139–169	154
5'3"	63	103–127	115	5'9"	69	144–176	160
5'4"	64	108–132	120	5'10"	70	149–183	166
5'5"	65	112–138	125	5'11"	71	155–189	172
5'6"	66	117–143	130	6'0"	72	160–196	178
5'7"	67	121–149	135	6'1"	73	166–202	184
5'8"	68	126–154	140	6'2"	74	171–209	190
5'9"	69	130–160	145	6'3"	75	176–216	196
5'10"	70	135–165	150	6'4"	76	182–222	202
5'11"	71	139–171	155	6'5"	77	187–229	208
6'0"	72	144–176	160	6'6"	78	193–235	214
6'1"	73	148–182	165	6'7"	79	198–242	220
6'2"	74	153–187	170	6'8"	80	203–249	226

[a]*Based on Females: 100 lb for first 5 feet and 5 lb for each inch over 5 feet; males: 106 lb for first 5 feet and 6 lb for each inch over 5 feet. Subtract 2–1/2 lb for each inch under 5 feet.*

[b]*kg = lb 2.2*

[c]*1 inch = 2.5 cm.*

comparing this with the patient's needs (see Appendix 35 for examples). Additional parameters to be evaluated include changes in serum albumin concentration, relation of present weight to IBW, and nonvolitional weight loss. The resulting nutrition-support plan reflects nutritional status, the sufficiency of oral intake and tolerance, and the presence or degree of GI function.

TABLE 53-2 FOOD COMPOSITION BY GENERAL FOOD CATEGORY

Food Category	Carbohydrate (g)	Protein (g)	Fat (g)	Calories
Starch/bread, 1 serving or approximately ½ c	15	3	trace	80
Meat, per oz, before added fat or breading				
Lean	—	7	3	55
Medium-fat	—	7	5	75
High-fat	—	7	8	100
Vegetable, ½ c nonstarchy veg or veg juice	5	2	—	25
Fruit or fruit juice, approximately, ½ c	15	—	—	60
Milk, 1c (8 oz)				
Skim	12	8	trace	90
Lowfat	12	8	5	120
Whole	12	8	8	150
Fat (1 tsp oil or margarine, approximately 2 tsp salad dressings, or 1 strip bacon)	—	—	5	45

Abbreviations: c, cup; veg, vegetable.

(Data from the American Diabetes Association and the American Dietetic Association.)

ORAL NUTRITION

Oral nutrition is certainly the preferred route to achieve nutritional homeostasis. Often overlooked, it can be extremely helpful in the early stages of diagnosis. As nutrition is one aspect of care over which the patient has influence, a plan of oral nutrition offers the individual the opportunity to participate positively in his on her own care. Assessed deficits of 300 calories or less, in our experience, respond best to dietary manipulation. Patients require instruction to maximize caloric intake in their food selection and preparation.

Popular, contemporary *low-fat, low-calorie cancer prevention regimens are contraindicated in patients with weight loss*. Rather, these patients benefit from low-volume, frequent feedings with calorie laden foods and fluids. The usefulness of oral supplements is contingent upon calorie contribution relative to nutritional deficits and volume tolerance. Products contributing 1 kcal/cc or less are often unable to be consumed in sufficient volume to meet calorie deficits. Moreover, the cost of these products given 3 to 4 times per day may be prohibitive as well as restrictive to the purchase of other items tolerated in the diet. Utility of supplements providing 1.5 to 2.0 calories per cc is generally better, resulting in less volume and a lower cost per calorie. Five hundred calories can be delivered with the use of a 2 calorie/cc product given in four 60-cc doses. This medication approach results in better compliance and lower cost, particularly in patients who experience taste dysfunction and volume intolerance. Moreover, the use of 60 cc as a dose generally will not interfere with usual meal consumption (see Appendix 35).

ENTERAL FEEDING SUPPORT

Alternate enteral feeding should *be considered if the patient is unable to meet 60% of the estimated nutritional requirement* in voluntary oral feeding (Fig. 53-1). The enteral feeding route should be used whenever the GI tract is functional and may include *nasogastric (NG), percutaneous endoscopic gastrostomy (PEG), or jejunostomy tube feedings*. Feeding tubes should be placed before treatment in patients in whom the need for nutritional support is predictable. PEG feeding is preferred over NG feeding for greater comfort and aesthetic appeal if support is likely to continue for more than several weeks. This is especially appropriate if the head and neck area is involved or there is increased risk for aspiration or patient removal of the NG tube.

Enteral support may be partial or total depending on the individualized needs of the patient (Fig. 53-2). Types of formulas for enteral nutrition support may be categorized as follows (Table 53-4 and Appendix 35):

Lactose-free formulas are indicated in lactose-intolerant patients, such as those with compromised GI function or those receiving *pelvic or abdominal radiation therapy*. There is also an increased incidence of lactose intolerance among the non-Caucasian population.

Calorically dense or high-protein formulas are indicated for patients with calorie or protein deficits, increased requirements, or low-volume tolerance.

Fiber-containing formulas promote normal bowel function in patients with either a tendency for frequent loose bowel movements or constipation by promoting a softer, bulkier stool. These formulas also offer the benefit of the inclusion of fiber for maintenance of bowel function in long-term total tube feeding.

Elemental formulas are indicated for some postsurgical or radiation patients with compromised gut function, who do not tolerate intact macronutrient composition.

Oncology patients require approximately 30% above normal basal energy expenditure (BEE) and activity needs overall or an estimated 30 to 35 kcal/kg. Protein needs range from .8 to 1.5 gm/kg body weight based on protein requirement (.8–1.2 gm/kg for nonprotein-depleted patients and 1.2–1.5 gm/kg for repletion). Dosage of nutritional formulas needed depends on estimated patient requirement, oral deficit, and formula composition (see Table 53-4 and Appendix 35 for examples).

PARENTERAL FEEDING

When the GI tract is functionally impaired and there are clear therapeutic goals, parenteral nutrition should be used, either partial or total. Enteral, or transitional, feeding is also used, sometimes combined with parenteral feeding. Parenteral nutrition is indicated to sustain life and prevent deterioration and potentially life threatening complications of progressive malnutrition in GI-compromised patients with opportunity for cure or palliation. Total parenteral nutrition (TPN) is also used extensively in bone marrow transplantation (BMT) patients because of the severe anorexia, nausea, and mucositis they experience.

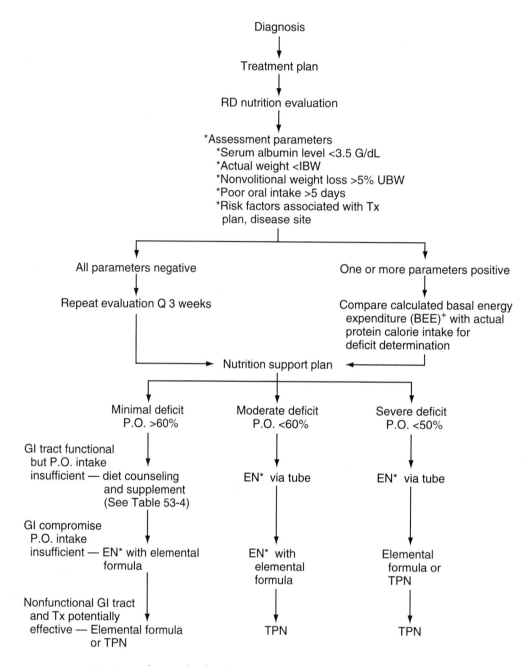

FIGURE 53-1 *Estimated or calculated energy and protein deficits in oncology patients exhibiting variable degrees of nutritional risk and requirement for nutrition support. (Guidelines formulated upon understanding of physiology of nutrition and not based on empirical trials.) (See also Appendix 35 for examples.) UBW, usual body weight; Ham's Benedict Equation: Male: BEE = 66 + (13.7 × W) + (5 × H) − (6.8 × A); Female: BEE = 655 + (9.6 × W) + (1.7 × H) − (4.7 × A): where W=weight in kg; H = height in cm; A = age in years; *Enteral Nutrition.*

Nutrition support continuum

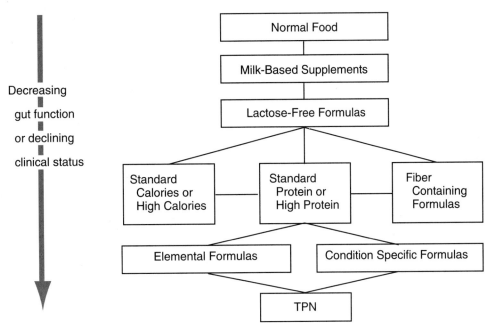

FIGURE 53-2 *Types of nutritional support required based on decreasing gastrointestinal function or clinical status. Recommendations formulated upon understanding of physiology of nutrition and are not based on empirical studies (See Appendix 35 and Table 53-4 for examples).*

TABLE 53-3 **FOOD COMPOSITION FOR COMMON FOODS**[a]

	Amount	Calories	Protein (g)	Fat (g)	CHO (g)	Ca (mg)	Na (mg)	K (mg)
Angel cake	1 sec(½ of 10 inch ck)	110	3	tr	24	4	113	35
Beer, average	1 12 oz bottle	147	1		12	17	24	87
Bouillon cubes	1 cube	3	.7		tr		840	3
Brandy, cognac	1 brandy glass (1 oz)	73						
Brownie with nuts	½ × 1½ × ⅞ inch	138	2	9	15	12	45	53
Cake, plain, no icing	3 × 2 × 1½ inch	200	2	8	31	35	165	44
Cake, plain, white icing	3 × 2 × 1¼ inch	290	4.0	10	46	36	175	45
Cake, chocolate chocolate icing	1-inch section (1/16 of 10 inch)	445	5	20	67	84	282	185
Cake, sponge	2-section (8 inch diameter)	120	3	2	22	12	67	35
Cupcake, chocolate, fudge icing	1	327	3	11	54			
Cupcake, plain, chocolate icing	2¾ inch diameter	185	2	7	30	32	115	57
Candy, caramels	1	41	1		8			
Candy, chocolate mint	1 small	37		1	7			
Candy, fudge	1 oz	115	1	3	21	22	53	41
Candy, hard	1 oz	110	0	tr	28	6	13	1.2
Candy, milk chocolate, sweetened	1 oz	162	2	10	16	76	32	128
Candy bar, average	3 oz	115	3	5	16.2	42	42	74

(Continues)

TABLE 53-3 *Continued*

	Amount	Calories	Protein (g)	Fat (g)	CHO (g)	Ca (mg)	Na (mg)	K (mg)
Cheese, American	1 oz	107	7	8	2	190	Var.	Var.
Cheese, swiss	1 oz	118	8	8	.5	295	389	34
Chocolate syrup	1 tablespoon	50	tr	tr	13	3	10	56
Coca-Cola, bottle	7 oz	92			23			
Cocoa, with milk	1 cup	235	9	11	26	286	123	351
Cookie, oatmeal[b]	One 3-inch diameter	63	3.9	2	10	3	23	52
Cookie, sugar[b]	One 3-inch diameter	89	1	3	13.6	16	64	15
Cookie, chocolate sandwich	1	49	.4	2	7	2	48	4
Cracker, Graham	3	96	2	2	18	22	126	67
Cracker, saltine	3	43	4.5	2	7	2	110	12
Cordials, liqueurs[b]	1 cordial glass (20 g)	74			7			
Custard, baked	1 cup	285	13	14	28	278	196	362
Daiquiri[b]	1 cocktail (100 g)	122	.1		5.2	4		
Doughnut, cake type	1	125	1	6	16	13	160	29
Gin	1 jigger	124			tr			
Gingerale	7 oz	70			18			
Hamburger in bun	1 (2 oz meat)	345	18	14	15	28	182	328
Hotdog in bun	1	251	9	15	18	NA	NA	NA
Ice cream, vanilla	½ cup	145	3	9	15	87	28	78
Ice milk	1 cup	285	9	10	42	292	127	365
Jams	1 tablespoon	55	tr	tr	14	4	2.4	18
Jellies	1 tablespoon	55	tr	tr	14	4	3.4	15
Jello	1 cup	140	4	0	34		122	
Lemonade	1 cup	110	tr	tr	28	2	tr	40
Malted milk	1 cup	280	13	12	32	364	246	540
Marshmallows	1 oz	90	1	tr	23	5	11	2
Martini[b]	1 cocktail (3½ oz)	140	.1	.3		5		
Milk, chocolate	1 oz	150	2	9	16	65	26	107
Milk shake, chocolate	1½ cups	421	11.2	17	58	363	194	433
Olives, ripe or green[b]	2 medium	13	.2	1	.4	9	240	6
Pickles, dill	1 large 4 × 1¾ inch	15	1	tr	3	35	1928	270
Pickles, sweet	1 (2¾ × ¾ inch)	30	tr	tr	7	2		
Pie, apple	⅐ of 9-inch pie	345	3	15	51	11	406	108
Pie, cherry	⅐ of 9-inch pie	355	4	15	52	19	410	142
Pie, chocolate cream	⅛ of med. pie	428	7.2	18	49	103	384	208
Pie, lemon meringue	⅐ of 9-inch pie	305	4	12	45	17	338	60
Pie, pumpkin	⅐ of 9-inch pie	275	5	15	32	66	278	208
Pizza, cheese	⅛ of 14 inch	185	7	6	27	107	527	98
Popcorn with oil	1 cup	65	1	3	8	1	Var.	
Potato chips	10 chips	115	1	8	10	8	Var.	226
Pretzel, small stick	5 sticks	20	tr	tr	4	1	Var.	6.5
Pudding, chocolate	½ cup	185	4	6	32	120	70	214
Pudding, rice with raisins	1 cup	365	9	8	67	245	178	443
Pudding, tapioca	1 cup	335	13	13	43	263	390	338
Rum	1 jigger (1½ oz)	133			tr			
Rye wafers	2	45	2	tr	10	7	115	78
Sandwich, roast beef-lettuce	1 (2 oz meat)	347	18	19	20	48	242	267
Sandwich, cheese-lettuce	1 (1 oz cheese)	223	10.4	9	22	204	Var.	Var.
Sherbet	1/2 cup	130	1	1	30	15	10	43
Sherry	1 sherry glass	38			2			
Seven-up	1 cup	97	0	0	24			
Spaghetti, meat	1 cup	335	19	12	39	125	1018	670

(Continues)

TABLE 53-3 *Continued*

	Amount	Calories	Protein (g)	Fat (g)	Cho (g)	CA (mg)	NA (mg)	K (mg)
Spaghetti, cheese	1 cup	260	9	9	37	80	955	408
Sugar, white	1 tablespoon	45	0	0	12	0	neg	neg
Sugar, powdered	1 tablespoon	30	0	0	8	0	neg	neg
Soup, bean with pork	1 cup	170	8	6	22	62	1008	395
Soup, beef noodle	1 cup	70	4	3	7	8	955	80
Beef bouillon, consomme	1 cup	30	5	0	3	tr	782	130
Soup, chicken noodle	1 cup	65	4	2	8	10	1020	58
Soup, clam chowder	1 cup	85	2	3	13	36	977	191
Soup, mushroom with water	1 cup	135	2	10	10	41	955	98
Soup, minestrone	1 cup	105	5	3	14	37	995	314
Soup, green pea	1 cup	130	6	2	23	44	899	196
Soup, tomato	1 cup	90	2	2	16	15	970	230
Soup, vegetable with beef	1 cup	80	3	2	14	20	863	245
Tom Collins[b]	1 cocktail (10 oz)	180.3			9	6		
Tomato catsup	1 tablespoon	15	tr	tr	4	4	177	62
Whiskey	1 jigger (1.5 oz)	133						
Wine, California red	1 wine glass (3 oz)	27			1.4	3	1.6	30
Wine, champagne, domestic[b]	1 wine glass (4 oz)	84.2			3.0			
Wine, port	1 wine glass (3 oz)	45			2.5	3	1	25
Wine, French vermouth[b]	1 wine glass (3.5 oz)	105			1.0			
Waffles	0.5 × 5.5 × 4.5 inch	210	7	7	28	85	355	109
Yogurt	1 cup	120	8	4	13	295	126	352

[a] All food values except those denoted by superscript b are taken from Watt BK, Merrill AL: *Composition of Foods Raw, Processed, Prepared, Revised USDA Agricultural Handbook No. 8, 1963,* or from *Nutritive Value of Foods. Revised. USDA Home and Garden Bulletin No. 72. 1964.*

[b] Data from Church CF, Church HN: *Food Values of Portions Commonly Used, Bowes and Church. 12th Ed.* Lippinocott-Raven, Philadelphia, 1975.

NUTRITIONAL REQUIREMENTS FOR TPN

The following facts are useful when initiating TPN (see also Table 53-5 and Appendix 35):

CARBOHYDRATE (CHO) REQUIREMENT

Dextrose = 3.4 kcal/g optimal amount for nitrogen retention, 2.5 to 4.0 mg/kg/min (or 0.4–1.4 g/kg/hr). In a 70-kg man, this would be 252 to 401 g of carbohydrate or 857 to 1,371 kcal/day. The remainder of calories needed would be provided as lipid.

Minimum of 100 to 150 g required daily to spare protein

Usually 100 to 150 nonprotein carbohydrate calories (NPC) per g nitrogen infused (1 g nitrogen = 6.25 g protein)

Maximum oxidative capacity, 5 to 7 mg/kg/min

The amount of dextrose and administration time should be adjusted as required. For example 7 mg/kg/min is equal to 706 g CHO or 2400 kcals (in a 70 kg man) and might be appropriate in a patient in whom lipids are contraindicated.

One should be careful to limit CHO to 180 to 200 g to initiate TPN in a diabetic patient. As stable blood sugar is demonstrated, CHO may be increased in 50 g/d increments to desired amount.

If insulin is required to control hyperglycemia, do not exceed 40 to 50 units regular insulin per liter.

PROTEIN REQUIREMENT

Maintenance	(1.2 g/kg)
Anabolic	(1.5 g/kg)

Protein needs vary up to 2.5 g/kg IBW for patients receiving anticancer therapy, protein-losing enteropathy, hypermetabolism, and extreme wasting.

FAT REQUIREMENT

Four to ten percent of daily NPC should be from lipids to prevent essential fatty acid deficiency (EFAD) (i.e., minimum of 1–3 bottles of 500 mL 10% lipids weekly).

TABLE 53-4 ENTERAL NUTRITION SUPPORT FORMULAS NUTRITIONAL ANALYSIS (NUTRIENTS/1000 mL)

Product	Cal/mL	Vol. for 100% U.S. RDA (mL)	Osmolality mOsm/Kg H₂O	Protein (g)	Fat (g)	Carbo-hydrate (g)	Dietary Fiber (g)	Sodium (mEg)	Sodium (mg)	Potassium (mEq)	Potassium (mg)
Lactose containing											
Meritene[a]	0.96	1250	510/570	58	32	110		38	880	41	1600
Meritine Powder[a,d]	1.06	1040	690	69	34	119		48	1100	72	2800
Carnation Inst. Bkf.[a]	1.0	a	N/A	61	32	144		44	1020	76	2960
Nutrashake[a]	1.67	a	N/A	50	50	258		20	458	47	1850
Intact protein, lactose-free											
Nutren 1.0 (vanilla)	1.0	1500	340	40	38	127		22	500	32	1252
Ensure[a]	1.06	1890	470	37	37	145		37	850	40	1560
Sustacal[a]	1.01	1060	650/690[a]	61	23	140		40	930	54	2100
Osmolite	1.06	1890	300	37	38	145		27	630	26	1010
Isocal	1.06	1890	270	34	44	135		23	530	34	1320
Resource Liquid[a]	1.06	1890	430	37	37	145		29	670	29	1140
Intact protein, lactose-free, high protein											
Osmolite HN	1.06	1320	300	44	37	141		40	930	40	1570
Jevity	1.06	1320	310	44	37	152	14.4	40	930	40	1560
Sustacal[a]	1.01	1060	650/690[c]	61	23	140		40	930	54	2100
Ensure HN[a]	1.06	1320	470	44	36	141		40	930	40	1560
Ensure Plus HN[a]	1.5	950	650	63	50	200		51	1180	47	1820
Replete	1.0	1500	350	63	34	113		22	500	40	1560
Promote	1.0	1000	350	62	26	130		40	928	51	1980
Intact protein, lactose-free, calorically dense											
Nutren 1.5	1.5	1000	410	60	68	169		33	752	64	2500
Nutren 2.0	2.0	750	710	80	106	196		44	1000	48	1872
Ensure Plus[a]	1.5	1420	690	55	53	200		50	1140	54	2100
Sustacal Plus[a]	1.52	1180	670	61	58	190		37	850	38	1480
Resource Plus[a]	1.5	1600	600	55	53	200		39	900	45	1730
Two Cal HN	2.0	950	690	84	91	220		46	1060	59	2300
Deliver 2.0	2.0	1000	640	75	102	200		35	800	43	1700
Magnacal	2.0	1000	590	70	80	250		43	1000	32	1250
Intact protein, lactose-free, high fiber											
Jevity	1.06	1320	310	44	37	152	14.4	40	930	40	1560
Nutren 1.0 with fiber	1.0	1500	373	40	38	127	14	22	500	32	1252
Ensure with fiber[a]	1.1	1390	480	40	37	162	14.4	37	840	43	1690
Ultracal	1.06	1180	310	44	45	123	14.4	40	930	41	1610
Replete with fiber	1.0	1000	300	63	34	113	14	22	500	40	1560
Promote with fiber	1.0	1000	370	63	28	139	14	57	1300	51	1980
Elemental											
Peptamen	1.0	2000	260	40	39	127		22	500	32	1250
Vivonex TEN	1.0	2000	630	38	2.8	210		20	460	20	780
Reabilan HN	1.33	1875	490	58	52	158		44	1000	42	1661
Vital HN	1.0	1500	500	42	10.8	185		20	470	34	1330

Abbreviation: N/A, not available; RTU, ready to use.

[a] Not preferred for tube feeding because of low micronutrient profile, higher sucrose, content, or hyperosmolality.

[b] 8 fl. oz = 240 ml.

[c] Osmolality of chocolate flavor.

[d] Meritene powder analysis when mixed with whole milk.

NOTE: Figures have been rounded.

H_2O (mL)	Calcium (mg)	Phosphorus (mg)	Magnesium (mg)	Form/How Supplied[b]	Product Description
850	1200	1200	320	RTU, 250-mL can	Protein, vitamin, mineral food
N/A	2200	1900	390	Powder, 1- & 4.5-lb. cans	Protein, vitamin, mineral food
N/A	1964	1632	452	Powder, 6–1.26 oz pkts	Calorie, protein food
N/A	1533	1533	200	RTU, 4-fl oz carton	Calorie, protein food
852	700	700	340	RTU, 250 ml can	Liquid nutrition
850	530	530	210	RTU, 8-fl oz, 32-fl oz bottle & can, quart can powder, 14-oz can	Liquid nutrition
840	1010	930	380	RTU, 8-, 12,- & 32-fl oz cans	Nutritionally complete liquid food
840	530	530	210	RTU, 8-fl oz bottle & can, 32-fl oz bottle & can	Isotonic liquid nutrition
840	630	530	210	RTU, 8-fl oz bottle, 8-, 12-&32-fl oz cans	Isotonic, complete liquid diet for tube feeding
N/A	550	550	210	RTU, 8-fl oz Tetra Pak	Nutritionally complete liquid food
840	760	760	300	RTU, 8-fl oz bottle & can, 32-fl oz can & bottle	High nitrogen isotonic liquid nutrition
830	910	760	300	RTU, 8-fl oz can, 32-fl oz bottle	Isotonic liquid nutrition with fiber
840	1010	930	380	RTU, 8-, 12,- & 32-fl oz can	Nutritionally complete liquid food
840	760	760	300	RTU, 8-fl oz, 32-fl oz cans	High-nitrogen liquid nutrition
770	1060	1060	420	RTU, 8-fl oz can	High-calorie, high-nitrogen liquid nutrition
860	1000	1000	400	RTU, 250 ml can	High-protein liquid nutrition
837	1200	1200	400	RTU, 8-fl oz can	High-protein liquid nutrition
776	1050	1050	510	RTU, 250 ml can	High-calorie nutritionally complete liquid food
700	1400	1400	680	RTU, 250 ml can	High-calorie nutritionally complete liquid food
770	710	710	280	RTU, 8-fl oz bottle & can, 32-fl oz can	High-calorie liquid nutrition
780	850	850	340	RTU, 8-fl oz can	High-calorie, nutritionally complete liquid food
NA	630	630	320	RTU, 8-fl oz Tetra Pak	High-calorie, nutritionally complete liquid food
710	1060	1060	420	Liquid, 8-fl oz can	High-calorie, high-nitrogen liquid nutrition
710	1000	1000	400	RTU, 8-fl oz can	High-calorie & nitrogen, nutritionally complete liquid diet for tube feeding
690	1000	1000	400	RTU, 120-mL bottle, 250-mL bottle, 250-mL can	High-calorie, nutritionally complete liquid food
830	910	760	300	RTU, 8-fl can, 32-fl oz bottle	Isotonic liquid nutrition with fiber
840	700	700	340	RTU, 250 mL can	Liquid nutrition with fiber
830	720	720	290	RTU, 8-fl oz, 32-fl oz can	Liquid nutrition with fiber
850	850	850	340	RTU, 8-fl oz can	Nutritionally complete liquid food with oat & soy fiber
836	1000	1000	400	RTU, 250 mL can	High protein nutritionally complete liquid food with fiber
830	1200	1200	400	RTU, 8-fl oz can	High protein nutritionally complete liquid food with fiber
850	600	500	300	RTU, 250 & 500-mL can	Liquid, isotonic, complete, semi-elemental diet
860	500	500	200	Powder, 80.4-g packet	Elemental high-nitrogen/high-BCAA Diet
800	451	500	330	RTU, 375 mL can	Semi-elementally high nitrogen complete liquid diet
870	870	670	270	Powder, 2.79-oz packets	Nutritionally complete partially hydrolyzed diet

TABLE 53-5 BASIC FORMULATION OF STANDARD TPN COMPONENTS IN A LITER OF STANDARD TPN

Routine Additives	Recommended adult-24-hr requirement
$D_{50}W^a$ (Final concentration 25%)	500 mL
8.5% Amino Acid[a] (Final concentration 4.25%)	500 mL
Sodium Chloride[b]	0–130 mEq (Sodium 60–125 mEq)
Sodium Phosphate[c]	0–20 mM (Phosphate 9–40 mM)
Potassium Chloride[d]	0–40 mEq (Chloride 40–229 mEq)
Magnesium Sulfate[e]	8–12 mEq (Magnesium 10–30 mEq)
Ca Gluconate[e,f]	4.5 or 9.0 mEq (Calcium 9–30 mEq)
MVI-12	10 mL
Multitrace[g]	5 mL
Optional Additives	
Sodium Acetate[b]	0–130 mEq
Potassium Acetate[d]	0–40 mEq (Potassium 60–180 mEq)
H_2 Antagonist[h]	See footnote
Regular Insulin[i]	0–40 units[h]
Vitamin K	10 mg twice weekly (2–4 mg/wk minimum)

ADMINISTRATION SCHEDULE FOR STANDARD TPN

Day of Therapy	Rate (mL/hr)
1	40
2	80
3	100–125[j]

FAT EMULSION INFUSION SCHEDULE

Infuse a 20% fat emulsion 500 mL intravenously per pump over a minimum of 8 hours at least 3 times per week via either an 18 gauge peripheral intravenous cannula or piggyback per the central infusion catheter.

[a] *The solution should be formulated to deliver 100–150 nonprotein carbohydrate calories per gram of nitrogen infused.*

[b] *Add sodium chloride if the serum CO_2 > 25m Eq/L. Add sodium acetate if the serum CO_2 ≤ 25mEq/L.*

[c] *The total phosphate dosage should not exceed 20 mM per liter or 60 mM daily.*

[d] *Add KCl if the serum CO_2 > 25 mEq/L. Add K Acetate if the serum CO_2 ≤ 25 mEq/L. The potassium dosage should not exceed 40 mEq per liter.*

[e] *Added to each liter.*

[f] *Add calcium gluconate 9 mEq to each liter if the serum calcium < 8.5 mEq/L. Add 4.5 mEq if the serum calcium ≥ 8.5 mEq/L.*

[g] *Administered in only one liter per day.*

[h] *Dosage variable. Consult the Physician's Desk Reference and add an equal dose to each liter.*

[i] *Total dosage should not exceed 40 units per liter.*

[j] *The final infusion rate depends on the patient's calculated daily caloric and protein requirements and overall cardiovascular status.*

(Modified from Hickey MS: Basic Guidelines for Nutritional Assessment, Enteral, Parenteral and AIDS Nutritional Therapy. Clintec, Deerfield, IL, 1992, with permission.)

TABLE 53-6   METHOD FOR TAPERING A STANDARD TPN INFUSION^a

An NPO patient or a patient consuming inadequate calories enterally may develop "rebound" hypoglycemia if the TPN infusion is suddenly discontinued. This potential problem can easily be avoided by immediately infusing $D_{10}NS$ at the same TPN infusion rate^a either via the TPN catheter or a peripheral intravenous cannula. Ideally, a TPN infusion should be tapered (gradually decreased) before discontinuing the infusion to prevent the possibility of "rebound" hypoglycemia. The actual taper schedule for a TPN infusion depends on the pretaper TPN infusion rate. An example taper schedule for an NPO patient receiving a pretaper TPN infusion rate of 125 mL/hour is listed below:

↓TPN infusion rate to 80 mL/hour and begin a simultaneous $D_{10}NS$ peripheral infusion at 40 mL/hour for 2 hours per pump

then

↓TPN infusion to 40 mL/hour and ↑$D_{10}NS$ peripheral infusion to 80 mL/hour for 2 hours per pump

then

Discontinue the TPN infusion, begin a $D_{10}NS$ infusion at 125 mL/hour per pump via the TPN catheter, and simultaneously discontinue the peripheral $D_{10}NS$ infusion.

^{a} Note: A standard TPN infusion may be discontinued without the fear of "rebound" hypoglycemia if the patient has adequate oral caloric intake.

(From Hickey MS: Basic Guidelines for Nutritional Assessment, Enteral, Parenteral, and AIDS Nutritional Therapy. Clintec, Deerfield, IL,

TABLE 53-7   MANAGEMENT OF STANDARD TPN THERAPY INDUCED METABOLIC COMPLICATIONS

Complication	Treatment
Hyperglycemia (> 160 mg%)	Algorithms (1) Maintain the current TPN infusion rate and begin adding regular insulin to the TPN solution in 10-unit increments until the serum glucose is maintained at ≤ 160mg%. (*Note: The maximum allowable insulin dosage per liter of TPN is 40 units.*) Until the hyperglycemia is controlled by adding insulin to the TPN solution, simultaneously administer intravenous regular insulin. (*Note: 1 unit of regular insulin results in approximately a 10 mg% decrease in the serum glucose. The maximum single intravenous dose of regular insulin should not exceed 15 units.*) If the serum glucose remains > 160 mg% despite the addition of a total of 40 units of regular insulin per liter of TPN and intravenous regular insulin therapy *then* (2) Maintain the current TPN infusion rate but begin gradually decreasing the dextrose concentration of the TPN solution. (*Note: The lower limit for the final dextrose concentration is 15%.*) In addition, begin adding regular insulin to the TPN solution in 10-unit increments until the serum glucose is maintained at ≤ 160 mg% or the maximum allowable insulin dosage (40 units) is reached. Regular insulin should also be simultaneously administered intravenously as in #1 above until the hyperglycemia is controlled by adding insulin to the TPN solution. If the serum glucose remains > 160 mg% despite adding 40 units regular insulin per liter of TPN solution, decreasing the final TPN dextrose concentration to 15% and administering intravenous regular insulin therapy *then* (3) Restart the original TPN solution (#1 above) but begin decreasing the TPN infusion rate. Also begin insulin therapy as discussed in #2 above while simultaneously increasing the frequency of fat emulsion therapy from q Mon., Wed. and Fri. to either qod or daily to provide adequate caloric intake.
Hypoglycemia (< 70 mg%)	May occur with the sudden discontinuance of TPN infusion. If the TPN infusion administered to either an NPO patient or a patient consuming inadequate oral calories is suddenly discontinued, immediately begin an infusion of $D_{10}NS$ at the previous TPN infusion rate per either the TPN catheter or a peripheral intravenous line to prevent "rebound" hypoglycemia.
Hypernatremia (>145 mEq/L)	Determine the etiology for the hypernatremia. Hypernatremia 2°-secondary to dehydration is treated by administering additional "free water" and providing only the daily maintenance sodium requirements (90–150 mEq/L) per the TPN infusion. Hypernatremia secondary to increased sodium intake is treated by reducing or deleting sodium from the TPN solution and all other intravenous fluids until the serum sodium ≤ 145 mEq/L.

(Continues)

TABLE 53-7 *Continued*

Complication	Treatment
Hyponatremia (<135 mEq/L)	Determine the etiology for the hyponatremia. Hyponatremia secondary to dilution is treated by fluid restriction and providing only the daily maintenance sodium requirements (90–150 mEq/L) per the TPN solution until the serum sodium ≥ 135 mEq/L. Hyponatremia secondary to inadequate sodium intake is treated by increasing the sodium content of the TPN solution until the serum sodium ≥ 135 mEq/L. (*Note: The maximum sodium content per liter of TPN should not exceed 154 mEq*).
Hyperkalemia (>5 mEq/L)	Immediately discontinue the current TPN infusion containing potassium and begin an infusion of $D_{10}NS$ at the previous TPN infusion rate. Then reorder a new TPN solution without potassium and continue to delete potassium from the TPN solution and all other intravenous fluids until the serum potassium ≤5 mEq/L.
Hypokalemia (<3.5 mEq/L)	A TPN solution should not be used for the primary treatment of hypokalemia. The potassium content per liter of TPN solution *should not exceed 40 mEq*. If additional potassium is necessary, it should be administered via another route (e.g. intravenous interrupts).
Hyperphosphatemia (>4.5 mg%)	Immediately discontinue the present phosphate-containing TPN infusion and begin an infusion of $D_{10}NS$ at the previous TPN infusion rate. Then reorder a new TPN solution without phosphate and continue to delete phosphate from the TPN solution and all other intravenous fluids until the serum phosphate ≤ 4.5 mg%.
Hypophosphatemia (<2.5 mg%)	Increase the phosphate content of the TPN solution to a maximum of 20 mM per liter. (*Note: The total daily phosphate dosage should not exceed 60 mM.*)
Hypermagnesemia (>2.7 mg%)	Immediately discontinue the present magnesium-containing TPN infusion and begin an infusion of $D_{10}NS$ at the previous TPN infusion rate. Then reorder a new TPN solution without magnesium and continue to delete magnesium from the TPN solution and all other intravenous fluids until the serum magnesium ≤ 2.7 mg%.
Hypomagnesemia (<1.6 mg%)	Increase the magnesium content of the TPN solution to a maximum of 12 mEq per liter. (*Note: The total daily dosage of magnesium should not exceed 36 mEq.*)
Hypercalcemia (>10.5 mg%)	Immediately discontinue the present calcium-containing TPN infusion and begin an infusion of $D_{10}NS$ at the previous TPN infusion rate. Then reorder a new TPN solution without calcium and continue to delete calcium from the TPN solution and all other intravenous fluids until the serum calcium ≤ 10.5 mg%.
Hypocalcemia (<8.5 mg%)	Increase the calcium content of the TPN solution to a maximum of 9 mEq per liter. (*Note: The total daily calcium dosage should not exceed 27 mEq.*)
High serum zinc: (>150 mcg%)	Discontinue the trace metal supplement (Multitrace 5 mL) in the TPN solution until the serum zinc ≤ 150 mcg%.
Low serum zinc: (<55 mcg%)	Add elemental zinc 2–5 mg daily to one liter of TPN only until the serum zinc ≥ 55mcg% (*Note: The elemental zinc is added in addition to the daily Multritrace 5 mL.*)
High serum copper: (>140 mcg%)	Discontinue the trace metal supplement (Multitrace 5 mL) in the TPN solution until the serum copper ≤ 140 mcg%.
Low serum copper: (<70 mcg%)	Add elemental copper 2–5 mg daily to one liter of TPN only until the serum copper ≥ 70 mcg%. (*Note: The elemental copper is added in addition to the daily Multitrace 5 mL.*)
Hyperchloremic metabolic acidosis (CO_2<22 mM/L and Cl>110 mEq/L)	Reduce the chloride intake by administering the Na and K in the acetate form as either Na/K acetate until the acidosis resolves (serum CO_2 ≥ 22 mM/L) and the serum chloride level returns to normal (<110 mEq/L).
Hypoalbuminemia (<2.5 gm%)	May cause decreased gut absorption, peristalsis, and gastric emptying (controversial issue). If a nasointestinal enteral feeding is to be administered, then 25% albumin 25 g supplements may be added to each liter of TPN solution until the albumin deficit is replenished, as calculated per the Andrassy Formula[a] in an attempt to enhance enteral diet tolerance. The goal of albumin therapy is to increase the serum albumin to ≥ 2.5 g%. (*Note: Albumin replacement therapy should be discontinued once the serum albumin ≥ 2.5 gm%.*)

Abbreviations: Ad, albumin deficit; ASA, actual serum albumin.

[a] $AD = (2.5\text{-}ASA) \times 0.3 \times 10 \times w + kg.$

(Modified from Hickey MS: Basic Guidelines for Nutritional Assessment, Enteral, Parenteral and AIDS Nutritional Therapy. Clinter, Deerfield, IL, with permission.)

Maximum = 60% of NPC; l g lipid = 10 kcal

10% lipid contains 1.1 kcal/cc

20% lipid contains 2.0 kcal/cc

Note: The safe upper limit for triglycerides is 500 mg/dl; clearance monitored via baseline and follow-up laboratory evaluation.

FLUID REQUIREMENTS

Fluids should equal 30 to 35 cc/kg or 1 cc/kcal fed.

ELECTROLYTES

Sodium, potassium, magnesium, chloride, calcium, and phosphorus are added to TPN when it is the sole source of nutrition (see Appendix 35 and Table 53-5 for suggested ranges).

VITAMINS

Adult RDA supplied by 10 mL MVI-12 added daily: vitamins A, C, D, E, B_{12}, pyridoxine, thiamine, niacin, riboflavin, pantothenic acid, biotin, and folic acid.

Vitamin K is not included and should be provided at a minimum of 2 to 4 mg/week. Use of anti-coagulants, such as warfarin sodium (coumadin), should be avoided.

TRACE ELEMENTS

Trace elements are usually supplied by 1 vial MTE-4 (zinc, copper, chromium, and manganese) or MTE-5 (all of the above plus selenium) added daily.

Iodine becomes essential after a year on TPN. (It is usually not included in standard trace mineral formulas.)

Iron is not routinely administered, but is usually given intramuscularly or intravenously as iron dextran (Imferon) when indicated.

HEPARIN

Functions to help prevent TPN catheter sepsis and clotting.

Is not routinely necessary as an additive.

Is a lipid clearance facilitator.

MONITORING RECOMMENDATIONS FOR TPN

Laboratory parameters are monitored according to patient condition and formula adjustment. Inpatient laboratory values are usually monitored daily or every other day. Nonhospitalized patient laboratory values may be monitored twice a week (first week), then weekly for 1 month, and then gradually reduced. All patients on parenteral feeding should be monitored at least every 30 days. Additional laboratory parameters may be required in acutely ill patients.

The following are recommended tests:

Chemistry profile (comprehensive SMA-18/SMA-24 varies according to laboratory)

Electrolytes, BUN/creatinine, glucose

Minerals (magnesium, phosphorus, calcium)

Liver enzymes (alkaline phosphatase, bilirubin, AST)

Triglycerides (safe upper limit of 500 mg/dl)

Protein levels (albumin, transferrin), retinal-binding protein, pre-albumin)

CBC and protime should be done weekly in the first month, then once every month

In patients with increased electrolyte losses, a weekly comprehensive chemistry profile should be done with SMA-7 (electrolytes, glucose, creatinine, BUN) monitored between comprehensive weekly chemistry profiles

For cyclic TPN, blood glucose should be drawn via fingerstick one hour after infusion onset and completion

A morning weight should be checked daily until stable, then at least weekly. Weight gains/losses greater than 5 lbs/week are significant and should be evaluated including intake/output.

Vital signs should be monitored for patients on TPN. Temperatures should be checked daily in late afternoon (more often if elevated). Blood pressure, pulse, and respirations are checked daily until stable, then weekly.

Note that the above recommendations are based on established practice and not on empirical trials demonstrating the superiority of this monitoring regimen over other regimens. They are formulated upon our understanding of the physiology and dynamics of TPN. Other practitioners may use guidelines that are slightly different.

SUGGESTED READINGS

Bloch AS (ed): Nutritional Management of the Cancer Patient. Aspen, Rockville, Maryland, 1990

Bloch AS: Nutritional management of patients with dysphagia. Oncology Suppl 7:127, 1993

Bozzetti F: Review: Nutritional support in the adult cancer patient. Clin Nutrition 11:167, 1992

Cella DF, Bonomi AE, Leslie WT et al: Quality of life and nutritional well-being: measurement and relationship. Oncology Suppl 7:105, 1993

Dewys WD, Becc C, Lavin PT et al: Prognostic effect of weight loss prior to chemotherapy in cancer patients. Am J Med 69:491, 1980

Halpert CR, Zahyma D: Nutritional intervention in the oncologist's office: a team approach. Oncology Suppl 7:79, 1993

Heber D, Tchekmedyian NS: Nutritional assessment of the cancer patient in the office. Oncology Suppl 7:71, 1993

Hickey MS: Basic guidelines for nutritional assessment, enteral, parenteral and AIDS nutritional therapy. Clintec, Deerfield, IL, 1992

Kaminski MV: Parenteral Nutrition and Cancer Chemotherapy. Hematology-Oncology, letter V-5

Klein S: Clinical efficacy of nutritional support the in patient with cancer. Oncology Suppl 7:87, 1993

Lopez M: Nutritional support for the cancer patient. p. 218. In Schein PS: Decision Making in Oncology. BC Decker Inc, Philadelphia, 1989

McCrae JD: Assessment and nutrition management of the patient receiving home nutrition support. p. 30. In: Suggested Guidelines for Nutrition and Metabolic Management of Adult Patients Receiving Nutrition. Support. 2nd Ed. The American Dietetic Association, Chicago, 1993

Skipper A: Monitoring and complications of parenteral nutrition. p. 351. In: Dietitian's Handbook of Enteral and Parenteral Nutrition. ASPEN, Rockville, MP, 1989

Winkler MF, Lyson LK: Assessment and nutrition management of the patient receiving parenteral nutrition support. p. 24. In: Suggested Guidelines for Nutrition and Metabolic Management of Adult Patients Receiving Nutrition Support. 2nd Ed. The American Dietetic Association, Chicago, 1993

54 Prevention and Treatment of Nausea and Vomiting

M. Jane Nolte

Prevention of chemotherapy-induced emesis (CIE) is critical to the physical and emotional well-being of the cancer patient. Nausea and vomiting are the top concerns of oncology patients about to undergo chemotherapy treatment. Patients report a significant impact of CIE on daily function, including the ability to complete household tasks, enjoy meals, spend time with family and friends, and recreational activities. Appropriate management of CIE can therefore substantially enhance the quality of life of patients undergoing chemotherapy.

Three distinct types of CIE are described in the literature: acute, delayed, and anticipatory. *Acute emesis* is defined as onset within the immediate 24 hours of emetogenic chemotherapy administration. *Delayed emesis* is a syndrome of nausea and/or vomiting that begins approximately 24 hours after the administration of certain chemotherapy, most commonly described following high-dose cisplatin. *Anticipatory emesis* is a learned behavior that develops over time, generally developing in patients who experience acute or delayed emesis. Although the exact cause of chemotherapy-induced emesis has not been completely determined, different mechanisms appear to be involved in the pathophysiology of each type of emesis, and the treatment of each should therefore be chosen accordingly.

PREVALENCE/INCIDENCE

Certain patient-related factors are highly predictive of the ability to control emesis with antiemetic therapy. Male patients can be expected to achieve at least a 7% to 10% higher response rate as compared with female patients. In general, the older the patient the better the expected control rate. Age greater than 65 years may result in significant protection, whereas age less than 12 years represents a group difficult to control. Heavy alcohol consumption provides protection from CIE; however, the particular amount of alcohol required has not been determined.

Of greatest importance in predicting the incidence of CIE is the emetogenic potential of the chemotherapy agent or combination of agents being administered. A classification system for the emetogenic potential of individual chemotherapy agents in various doses is presented in Table 54-1. This table, which categorizes emetogenic potential of chemotherapy regimens into five classifications, is based on the percentage of patients who experience emesis if antiemetic prophylaxis was not administered. For combination chemotherapy regimens, an example algorithm is provided in Table 54-2 in which emetogenic level is determined by the most emetogenic agent in the combination, and the combination of agents increase the emetogenic level above that of any individual agent. Such a classification schema provides a framework for the development of antiemetic treatment recommendations for common chemotherapy regimens based on level of emetogenicity.

TREATMENT AND PROGNOSIS

The methodology to study antiemetic drugs was established by Gralla et al. in 1981, with an evaluation of intravenous metoclopramide for cisplatin-induced emesis. The clinical efficacy of antiemetic therapy for prevention of acute CIE is assessed by number of emetic episodes and degree of nausea within the immediate 24 hours after chemotherapy administration. Complete response is generally defined as no vomiting and mild nausea; in contrast, total control is defined as no nausea and no vomiting.

Metoclopramide was the first serotonin-receptor antagonist antiemetic, which when given in high doses blocks both dopamine and serotonin receptor sites. High-dose metoclopramide plus dex-

377

TABLE 54-1 EMETOGENIC POTENTIAL OF INDIVIDUAL CHEMOTHERAPY AGENTS

Class V—High (> 90%)

Carboplatin	≥ 1 gm/m²
Cisplatin	≥ 70 mg/m²
Cyclophosphamide	≥ 1000 mg/m²
Cytarabine	≥ 1 gm/m²
Carmustine	≥ 200 mg/m²
Dacarbazine	≥ 500 mg/m²
Ifosfamide	≥ 3 gm/m²
Lomustine	≥ 60 mg/m²
Mechlorethamine	
Melphalan	≥ 140 mg/m²
Streptozocin	
Thiotepa	(high dose)

Class IV—Moderate (60%–90%)

Carboplatin	500–< 1000 mg/m²
Cisplatin	< 70 mg/m²
Dacarbazine	< 500 mg/m²
Cyclophosphamide	≥ 750–< 1000 mg/m²
Cytarabine	250 mg/m²–1000 mg/m²
Carmustine	200 mg/m²
Daunorubicin	≥ 75 mg/m²
Doxorubicin	≥ 45 mg/m²
Ifosfamide	≥ 1200–< 3000 mg/m²
Lomustine	< 60 mg/m²
Methotrexate	≥ 1000 mg/m²
Procarbazine	100 mg/m²

Class III—Mild (30%–60%)

Carboplatin	< 300 mg/m²
Cisplatin	< 60 mg/m²
Methotrexate	250–< 1000 mg/m²
Doxorubicin	< 45 mg/m²
Cytarabine	20–< 250 mg/m²
Bleomycin	
Etoposide	
Ifosfamide	< 1200 mg/m²
Cyclophosphamide	< 750 mg/m²

Class II—Low (10%–30%)

Bleomycin	
Cytarabine	< 20 mg/m²
Doxorubicin	< 20 mg/m²
5-Fluorouracil	< 1000 mg/m²
Hydroxyurea	1000–6000 mg/m²
Mercaptopurine	100 mg/m²
Methotrexate	< 250 mg/m²
Mitomycin	
Mitoxantrone	10–14 mg/m²

Class I—Minimal (< 10%)

Asparaginase	
Busulfan	
Chlorambucil	
Cladribine	
Cyclophosphamide (PO)	
Docetaxel	
Floxuridine	
5-Fluorouracil	

(Continues)

TABLE 54-1 *(Continued)*

Interferon
Goserelin
Leuprolide
Paclitaxel
Pegaspergase
Thioguanine
Vincristine
Vinblastine
Vinorelbine

amethasone and lorazepam became the standard antiemetic regimen in patients receiving highly emetogenic chemotherapy. With the development of selective serotonin-antagonists, more specific treatment with fewer side effects and greater convenience became the standard. Studies comparing metoclopramide regimens with different serotonin antagonists have revealed either similar or superior efficacy for the later agents. *Ondansetron (Zofran) and granisetron (Kytril), the two serotonin antagonists currently approved for use in the United States, are now routinely used as first-line therapy in the prevention of acute emesis secondary to highly and moderately emetogenic chemotherapy.*

Combining dexamethasone with ondansetron or granisetron has been demonstrated in numerous studies to be superior in efficacy to either of these serotonin-receptor antagonists alone. Total control rates are improved by approximately 10% to 15%, with the greatest contribution in those patients at highest risk for emesis. Whenever possible, dexamethasone should be added to serotonin-antagonist therapy. Exceptions exist for chemotherapy protocols that specifically prohibit the use of steroids, or for protocols in which a steroid is already in use. Limited data are available regarding their use for mild (30% to 60% incidence) or low (10% to 30% incidence) emetogenic chemotherapy regimens, for which it appears prudent to use less expensive regimens of prochlorperazine and dexamethasone.

RATIONALE FOR ACUTE ANTIEMETIC REGIMEN SELECTION

Recommended antiemetic treatment regimens (Table 54-3) are based upon efficacy as reported in the literature (and summarized below), ease of administration schedule and route, and cost. If possible, an alternative regimen is included when oral therapy is not feasible or patient failure to the first-line regimen occurs. It is of utmost importance to use the most effective acute antiemetic regimen possible because poor control of emesis pre-

TABLE 54-2 GUIDELINES FOR DETERMINATION OF EMETOGENIC POTENTIAL OF CHEMOTHERAPY COMBINATION REGIMENS

1. Discount antineoplastic combinations in Class I.
2. Any number of Class II agents are considered only once.
3. Combining two agents in Class II and above increases the emetogenic potential of the combination one class higher than the most emetogenic agent in the combination. (Example: Low + Mild = Moderate; Mild + Moderate = High)
4. Combining three agents from Class III and above raises the emetogenic level two classes higher than the most emetogenic agent in the combination. Combining three agents in which two are from Class II, follow rule # 3. (Example: Low + Low + Mild = Moderate) (Example: Mild + Mild + Mild = High)

(Adapted from Hesketh P et al: J Clin Oncol 13:2117–2122, 1995, with permission.)

disposes the patient to anticipatory emesis and unsatisfactory results on subsequent chemotherapy courses. Generally, ondansetron and granisetron are considered to be therapeutically equivalent, and the decision for use of one agent over another for moderate to highly emetogenic chemotherapy is therefore based on cost.

Intravenous therapy Several comparative trials between intravenous (IV) ondansetron and granisetron have been conducted in European countries where approved doses of both drugs differ from doses approved for use in the United States. Results from a comparative trial between IV ondansetron and IV granisetron designed to assess these agents at Food and Drug Administration (FDA) approved

doses substantiate findings of earlier dose-ranging studies that showed comparable antiemetic efficacy between 10 μg/kg and 40 μg/kg doses of granisetron and demonstrate that a single 10 μg/kg dose of granisetron is as effective as three doses on ondansetron 0.15 mg/kg for moderate- and high-dose cisplatin-containing chemotherapy regimens.

While the minimally effective dose of granisetron of 10 μg/kg has been well defined as the optimal dose for moderate and highly emetogenic regimens, the minimally effective dose of ondansetron is less clear. An open-label study of variable-dose ondansetron assigned according to emetogenicity of the chemotherapy regimen in use demonstrated the maintenance of efficacy for highly, moderately, and mildly emetogenic

TABLE 54-3 SUGGESTED ANTIEMETIC REGIMENS BASED ON EMETOGENIC POTENTIAL OF CHEMOTHERAPY

Class	Incidence	First-Line Oral Therapy	If Unable to Take Oral	Evidence Level/Grade
V	High (> 90%)[a]	Granisetron 2 mg p.o. (II/B)[b] Dexamethasone 20 mg p.o.	Granisetron 10 μg/kg IV Dexamethasone 20 mg IV	(I/A)[b] OR Ondansetron 32 mg IV (I/A)[b] Dexamethasone 20 mg IV
IV	Moderate	Granisetron 2 mg p.o. (II/A)[b]	Granisetron 10 μg/kg IV	(I/A)[b] OR Ondansetron 24 mg IV (II/B)[b]
	(60%–90%)	Dexamethasone 20 mg p.o. OR Ondansetron 8 mg p.o. b.i.d. (II/A)[b] Dexamethasone 20 mg p.o.	Dexamethasone 20 mg IV	Dexamethasone 20 mg IV
III	Mild (30%–60%)	Prochlorperazine 15 mg b.i.d. (II/A)[b] Dexamethasone 20 mg p.o. W Dexamethasone 20 mg p.o. (II/A)[b]	Ondansetron 8 mg IV Dexamethasone 20 mg IV	(II/B)[b]
II	Low (10%–30%)	Dexamethasone 20 mg p.o. (II/A)[b]	Dexamethasone 20 mg IV	(II/A)
I	Minimal (< 10%)	p.r.n. antiemetics only[c] (V)[b]		

Abbreviation: IV, intravenous.

[a] Incidence of emesis if prophylactic antiemetics not given.

[b] Evidence level/grade (see Table 1-7).

[c] PRN antiemetics include: lorazepam 1–3 mg p.o. every 4–6 hours (maximum 4 mg daily); prochlorperazine 15 mg spansule b.i.d., plus diphenhydramine 50 mg every 4 hours p.r.n. for restlessness; or metoclopramide 30 mg IV/p.o. q.i.d. plus diphenhydramine 50 mg every 4 hours p.r.n. for restlessness.

chemotherapy regimens when using 32 mg, 24 mg, and 8 mg ondansetron, respectively, in combination with a fixed 20 mg IV dose of dexamethasone.

Oral therapy Oral serotonin-receptor antagonists have proven highly effective for the control of chemotherapy-induced emesis, with a similar side effect profile to that seen with IV administration. Direct comparative studies with IV agents have not been completed; in theory, oral administration may be more effective because of direct contact with the primary site of action, the gastrointestinal tract. The convenience of oral therapy benefits both patient and staff and translates into a reduction in the overall cost of chemotherapy treatment.

Both ondansetron and granisetron are commercially available in tablet formulation. The indications for these preparations differ; oral granisetron, but not oral ondansetron, is indicated for highly emetogenic chemotherapy regimens. This is principally due to the amount of drug delivered systemically as a function of tablet strength (Table 54-4). Both agents have the same bioavailability at approximately 60% (Zofran package insert, Glaxo-Wellcome; Kytril package insert, SmithKline Beecham). However, oral ondansetron delivers only 30% the amount of drug as compared with its approved IV dose, whereas oral granisetron delivers over 120% as compared to its approved IV dose.

Oral ondansetron Evaluative studies of oral ondansetron have primarily been conducted for moderately emetogenic chemotherapy, in which a dose of 8 mg b.i.d. for a duration of 3 days results in 0 emetic episodes in 61% of treated patients. Identical results were achieved in a randomized, double-blind study that evaluated ondansetron 8 mg b.i.d. for 3 days in a placebo-controlled study of patients receiving similar moderately emetogenic chemotherapy. These results are difficult to put into context as efficacy was assessed for only 3 days;

subset analysis of acute emesis (24 hours) control is not provided, and assessment of nausea is excluded from the definition of response.

Oral granisetron Data from prospective, randomized trials on the efficacy and safety of oral granisetron in patients receiving both moderately and highly emetogenic chemotherapy regimens are available. A dose-finding study in patients receiving moderately emetogenic chemotherapy reported 24-hour total control (defined as no vomiting, no nausea, and no rescue medication) to be 60% at a granisetron dose of 1 mg b.i.d. A comparative study of granisetron 1 mg b.i.d. versus prochlorperazine 10 mg b.i.d. demonstrated that 57.6% and 33.3% of patients, respectively, had total control at 24 hours.

Evaluation of oral granisetron for highly emetogenic chemotherapy was undertaken in 357 patients stratified into one of three treatment groups: granisetron 1 mg b.i.d., granisetron 1 mg b.i.d. plus dexamethasone 12 mg IV, or high-dose IV metoclopramide plus dexamethasone 12 mg IV. Total control was achieved in 54.7%, 43.7%, and 37.2% of patients receiving granisetron plus dexamethasone, granisetron alone, or metoclopramide plus dexamethasone, respectively. These results demonstrate that oral ondansetron alone is as effective as high-dose metoclopramide plus dexamethasone in preventing cisplatin-induced emesis, and that oral granisetron plus dexamethasone provided control of symptoms superior to conventional regimens.

Documentation of the efficacy of a once-daily dose of oral granisetron 2 mg versus 1 mg b.i.d. was confirmed in a study in 697 patients receiving moderately emetogenic chemotherapy; total control was achieved in 50% of patients in each treatment arm. The once daily dosing schedule is beneficial for its ease of administration and patient compliance.

SEROTONIN ANTAGONISTS FOR DELAYED EMESIS

Delayed emesis remains one of the most persistent and difficult to control situations for CIE. Studies designed to characterize the syndrome have found it to occur in most patients given high-dose cisplatin; despite the use of combination antiemetics for acute emesis, peak emesis occurs between 48 and 72 hours, and, perhaps most importantly, complete control of acute emesis is associated with greater control of delayed emesis. *While the serotonin antagonists have greatly improved acute emesis, studies have failed to demonstrate improved efficacy of serotonin antagonists for the prevention of delayed emesis.* Randomized trials of ondansetron

TABLE 54-4 COMPARISON OF ORAL AND INTRAVENOUS SEROTONIN ANTAGONISTS

	Ondansetron	*Granisetron*
Tablet strength	8 mg	1 mg
Daily dose	8 mg b.i.d.	1 mg b.i.d.
Total daily dose	16 mg	2 mg
Bioavailability (60%) (systemic dose)	9.6 mg	1.2 mg
Intravenous dose	32 mg	0.7–1 mg
% p.o. vs. intravenous	30%	120%–170%

versus placebo have shown only a 10% complete control rate advantage for the drug over placebo. One study specifically excluded those patients with lack of acute emesis control, the group at greatest risk for delayed emesis. A comparison of ondansetron with metoclopramide found efficacy to be nearly identical. Similar findings have been observed in trials of granisetron. Based on the studies conducted to date, the serotonin antagonists have not proven to prevent or lessen delayed emesis after high-dose cisplatin. Thus far, the best results for delayed emesis secondary to high-dose cisplatin have been attained with a combination regimen of oral metoclopramide plus dexamethasone.

MANAGEMENT OF BREAKTHROUGH AND ANTICIPATORY EMESIS

The treatment of breakthrough emesis has not been well studied. Antiemetic clinical trials often use the need for "rescue" antiemetics as a measure of drug failure; however, the effectiveness of rescue regimens has not been evaluated. The recommended treatment for breakthrough antiemetics is based upon assumed failure to the serotonin antagonist and the need for patient sedation. Anecdotally, one or two doses of IV lorazepam 1 to 2 mg has often been found to sedate the patient sufficiently and provide a satisfactory level of antiemetic control. High-dose metoclopramide (2 mg/kg, plus diphenhydramine 50 mg IV p.r.n. for dystonic reactions) is generally necessary for intractable cases.

Anticipatory emesis, defined as emesis occurring before chemotherapy is given, has not been well studied. It has been demonstrated that the incidence of anticipatory emesis is directly related to the amount of nausea and vomiting observed immediately after previous chemotherapy courses and highlights the need for appropriate control of acute emesis. Studies have indicated that behavioral therapy can be helpful for patients with anticipatory emesis. Patients exhibiting anticipatory nausea and vomiting exhibit some degree of anxiety, which may best be managed with an oral benzodiazepine, administered before the patients arrival for chemotherapy. With more effective control of acute CIE, the incidence of anticipatory emesis is expected to decrease.

Figure 54-1 summarizes recommended strategy for prevention and treatment of nausea and vomiting. Recommendations for management of acute emesis are based on high-quality data (level I/grade A evidence); evidences for management of delayed and anticipatory emesis are also based on high-level evidence, although the best regimen is still not identified; data on management of anticipatory emesis are of anecdotal character (level V evidence).

SUGGESTED READINGS

Beck T, York M, Chang A et al: Oral ondansetron 8 mg B.I.D. as effective as 8 mg T.I.D. in the prevention of nausea and vomiting associated with cyclophosphamide-based chemotherapy. Proc ASCO 14:538, 1995

Coates A, Abrahams, S, Kaye S et al: On the receiving-end patient perception of the side effects of cancer chemotherapy. Eur J Cancer Clin Oncol 19:203–208, 1983

De Mulder PHM, Seynaeve C, Vermoreker JB et al: Ondansetron compared with high-dose metoclopramide in prophylaxis of acute and delayed cisplatin-induced nausea and vomiting: a multicenter, randomized, double-blind cross over study. Ann Intern Med 113:834–840, 1990

Dibenedetto J, Cubeddu LX, Ryan R et al: Ondansetron 8 mg twice daily effectively prevents nausea and vomiting associated with moderately emetogenic cancer chemotherapy. Proc Am Soc Clin Oncol 14:538, 1995

Dilly SG, Friedman C, Yocum K: Contribution of dexamethasone to antiemetic control with granisetron is greatest in patients at high risk of emesis. Proc Am Soc Clin Oncol 13:436, 1994

Gandara DR: Progress in the control of acute and delayed emesis induced by cisplatin. Eur J Cancer 27:509–511, 1991

Gebauer A, Merger M, Kilbinger H: Modulation by 5-HT-3 and 5-HT-4 receptors of the release of 5-hydroxytryptamine from the guinea-pig small intestines. Arch Pharmacol 347:137–140, 1993

Gralla RJ, Itri LM, Pisko SE et al; Antiemetic efficacy of high-dose metoclopramide: randomized trials with placebo and prochlorperazine in patients with chemotherapy-induced emesis. N Engl J Med 305:905–909, 1981

Gralla RJ: Adverse Effects of Treatment. Chapter 63. In DeVita VT, Hellman S, Rosenberg SA Cancer: Principles and Practice of Oncology. 4th Ed. Lippincott-Raven, Philadelphia, 1993

Granisetron Study Group: The antiemetic efficacy and safety of granisetron compared with metoclopramide plus dexamethasone in patients receiving fractionated chemotherapy over 5 days. J Cancer Res Clin Oncol 119:555–559, 1993

Grunberg SM, Gala KV, Lampenfeld M et al: Comparison of the antiemetic effect of high-dose intravenous metoclopramide and high-dose intravenous haloperidol in a randomized double-blind crossover study. J Clin Oncol 2:782–787, 1984

Hacking A: Oral granisetron simple and effective: a preliminary report. Eur J Cancer 28A(suppl 1):528–532, 1992

Hainsworth J, Harvey W, Pendergrass K et al: A single-blind comparisons of intravenous ondansetron, a selective serotonin antagonist with intravenous metoclopramide in the prevention of nausea and vomiting associated with high-dose cisplatin chemotherapy. J Clin Oncol 9:721–728, 1991

Heron JF, Goedhals L, Jordan JP et al: Oral granisetron alone and in combination with dexamethasone: a double-blind randomized comparison against high-dose metoclopramide plus dexamethasone in prevention of cisplatin-induced emesis. Ann Oncol 5:579–584, 1994

Hesketh PJ, Harvey WH, Harker HG et al: A randomized double-blind comparison of intravenous ondansetron alone and in combination with intravenous dexamethasone in the prevention of high-dose cisplatin-induced emesis. J Clin Oncol 12:596–600, 1994

Hesketh P, Beck T, Uhlenhopp M et al: Adjusting the dose of intravenous ondansetron plus dexamethasone to the emetic potential of the chemotherapy regimen. J Clin Oncol 13:2117–2122, 1995.

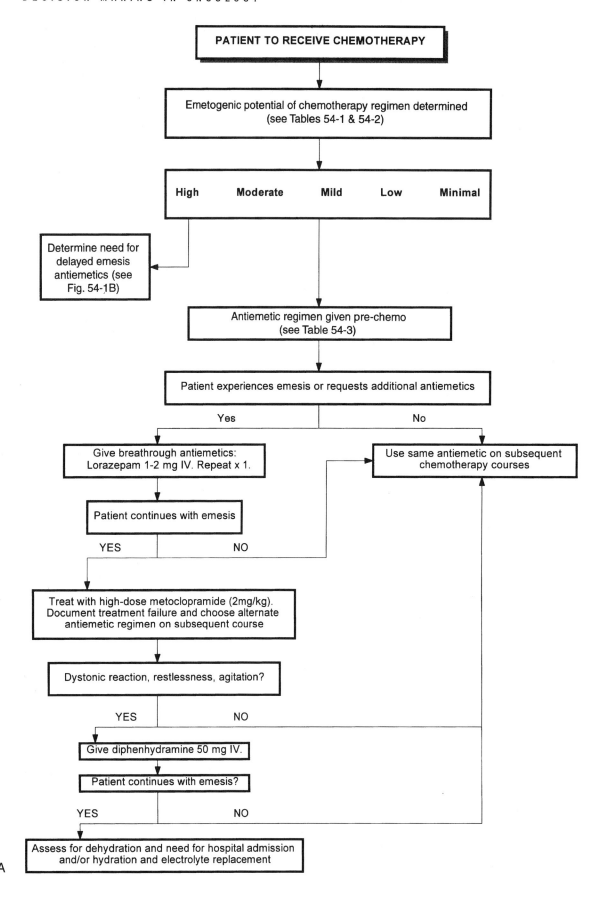

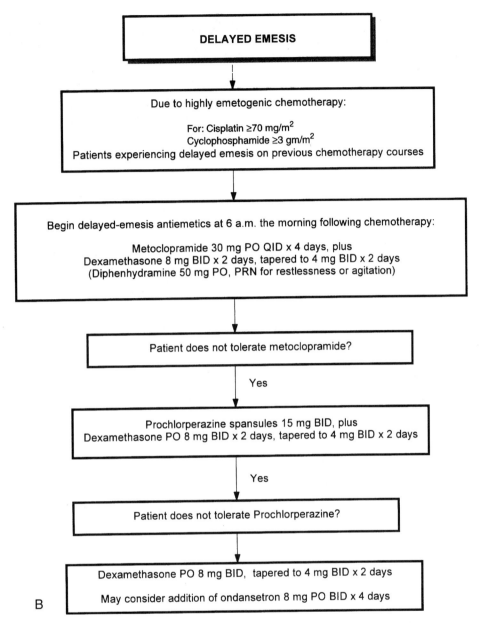

FIGURE 54-1 (A & B) *Algorithms for prevention and treatment of nausea and vomiting. Recommendations for management of acute emesis are based on high-quality data (level I/grade A evidence); evidences for management of delayed and anticipatory are also based on high-level evidence (level I/B), although the best regimen is still not identified; data on management of anticipatory emesis are of anecdotal character (level V evidence).*

Italian Study Group for Antiemetic Research. Dexamethasone, granisetron, or both for the prevention of nausea and vomiting during chemotherapy for cancer. N Engl J Med 332:1–5, 1995

Johnsonbaugh RE, Mason BA, Friedman CJ et al: Oral granistron is an effective antiemetic in patients receiving moderately emetogenic chemotherapy. Proc ASCO 1994

Johnsonbaugh RE, Mason VA, Friedman CJ, Pellier P: Acute antiemetic response to oral granisetron superior to oral prochlorperazine in patients receiving moderately emetogenic chemotherapy. Ann Oncol 5(suppl 8):205, 1994

Kris MG, Gralla RJ, Clark RA et al: Incidence, course, and severity of delayed nausea and vomiting following the administration of high-dose cisplatin. J Clin Oncol 3:1379–1384, 1985

Kris MG, Gralla RJ, Clark RA et al. Antiemetic control and prevention of side effects of anti-cancer therapy with lorazepam or diphenhydramine when used in combination with metoclopramide plus dexamethasone: a double-blind randomized trial. Cancer 60:2816–2822, 1987

Kris MG, Gralla RJ, Lyson L et al: Controlling delayed vomiting: double-blind, randomized trial comparing placebo, dexamethasone alone, and metoclopramide plus dexamethasone in patients receiving cisplatin. J Clin Oncol 7:108–114, 1989

Lindley CM, Bernard S, Fields SM: Incidence and duration of chemotherapy-induced nausea and vomiting in the outpatient oncology population. J Clin Oncol 7:1142–1149, 1989

Lindley CM, Hirsch JD, O'Neill CV et al: Quality of life consequences of chemotherapy induced emesis. Qual of Life Res 1:331–340, 1992

Markman M, Sheilder V, Ettinger DS et al: Antiemetic efficacy of dexamethasone: randomized double-blind crossover study with prochlorperazine in patients receiving cancer chemotherapy. N Engl J Med 311:549–552, 1984

Miner WD, Sanger GJ: Inhibition of cisplatin-induced vomiting by selective 5-hydroxytryptamine M-receptor antagonism. Br J Pharmacol 88:497–499, 1986

Navari R, Gandara D, Hesketh P et al: Comparative clinical trial of granisetron and ondansetron in the prophylaxis of cisplatin-induced emesis. J Clin Oncol 13:1242–1248, 1995

Navari RM, Kaplan HG, Gralla RJ et al: Efficacy and safety of granisetron, a selective 5-HT3 receptor antagonist in the prevention of nausea and vomiting induced by high-dose cisplatin. J Clin Oncol 12:2204–2210, 1994

Navari RM, Madajewicz S, Anderson M et al: Oral ondansetron for the control of cisplatin-induced delayed-emesis: a large, multicenter, double-blind, randomized comparative trial of ondansetron versus placebo. J Clin Oncol 13:2408–2416, 1995

Roila F, Tonato M, Cognetti F et al: Prevention of cisplatin-induced emesis: a double-blind multicenter randomized crossover study comparing ondansetron and ondansetron plus dexamethasone. J Clin Oncol 9:675–678, 1991

Smyth J: Delayed emesis after high-dose cisplatin: the residual problem. Proc Eur Soc of Med Oncol Lyon, France, 1992

Tonata M, Roila F: Ann Oncol 2:107–114, 1991

Wilcox PM, Fetting JH, Nettesheim KH et al: Anticipatory vomiting in women receiving cyclophosphamide, methotrexate, and 5-FU (CMF) adjuvant chemotherapy for breast carci-

55 Pain Management

William R. Dinwoodie
Jacqueline A. LaPerriere
Carol Rodriguez
Maribeth Brune

Prevalence: Cancer pain occurs in 60%–90% of patients with advanced incurable cancer (~400,000/year)

Key management principle: Selection of the medication depends on the evaluation of the quality (neuralgic vs. neuropathic vs. somatic/visceral) and intensity of the pain (mild, moderate, severe)

Goal of treatment: Improvement of the quality of life through adequate analgesia

Main modality of treatment: Oral analgesics

Outcome: Adequate pain control can be achieved in up to 90% of patients

In 1996, over half a million people will die as a result of cancer in the United States. Estimates are that 75% of patients with advanced cancer experience pain in association with their disease. While occurring less frequently at the time of diagnosis, cancer pain has been reported to be present in up to 90% of hospitalized cancer patients. Relatively simple means, predominantly oral medications, exist for controlling cancer pain in approximately 85%–90% of patients, but data indicate that patients often receive inadequate analgesia. When a large group of physicians in the Eastern Cooperative Oncology Group (ECOG) was questioned about cancer pain management, 86% of those responding felt that the majority of cancer patients with pain were undermedicated, and only 51% rated pain control in their own practice setting as good or very good.

Adequate analgesia can allow patients with incurable cancers to function more normally and allow them to enjoy more fully the time remaining to them. For patients with potentially curable malignancies, controlling the pain that is often associated with cancer therapies can allow patients to complete potentially life-saving therapy instead of stopping such therapy early because of excessive discomfort.

BARRIERS TO ADEQUATE PAIN CONTROL

Many barriers can interfere with the achievement of adequate analgesia for cancer pain. Physicians, nurses, pharmacies, the legal system, and even patients and their families may contribute to the barriers that make adequate pain relief more difficult to achieve. The major barriers are listed in Table 55-1. When physicians in the ECOG were questioned about the reasons for inadequate pain relief, the main causes reported were as follows:

Inadequate pain assessment

Patient reluctance to report pain

Patient reluctance to take opioids

Physician reluctance to prescribe opioids

Inadequate staff knowledge about pain management

COMMON PAIN PROBLEMS IN CANCER PATIENTS

Patients with cancer can experience pain that is acute or chronic in nature. The pain may be related to their disease or its treatment or can be related to other preexisting, chronic, nonmalignant, painful conditions. These pain syndromes can thus be divided into three categories:

1. Pain associated with direct tumor involvement

2. Pain associated with cancer treatment

3. Pain unrelated to the cancer or its treatment

Metastatic bone pain, nerve compression or infiltration by tumor, or hollow viscus encroachment are the most common causes of pain from direct tumor involvement. Pain syndromes associated with cancer treatment include pain occurring during, or as a result of chemotherapy, surgery, or radiation therapy. The third category of pain syndromes includes those that are unrelated to the cancer or its treatment, such as arthritis.

Table 55-2 summarizes the types of pain commonly encountered in patients with cancer as well as the descriptors most often used by patients for each type of pain. The etiology and descriptor(s) given by the patient can provide valuable clues to selecting the most appropriate medication(s).

PAIN ASSESSMENT

Recently, guidelines were released by the Agency for Health Care Policy and Research (AHCPR) to assist health care consumers and providers in decision making regarding cancer pain and its management. The guidelines reflect the need for a multimodal approach to the management of pain and emphasize the need for careful and continuous assessment.

Accurate assessment is critical in identifying appropriate interventions for cancer pain as well as in evaluating treatment outcomes. In this section, assessment of pain in the general cancer population will be discussed.

In evaluating an individual, the patient's self-report of pain should be the primary source of the assessment and neither the patient's behavior nor

---

TABLE 55-1   BARRIERS TO RELIEF OF CANCER PAIN

Patient/family
  Fear of addiction
  Fear of analgesic toxicities (constipation, nausea, vomiting, mental clouding)
  Fear that discussing pain will take time away from treatment of cancer
  Fear that nothing will help
  Fear that too early use of analgesics will make them ineffective later
  Poor compliance caused by misunderstanding
  Reluctance to take medicines
  Reluctance to increase medications because it indicates worsening cancer
Physician/health care provider
  Inadequate pain assessment
  Lack of training in analgesic use
  Concern about addiction and toxicities
  Limited time because of busy schedule
  Fear about legal scrutiny
  Failure to recognize own limitations
Pharmacy
  Reluctance to stock opioids because of concerns about burglary, record keeping, or legal scrutiny

---

TABLE 55-2   COMMON PAIN TYPES

Etiology	Usual Pain Quality
Bone/muscle infiltration	Aching, dull, boring, nagging, usually localized
Nerve compression/infiltration	
Neuropathic	Burning, tingling, usually continuous
Neuralgic	Sharp shooting, jabbing, electrical, shock-like, intermittent
Mucositis	Raw, burning, scratchy, stinging
Visceral	
Pleural/peritoneal, pericardial	Sharp stabbing; may worsen with respiration or movement
Organ involvement	Deep, gnawing, vague, poorly localized

vital signs should be used in lieu of a self-report. A person's complaint of pain is not simply a report of physical injury. In reality pain is a complex, multidimensional experience influenced by multiple factors including age, sex, coping mechanisms, past pain experiences, cultural and socioeconomic issues as well as medical history and various psychological factors. Because of the multiple facets of pain, an appropriate pain evaluation may be time consuming and must be detailed. The initial assessment should always be followed up with frequent and repeated reassessments, as long as the pain persists, to determine effectiveness of the prescribed treatment plan and need for treatment changes or adjustments.

Initial pain assessment should always include use of a pain scale to measure pain intensity at *all* sites of pain. Several pain scales are available for use. The scale selected should be appropriate for the patient's age and cognitive abilities, and the same scale should be used consistently throughout each reassessment. Documentation not only of the scale used but of pain scores obtained is important in determining the overall effectiveness of the treatment plan. Pain scales allow patients to identify subjective pain levels at all sites. In our practice, the numeric rating scale (NRS) is the preferred rating system. This scale is verbal in nature. Patients rate their pain from zero to ten with zero being "no pain" and ten being "the worst imaginable pain." The number selected by the patient represents their pain intensity. The NRS is easy to administer, and validity has been well documented. However, there is lack of research comparing the sensitivity of the NRS to that of other measures, particularly the visual analogue scale (VAS) (Fig. 55-1). Other available scales include the behavior rating scale (BRS), the faces scale, and the descriptor differential scale (DDS). Pain ratings should be obtained at each reassessment, compared with previous pain scores, and used as a guide to therapy. Table 55-3 lists the components of a complete pain assessment.

After a detailed pain history is obtained, a thorough physical examination should be performed. Special attention should be directed to those areas identified by the patient as being painful. Palpation and inspection of the painful area(s) may reveal visible masses or inflammatory lesions, for example, that provide a ready explanation for the pain. Palpation will indicate whether light or deep palpation exacerbates the pain. Tenderness to palpation of a bony area may indicate bone metastasis. Excess sensitivity to light touch is often seen with neuropathic pain, such as that seen with chemotherapy-

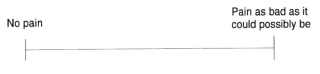

A 10 cm. baseline is recommended for VAS scales

FIGURE 55-1 *Visual analogue scale (VAS) for pain.*

induced paresthesias or postherpetic neuralgia. When the patient complains of numbness or weakness, a detailed neurologic examination is indicated. The presence of objective neurologic deficits indicates the possibility of CNS metastasis or nerve or cord compression, depending upon location.

ANALGESICS

Figure 55-2 provides suggestions for initial analgesic therapy depending on the suspected etiology of pain. Clues to the etiology of pain are based on the patient's description of the pain as well as physical findings and/or radiographic studies. For some categories in Figure 55-2 you will be referred to the analgesic algorithm (Fig. 55-3). Patients may at times have several pains or several types of pain with different causes. In such cases, select the one or two most severe pains and begin only a few medications rather than giving multiple new medications, which often share similar toxicities. If toxicities occur, it is easier to determine the offending medications if only a few are initiated at one time. Additional medications can be added later in a stepwise fashion if indicated.

At times, it is difficult to determine the precise nature of the pain from clinical findings or from the patient's description. In such cases, decide on the most likely etiology to help select initial therapy. If the patient fails to respond as expected, reevaluate and consider a trial of a medication from a different class of analgesics.

TABLE 55-3 **COMPONENTS OF A COMPLETE PAIN ASSESSMENT**

Location(s) of pain(s)
Date of onset of pain(s)
Pain characteristics
Aggravating or alleviating factors
Pain intensity
Psychosocial evaluation
Physical examination
Laboratory and/or radiologic studies if appropriate

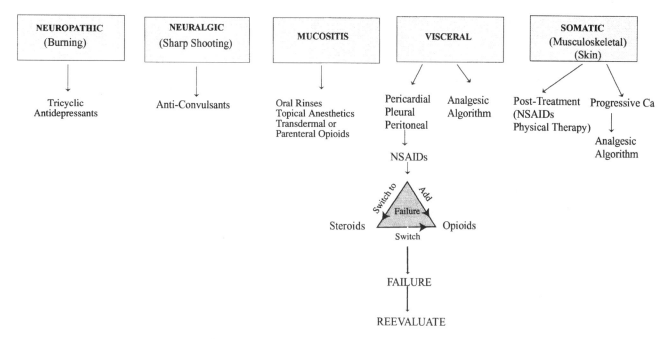

FIGURE 55-2   *Cancer-related pain: etiology-based algorithm. The key principle in the management of pain in the cancer patient is based on the evaluation of the quality and intensity of the pain. Pharmacologic agents with different pharmacodynamic properties are selected depending on whether the pain is neuropathic, neuralgic, or somatic/visceral in nature (with special considerations for mucositis). While opioids and NSAIDs/acetaminophen work well for somatic/visceral type pains, other agents are more effective (long term) for neuropathic or neuralgic pain. These recommendations are based on level I (opioids), II (NSAIDs), and III (adjuvant drugs) evidence.*

Once a treatment has been started, periodic reevaluation is necessary. When the medication does not have the desired result, always consider the possible causes for failure, which may include improper selection of analgesic type, inadequate dose or improper dose scheduling, lack of patient compliance, or a different or additional etiology to the pain not previously considered.

NONSTEROIDAL ANTI-INFLAMMATORY DRUGS AND ACETAMINOPHEN

Nonsteroidal anti-inflammatory drugs (NSAIDs) are the front-line therapy for patients with mild to moderate somatic and visceral pain. NSAIDs decrease levels of inflammatory mediators generated at the site of injury, leading to their analgesic and anti-inflammatory properties. In contrast to opioids, NSAIDs do not produce tolerance or physical dependence, and a ceiling effect to the analgesic properties exists. A wide variety of NSAIDs are currently available, with subtle differences existing

between side-effect profiles, administration, and half-life (Table 55-4). Selection of an NSAID should be based on dosing considerations, side effect profile, and clinical experience. Dosages of agents should be adjusted based on patients renal and hepatic function, as well as their age.

Acetaminophen is often used in patients with contraindications to treatment with the nonsteroidal drugs. Its mechanism of action results in more antipyretic and analgesic action, with poor anti-inflammatory activity. Additionally, acetaminophen can be used safely in patients with thrombocytopenia (as it has no antiplatelet effects) and it has very little gastrointestinal effects. The dose of acetaminophen should be adjusted in patients with hepatic insufficiency. The drug is metabolized in the liver and if accumulation occurs can be hepatotoxic. Acetaminophen should be used cautiously in patients with a history of hepatic disease or failure. The use of single-agent NSAIDs or acetaminophen in cancer pain is based on level I evidence and, for use in combination with opioids, level II.

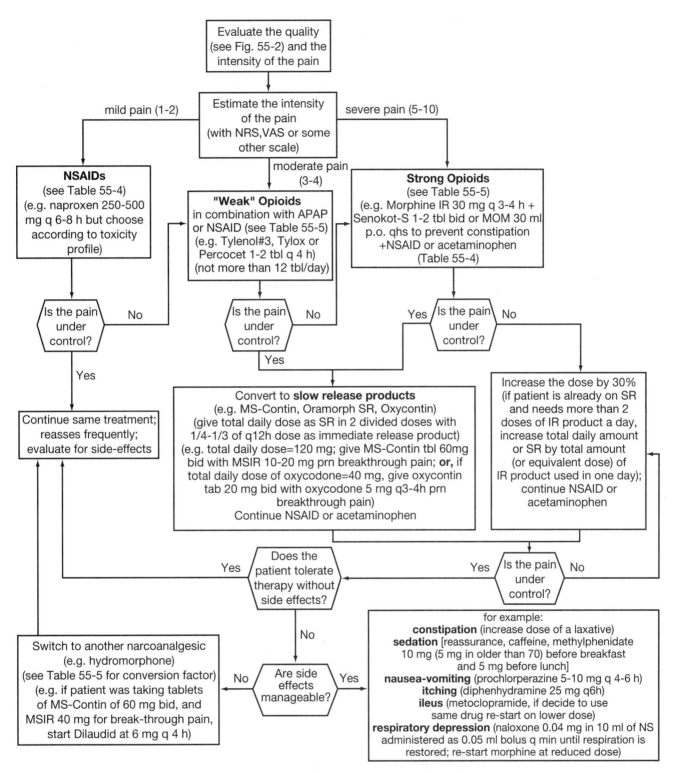

FIGURE 55-3 *Analgesic algorithm. This figure is based on World Health Organization Guidelines for the treatment of cancer pain, with recommendations also dependent on pain intensity. It includes modifications based on response to therapy or ability to control toxicities of analgesics. The goal of treatment is to improve quality of life in the patient through adequate analgesia, which is possible in approximately 80%–90% of patients using oral medications. These recommendations are based on level I (opioids) and II (NSAIDs) evidence.*

TABLE 55-4   SELECTED NSAIDs AND ACETAMINOPHEN DOSING RECOMMENDATIONS FOR MILD TO MODERATE PAIN

Agent (Brand)	Dosing range[a]	Max. dose (mg/day)	Comments
Aspirin	500–1000 mg q4–6 hours	4000 mg	Irreversibly inhibits platelet aggregation; available in suppository form; available OTC
Ibuprofen	400–600 mg q6 hours	2400 mg	Inhibits platelet aggregation; available in suspension; some strengths available OTC
Naproxen (Naprosyn)	250–500 mg q6–8hours	1250 mg	Inhibits platelet aggregation; available in suspension; some strengths available OTC
Ketoprofen (Orudis)	25–50 mg q6–8hours	300 mg	Inhibits platelet aggregation; available OTC
Ketorolac (Toradol)	15–30 mg IV q6hours 10 mg p.o. q6hour	120 mg IV 40 mg p.o.	Available in IV and p.o. formulation; use limited to 5 days IV + PO total
Magnesium choline Trisalicylate (Trilisate)	750–1500 mg q12hours	3000 mg	Minimal antiplatelet activity; less gastrointestrial irritation
Salsalate (Disalcid)	500–1000 mg q8–12hours	4000 mg	Minimal antiplatelet activity; less gastrointestinal irritation
Acetaminophen	500–1000 mg q4–6hours	4000 mg	No antiplatelet activity; less gastrointestinal irritation; poor antiinflammatory action; available in suspension and suppository form; OTC

Abbreviations: IV, intravenous; OTC, over the counter; p.o., per os

[a] Doses recommended for patients with normal renal function; adjust doses in patients with renal/hepatic impairment and in the elderly.

OPIOID ANALGESICS

If a nonopioid medication is not effective or is poorly tolerated, opioid analgesics are added to manage acute pain and chronic cancer-related pain. Although propoxyphene, codeine, and oxycodone are often thought of as "weak" opioids, they all share the same pharmacologic properties as morphine (Table 55-5). They are available as single-entity agents but are most frequently prescribed in fixed oral dose combinations with nonopioid medications. Propoxyphene and codeine do possess analgesic properties that make them more efficacious when combined with a nonopioid, but as the dose is increased to achieve this potential benefit, the incidence of opioid side effects increases, thus limiting their usefulness. Additionally, the nonopioid component of the fixed combination analgesic does have a maximum dose, or ceiling effect, and caution must be taken not to exceed this dose when dose escalation is required to minimize or prevent toxicity.

Oxycodone hydrochloride is an oral opioid analgesic that has been used for the relief of pain for more than 75 years. Its duration of action is similar to morphine, in the range of 3 to 5 hours. A new, sustained-release formulation of oxycodone (Oxycontin) is now available and approved for the management of moderate to severe pain when use of an opioid analgesic is appropriate for more than a few days. This formulation allows for biphasic absorption, resulting in an immediate release of oxycodone after ingestion, followed by a slow release of the remaining oxycodone. This immediate-release effect is a major difference between this product and other sustained-release oral opioid products that have been commercially available for some time (MS Contin and Oramorph). The dosing interval of Oxycontin is every 12 hours.

While morphine is the gold standard, all morphine-like agonists provide similar qualities of analgesia, with similar side effect profiles. In clinical practice, however, individual patients will

TABLE 55-5   OPIOID ANALGESICS COMMONLY USED FOR CANCER PAIN MANAGEMENT

Agent	Route	Equianalgesic Dose (mg)	Usual Starting Dose (mg)	Dosing Interval (hours)	Available Forms	Comments
Propoxyphene (Darvon)	PO		65	3–4	Tablets	Weak analgesic, may be combined with NSAIDs,
Propoxyphene napsylate (Darvocet)	PO		100	3–4	Tablets	Potentially toxic metabolite, norpropoxyphene; accumulates with repetitive dosing; may cause seizures; not recommended in cancer patients
Codeine	IM/SC	130	60	3–4	IM/SC	Metabolized to morphine, available alone or in combination products with acetaminophen
	PO	200	60	3–4	Tablets	
Hydrocodone	PO	30	10	3–4	Tablets Liquid	Available only in combination with acetaminophen
Meperidine (Demerol)	IV	75	100	2–3	IV	Metabolized to normeperidine, which may accumulate with repetitive dosing causing CNS stimulation; avoid chronic use (<48 hours only) or use in patients with renal dysfunction; Oral dosing not recommended
	PO	300	300	2–3	Tablets	
Oxycodone	PO (IR)	30	10	3–5	IR tablets, liquid	Short acting; now available as a sustained release product; also available in combination with acetaminophen and aspirin, which limits the maximum daily dose (Tylox, Percocet)
	PO (SR)	30	10	12	SR tablets	
Morphine	IV/SC	10	10	3–4	IV	Standard, available in sustained release tablets; starting oral dose 30–60 mg every 3–4 hours; active metabolite may accumulate in renal failure
	PO (IR)	30–60	30	3–4	IR tablets Liquid	
	PR	30–60	30–60	3–4	Suppository	
	PO (SR)	30–60	60–90	8–12	SR tablets	
Hydromorphone (Dilaudid)	IV/SC	1.5	1	3–4	IV, tablets, Liquid, suppository	Slightly shorter half-life than morphine; may be an alternative in those patients who do not tolerate morphine; no active metabolites
	PO	7.5	4	3–4		
Fentanyl	IV	0.1	—	—	IV	Much shorter half-life than morphine necessitates IV be given as an infusion, not p.r.n; up to a 12–18-hour delay in onset of pain relief with the patch because of drug reservoir; fever and heat may increase drug delivery from patch; extended duration of side effects even when patch removed
	Transdermal		25 mcg	48–72	Patch	
Methadone (Dolophine)	IV	10	10	6–8	IV	Good potency; accumulates with repetitive dosing (by days 2–5); use carefully in opioid naive and elderly patients; requires frequent reassessment
	PO	20	20	6–8	Tablets, liquid	
Levorphenol (Levo-Dromoran)	IV	2	2	6–8	IV	May accumulate with repetitive dosing (days 2–3); requires frequent reassessment
	PO	4	4	6–8	Tablets	

Abbreviations: CNS, Central nervous system; immediate release; IM, intramuscular; IV, intravenous; PO, per os; PR, per rectum; SC, subcutaneous; SR, sustained release.

respond differently to different opioids. The oral route is the preferred route for administration of opioid analgesics, as this route remains the most convenient, flexible, and cost-effective choice for the chronic treatment of pain. With the availability of sustained-release oral formulations of oxycodone and morphine, dosing every 12 hours is possible, leading to increased compliance and optimal pain control for patients. A sustained-release transdermal fentanyl patch is also available, but it has a relatively slow onset of action, is difficult to titrate because of the lag time from each dose change until the peak effect, and is expensive when compared with other options.

Agents to be avoided in the management of cancer pain include meperidine and the partial agonist or agonist/antagonist opioid preparations. Meperidine is extremely short-acting, with a duration of effect of approximately 2 hours. Meperidine is metabolized in the liver to normeperidine, a weak analgesic with a long half-life that accumulates with chronic dosing. Normeperidine is a central nervous system excitotoxin that can produce anxiety, tremors, myoclonus, and generalized seizures. Normeperidine is cleared renally, placing patients with renal impairment at greater risk. For these reasons, meperidine should not be used for more than 48 hours, in patients with renal or central nervous system disease, or at doses greater than 600 mg/day. Partial agonist and mixed agonist/antagonist opioids display a ceiling effect to their analgesia and may precipitate opioid withdrawal if given to a patient already on an opioid analgesic. These properties limit their usefulness in chronic cancer pain management. The use of oral opioids in cancer pain is based on level I evidence.

INITIATION OF PHARMACOLOGIC THERAPY

A simple model that can be followed to initiate analgesic therapy in the treatment of pain has been created by the World Health Organization (WHO). Figure 55-3, which was constructed based on WHO recommendations, shows one possible approach to pain control in opioid naive patients. The WHO "step ladder" was designed to treat cancer pain in a step-wise fashion, beginning with the least toxic/least potent analgesics for intitial treatment and progressing to combination drugs for patients not responding to the initial step. The third, or highest step, uses "strong opioids" and is often needed for those patients with more severe pain. Patients often progress from mild to severe pain in a step-wise fashion, but, at times, patients develop

severe pain early on and NSAIDs or combination drugs (which have a ceiling effect) may not be potent enough as an initial step for such patients. Following the steps of the WHO Guidelines is suited for use in most patients, but it may at times be appropriate for cancer patients with severe pain to receive an opioid, such as morphine or oxycodone, as their initial analgesic to prevent delays in achieving pain relief. Adjuvant medications can be used initially, or in later steps as needed, to enhance analgesia or treat neuropathic pain.

When pain persists or increases, an opioid medication should be added to the NSAID. It is important to continue the patient's NSAID therapy along with the opioid. When NSAIDs are prescribed in addition to opioids, an opioid-sparing effect is seen, which often allows for a reduction in the opioid dose as the pain lessens in intensity. Overall this results in a better quality analgesia, with less opioid side effects. This is considered step 2 of the WHO ladder. Although the WHO approach advocates the use of a weak opioid for mild to moderate pain at this point, in clinical practice there is no reason why stronger opioids cannot be used in the opioid naive patient. In our practice, appropriate doses of single-entity oxycodone tablets or liquid and the available morphine preparations are the initial drugs of choice when starting patients on oral opioid therapy (see Table 55-5).

When initiating opioid therapy with a short-acting (or immediate-release) medication on an "as needed" basis, normal starting doses should be used at a dosing interval that is appropriate for the medication selected. If the initial dose selected does not adequately relieve the patient's pain and the patient is suffering no significant toxicities, the dose can be safely escalated by 33% without undue concern about untoward side effects. Once an appropriate dose of opioid medication has been prescribed, an around-the-clock dosing schedule should be considered if the pain persists. Converting the patient to a sustained-release opioid, such as oxycodone or morphine, that can be dosed every 12 hours can increase patient compliance and reduce the incidence of breakthrough pain. An additional "as needed," short-acting opioid should be prescribed on a q4h p.r.n. basis to help alleviate any breakthrough pain. The dose of the immediate release medication is 25% to 33% of the scheduled 12-hour dose of the long-acting opioid. The need for frequent breakthrough doses throughout the day may indicate a need for dose escalation of the long-acting opioid. The new dose of long acting opioid can be determined by adding up the approximate amount of short-acting opioid the patient has been averaging per day. This daily amount should be converted to an equianalgesic dose of the drug in the long-acting preparation and is then divided by the number of long-acting doses currently being given (usually two or three). This amount is then added to each dose of long-acting medicine. Using long-acting and short-acting medications that are the same basic drug (e.g., long-acting morphine with short-acting morphine) helps simplify the task of adjusting the long-acting dose when necessary. Frequent follow-up and reassessment are recommended during the titration period. This will assist the clinician in getting the patient's pain under control quickly, while making sure that any side effects are addressed and treated promptly.

Patient diaries can assist in managing a patient's pain effectively at home. Diaries are used by patients or other support persons to record pain intensity as well as use of scheduled and breakthrough pain medication. These logs assist to direct treatment changes based on the information recorded and are very useful, especially with follow-up telephone evaluations. Diaries also assist in assessing pain and treatment outcomes between clinic visits.

OPIOID TOXICITIES AND THEIR MANAGEMENT

Concern about potential toxicities often results in underusage of opioids by health care providers and patients. With proper utilization of opioids and management of toxicities, opioids can be employed with relative safety, even when large doses are necessary. Awareness of opioid toxicities and their management can help to assure adequate analgesia.

Common toxicities associated with opioids include the following.

CONSTIPATION

Constipation will occur in almost all patients on opioids unless adequate prophylactic measures are utilized. Stool softeners and/or mild stimulants can be used and should be instituted when opioids are started, especially when the opioids are used on an "around the clock" schedule. Commonly used agents include docusate sodium in combination with senna; bisacodyl; milk of magnesia; and nonabsorbable sugars (lactulose or sorbitol).

In our practice, we prefer to use docusate sodium and senna in combination and adjust the dose to maintain soft bowel movements every other day (on the average). These two medications are available separately or in combination. When using the combination, up to 18 tablets per day in three or four divided doses may be required to prevent constipation, although one tablet two to three times daily is usually sufficient for smaller doses of opioids. For patients in whom this is not effective, sorbitol (70% solution) or lactulose can be added as needed at a dose of 15 to 30 cc up to four times daily. It is important to educate patients about the need to use medications prophylactically for constipation. Once severe constipation develops, it can lead to anorexia, cramping, and even nausea or vomiting and may take several days to correct. Dietary factors, such as fruits, and fiber, may help in preventing constipation, but generally, these are not sufficient by themselves.

NAUSEA AND VOMITING

Nausea and vomiting have been reported to occur in approximately 40% of patients upon their initial exposure to opioids. Many patients develop tolerance to this side effect (usually within 5–7 days), but for patients to continue taking their oral opioid until tolerance develops, antiemetics should be used. If nausea and vomiting develop upon first exposure to opioids, an antiemetic should be prescribed on a regular basis for one to two days and subsequently on a p.r.n. schedule. Prochloperazine 5 or 10 mg every 4 to 6 hours or phenergan 25 mg every 6 hour orally are often effective in this situation. Lorazepam 0.5 to 1 mg every 6 hour orally can also be used, but cautiously, because of the sedative effects that can occur when opioids and benzodiazepines are used concomitantly. If these measures are ineffective, switching to an alternate opioid may be tried. Occasionally, patients tolerate some opioids and not others. Nausea and vomiting caused by opioids are not an allergy and patients should not be told that such is the case. They should be instructed that nausea and emesis are common toxicities of opioids that can be controlled in most patients.

SEDATION

Sedation of some degree often occurs in patients (precise data on percentage of patients affected is not available) starting opioid medications for the first time or when opioid doses are increased. Like nausea and emesis, this side effect often subsides after several days and at steady doses. Patients often have the misconception that all people who are on opioids feel drowsy or "foggy-headed." Explaining that this side effect is often transient can allow the patient to give the opioid an adequate trial before refusing to take a potentially useful medication. Other medications with sedative properties may lead to excess sedation when used in combination with opioids. Limiting the use of other potentially sedating medications can help minimize the risk of excess drowsiness. A recent study indicates that methylphenidate may, to a degree, relieve the daytime drowsiness associated with opioid use. The authors of that study used methylphenidate 10 mg before breakfast (5 mg in those over 70 years of age) and 5 mg before lunch.

If excess sedation or respiratory depression does occur (no definite data on frequency of this complication — it depends on presence or absence of contributing factors), temporary discontinuation of the opioid agent and careful monitoring are recommended until the problem resolves. If felt to be severe, naloxone can be used. Remember, however, that naloxone can reverse the analgesic effects of opioids and may result in the return of severe pain. For patients on longstanding or high-dose opioids, naloxone may precipitate withdrawal seizures. If naloxone is used, the following are recommended:

1. Administer naloxone in titrated doses—only to reverse respiratory depression but not completely reverse analgesia—0.4 mg in 10 ml of saline administered as 0.5 ml (0.02 mg) boluses every minute or give as an infusion of two ampules (0.8 mg) in 250 cc. D5W continuously titrated.

2. Remember that naloxone effects may last only about 45 minutes. Even if naloxone administration successfully reverses the respiratory depression, the patient will require careful monitoring, possibly requiring additional doses of naloxone.

3. After the patient is stabilized and monitoring procedures are established, evaluate the patient for the other factors, which can lead to excess sedation in a patient receiving opioids.

PRURITIS

Pruritus can occur with opioid use in some patients (occurrence rates are not well documented in the literature, but personal experience suggests a rate of ~5%–10%). In the absence of rash or other symptoms, this probably does not represent an allergic reaction. Diphenhydramine 25 mg orally every 6 hours or hydroxyzine HCl 25 mg orally every 6 hours may help control the pruritus. The use of an alternate opioid may lead to less pruritus.

MYOCLONIC JERKING

Myoclonic jerking can occur (occurrence rates are not well documented in the literature, but personal experience suggests a rate of ~5%–10%) in some patients on opioids, especially at larger doses. Clonazepam is a benzodiazepine used for myoclonic seizure, and we have occasionally found it useful in treating myoclonic jerks secondary to opioids. We use 0.5 mg orally, one to three times daily. Caution should be used when giving clonazepam or other benzodiazepines because of the potential for central nervous system depression that can occur when these drugs are used in combination with opioids.

ILEUS

Ileus rarely occurs with the use of proper prophylactic measures. Once other etiologies are excluded, the dose of opioid can be reduced somewhat or an alternative opioid, at equianalgesic doses, can be tried. Metaclopramide or an osmotic laxative (i.e., sorbitol or lactulose) may be helpful in less severe cases.

ADDICTION

Finally, there is a concern about the risk of addiction with opioid usage. Available information indicates that addiction in cancer patients receiving opioids is a very uncommon problem (only 4 of 11,882 patients in one retropsective review). It is important to educate and reassure patients and health care providers that addiction is an uncommon problem in patients with malignancies.

ADJUVANT ANALGESICS

Tricyclic Antidepressants Antidepressant drug therapy, used in the treatment of a wide range of chronic pain syndromes for many years, is particularly useful in the treatment of neuropathic pain. Described by patients as "burning pain," "pins and needles," "tingling," or "numbness" pain associated with peripheral neuropathies and postoperative syndromes (e.g., postmastectomy syndrome, postthoracotomy syndrome) is typically difficult to control and is not optimally managed with opioid analgesics. Studies examining the effectiveness of the tricyclic antidepressants (TCAs) have primarily focused on amitriptyline, nortriptyline, and desipramine with anecdotal reports suggesting imipramine, doxepin, trazadone, and others may be as efficacious. Data are limited on the efficacy of the newer serotonin antagonists (fluoxetine, sertraline, paroxetine), and these newer antidepressants are not typically used for the management of pain. Side effects, similar among the various TCAs, include anticholinergic side effects (particularly dry mouth, urinary retention, and constipation), worsening or exacerbation of glaucoma, drowsiness, appetite stimulation and weight gain, confusion, lowering of seizure threshold, and cardiovascular side effects (postural hypotension, tachycardia). TCAs should therefore be used cautiously with patients with a history of seizures, preexisting glaucoma, or cardiac disease. Choice of an antidepressant should be based on the individual agent side-effect profile, as some agents have less anticholinergic activity than others. Doses should be adjusted in elderly patients or in those with decreased renal or hepatic dysfunction. To minimize side effects, low doses should be initiated and increased by 10 mg or 25 mg increments every five to seven days until pain control is achieved or side effects occur (Table 55-6). Plasma levels can be drawn and may be used to monitor compliance or to confirm therapeutic failure; however, no therapeutic range for pain management has been established.

The use of tricyclic antidepressants for cancer pain is supported by level II and III evidence.

Anticonvulsant Therapy As with the tricyclic antidepressants, anticonvulsant agents are also found to be useful in the treatment of neuropathic pain, specifically neuralgias. These agents appear especially useful in pain described by patients as "sharp," "shooting," "lancinating," or "knife-like." These agents are most active against paroxysmal nerve firing. Carbamazepine and phenytoin have been used for the treatment of neuralgic pain, with most studies examining the effectiveness of carbamazepine. Optimal doses for these agents are not known, and typically in practice one follows the recommendations for the treatment of seizures. These agents should be initiated at low doses and titrated slowly until effective to minimize adverse effects (Table 55-7). Carbamazepine is the drug of choice in patients with neuralgic pain, but use is limited in some patients because of adverse effects (including drowsiness, dizziness, nausea, and vomiting). In less than 1% of patients receiving carbamazepine, the drug may cause bone marrow suppression and aplastic anemia. This adverse effect has limited the use of carbamazepine in patients with bone marrow suppression. A new antiepileptic agent, gabapentin (Neurontin), has recently been studied with regard to pain management. Case studies have examined the effectiveness of gabapentin in patients with reflex sympathetic dystrophy, and results have been promising. Gabapentin is well tolerated; the most common side effects are listed in Table 55-7. Additional studies are ongoing to assess the effectiveness of this agent in other painful syndromes. The use of anticonvulsants in cancer pain is supported by level III evidence in the literature.

Corticosteroids Other useful agents for the treatment of cancer-related pain are in the corticos-

TABLE 55-6   SELECTED TRICYCLIC ANTIDEPRESSANT THERAPY DOSING RECOMMENDATIONS FOR THE TREATMENT OF NEUROPATHIC PAIN

Agent (Brand)	Starting Dose[a]	Maximum Dose (mg/day)	Possible Side Effects
Amitriptyline (Elavil)	25 mg p.o. q.h.s.	300	High anticholinergic, sedative, and conduction abnormality SE
Nortriptyline (Pamelor)	25 mg p.o. q.h.s.	300	Moderate anticholinergic SE and sedation, very low orthostatic hypotension; available as liquid
Desipramine (Norpramin)	25 mg p.o. q.h.s.	300	Low anticholinergic SE and sedation; moderate orthostatic hypotension and conduction abnormalities; can be used in patients with seizure disorder
Imipramine (Tofranil)	25 mg p.o. q.h.s.	300	High incidence of orthostatic hypotension and conduction abnormalities; moderate anticholingeric effects
Trazodone (Desyrel)	50 mg p.o. q.h.s.	600	No anticholinergic SE, can cause moderate sedation and orthostatic hypotension; can be used safely in patients with seizure disorder; associated with priapism

Abbreviation: SE, side effects

[a]Lower dose and slower titration recommended in elderly patients.

TABLE 55-7   SELECTED ANTICONVULSANTS FOR THE MANAGEMENT OF NEURALGIA:
DOSING RECOMMENDATIONS

Agent (Brand)	Dosing Range[a] (mg/day)	Comments
Carbamazepine (Tegretol)	200–1200	Side effects include dizziness, nausea and vomiting, aplastic anemia, and bone marrow suppression; therapeutic levels for seizure control 4–12 mcg/ml
Phenytoin (Dilantin)	300–400	Side effects include dizziness, nausea and vomiting, gingival hyperplasia and peripheral neuropathy. Use abandoned secondary to side effect profile. Therapeutic levels for seizure control 6–20 mcg/ml
Gabapentin (Neurontin)	900–2400	Side effects include dizziness, drowsiness, nausea, vomiting, fatigue, and ataxia. No therapeutic levels have been established.

[a] *Recommend low starting dose, titrating slowly to minimize side effects; range provided is dosing recommendations for the treatment of seizures.*

teroid drug class. Corticosteroids appear to be most effective in the treatment of pain secondary to edema or pressure on surrounding nerves. Especially useful in conditions such as bone pain, spinal cord compression, plexopathies, and brain metastases, corticosteroids, such as dexamethasone and prednisone, are generally used for short treatment courses. Typically, low doses are used when treating bone pain and higher doses in acute pain episodes secondary to spinal cord compression, plexopathies, and brain metastases. While some side effects of this drug class are beneficial for some patients (e.g., weight gain and mood elevation), prolonged use can be associated with undesirable adverse effects such as adrenal and immune suppression, myopathy of large muscle groups, mentation changes, and gastritis. The use of corticosteroids in the treatment of cancer pain is supported by level II evidence.

REASSESSMENT

Pain is a dynamic process and treatment must consistently be reevaluated to determine effectiveness. The frequency of reassessment varies depending on the individual situation. We recommend that inpatients be assessed at least once each shift. If frequent pain medication adjustments or titrations are made, pain should be reassessed after *each* intervention (i.e., 15–30 minutes after parenteral adjustments and 60 minutes after oral). In an outpatient setting, reassessment varies from monthly, to weekly, to daily, depending on the severity of the pain and aggressiveness of the treatment plan.

EDUCATION

Despite marked expansion in the area of pain management, undertreatment of pain continues to be a widespread problem. Over the last two decades, numerous studies have documented that physicians and nurses lack knowledge about pain management, particularly in the area of opioid use and addiction.

Educating patients and health care professionals and controlling cancer pain and its associated suffering can vastly improve the quality of life for patient. This improved quality of life provides patients the opportunity, as well as the right, to enjoy family and friends for the remainder of their lives, instead of focusing on uncontrolled cancer pain.

SUGGESTED READINGS

Agency for Health Care Policy and Research. Clinical Practice Guideline, Number 9. Management of Cancer Pain. Publication No. 94-0592:8, 1994

American Pain Society. Principles of Analgesic Use in the Treatment of Acute Pain and Cancer Pain. American Pain Society, Skokie, IL, 1992

Bonica JJ: Cancer Pain. p. 422. In Bonica JJ (ed): The Management of Pain. Vol 1, 2nd Ed. Lea & Febiger, Philadelphia, 1990

Brooks PM, Day RO: Nonsteroidal antiinflammatory drugs—differences and similarities. N Engl J Med 324:1716–1725, 1991

Cleeland CS, Gonin R, Hatfield AK et al: E Pain and its treatment in outpatients with cancer. N Engl J med 330:592–596, 1994

Ellison NM: Opioid analgesics for cancer pain: twoxicities and their treatments. p. 188. In Pratt (ed): Cancer Pain. Lippincott-Raven, Philadelphia, 1993

Foley KM: Pain syndromes in patients with cancer. Vol. 2:59–75. In Bonica JJ, Ventafridda V (eds): Advances in Pain Research and Therapy. Raven Press, New York, 1979

Foley KM: The treatment of cancer pain. N Engl J Med 313:84–95, 1985

Foley KM: Assessment of pain in patients with cancer. pp. 37–44. In Swerdlow M, Ventafridda V (eds): Cancer Pain. MTP Press, Boston, 1987

Foley KM: Pain syndromes in patients with cancer. Med Clin N arth Am 71:169–184, 1987

Foley KM, Inturrisi CE: Analgesic drug therapy in cancer pain: principles and practice. Med Clin North Am 71:207–232, 1987

Foley KM: Supportive care and the quality of life of the cancer patient. p. 2434. In DeVita V, Hellman S, Rosenberg SA (eds) Cancer: Principles and Practice of Oncology. Lippincott-Raven, Philadelphia, 1993

Fromm GH: Physiological rationale for the treatment of neuropathic pain. APS Journal 2:1–7, 1993

Hill CS: Effective treatment of pain in the cancer patient. pp. 657–669. In Murphy GP, Lawrence W, Lenhard RE. (eds): Textbook of Clinical Oncology, 2nd Ed. American Cancer Society, Atlanta, 1995.

Insel PA: Analgesic-antipyretic and antiinflammatory agents and drugs employed in the treatment of gout. pp. 617–657. In Hardman JG, Goodman Gilman A, Limbird LE (eds): Goodman and Gilman's The Pharmacologic Basis of Therapeutics. 9th Ed. McGraw-Hill, New York, 1996

Jaffe JH, Martin WR: Opioid analgesics and antagonists. pp. 485–525. In Gilman AG, Rall TW, Nies AS, Taylor P (eds): The Pharmacologic Basis of Therapeutics. 8th Ed. Pergamon Press, Elmsford, NY, 1990

Jensen MP, Karoly P: Measurement of cancer pain via patient self-report. pp. 193–218. In Chapman CR, Foley KM (eds): Current and Emerging Issues in Cancer Pain. Raven Press, New York, 1993

Kaiko RF, Foley KM, Grabinski PY et al: Central nervous system excitatory effects of meperidine in cancer patients. Ann Neurol 13:180–185, 1983

Levy MH: Pain Management in Advanced Cancer. Semin Oncol 12:394–410, 1985

Magni G: The use of antidepressants in the treatment of chronic pain. A review of the current evidence. Drugs 42:730–748, 1991

McNamara JO: Drugs effective in the therapy of the epilepsies. In pp. 461–486. Hardman JG, Goodman Gilman A, Limbird LE (eds): Goodman and Gilman's The Pharmacologic Basis of Therapeutics. 9th Ed. McGraw-Hill, New York, 1996

Mellick GA, Mellick LB. Gabapentin in the management of reflex sympathetic dystrophy. J Pain Symp Manage 10:265–266, 1995

Mellick LB, Mellick GA: Successful treatment of reflex sympathetic dystrophy with gabapentin. Am J Emergency Med 13:96, 1995

Mellick GA, Seng ML: The use of gabapentin in the treatment of reflex sympathetic dystrophy and a phobic disorder. Am J Pain Manage 5:7–9, 1995

Parker SL, Tong T, Bolden S, Wingo PA: Cancer Statistics, CA Cancer J Clinician 65:5–27, 1996

Porter J, Jick H: Addiction rare in patients treated with narcotics (letter). N Engl J Med 302:123, 1983

Schug SA, Zech D, Dorr U: Cancer pain management according to WHO analgesic guidelines. J Pain Symptom Manage 5:27–32, 1990

Swerdlow M: Anticonvulsant drugs and chronic pain. Clin Neuropharm 7:51–82, 1984

Ventafridda V, Tamburini M, Caraceni A et al. A validation study of the WHO method for cancer pain relief. Cancer 59:850–856, 1987

Von Roenn JH, Cleeland CS, Gonin R, Hatfield AK, N Engl J Med Pandya KJ: Physician attitudes and practice in cancer pain management: a survey from the Eastern Cooperative Oncology Group. Ann Intern Med 119:121–126, 1993

Watson CPN: Antidepressant drugs as adjuvant analgesics. J Pain Symp Manage 9:392–405, 1994

Wells BG, Hayes PE: Depressive disorders. pp. 1065–1083 In DiPiro JT, Talbert RL, Hayes PE et al (eds): Pharmacotherapy: A Pathophysiologic Approach. 2nd Ed. Elsevier Science, New York, 1992

Wilwerding MB, Loprinzi CL, Mailliard JA et al: A randomized crossover evaluation of methylphenidate in cancer patients receiving strong narcotics. Support Care Cancer 3:135–138, 1995

56 Infections in the Patient With Cancer

A. K. Huang

Infections in patients with cancer are potentially life-threatening. The so-called "3 + 3 + 2 rule" can help us remember that 85% of severe infections are due to eight pathogens: three gram positive cocci (α-hemolytic streptococci, *S. aureus*, *S. epidermis*), three gram-negative bacilli (*E. coli*, *Klebsiella pneumonia*, *Pseudomonas aeruginosa*) and two fungal infections (*Candida*, *Aspergillus*).

Goal of treatment: Eradication of infections

During the past 30 years, intensive cancer research has led to the development of aggressive chemotherapeutic regimens and increased clinical response rates in patients with malignancies. Significant attention turned to the diagnosis and treatment of infection because of subsequent studies of mortality rates. These demonstrated that as many as 70% of deaths were due to infection, often in a rapidly progressive fashion and with atypical clinical presentations. The major risk factor leading to infection in patients with neoplasms is therapy-induced neutropenia, as defined by an absolute neutrophil count (ANC) less than 500 cells per cubic millimeter. A subpopulation with the greatest infection risk are those who experience more profound (ANC < 100 cells per cubic millimeter) and prolonged (> 7 days) neutropenia. These patients often have lymphoreticular malignancies or undergo bone marrow transplantation and receive high doses of immunosuppressive agents.

In 30% to 60% of people with fever and neutropenia, an infection can be documented clinically or microbiologically. A predominance of gram-negative aerobic bacillary infections (e.g., *Pseudomonas*, *Escherichia coli*, and *Klebsiella*) was identified in the first surveillance studies. The large number of deaths often occurred before culture results were known and appropriate antibiotic ther-

apy instituted. Resultant clinical trials proved the efficacy of empiric antibiotic therapy for the febrile neutropenic patient. Success was measured by the proportion of patients defervescing during the first 72 hours when mortality was likeliest and whose identified infections required no change in antimicrobial regimen. In the past 10 to 15 years, physicians have had to make a number of modifications in antibiotic therapy for individual patients before the resolution of neutropenia. This has occurred mainly because of a shift in retrievable pathogens, such as *Staphylococcus aureus* and *S. epidermidis*, yeast and fungi, and viruses from the herpes family. Research protocols of empiric antibiotic therapy now measure success rates by the proportion of patients who survive the neutropenic episode, regardless of the therapies used outside of the investigational regimens.

Currently over 50% of microbiologically confirmed infections are due to gram-positive bacteria. Contributing factors include empiric antimicrobial regimens with good coverage against gram-negative organisms, greater utilization of central venous access catheters, and the emergence of multidrug-resistant organisms (such as pneumococcus, methicillin-resistant *S. aureus*, and enterococcus). There has been greater recognition of the pathogenic nature of certain organisms, such as *S. epidermidis*

399

and *Corynebacterium jeikeium*, because of their eradication and the clinical response of neutropenic patients following appropriate antibiotic therapy. Some investigators have argued for the early empiric use of vancomycin; however, there is good evidence that mortality is not affected if the institution of vancomycin is delayed until a specific pathogen is identified or fever persists despite routine empiric antibiotics. In addition, recent outbreaks of vancomycin-resistant enterococcus in oncology units point to the need to control indiscriminate use of this agent.

Intensive chemotherapeutic protocols, especially for hematopoietic malignancies, and bone marrow transplantation have led to longer periods of profound neutropenia. Patients then develop serious infections from a wide variety of pathogens, including *Candida* species, *Aspergillus* species, other opportunistic fungi, *Legionella*, *Pneumocystis carinii*, herpes simplex, herpes zoster, and cytomegalovirus. With the routine empiric use of broad-spectrum antibiotics, postmortem studies of cancer patients revealed disseminated candidal infections. Well-designed studies have demonstrated the efficacy of adding empiric low-dose (0.3–0.6 mg/kg/day) amphotericin B to control occult yeast infections after 7 days of antibiotic therapy and persistent fever. If fever still persists after several days, the clinician is faced with a broad differential diagnosis for possible pathogens. It is worth remembering that 85% of severe infections are due to eight pathogens. We have, therefore named this, the "3+3+2 rule": three gram-positive cocci (hemolytic streptococci, *S. aureus*, *S. epidermidis*), three gram-negative bacilli (*E. coli*, *Klebsiella pneumoniae*, *pseudomonas aeruginosa*) and two Fungal infections (*Candida*, *Aspergilus*).

In the management of all febrile neutropenic patients, the clinician is directed to careful and repeated evaluation for specific signs and symptoms of a focus or type of infection (e.g., the nasal pain and discharge that may herald *Aspergillus* rhinosinusitis). The lack of neutrophils leads to minimal signs of inflammation at the site of infection. The central venous access catheter with an exit site infection may only exhibit slight erythema, tenderness, and nonspecific drainage. Pneumonia in the profoundly neutropenic patient may be visible as a small area of atelectasis or pleural effusion on plain chest radiograph. The new appearance of or any change in focal symptoms should raise the suspicion of developing infection and indicate the need for aggressive microbiologic, pathologic, or radiographic evaluation. Recognition of presenting syndromes for unusual pathogens will guide the clinician in the initial choice of diagnostic modalities. For example, persistent fever, even as neutropenia is resolving, has been strongly associated with hepatosplenic candidiasis, which may not yield positive blood cultures but can be diagnosed with abdominal computed tomography (CT). Other sensitive microbiologic and radiographic methods are being developed and will aid in the earlier diagnosis and treatment of the high-risk patient with the goal of increased survival. Table 56-1 lists pathogens that have been associated with specific sites of infections in neutropenic patients.

Medical literature contains many other adjunctive therapies (e.g., colony-stimulating factors, prophylactic antibiotics or antifungal agents, granulocyte transfusions) for the prevention and treatment of infection in the febrile neutropenic patient (Table 56-2). In various controlled studies to date, these interventions appear to reduce the incidence

TABLE 56-1 COMMON PATHOGENS BY SITE OF INVOLVEMENT

Oral or mucous membranes, skin	*Candida* species, herpes simplex, *Actinomyces*, *Histoplasma*, group A *Streptococcus*, *Staphylococcus aureus*
Central venous access	*Staphylococcus aureus*, *Staphylococcus epidermidis*, enterococcus, *Candida* species, *Corynebacterium jeikeium* (JK diphtheroids)
Gastrointestinal tract	*Enterobacteriaceae*, anaerobes, cytomegalovirus, *Clostridium difficile*
Respiratory system	pneumococcus, *Staphylococcus aureus*, *Pseudomonas aeruginosa*, *Legionella*, *Nocardia*, *Actinomyces*, *Mycobacterium tuberculosis*, *Aspergillus* species, *Pneumocystis carinii*, cytomegalovirus, influenza.

TABLE 56-2 CONTROVERSIAL PROPHYLACTIC AND THERAPEUTIC INTERVENTIONS

Intervention	Evidence-Based Recommendations	Concerns
Prophylactic oral antibiotics, antifungal agents	Level I evidence May be used at the discretion of the clinician Will reduce number of infections in a neutropenic episode. No survival benefit demonstrated.	Empiric antibiotics for fever are still required in a most cases, but initiation is delayed Emergence of resistant organisms with subsequent superinfection
Granulocyte transfusions	Level III/IV evidence No therapeutic indications at present Well-designed studies needed to compare with current management strategies	Inability to obtain sufficient quantities Serious potential and reported side effects (pulmonary edema, viral transmission, alloantibodies)
Colony-stimulating factors	Level I/II evidence May be useful in protocols in which 40% of patients are expected to have profound neutropenia (ANC < 100/mm³) May be useful in patients with neutropenia during primary treatment cycle to avoid dose reduction in chemotherapy during subsequent cycles	Cost-effectiveness has not been proven
Immunoglobulins	Level III/IV evidence No therapeutic indications at present	
Antiendotoxin antibodies	Level I/II evidence No therapeutic indications at present	
Protective isolation environment	Level IV evidence May be beneficial in cases in which prolonged periods of profound neutropenia are expected	Cost-effectiveness has not been proven

of infection but not to change the survival rate to bone marrow recovery nor significantly decrease the use of empiric antimicrobial therapy. Table 56-2 presents situations when adjunctive therapies may be beneficial. Several detailed analyses of these modalities are referenced for the interested reader. Ongoing studies are examining the effectiveness, from the standpoint of both outcome and cost, of antimicrobial/antifungal prophylaxis and of the use of colony-stimulating factors. This data should result in better-defined indications for their use in high-risk neutropenic populations.

Recently published studies have examined characteristics within patients populations that define low-risk neutropenia. It is felt that such a status may indicate the potential for a less aggressive approach to the treatment of fever and neutropenia following chemotherapy. This may take the form of shorter hospitalizations or the conversion from intravenous to oral medications without subsequent medical complications. For example, Talcott et al. have identified low risk patients as those who (1) are not hospitalized at the onset of fever and neutropenia, (2) do not have significant accompanying medical illness requiring hospitalization (e.g., hypotension, dehydration, vomiting), and (3) do not have uncontrolled neoplastic disease. Initial studies validating various risk assessments and attempting outpatient antibiotic management have been successfully performed; however, the lack of larger prospective evaluation precludes routine implementation.

Figure 56-1 and Table 56-3 detail the management of the febrile neutropenic patient and are applicable to those with solid tumors and hematopoietic malignancies since the neutropenia, and not the cell type, conveys the risk for infection. ANC has been defined as less than 1,000 cells per cubic millimeter (rather than less than 500 cells per cubic millimeter as in many clinical trials) to give clinicians greater flexibility in applying these algorithms. Table 56-4 lists the common empiric antimicrobial therapies that are mentioned in the algorithms. There are no guidelines to the duration of antibiotic therapy if no source or pathogen is identified and the patient is responding clinically. Most investigators have chosen to treat for 7 days or until neutropenia is clearly resolving, whichever

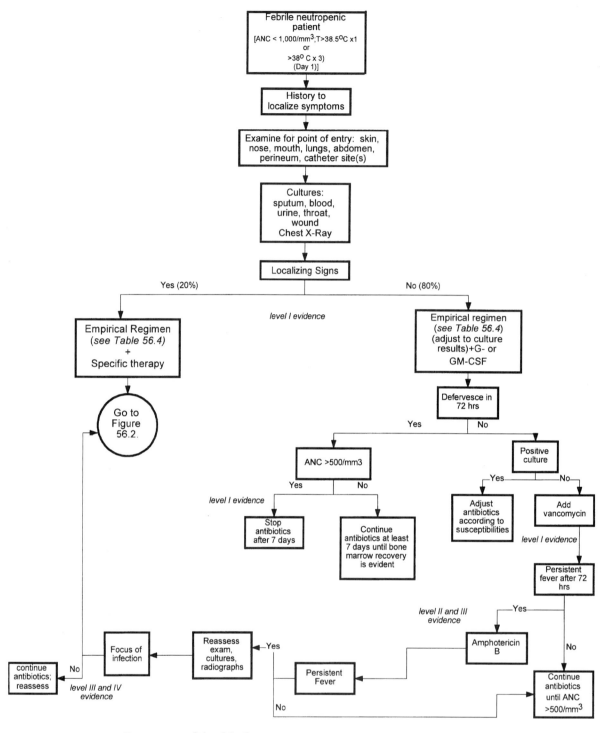

FIGURE 56-1 *Treatment of the febrile neutropenic patient. Reasoning strategy is highly probabilistic, based upon the premise that early demise (sepsis) will follow if empiric treatment is not started urgently ("diagnosis you can't afford to miss"). Sequential choice of therapies is also based upon estimates of likely specific etiologic agent causing infection in question. For example, initial treatment is targeted against bacterial agents, first to cover a broad spectrum of gram-positive and gram-negative bacteria (especially Pseudomonas aeruginosa), then against gram-positive bacteria such as Staphylococcus (vancomycin added), then to cover fungi, as the likelihood of these infections increases with duration of neutropenia. Obviously, this empirical (probabilistic) strategy will be modified as specific agents are isolated or a particular set of symptoms suggests a culprit causing the infection.*

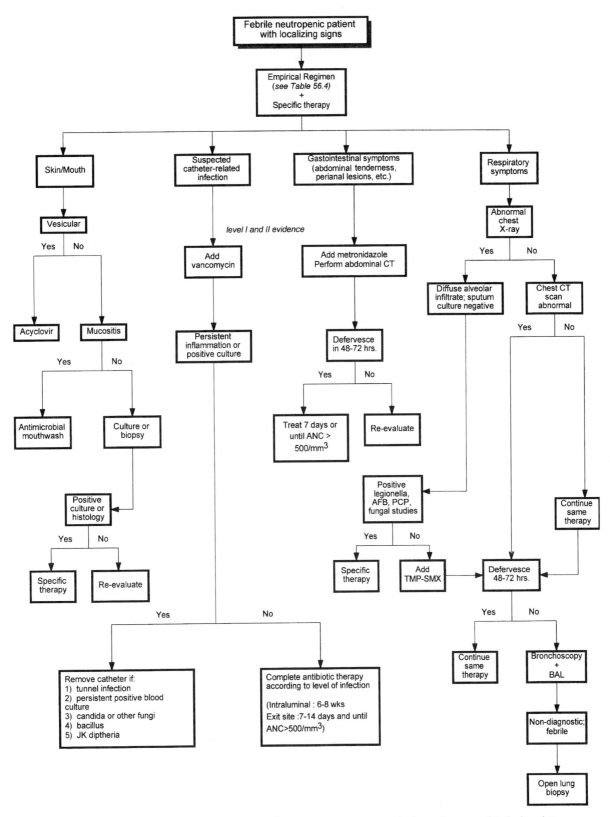

FIGURE 56-2 *Recommended strategy for empiric treatment is based on multiple level I evidences; etiologic (cause-effect) principles are employed when microbiologic agents are uncovered. (Modified from Joseph G, Herzig R, Djulbegović B: Treatment of immunocompromised neutropenic patients. In Djulbegović B (ed): Reason and Decision Making in Hematology. Churchill Livingstone, New York, 1992, with permission.)*

TABLE 56-3   **GENERAL PRINCIPLES FOR THE MANAGEMENT OF FEVER IN PATIENTS WITH NEUTROPENIA**

1. Instruct the patient to seek medical help if a fever develops when the neutrophil count is low or declining.
2. Evaluate the patient at least daily.
3. Initiate prompt therapy with broad-spectrum antibiotics when a patient with neutropenia (neutrophil count, <500/mm³) becomes febrile (single elevation in oral temperature to >38.5°C, or three elevations to >38°C during a 24-hour period).
4. If the patient has an indwelling intravenous catheter, obtain cultures from each catheter port and lumen as well as from a peripheral vein. Rotate antibiotic therapy through each lumen of multiple-lumen catheters.
5. Monitor the patient closely for secondary infections requiring additions or modifications to the initial antibiotic regimen.
6. Continue empirical antibiotic therapy if the patient has prolonged (>1 week) neutropenia, particularly if there is persistent fever.
7. Add empirical antifungal therapy if a patient with neutropenia remains febrile after a week of broad-spectrum antibiotic therapy or has recurrent fever.
8. Discontinue antibiotic therapy when the neutrophil count rises above 500/mm³ in a patient at high risk or is increasing in a patient at low risk.
9. Although 10 to 14 days of treatment is adequate in most patients with neutropenia, prolonged therapy is necessary for a patient with a residual focus of infection or invasive mycoses (e.g., hepatosplenic candidiasis).
10. All those caring for a febrile patient with neutropenia should wash their hands carefully before any contact with the patient.

(From Pizzo, N Engl J Med 1993, with permission.)

TABLE 56-4   **ANTIMICROBIAL REGIMENS**

Indication	Drug/Dosing	Comments
Empiric antibiotics	Anti-pseudomonal penicillin (e.g. pipercillin 3 gm IV 6 hours) plus Aminoglycoside (e.g. amikacin 55 mg/kg q8h) (adjust dose for adequate serum levels) (check peak and trough levels after 4th dose) Ceftazidime 2 g IV 8 hours Imipenem 1 g IV 6 hours	Once-daily dosing of aminoglycoside may be a cost-effective alternative
Empiric or documented gram-positive antibiotic therapy	Vancomycin 1 g IV 12 hours (adjust dose for adequate serum levels)	
Empiric antifungal therapy	Amphotericin B 0.3–0.6 mg/kg qd over 1–3 hours (must be given in D5W)	Monitor serum creatinine, potassium, magnesium levels 1-2x weekly
Documented *Aspergillus* or fungal infection	Amphotericin B 1.0–1.5 mg/kg qd to a cumulative dose of 2–3 gm	Liposomal amphotericin B may be considered for those intolerant of amphotericin B
	Give 1 mg test dose with first infusion (in 50 ml of D5W over 10 min) to detect anaphylaxis or idiopathic hyperthermia. Premedicate and repeat every 4 hours with acetaminophen 650 mg and diphenhydramine 25–50 mg p.o. if symptomatic with infusions. Hydrocortisone 20–50 mg IV can be added if phlebitis occurs. Give meperidine 25–50 mg IV p.r.n. during infusion	
Herpes simplex	Acyclovir 5.0–7.5 mg/kg IV q 8 hours or 200 mg PO 5x qd for 7–10 days or until lesions scab over	Monitor renal function
Herpes zoster	Acyclovir 10.0–12.5 mg/kg IV q 8 hours or 800 mg p.o. 5x qday until lesions scab over.	High doses may cause encephalopathy
Legionella pneumophila	Erythromycin 1 g IV or p.o. q 6 hours for 21 days	Fluoroquinolones +/– rifampin has been used in intolerant patients
Pneumocystis carinii pneumonia	Trimethoprim-sulfamethoxazole 15–20 mg (trimethroprim component)/kg p.o. or IV qd **or** Pentamidine 4 mg/kg IV qday for 21 days	Monitor renal function; can cause leukopenia Causes pancreatitis with hyperinsulinemia after 7 days. Monitor blood sugars. Can cause leukopenia and thrombocytopenia

is longer. At the present time there is little data to support stopping antibiotic therapy in the well-appearing febrile, neutropenic patient.

SUGGESTED READINGS

American Society of Clinical Oncology. Recommendations for the use of hematopoietic colony-stimulating factors: evidence-based, clinical practice guidelines. *J Clin Oncol* 12:2471–2508, 1994

Buchanan GR: Approach to treatment of the febrile cancer patient with low-risk neutropenia. *Hematol Oncol Clin North Am* 7:919–935, 1993

Freifeld AG, Walsh T, Marshall D et al: Monotherapy for fever and neutropenia in cancer patients: a randomized comparison of ceftazidime versus imipenem. *J Clin Oncol* 13:165–176, 1995

Giamarellou H: Empiric therapy for infections in the febrile, neutropenic, compromised host. *Med Clin North Am* 79:559–580, 1995

Hathorn JW: Critical appraisal of antimicrobials for prevention of infections in immunocompromised hosts. *Hematol Oncol Clin North Am* 7: 1051–1098, 1993

Malik IA, Khan WA, Karim M et al: Feasibility of outpatient management of fever in cancer patients with low-risk neutropenia: results of a prospective randomized trial. *Am J Med* 98:224–231, 1995

Pizzo PA: Management of fever in patients with cancer and treatment induced neutropenia. *N Engl J Med* 328:1323–1332, 1993

Sanders JW, Powe NR, Moore RD: Ceftazidime monotherapy for empiric treatment of febrile neutropenic patients: a meta-analysis. *J Infect Dis* 164:907–916, 1991

Talcott JA, Siegel RD, Finberg R, Goldman L: Risk assessment in cancer patients with fever and neutropenia: a prospective, two-center validation of a prediction rule. *J Clin Oncol* 10:316–322, 1992

Joseph G, Herzig R, Djulbegovic B: Treatment of immunocompromised (neutropenic) patients. In Djulbegovic B (ed): Reason and Decision Making in Hematology. Churchill Livingstone, New York, 1992

57 Oral Care of the Cancer Patient

C. Edgar Davila

Most of the time, the integrity of the oral cavity is taken for granted by primary caregivers until it is compromised by cancer therapy. Then, oral complications associated with pain and dysphagia become a vivid reality. This chapter discusses principles of prevention and management of oral complications during cancer chemotherapy as detailed in Figure 57-1.

Oral pain is a very common complaint of cancer patients. Despite technologic developments and the therapeutic success of cancer treatment, it is estimated that 400,000 or more episodes of adverse oral and dental sequela occur each year in the United States among patients receiving chemotherapy, radiation therapy, and bone marrow transplantation. Complications of cancer chemotherapy can be *direct* (mucositis), resulting from the toxic action of antineoplastic agents on the proliferative mucosal lining of the mouth, or *indirect* (infection, bleeding), the result of hematopoietic shutdown. The biologic effect is transient, lasting during the period of immunosuppression. *Infections account for the majority of oral complications*, which can disseminate systemically and increase morbidity and mortality. The frequency and severity of oral complications vary with the patient, malignancy, modality of therapy, agents used, sequencing of agents, rate of delivery of the anticancer treatment, and local oral factors. Oral complications occur two to three times more frequently during chemotherapy for leukemia and myeloproliferative disease than in drug therapy for solid tumors.

Oral complications associated with cancer chemotherapy can be classified into the three following types: *mucositis, infection, and bleeding*. The majority are associated, both in occurrence and severity, with preexisting conditions that significantly affect their initiation, augmentation, and persistence. It is unfortunate when a patient develops an oral complication that a preventive measure or simple hygiene and oral care could have prevented or reduced.

PREVENTION

The primary goals of oral and dental care are to prevent oral and dental disorders and to modify the acute complications and long-term consequences of cancer therapy. The first step in prevention is a comprehensive oral and dental examination by the dental oncologist before or early in the patient's medical therapy. Therefore, procedures have to be established to ensure early referral of these patients to the dental clinic for an oral evaluation and dental treatment. Chronic periodontal and dental pulp sources of infection must be examined thoroughly and removed before cancer therapy. Local irritants, such as calculus on teeth or prostheses, should be smoothed and polished. As denture surfaces are commonly colonized with *Candida* species, attention to denture hygiene and removal of the appliance at least at night is recommended. When the denture is not in the mouth, it should be soaked in an antiseptic solution. Patients with no dental plaque present during cancer chemotherapy treatment develop significantly less mucositis for a shorter period (Lindquist S et al.). Professional dental prophylaxis, scaling, and root planing of all dentition and good oral hygiene are important preventive measures to reduce the risk of oral complications during chemotherapy.

Oral hygiene instructions, such as adequate toothbrushing technique, flossing, and the daily use of 1.1% sodium fluoride (Thera-Flur Gel Drops, Colgate Oral Pharmaceuticals) should be discussed and explained to the patient. In some instances, when mucositis is severe, a chemobrush (Ultrasoft toothbrush, Periodontal Health Brush, Inc., Rx Ultrasuave) is recommended.

407

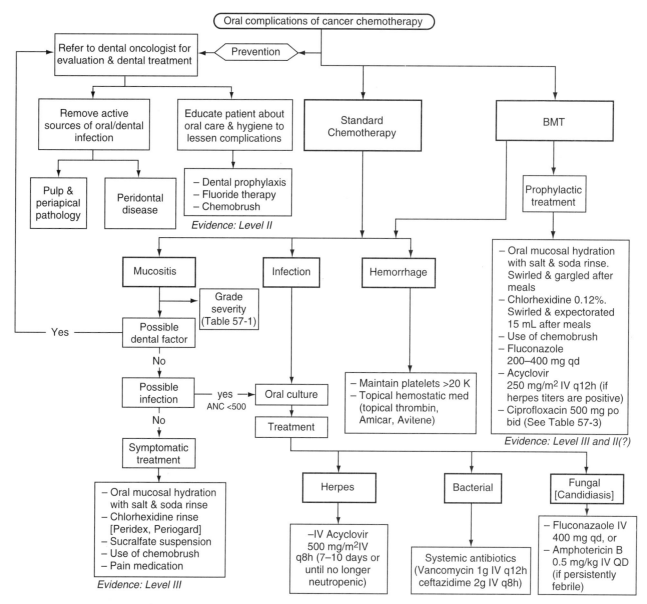

FIGURE 57-1 *Algorithm for the prevention and management of oral complications of cancer chemotherapy. A pretreatment evaluation by a dental oncologist is important for patients receiving either a standard dose or high-dose bone marrow transplantation chemotherapy. Patients receiving high-dose chemotherapy and either autologous or allogeneic stem cell transplants are treated prophylactically with antifungal, antiviral, and antibacterial drugs. The treatment of oral infections in nonneutropenic patients may be specifically directed by culture results or clinical suspicions; however, neutropenic patients (ANC <500) with a fever are empirically treated with intravenous acyclovir, broad spectrum antibiotics, and antifungal agents; the treatment may later be modified depending on culture results. The level of evidence supporting this algorithm is generally level III.*

MUCOSITIS

Mucositis is the most frequent oral complication of chemotherapy that has clinical significance. Mucositis, evidenced by thinning or ulceration of the mucosal barrier, may occur within five to seven days after drug administration. The resulting mucositis occurs in approximately 20% of patients treated for adult leukemia or breast cancer. Painful ulcerative lesions primarily occur on nonkeratinized tissues and will continue to develop as long as the drug is administered. Oral sites most commonly involved include the buccal and labial mucosa, ventral and lateral surfaces of the tongue, soft palate, and floor of the mouth. The severity varies with the type and dose of the chemotherapeutic agent administered and the patient's ability to tolerate the drug. Use of a grading score of severity for mucosal reactions during each course of the therapy allows clinicians to take appropriate preventive and therapeutic measures during current and future treatment courses (Table 57-1). Certain agents are more stomatotoxic than others; however, large doses of less potent agents prescribed for long periods may cause mucositis (Table 57-2). Patients who develop mucositis during the initial course of chemotherapy will almost certainly react in the same way during subsequent course unless the drug is changed or doses reduced. Although mucositis may occur in healthy mouths, the literature suggests that a patient's oral/dental status plays a significant role in the incidence, severity, and duration of mucosal lesions. Palliative treatment is aimed at minimizing mucosal trauma and increas-

TABLE 57-2 CHEMOTHERAPEUTIC DRUGS THAT PRODUCE DIRECT STOMATOTOXICITY

Alkylating Agents
  Mechlorethamine
Antimetabolics
  Cytarabine hydrochloride
  Floxuridine
  Fluorouracil
  Mercaptopurine
  Methotrexate
  Thioguanine
Natural Products
  Bleomycin
  Dactinomycin
  Daunorubicin
  Doxorubicin
  Mithramycin
  Mitomycin
  Vinblastine sulfate
  Vincristine sulfate
Other Synthetic Agents
  Hydroxyurea
  Procarbazine hydrochloride

(From DeVita VT, Hellman S, Rosenberg SA et al. Cancer. Principles and Practice of Oncology. pp. 2385–2394. Lippincott-Raven, 1993, with permission.)

TABLE 57-1 MUCOSITIS GRADING

Grade	Criteria
0	Normal
	No mucositis
I	Mild tissue changes (focal)
	White anemic changes
	Erythematous patches
	Mucosal thinning
	No sensitivity
	Normal eating
II	Mild tissue changes (focal)
	Erythematous/thinning mucosa
	Small ulceration (<2 mm)
	Slight sensitivity
	Normal eating
III	Moderate tissue changes (focal/diffuse)
	Erythematous/denuded/ulcerated
	<½ mucosal area involved
	Blood clots, no active hemorrhage
	Moderate sensitivity
	Eating/drinking with difficulty
IV	Marked tissue changes (diffuse)
	Erythematous/denuded/ulcerated
	>½ mucosal area involved
	Active oozing/bleeding
	Marked pain
	No eating

(Adapted from Toth B, Chambers M, Fleming T et al: Minimizing oral complications of cancer treatment. Oncology 9:851–858, 1995, with permission.)

ing patient comfort. Mouth rinses are recommended as mucositis therapy to cleanse the mouth and provide mucosal hydration. We recommend the frequent use of a diluted salt and baking soda solution (½ teaspoon of each added to 1 quart of water), which is soothing to irritated tissues and helps to dislodge mucinous salivary secretions. The use of chlorhexidine gluconate 0.12% (Peridex, Periogard) along with a sucralfate suspension is also recommended to reduce mucositis. The patient must practice good oral hygiene to help prevent bacterial or fungal superinfections. Unidentifiable pain associated with chemotherapy is controlled with analgesics or intravenous pain medication (see Ch. 55).

BLEEDING

Approximately 88% of the oral hemorrhagic complications observed in chemotherapy patients result from thrombocytopenia secondary to myelosuppression. Hemorrhage can manifest as petechiae on the lips, soft palate, and floor of mouth, or as larger submucosal hematomas that are commonly seen in the buccal mucosa and lateral borders of the tongue. Bleeding episodes may be spontaneous or may be precipitated by trauma or existing disease. When inflammation or ulceration from periodontal disease is present, the gingival crevice is prone to either spontaneous or traumatic bleeding. This is the most common, yet difficult to manage, source of hemorrhage. All oral hygiene measures, including rinsing, should be discontinued when spontaneous bleeding occurs. Debridement of large clots and pressure applied to the area with 2 × 2 inch sponges soaked in topical thrombin is recommended. If ineffective, the use of amino caproic acid (EACA, Amicar) in the same manner is indicated. If the platelet count is below 20,000/mm³, platelet transfusions should be administered to achieve a goal of 50,000/mm³ (see Ch. 56). Removable dental appliances should be removed to avoid harmful irritation. If extractions must be performed on patients with thrombocytopenia, debridement of all granulation tissue, careful closure of wounds with absorbable sutures, and the use of hemostatic agents, such as microfibrillar collagen (Avitene), are indicated. Packing agents, such as oxidized cellulose (Surgicel) or absorbable gelatin sponge (Gelfoam), must be avoided because they may act as a nidus of infection in severe granulocytopenia.

INFECTION

The majority of patients who die after chemotherapy do so because of infections, and the oral cavity is the most frequently identified source of sepsis in patients with granulocytopenic fever. More infections of oral origin are expected in patients with leukemia than in those with solid tumors. The three major types of oral infections are bacterial, fungal and viral.

BACTERIAL INFECTION

The gingival tissues are a common site of bacterial infection, especially in patients with preexisting periodontal disease, with the most common clinical manifestation resembling acute necrotizing ulcerative gingivitis (ANUG). The treatment includes debridement with cotton pellets soaked with 3% hydrogen peroxide, maintenance of good oral hygiene, and systemic antibiotics. Mucosal bacterial infections are usually secondary to ulcerations produced by direct stomatoxicity or trauma and may present clinically as ulcerations with a yellow-white necrotic center with the borders slightly raised and indurated. If fever and a low white blood cell count (<500/mm³ granulocytes) are present, systemic antibiotics are indicated.

Odontogenic bacterial infections in the myelosupressed patient may be difficult to diagnose because the patient cannot produce an inflammatory response. Tooth pain and fever may be the only signs of periapical infection, and a thorough dental examination, including dental radiographs, is needed for a diagnosis.

It is very important to treat or remove any questionable teeth before chemotherapy. If teeth are the cause of infection during chemotherapy, removal should be accomplished in close coordination between the dentist and the medical oncologist.

FUNGAL INFECTIONS

Fungal infections, primarily *Candida*, are common in patients undergoing cancer chemotherapy. Most candidal lesions appear as superficial, raised white patches with a hemorrhagic base and can be difficult to differentiate clinically from mucositis. The prophylactic use of topical antifungal agents, such as Mystatin lozenges or clotrimazole troches, begun at the time of chemotherapy reduces the frequency and severity of infection as does the systemic use of fluconazole. Use of topical antiseptic rinses with 0.2 percent chlorhexidine, in conjunction with other topical and systemic antimicrobial agents, can be helpful. Be alert to any spread of infection into the esophagus or bronchus, which can lead to fatal systemic disseminations. Amphotericin B is administered if the patient is persistently febrile.

VIRAL INFECTIONS

Viral infections affecting the oral cavity and head and neck region in the immunocompromised patient are commonly caused by herpes simplex and varicella zoster viruses, in addition to the less frequent involvement of cytomegalovirus and Epstein-Barr virus. Nearly 50% of leukemia patients undergoing chemotherapy develop oral herpes simplex infections. Oral viral infections usually present as a small cluster of round ulcers that spread and coalesce to form longer irregular ulcerations, which have a central gray or white area of necrosis and a surrounding band of erythema. The treatment is the administration of acyclovir. Patients with viral infections should be monitored closely to ensure they are eating properly and that no systemic spread of the virus occurs.

ORAL COMPLICATIONS OF BONE MARROW TRANSPLANTATION

Allogeneic bone marrow transplantation (BMT) is used frequently in the treatment of acute leukemia, chronic myelogenous leukemia, aplastic anemia, and

TABLE 57-3 PROPHYLACTIC PROTOCOL FOR BONE MARROW TRANSPLANTATION PATIENTS

Rinses
    Salt and baking soda rinse (1/2 teaspoon each of salt and baking soda added to 1 quart of water). Swirled and gargled to remove residual debris after meals.
    Chlorhexidine gluconate 0.12% rinse (Peridex, Periogard, 15 ml swirled and expectorated three times daily after meals).
Regular plaque removal with "chemobrush" (Ultrasoft toothbrush, Periodontal Health Brush, Inc., Rx Ultrasuave), which is rinsed with hydrogen peroxide and water after use. Change of brush weekly.
Drugs (general antimicrobial prophylaxis in allogeneic BMT setting)
    Fluconazole 200–400 mg q day (from 7 days before transplantation until marrow engraftment)
    Acyclovir 250 mg/m^2 IV q8hours (from 1 day before transplantation until engraftment)
    Ciprofloxacin hydrochloride 500 p.o. b.i.d. (from 7 days before transplantation until marrow engraftment)
    Bactrim DS, 2 tablets twice weekly (from marrow engraftment until 180 days after transplantation or for duration of immunosuppression)
    Penicillin 250 mg b.i.d.

(From Momin F, Chandrasekar P: Antimicrobial Prophalaxis in Bone Marrow Transplantation Ann Intern Med 123:205–215, 1995, with permission.)

severe combined immunodeficiency. In general, bone marrow transplantation patients are conditioned with chemotherapy and total body irradiation to eliminate malignant cells and prevent graft rejection. As part of the treatment, immunosuppressive therapy is used to prevent or manage graft-versus-host disease (GVHD). If oral complications occur after BMT, they are associated with either the conditioning chemoradiation therapy, postgrafting immunosuppression, or the effects of chronic GVHD.

Early changes of the oral mucosa secondary to chemoradiationtherapy include erythema, atrophy, and ulceration. *The incidence of mucositis in the BMT patient is close to 100%.* The post-transplant use of drugs such as methotrexate, cyclosporin A, and steroids can cause severe mucositis, gingival hypertrophy, and susceptibility to oral infections,

and those effects can be complicated by xerostomia. During these periods of severe immunosuppression, evidence of head and neck infections or febrile episodes must be treated with broad spectrum antibiotic therapy. Antifungal rinses or troches and antiviral chemotherapy have proven to be effective when used prophylactically. Different from patients receiving standard chemotherapy, BMT patients must follow a prophylactic protocol to reduce the risk of oral and systemic infection (Table 57-3).

GVHD occurs in 25% to 40% of long-term survivors of allogeneic transplantation and can generally be seen anytime beyond day 20 after transplantation. The oral changes of chronic GVHD include generalized mucosal atrophy, erythema, and lichen planus-like lesions. GVHD can also causes changes in the salivary flow rate with resultant xerostomia.

SUGGESTED READINGS

Berkowitz R, Berg J, Ferreti G: Oral complications of bone marrow transplantation. pp. 413–425. In: Bone Marrow Transplantation in Children. Lippincott-Raven New York, 1990.

De Paola L, et al: Dental care for patients receiving chemotherapy. JADA 112:198, 1986

DeVita V, Hellman S, Rosenberg SA et al: Cancer principles and practices of oncology. Lippincott-Raven Philadelphia, 1993, 2385–2394

Ferreti G, Ash RC, Brown AT, et al: Control of oral mucositis and candidiasis in marrow transplantation. A prospective, double-blind trial of chlorhexidine digluconate oral rinse. Bone Marrow Transplant 3:483–493, 1988

Lindquist S, Hickey A, Drane J: Effect of oral hygiene on stomatitis in patients receiving cancer chemotherapy. J Prosth Dent 40:312–314, 1978

Momin F, Chandrasekar P: Antimicrobial prophylaxis in bone marrow transplantation. Ann Intern Med 123:205–215

Prada A, Chiesa F: Effects of benzydamine on oral mucositis during antineoplastic radiotherapy and/or intra-arterial chemotherapy. Int J Tiss React 9:115–119, 1987

Toth B, Chambers M, Fleming T, Lemon J, Martin J: Minimizing oral complications of cancer treatment. Oncology 9:851–858, 1995

Toth B, Martin J, Fleming T: Oral complications associated with cancer therapy. J Clin Periodontal 17:508–515, 1990

Toth B, Martin J, Fleming T: Oral and dental care associated with cancer therapy. Cancer Bull 43:397–402, 1991

Wright W, Hallen J, Harlow S, Pizzo P: An oral disease prevention program for patients receiving radiation and chemotherapy. JADA 110:43, 1985

58 Red Blood Cell Transfusion and Platelet Transfusion

Donald R. Fleming

The principles involving red blood cell and platelet transfusions are similar during both conventional and high-dose chemotherapy. Even the amount of required blood-product support can be similar in both situations. One report reviewed the actual amounts of platelet and packed red cell transfusions required among a group of conventionally treated and "high-dose" treated patients. The latter group included a separation of the autologous and allogeneic transplant patients. Basically, an average of 150 and 15 units of platelets and packed red blood cells, respectively, were required with no significant difference among the various groups. This chapter discusses basic parameters to guide physicians in transfusing patients undergoing cancer therapy as well as those patients in whom therapy is no longer indicated.

As to the acceptable level of hemoglobin (Hb) to maintain, there has been some controversy. Previous levels of 10 g/dl were believed to be the universally optimal level for cardiovascular support. In addition, some have felt lower levels of Hb may stimulate erythropoiesis at the expense of delayed platelet and leukocyte recovery. In reality, red blood cell transfusions may transiently cause a decrease in platelets because of dilution and/or a microaggregation effect. While factors such as patient age, cardiovascular status, and time factors in anemia development are considered in transfusion decisions, symptoms related to anemia should take priority. Dyspnea, confusion, or just generalized fatigue are by far the best indicators of transfusion requirements. Generally, young, sedentary, and/or otherwise healthy individuals may not become symptomatic until a gradual decline in Hb falls below 7 to 8 g/dl. Other patient populations, such as an elderly patient with a history of coronary artery disease can have a one in two and one in twenty chance of sustaining angina pectoris and myocardial infarction respectively, if the hematocrit falls below 28 percent.

Despite the constant measures to improve the volunteer donor pool of blood products, a significant number of patients as well as health professionals remain concerned about the safety of the blood supply in regard to viral infection transmission. One solution, "designated donors," usually with family members, has been practiced in response to this concern. Transfusion-associated graft-verses-host disease becomes an issue in this situation. There is an increased risk of homozygote donor reactivity in a healthy heterozygote recipient, especially among related donor/recipient situations. Blood products should be irradiated with 1,500 to 2000 cGy in these situations.

A more controversial area, concerning platelet transfusion requirements, is the potential alloimmunization associated with donor platelets. The traditional transfusion threshold of $20 \times 10^9/L$ is based on antiquated studies using leukemia patients, some of whom were receiving aspirin during remission-induction chemotherapy. Nevertheless, most institutions have adopted the traditional platelet transfusion threshold of $20 \times 10^9/L$ in uncomplicated cancer patients destined to soon recover platelet production. An even more controversial issue involves clinically stable patients with no evidence of chronic hypoproliferative states, such as myelodysplasia or aplastic anemia. These patients may only be transfused when clinical situations demand platelet transfusions. Some, however, suggest transfusion thresholds of $5 \times 10^9/L$ in this patient population as opposed to waiting on clinical indications (i.e., bleeding) to determine the necessity of platelet transfusions. Again, alloimmunization may cause platelet refractoriness when

413

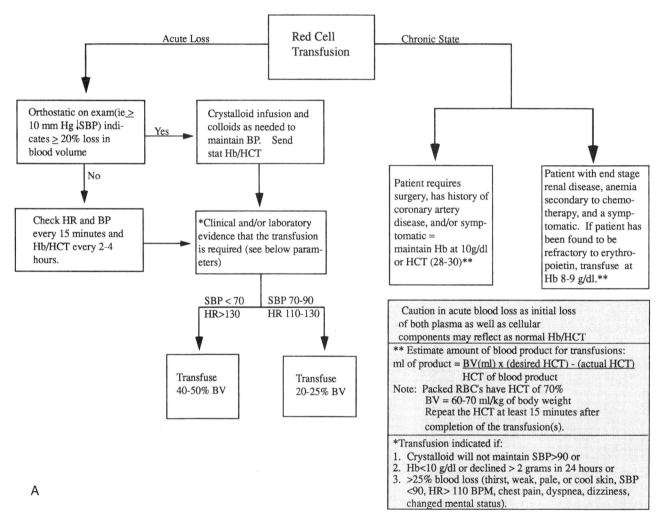

A

FIGURE 58-1   *Red blood cell (A) and platelet transfusion (B) guidelines depend on the dynamics of anemia and thrombocytopenia respectively. While prompt action in cases of acute loss or destruction is necessary, the judicious application of transfusion therapy during chronic disease states or production defects are just as crucial. Recommendations on transfusion parameters are generally based on evidence from multiple time series, both with and without intervention. Generally, data supporting platelet transfusion guidelines are based on level I and II prospective, randomized trials. Use of RBC products is based on solid non-experimental clinical studies (level III evidence). HR, heart rate; SBP, systolic blood pressure; BV, blood volume; TTP, thrombotic thrombocytopenia purpura; MPV, mean platelet volume; HIT, heparin-induced thrombocytopenia; CNS, central nervous system; BT, bleeding time; PTP, post-transfusion purpura; CMV, cytomegalovirus.*

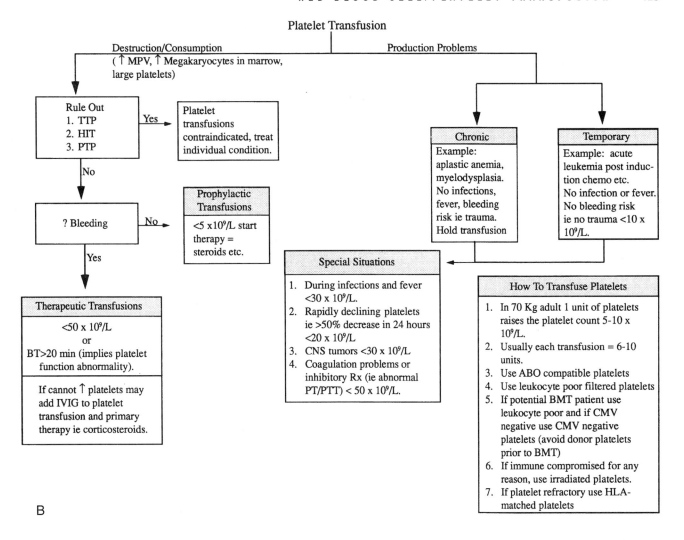

Platelet Transfusion

Destruction/Consumption
(↑ MPV, ↑ Megakaryocytes in marrow, large platelets)

Production Problems

Rule Out
1. TTP
2. HIT
3. PTP

→ Yes → Platelet transfusions contraindicated, treat individual condition.

↓ No

? Bleeding → No → **Prophylactic Transfusions**
<5 x10⁹/L start therapy = steroids etc.

↓ Yes

Therapeutic Transfusions

<50 x 10⁹/L
or
BT>20 min (implies platelet function abnormality).

If cannot ↑ platelets may add IVIG to platelet transfusion and primary therapy ie corticosteroids.

Chronic
Example: aplastic anemia, myelodysplasia. No infections, fever, bleeding risk ie trauma. Hold transfusion

Temporary
Example: acute leukemia post induction chemo etc. No infection or fever. No bleeding risk ie no trauma <10 x 10⁹/L.

Special Situations
1. During infections and fever <30 x 10⁹/L.
2. Rapidly declining platelets ie >50% decrease in 24 hours <20 x 10⁹/L
3. CNS tumors <30 x 10⁹/L
4. Coagulation problems or inhibitory Rx (ie abnormal PT/PTT) < 50 x 10⁹/L.

How To Transfuse Platelets
1. In 70 Kg adult 1 unit of platelets raises the platelet count 5-10 x 10⁹/L.
2. Usually each transfusion = 6-10 units.
3. Use ABO compatible platelets
4. Use leukocyte poor filtered platelets
5. If potential BMT patient use leukocyte poor and if CMV negative use CMV negative platelets (avoid donor platelets prior to BMT)
6. If immune compromised for any reason, use irradiated platelets.
7. If platelet refractory use HLA-matched platelets

B

and if further bleeding episodes require platelet transfusions.

Methods to prevent or delay refractoriness to platelet transfusions caused by alloimmunization have been attempted. Despite leukofiltration, use of HLA-matched platelets, and investigational methods, such as ultraviolet radiation exposure, 25%–50% of those patients requiring repeated and frequent platelet transfusions will develop clinically significant alloimmunization. Basically, in these situations the one-hour host platelet transfusion level is generally less than 20×10^9/L.

In summary, the crucial information in transfusing oncology patients is to utilize blood components judiciously and become aware of alternative measures, such as the use of recombinant erythropoietin, to circumvent the need for transfusions. Guidelines for both red cell and platelet transfusions are presented in Figure 58-1.

SUGGESTED READINGS

Djulbegović B. Reasoning and decision making in hematology. Churchill Livingstone, New York; 1992:239–242

George CD, Morello PJ: Immunologic effect of blood transfusion upon renal transplantation, tumor operations and bacterial infections. Am J Surg 159:329, 1986

Klein HG (ed): Standards for blood banks and transfusion services, 16th Ed. American Association of Blood Banks, Bethesda, 1994

Murphey MF, Brozovic B, Murphy W et al: British Committee for Standards in Hematology; Working Party of the Blood Transfusion Task Force. Guidelines for platelet transfusions. Transfus Med 4:311, 1992

Salem-Schatz SR, Avovn J, Soumerais B: Influence of clinical knowledge, organizational context, and practice style on transfusion decision making. Implications for practice change strategies. JAMA 264:471, 1990

Schreiber GB, Busch MP, Kleinman SH, Korelitz JJ: The risk of transfusion-transmitted viral infections. N Engl J Med 334:1685, 1996

Task Force of the College of American Pathologists: Practice parameters for the use of fresh-frozen plasma, cryoprecipitate and platelets. JAMA 10:777, 1994

van Marwijk: Use of leukocyte-depleted platelet concentrates for the prevention of refractoriness and primary HLA alloimmunization. A prospective, randomized trial, Blood 77:201, 1991

59 | Transfusion Reaction

Donald R. Fleming

Despite the frequent occurrence of adverse transfusion reactions, most have minimal sequela for the patients. In addition to managing the commonly seen reactions, this chapter will address the more infrequent and severe reactions, which at times are difficult to recognize. Basically adverse reactions can be segregated into two categories, immune and nonimmune-mediated types. The former includes febrile transfusion reactions, both acute and delayed hemolytic transfusion reactions, urticaria, anaphylaxis secondary to IgA deficiency, transfusion-associated lung injury, transfusion-associated graft-versus-host disease, and post-transfusion purpura. The latter category includes transfusion sepsis, congestive heart failure, iron overload, and various metabolic abnormalities. The mortality rate for these reactions can be as high as 90% to 100% for transfusion-associated graft-versus-host disease to as low as less than 1% for febrile transfusion reactions. Other mortality rates are 10% to 20% for ABO incompatible hemolytic transfusion reaction and 6% for transfusion-associated acute lung injury.

Within the immune category lies a recently defined concept of transfusion-associated immunosuppression. While initially believed to serve primarily an advantage to graft survival in renal transplant patients, now there is evidence of transfusion-associated immunosuppression leading to increased cancer relapse rates, increase in autoimmune disease activity, and increased viral replications.

While not usually considered among transfusion reactions, transfusion-transmitted infections have been of major concern. Despite the concern, the blood supply has a greater safety profile than anytime since the development of organized volunteer blood distribution. The risk of HIV infection remains approximately 1:225,000 to 1:400,000, while the risk of HTLV I/II is 1:50,000. The risk of hepatitis B and hepatitis C is approximately 1:200,000 and 1:3,300 respectively. Despite the ever increasing scrutiny of the blood supply, the remote possibility of life-long affliction must be considered when assessing patients need for transfusions.

This Figure 59-1 and Table 59-1 delineate the treatment options for the one in five patients who develops one of the various transfusion reactions. A major focus has been on management based on clinical symptoms. This approach will allow for the quick response time necessary to manage transfusion reactions while awaiting confirmatory laboratory results.

TABLE 59-1   MEDICATION DOSING FOR ADVERSE TRANSFUSION REACTION

Dopamine (renal perfusion), 2.5–5.0 µg/kg/minutes continuous infusion
Lasix, 1mg/kg IV
Hydrocortisone, 100–500 mg IV q 4–6 hours
Epinephrine, 0.3–0.5 mg of a 1:1000 solution q 20–30 minutes
Aminophyline, 6 mg/kg loading dose over 30 minutes followed by 0.6 mg/kg/hour
IVIG, 500 mg/kg/day IV over 3–4 hours x 3–4 days

Abbreviation: IV, intravenous.

SUGGESTED READINGS

Barbara JA, Coutieras M: Infectious complications of blood transfusion. Bacteria and Parasites. BMJ 300:386, 1990

Djulbegović B: Reasoning and decision making in hematology. Churchill Livingstone, NY 1992:243–246

Heddle NM, Klama LN, Griffith L et al: A prospective study to identify the risk factors associated with acute reactions to platelet and red cell transfusions. Transfusion 10:794, 1993

Sandler JG, Mallory D, Malamut et al: IgA anaphylactic transfusion reactions. Transfus Med Rev 1:1, 1995

Schreiber GB, Busch MP, Kleiman SH, Korelitz JJ: The risk of transfusion transmitted viral infections. N Engl J Med 334:1685, 1996

Tipple MA, Bland LA, Murphy JJ et al: Sepsis associated with transfusion of red cells contaminated with *Versinia enterocolitica*. Transfusion 30:207, 1990

Walker RH (ed): Technical Manual. 11th Ed. American Association of Blood Banks. Bethesda, 1993

Transfusion Reactions

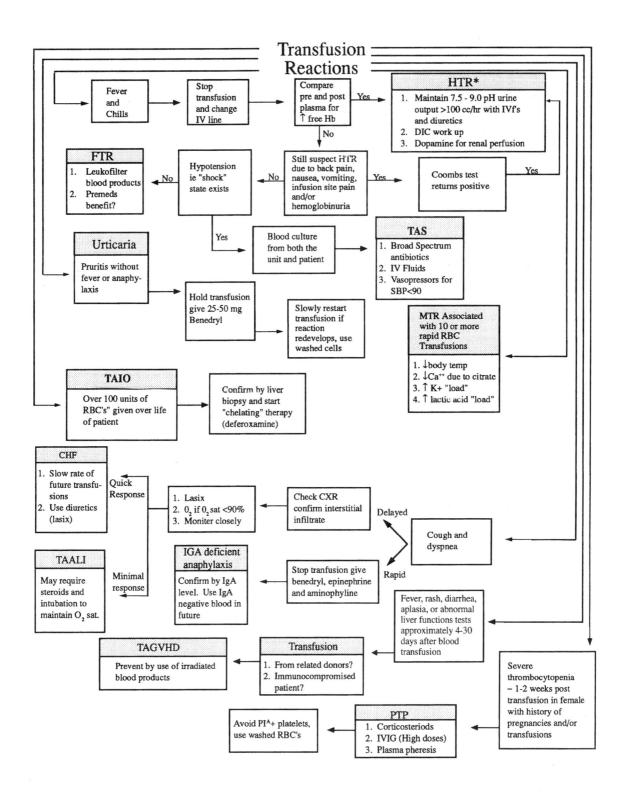

Fever and Chills → **Stop transfusion and change IV line** → **Compare pre and post plasma for ↑ free Hb** —Yes→ **HTR***
1. Maintain 7.5 - 9.0 pH urine output >100 cc/hr with IVf's and diuretics
2. DIC work up
3. Dopamine for renal perfusion

No ↓

Still suspect HTR due to back pain, nausea, vomiting, infusion site pain and/or hemoglobinuria —Yes→ **Coombs test returns positive** —Yes→

FTR
1. Leukofilter blood products
2. Premeds benefit?
←No— **Hypotension ie "shock" state exists** ←No—

Urticaria
Pruritis without fever or anaphylaxis

Yes ↓

Blood culture from both the unit and patient → **TAS**
1. Broad Spectrum antibiotics
2. IV Fluids
3. Vasopressors for SBP<90

Hold transfusion give 25-50 mg Benedryl → **Slowly restart transfusion if reaction redevelops, use washed cells**

MTR Associated with 10 or more rapid RBC Transfusions
1. ↓body temp
2. ↓Ca++ due to citrate
3. ↑ K+ "load"
4. ↑ lactic acid "load"

TAIO
Over 100 units of RBC's given over life of patient → **Confirm by liver biopsy and start "chelating" therapy (deferoxamine)**

CHF
1. Slow rate of future transfusions
2. Use diuretics (lasix)
←Quick Response— **1. Lasix 2. O₂ if O₂ sat <90% 3. Moniter closely** ← **Check CXR confirm interstitial infiltrate** ←Delayed— **Cough and dyspnea**

TAALI
May require steroids and intubation to maintain O₂ sat.
←Minimal response—

IGA deficient anaphylaxis
Confirm by IgA level. Use IgA negative blood in future
← **Stop tranfusion give benedryl, epinephrine and aminophyline** ←Rapid—

Fever, rash, diarrhea, aplasia, or abnormal liver functions tests approximately 4-30 days after blood transfusion

TAGVHD
Prevent by use of irradiated blood products
← **Transfusion**
1. From related donors?
2. Immunocompromised patient?
←

Severe thrombocytopenia ~ 1-2 weeks post transfusion in female with history of pregnancies and/or transfusions

Avoid PIᴬ+ platelets, use washed RBC's ← **PTP**
1. Corticosteriods
2. IVIG (High doses)
3. Plasma pheresis
←

FIGURE 59-1 *Although transfusion reactions are traditionally designated as either immune- or nonimmune-mediated, the clinical separation is often difficult. Presented is an algorithm to help make this distinction and further delineate the most likely occurring transfusion reaction. Because of the infrequent occurrence and urgency associated with such reactions, most recommendations are based on opinions of respected authorities. Main practice point: Initial response to a transfusion reaction needs to be a prompt assessment based on clinical parameters, which is later confirmed by laboratory methods. Due to the low number of anticipated and experienced serious transfusion reactions, the recommendations for management are often based on level III, IV, or V evidence. FTR, febrile transfusion reaction; HTR, hemolytic transfusion reaction; TAS, transfusion-associated sepsis; TAIO, transfusion-associated iron overload; CNF, congestive heart failure; TAALI, transfusion-associated acute lung injury; MTR, metabolic transfusion reaction; TAGVHD, transfusion-associated graft-versus-host disease; PTA, post-transfusion purpura. ∗-delayed HTR approximately 1–2 wks post-transfusion, few symptoms, observe renal function.*

60 Use of Growth Factors

Donald R. Fleming

Hematopoiesis requires progenitor cells in a properly balanced combination of stromal cells and matrix proteins. By products of these various cellular components are the numerous growth factors involved in transcellular signaling. The past decade has seen the development of recombinant growth factors leading to the commercial availability of such factors as erythropoietin, granulocyte-macrophage colony stimulating factor (CM-CSF), granulocyte colony stimulating factor (G-CSF), and interleukin-2.

This chapter focuses on the clinical use of both G-CSF and GM-CSF in today's oncology patients Fig 60-1. These two factors are widely accepted in supporting such patients, both in and out of the setting of cancer therapeutics. Despite the expansive and often empirical use of these two agents, the only definite benefit has been established in patients receiving "high doses" of chemotherapy with or without hematopoietic stem cell support. Only recently have randomized prospective trials demonstrated benefit among elderly acute myelogenous leukemia patients receiving a growth factor after induction chemotherapy. Other trials, also randomized and prospective, have demonstrated neither harm nor benefit in these patients. The role of GM-CSF and G-CSF in allogeneic transplant patients is being defined thus far, with evidence that supports their use based on a significantly shorter neutropenic period. In situations involving autologous stem-cell support, the role for G-CSF and GM-CSF has been well established.

In patients receiving conventional chemotherapy, the use has primarily been recommended in those patients demonstrating a past history of a neutropenic febrile episode necessitating attenuation as well as delay in administering therapy. In oncology patients not receiving chemotherapy and demonstrating a chronic state of neutropenia because of a hypoproliferative marrow, the use has been somewhat less established. It is also potentially risky because of acceleration of a leukemic state as is the case in advanced forms of myelodysplastic syndromes. Another potential benefit of both G-CSF and GM-CSF has been in patients requiring life preserving and often life-long medications, which unfortunately have marrow suppression as a therapeutic dose side effect. Patients being followed after bone marrow transplantation and during human immunodeficiency virus therapy represent a large segment of this patient population.

While in most situations GM-CSF and G-CSF can be used interchangeably, there are exceptions. GM-CSF not only quantitatively enhances granulocyte production but also qualitatively stimulates phagocytic activity. Limited randomized studies have indicated improvement in outcome among bone marrow transplant patients when given GM-CSF in addition to antifungal agents.

Both GM-CSF and G-CSF are well tolerated; myalgias and arthralgias are the only commonly reported side effects. Rarely, some patients receiving CM-CSF experience an acute lung toxicity, necessitating corticosteroids and possibly intubation with respirator support.

Despite randomized clinical trials demonstrating efficacy, clinical applications of erythropoietin in cancer chemotherapy patients is somewhat less established than previously mentioned recombinant growth factors. Manufacturer's recommendations to utilize recombinant erythropoietin in such patients with an endogenous erythropoietin level of less than 200 mU/mL is primarily based on data demonstrating lower levels of endogenous erythropoietin in cancer chemotherapy patients and not on clinical trials demonstrating predictive response value in those patients. Our recommendations are based on both myeloma and non-Hodgkin's lymphoma patient models and are likely to be more predictive of response in the oncology patient population (Fig. 60-2).

G-CSF/GM-CSF

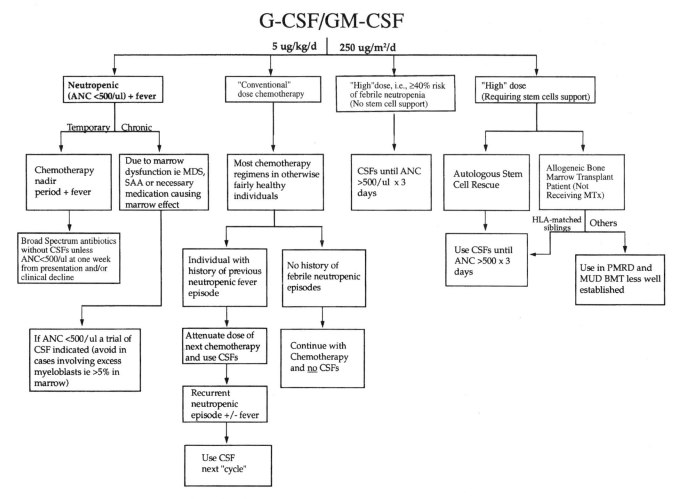

FIGURE 60-1   *An algorithm for the clinical application of both GM-CSF and G-CSF. It emphasizes the general acceptance of growth factors in settings of "high dose" cancer patients, while decisions on their use in other patients depend on individual situations. Evidence of their efficacy is based on level I and II prospectively randomized controlled trials. Caution should be observed in patients diagnosed with acute myelogenous leukemia receiving CSFs prior to being determined aplastic on marrow exam, especially if high-dose cytarabine is not utilized for induction therapy. MDS, myelodysplastic syndrome; SAA, severe aplastic anemia; PMRD, partially HLA-matched related donor; MUD, HLA-matched unrelated donors; ANC, absolute neutrophil count; CSF, colon-stimulating factor. Main practice point: General use of growth factors such as GM-CSF and G-CSF represents a standard of care that is primarily "cost effective" for only "dose intensive" chemotherapy patients.*

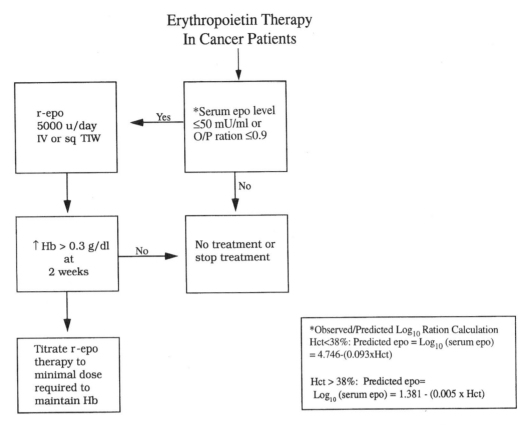

FIGURE 60-2   *An algorithm for the use of erythropoietin in cancer patients determines which patients can forego precious red cell transfusions by using recombinant erythropoietin. Evidence of its effectiveness is based on level II properly randomized controlled trials as well as level III matched cohort and cased controlled studies.*

While the properly applied use of growth factors, such as G-CSF and GM-CSF, can be cost effective, their use can also be just as improvident. At the present time, the empiric use of these growth factors during conventional cancer chemotherapy and resultant periods of brief neutropenic fever are not indicated as an adjunct to broad-spectrum antibiotic therapy.

SUGGESTED READINGS

Adamson JW, Spivak JL: Physiologic basis for the pharmacologic use of recombinant human erythropoietin in surgery and cancer treatment. Surgery 115:7, 1994

American Society of Clinical Oncology Update of Recommendations for the Use of Hematopoietic Colony Stimulating Factors: Evidence-based clinical practice guidelines. J Clin Oncol 14:1957, 1996

Cazzola M, Messinger D, Battistel V et al: Recombinant human erythropoietin in the anemia associated with multiple myeloma or non-Hodgkin's lymphoma: dose finding and identification of predictors of response. Blood 86:4446, 1995

Dombret H, Chastang C, Fenaux P et al: A controlled study of recombinant human granulocyte colony-stimulating factor in elderly patients after treatment for acute myelogenous leukemia. N Engl J Med 332:1678, 1995

Goodnough LT, Anderson KL, Kurtz S et al: Indications and guidelines for the use of hematopoietic growth factors. Transfusion 33:944, 1993

Nemunaitis J, Shannon-Dorey K, Appelbaum FR et al: Long term follow-up of patients with invasive fungal disease who received adjunctive therapy with recombinant human macrophage colony stimulating factor. Blood 82:1422, 1993

Petros WP: Pharmacokinetics and administration of colony-stimulating factors. Pharmacotherapy 12:325, 1992

Rowe JM, Anderson JW, Mazza JJ et al: A randomized placebo-controlled phase III study of granulocyte-macrophage colony stimulating factor in adult patients (>55 to 70 years of age) with acute myelogenous leukemia: a study of the Eastern Oncology Group (El490). Blood 86:457, 1995

Stone RM, Berg DT, George SL et al: Granulocyte macrophage colony stimulating factor after initial chemotherapy for elderly patients with primary acute myelogenous leukemia. N Engl J Med 332:1671, 1995

61 Superior Vena Cava Syndrome

Leela Bhupalam

INCIDENCE AND ETIOLOGY

Superior vena cava (SVC) syndrome is the clinical expression of obstruction of the superior vena cava. Symptoms and signs can occur acutely or gradually when this thin-walled vessel is compressed, invaded, or thrombosed by a process in the superior mediastinum.

Superior vena cava syndrome has been recognized since 1757 when William Hunter reported the syndrome as a complication of syphilitic aortic aneurysm. During this early period syphilis and tuberculosis were the most common causes of superior vena cava syndrome. Before the advent of antibiotic therapy, a high percentage of SVC syndrome had infectious etiologies. Since then, *malignant disease is the most common cause of SVC syndrome*. Today malignant causes represent 85% to 97% of all cases of which 67% to 82% are primarily broncogenic carcinomas. While lung cancer is the leading cause of SVC syndrome, the incidence of this syndrome in patients with lung cancer ranges from 3% to 30%. Small-cell cancer is the most common histology. Refer to Table 61-1 for frequency of causes of SVC.

Non-Hodgkin's lymphoma is the second leading cause of SVC syndrome. Among different histologic subsets of lymphoma, SVC obstruction is most commonly observed with the diffuse large cell and lymphoblastic lymphomas. The incidence of SVC obstruction in these categories of non-Hodgkin's lymphoma is reported to be 7% and 20%, respectively.

Metastatic disease accounts for 5% to 10% of SVC obstruction. The most common primary tumors are, in order of frequency, breast cancer, germ cell malignances, and gastrointestinal cancers. Less common primary tumors are sarcomas, transitional cell carcinomas, and melanomas. Benign causes of SVC are less commonly seen because of progressive antibiotic therapy. However, with increasing numbers of patients presenting with autoimmune deficiency syndrome AIDS and the corresponding increase in tuberculosis and syphilis, infectious etiologies must be considered in the differential diagnosis. SVC obstruction caused by histoplasmosis may be seen in patients in areas where infection is endemic. Rare causes resulting from goiter, benign idiopathic mediastinal fibrosis, aortic valve replacement, and congestive heart failure have been reported.

SVC obstruction may be iatrogenic, caused by thrombus formation in the presence of pacemaker wires, indwelling central lines, Le-Veen shunts, Swan-Ganz catheters, and hyperalimentation catheters. In the pediatric population, iatrogenic SVC obstruction is usually secondary to cardiovascular surgery for congenital heart disease or ventriculoatrial shunts for hydrocephalus. Most common causes of SVC obstruction in children are non-Hodgkin's lymphomas, acute lymphoid leukemia, Hodgkin's disease, neuroblastomas, and yolk sac tumors.

ANATOMY AND PHYSIOLOGY

The SVC, formed by the union of the right and left brachiocephalic veins, empties into the superior-posterior right atrium. It is the major drainage system for blood returning from the upper extremities, head, and neck. The azygos vein, the only major vein that enters the SVC, carries blood returned from the posterior torso. The SVC is relatively thin-walled and lies within a nondistensible space in the mediastinum, making it susceptible to extrinisic compression by primary tumors or lym-

TABLE 61-1   CAUSES OF SUPERIOR VENA CAVA SYNDROME

Cause	Purish	Yellin	Lochridge	Davenport	Bell	Armstrong	Sca niotino	Little
Total patients	86	63	66	35	159	125	60	42
Lung cancer	45	30	52	26	129	99	36	35
Non-small cell	33	26	44	6	64	57	23	28
Small cell	12	4	8	20	65	42	13	7
Lymphoma	8	13	8	1	3	18	8	3
Metastases	12	4	4	4	4	3	4	3
Thymoma/thyroid	2	4	—	1	—	—	—	1
Benign	19	11	2	—	2	—	—	—
Not biopsied	—	—	—	3	21	—	12	—

(From Murray MJ, Stewart JR, Johnson DR: Superior vena cava syndrome. pp. 609–618. In Abeloff MD, Armitage JA, Lichter AL, Niederhuber JN [eds]: Clinical Oncology. Churchill Livingstone, New York, 1995, with permission.)

phadenopathy. Intraluminal thrombus formation may be exacerbated by the low-pressure blood flow within the SVC.

The appearance of the SVC on computed tomography (CT) scans has been reviewed by Raptopoulos. The SVC measures 6 to 8 cm long and 1.5 to 2.0 cm wide and is located to the right of the ascending aorta. The azygos vein enters the SVC at the level of the right main stem bronchus. The inferior portion of the SVC is covered by pericardium.

SIGNS & SYMPTOMS

The clinical presentation of SVC syndrome may be acute or subacute. As the result of diminished blood return from head, neck, arms, and upper torso, patients frequently complain of a sense of head "fullness," mild dyspnea, cough, chest pain, and occasional dysphagia. Refer to Table 61-2 for signs and symptoms. They also complaint of arm swelling, facial edema, hoarseness, headache, dizziness, lethargy, and alteration of mental status. If

SVC syndrome is untreated, increased intracranial pressure, intracerebral bleeding, and airway compromise can develop. Duration of symptoms may range from a few days to several weeks, but most patients present with symptoms of four weeks' duration or less. Symptoms may be aggravated by positional changes, particularly those associated with lowering of the head. Life-threatening neurologic symptoms such as seizures, syncope, and coma can occur.

DIAGNOSIS

If patients present with overt SVC syndrome, they may be diagnosed by physical examination alone. But most subtle presentations require diagnostic imaging, as outlined below.

1. Chest x-ray may show mediastinal widening, mass in superior mediastinum or mass in right upper lobe of lung, and pleural effusion (see Table 61-3).

TABLE 61-2   COMMON SYMPTOMS AND PHYSICAL FINDINGS OF SUPERIOR VENA CAVA SYNDROME

Symptoms	Patients Affected[a] (%)	Physical Findings	Patients Affected (%)
Dyspnea	63	Venous distention of neck	66
Facial swelling or head fullness	50	Venous distention of chest wall	54
Cough	24	Facial edema	46
Arm swelling	18	Cyanosis	20
Chest pain	15	Plethora of face	19
Dysphagia	9	Edema of arms	14

[a]Analysis based on data from 370 patients

(From Yamalon J: Superior vena caval syndrome. pp. 2111–2118. In Devita VT [ed]: Cancer Principles and Practice of Oncology. 4th Ed. Lippincott-Raven, Philadelphia, with permission.)

TABLE 61-3 CHEST RADIOGRAPHIC FINDINGS FOR 86
PATIENTS WITH SUPERIOR VENA CAVA SYNDROME

Finding	No. of Patients (%)
Superior mediastinal widening	55 (64)
Pleural effusion	22 (26)
Right hilar mass	10(12)
Bilateral diffuse infiltrates	6 (7)
Cardiomegaly	5 (6)
Calcified paratracheal nodes	4 (5)
Mediastinal (anterior) mass	3 (3)
Normal	14 (16)

(From Parish JM et al: Etiologic considerations in SVCS. Mayo
Clin Proc 56:407–413, 1981, with permission.)

2. Contrast-enhanced CT scanning provides
more detailed evaluation of SVC syndrome. Its
advantages are that it provides more acurate information on the location of the obstruction and may
guide attempts at biopsy by mediastinoscopy, bronchoscopy, and percutaneous fine-needle aspiration.

3. Magnetic resonance imaging (MRI) studies
of mediastinum have potential advantages over CT
including the ability to image in several planes of
view and directly visualize blood flow. MRI does not
require iodinated contrast material. Disadvantages
are increased scanning time with attendant problems in patient compliance and increased cost.
Hansent et al. studied the ability of MRI to diagnose thoracic venal obstruction with 94% sensitivity and 100% specificity.

4. Contrast venography was occasionally obtained before CT and still has an occasional role in
determining management strategy, particularly
when surgical bypass is being considered.

5. Radionuclide studies have advantages over
contrast venography. The tracer is not thrombo-
genic.

6. Gallium single photon emission computed
tomography (SPECT) can be useful in some cases.

SVC syndrome was long considered a medical
emergency, and treatment before histologic evaluation was common. Treatment without an established diagnosis should be withheld only in those
patients with rapidly progressing symptoms or
those in whom multiple attempts to attain tissue
diagnosis have been unsuccessful. Histologic diagnosis before treatment is desirable when SVC
syndrome is the presenting manifestation of the
disease process. In many cases, the development of

SVC obstruction occurs in individuals with an
established diagnosis of cancer. In such circumstances, attempts to reestablish histology of underlying cause is not productive.

Fortunately, relatively noninvasive measures
establish diagnosis in a high percentage of SVC
syndrome. The most common procedures used to
establish diagnosis are sputum cytology, bronchoscopy, lymph node biopsy, mediastinoscopy, fine
needle aspiration biopsy of the lung, and thoroco-
tomy (Table 61-4) The diagnostic yield from various
noninvasive and invasive procedures varies from
20% for cytology, 100% for thoracotomy. The complication rate of invasive procedures for SVC syndrome is modest. Thus, only in rare cases with rapid
progression of symptoms associated with severe respiratory distress should irradiation be undertaken
without tissue confirmation of underlying cause. On
the other hand, prolonged attempts at histologic
diagnosis should be discouraged in the presence of
severe dyspena caused by tracheal compression or
rapidly progressing neurologic symptoms.

TREATMENT

Conservative measures include bed rest, elevation
of the head of the bed, and supplemental oxygen.
Patients may gain significant symptomatic improvement from these measures. Corticosteroids and
diuretics are often used, although documentation
of their efficacy is lacking.

Treatment of SVC obstruction depends on
underlying causes. The goals of treatment are to
relieve symptoms and to attempt to kill the primary
malignant process. In the absence of known cause
of SVC obstruction, every effort should be made
to obtain histologic diagnosis before initiation of

TABLE 61-4 POSITIVE YIELD OF DIAGNOSTIC PROCEDURES
FOR PATIENTS WITH SUPERIOR VENA CAVA SYNDROME

Procedure	No. of Procedures	No. Positive	Percent Positive
Sputum cytology	59	29	49
Thoracocentesis	14	10	71
Bone marrow biopsy	13	3	23
Lymph node biopsy	95	64	67
Bronchoscopy	124	65	52
Mediastinoscopy	54	44	81
Thoracotomy	49	48	98

(From Yamalon J: Superior vena Caval Syndrome. In Devita VT
(ed): Cancer: Principles and Practice of Oncology. 4th Ed. Lippincott-Raven, Philadelphia, 1993, with permission.)

treatment. In rare cases, a definite tissue diagnosis cannot be made in a timely manner. It is then appropriate to proceed with radiation therapy since this therapy is effective for most underlying causes of SVC obstruction.

CHEMOTHERAPY

Chemotherapy with or without thoracic radiation therapy is the preferred initial treatment of *small-cell lung cancer*, since up to 20% of such patients may survive for two years from diagnosis and a smaller percentage may be cured. Patients experience a resolution of symptoms in seven days of treatment and complete resolution can occur in two weeks. The addition of radiation treatment to chemotherapy in limited stages of small-cell lung cancer imparts a survival benefit. Three randomized trials have shown that there is an advantage for combining radiation treatment to chemotherapy alone in treatment of limited disease small-cell cancer of the lung.

In *non-Hodgkin's lymphoma* the choice of treatment should be based on histologic diagnosis, and the patient should undergo a complete staging workup before therapy. Chemotherapy is the treatment of choice as it provides local and systemic therapeutic activity. Local recurrences tend to occur in patients with large-cell lymphoma and mediastinal masses greater than 10 cm. On the other hand, lymphoblastic lymphoma recurrences are usually systemic, obviating the need for radiation therapy in this histologic type of non-Hodgkin's lymphoma.

Radiation therapy is the preferred initial treatment of SVC obstruction in non-small-cell lung cancer.

SURGERY

Operation is reserved most often for patients with SVC obstruction caused by a benign cause: granulomatous disease, aortic aneurysm, or retrosternal goiter. When symptomatic malignant obstruction is refractory to radiation therapy, chemotherapy, or both, and when anticipated survival approaches 6 months or greater, operation may be considered. Surgical intervention may prove beneficial in the setting of recurrent SVC obstruction after chemotherapy and irradiation, and when caval thrombosis is the primary problem and fails to improve symptomatically with anticoagulants or thrombolytic therapy.

Surgical bypass of the obstructed SVC may be accomplished with synthetic grafts (Dacron or Gore-Tex), autologous pericardium, or autogenous vein graft, with a preference for the latter because of its better potential for long-term patency. The bypass is constructed between the brachiocephalic or left internal jugular vein and the right atrial appendage. Long-term relief of symptoms may be achieved.

As stated, treatment of venal caval obstruction caused by malignancy is usually with radiation and chemotherapy. Success occurs in 90% of patients. SVC syndrome reoccurs in 10% to 20% of these patients. If conventional treatment does not reduce the tumor volume or relieve caval compression, *intraluminal stenting* can provide sufficient force to reopen the vessel lumen and prevent tumor and thrombotic occlusion. The application of Z-type metal stents in patients with recurrent malignant obstruction of the SVC appears to be a useful palliative procedure. Refer to Table 61-5 for complications of stents. The Palmaz balloon expandable stent has been used successfully in cancer patients

TABLE 61-5   COMPLICATIONS OF VENA CAVAL STENTING

Complication	SVC	IVC	Total
No complications	10 (45%)	4 (18%)	14 (64%)
Complications	4 (18%)	4 (18%)	8 (36%)
Stent migration		1[a]	1 (4%)
Cardiac arrhythmias		3[a]	3 (14%)
Chest pain		1	1 (4%)
Stent occlusion	3[a]		3 (14%)
No. of procedures	14 (64%)	8 (36%)	22

Abbreviations: SVC, superior vena cava, IVC, inferior vena cava.

[a]Stent breakage (three patients. One in each category)

(From Oudkerk MD, Heystraten FMJ, Stoter G: Stenting in malignant vena caval obstruction. Cancer 71:142–146, 1993, with permission.)

TABLE 61-6   MANAGEMENT OF SVC SECONDARY TO A CLOT: SEQUENCE OF CHOICES

Urokinase 10,000 units IV injected periodically to keep the catheter patent.

During Acute Thrombosis

IV heparin 5,000 bolus followed by infusion PTT 1.5–2 times control. If lack of clinical response, a peripheral infusion of 80 mg recombinant rtPA should be administered (1.25 mg/kg) 60% of dose given in the first hour (inclusive of bolus and infusion). The remaining 40% infused continuously over 2 hours.

Resolution of clot is usually seen within 24 hours.

Implanted port is removed

Continue anticoagulation with oral coumadin.

Abbreviations: IV, intravenous; PTT, partial thrombin time.

(From Greenberg S, Kosinski, Daniels J: Treatment of superior vena cava thrombosis with recombinant tissue type plasminogen activator. Chest 99:1298–1300, 1991, with permission.)

with superior venal caval obstruction. Potential risks associated with intravascular stents are not trivial, including thrombosis, migration, embolization, and infection of the device. For this reason, persons requiring metallic stents require systemic anti coagulation and antiplatelet therapy. Restenosis of a stented area is a concern.

Reconstruction of large mediastinal veins has been tried with sythetic grafts (Dacron or Gore-Tex), autogenous pericardium, or autogenous vein grafts with a preference for the latter because of its better potential for long-term patency.

CATHETER-INDUCED OBSTRUCTION

In catheter-induced superior vena cava obstruction, the mechanism of obstruction is usually thrombosis. This complication may be life threatening, with the complete obstruction of the SVC. Heparin administration may arrest the propagation of the thrombus, but it is ineffective for clot lysis. Streptokinase, urokinase, or recombinant tissue plasminogen activator (tPA) may cause lysis of the thrombus early in its formation. The success of clot lysis depends less on duration of thrombosis. Its higher rate of early clot lysis with earlier recanalization may potentially reduce the high morbidity associated with the disease by diminishing the duration of the SVC occlusion. Removal of the catheter, another option, should be combined with anticoagulation therapy to avoid embolization. Percutaneous transluminal angioplasty with or without thrombolitic therapy has been successful in opening catheter-induced SVC obstruction. See Table 61-6 for management of SVC secondary to a clot.

Figure 61-1 summarizes a management approach to SVC. The algorithm is based on understanding the urgency of this syndrome and the principle that treatment has to be directed toward the underlying cause of the syndrome. Data shown in Tables 61-1 to 61-6 are all retrospective in nature.

SUGGESTED READINGS

Ahmann FR: A reassessment of the clinical implications of the superior vena caval syndrome. J Clin Oncol 8:961–969, 1984

Dodds AG, Harrison JK, O'Laughlin MP et al: Relief of superior vena cava syndrome due to fibrosing mediastinitis using the palmaz stent. Chest 106:315–318, 1994

Gaines PA, Belli AM, Anderson PB, McBride K, Hemingway AP: Clinics in interventional radiology: Superior vena caval obstruction managed by the gianturco Z stent. Clin Radiol 49:202–208, 1994

Greenberg S, Kosinski R, Daniels J: Treatment of superior vena cava thrombosis with recombinant tissue type plasminogen activator. Chest 99:1298–1300, 1991

Hansen ME, Spritzer CE, Sostman MD: Assessing the patency of mediastinal and thoracic inlet veins: value of MR imaging. Am J Radiol 155:1172–1182, 1990

Jahangiri M, Taggart DP, Goldstraw P: Role of mediastinoscopy in superior vena cava obstruction. Cancer 71:3006–3008, 1993

Larsson S, Lepore V: Technical options in reconstruction of large mediastinal veins. Surgery 2:311–317, 1992

Loeffler JS, Leopold KA, Recht A et al: Emergency prebiopsy radiation for mediastinal masses: impact on subsequent pathologic diagnosis and outcome. J Clin Oncol 4:716–721, 1986

Murray MJ, Stewart JR, Johnson DH: Superior vena cava syndrome. pp. 609–618. In Abeloff MD (ed): Clinical Oncology. Churchill Livingstone, New York, 1995

Oudkerk M, Heystraten FMJ, Stoter G: Stenting in malignant vena caval obstruction. Cancer 71:142–146, 1993

Painter TD, Karpf M: Superior vena cava syndrome: diagnostic procedures. Am J Med Sci 285:2–6, 1983

Perez-Soler R, McLaughlin P, Velasquez WS et al: Clinical features and results of management of superior vena cava syndrome secondary to lymphoma. J Clin Oncol 2:260–266, 1984

Raptopoulos V: Computed tomography of the superior vena cava, CRC Crit Rev Diagn Imaging 25:373–429, 1986

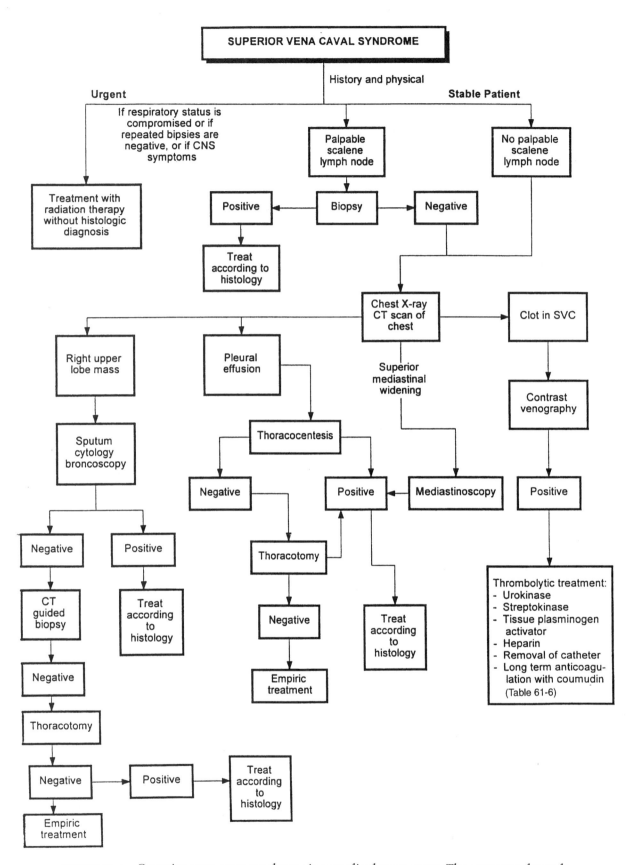

FIGURE 61-1 *Superior vena cava syndrome is a medical emergency. The outcome depends on the underlying cause of the syndrome. Understanding the emergency of the situation and distinguishing between a benign or malignant nature for the process constitutes the basic elements of clinical approach to the patient presenting with this syndrome.*

62 Spinal Cord Compression

Rambabu Tummala

Incidence: In 5% of cancer patients at autopsy, with an annual incidence of 20,000 new cases.

Goals of treatment: Preservation and restoration of neurologic function is possible if detected early.

Main modality of treatment: Depends upon the stability of spine (surgery for unstable spine) and radiosensitivity of the tumor (radiation therapy for sensitive tumor).

Prognosis: Depends upon the neurologic status at diagnosis. Median survival varies from 3 to 6 months, and up to 30% of patients are alive 1 year from diagnosis.

Compression of the spinal cord and cauda equina is a major cause of morbidity and mortality in a cancer patient. This is one of the few oncologic emergencies, as delay in therapy leads to frank paralysis. It is classified as epidural, leptomeningeal, or intramedullary. This discussion will focus on epidural cord compression.

INCIDENCE

Cord compression is found in 5% of cancer patients at autopsy and approximately 20,000 new cases per year. The incidence is expected to increase with improvement in palliative therapy for metastatic disease. About half the cases in adults arise from breast, lung, and prostate cancer (Table 62-1). Other frequent cancers include lymphoma, sarcoma, kidney, and multiple myeloma. This is the first manifestation of disease in about 10% of cases. In one series from Denmark, the mean period from primary malignant diagnosis to cord compression varied considerably according to the primary tumor e.g., lung, 0.5 years; prostate, 1.7 years; kidney, 2.2 years; and breast, 4.6 years. In children, epidural metastasis occurs in 3% to 5% of solid tumors, commonly from sarcoma, neuroblastoma, and germ cell tumors. The site of the compression is at the thoracic level in 70% of cases, lumbar in 20%, and cervical in the remaining 10%.

CLINICAL PRESENTATION

Any new pain in a cancer patient should be viewed with suspicion. Progressive axial or radicular pain, worse on recumbency, is the presenting symptom in more than 90% of patients. The next most common symptom is weakness, often associated with or preceded by sensory loss. Autonomic dysfunction usually appears late and is seen in 12% to 77% of cases. About 11% to 48% of the patients are ambulatory, 32% to 63% are paraparetic, and 10% to 48% are paraplegic at the time of presentation. Once weakness is present, progression is often rapid and urgent diagnosis is crucial.

DIAGNOSIS

This is an oncologic emergency and requires prompt evaluation and treatment (Fig. 62-1). There is local bony tenderness to percussion in 32% to

TABLE 62-1   PRIMARY SITE OF NEOPLASM IN DIFFERENT SERIES

Primary Site	United States n=439 (%)	France/Italy n=600 (%)	Denmark n=345 (%)	United Kingdom n=131 (%)	Total n=1432 (%)
Breast	18	26	13	28	21
Lung	14	12	19	32	19
Prostate	10	8	18	4	10
Unknown	3	11	11	14	10
Lymphoma	10	6	9	a	8
Myeloma	4	a	5	a	4.5
Gastrointestinal	4	5	3	5	4
Others	16	18	10	9	18.5

aUnavailable.

(Adapted from Grant R, Papadopoulos SM, Greenberg HS: Metastatic epidural spinal cord compression. Neurol Clin 9:825–840, 1991, with permission.)

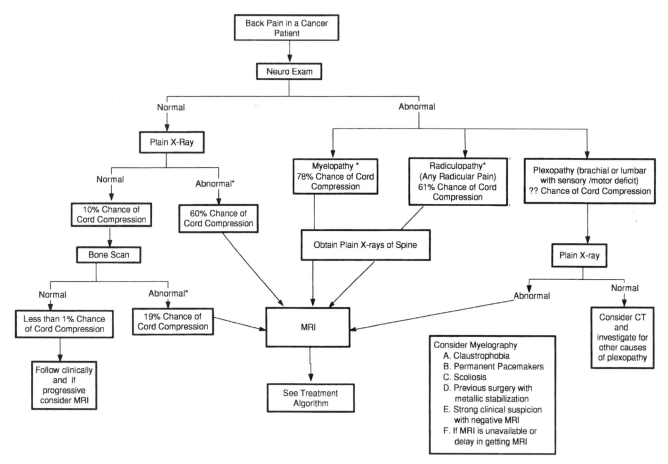

FIGURE 62-1   *Algorithm for evaluation of back pain in a patient with cancer. Always consider rebiopsy if the disease-free interval is more than two years or if the tumor is solitary. The key reasoning principle is to define anatomically the extent of cord involvement. The goal is to make an early diagnosis to prevent paralysis. Note that all cancer patients with back pain do not need MRI for evaluation, especially with a normal neurologic examination, x-rays, and bone scan. Level of evidence III. (Asterisks indicate start of Decadron, 10 mg IV, followed by 4 mg IV/po q6h whenever there is suspicion of cord compression.) (Modifed from Rodichok LD, Harper GR, Ruckdeschel JC et al: Early diagnosis of spinal epidural metastates. Am J Med 70:1181–1187, 1981, with permission.)*

74% of patients, usually aggravated by neck flexion or a straight leg raising test. Motor weakness and abnormal reflexes are also present in many patients. The sensory examination usually reveals losses indicating the level of cord compression. In cases of autonomic dysfunction, a palpable bladder and decreased anal tone may be seen. The nature and the tempo of the work-up depends upon the neurologic status at presentation. The following are the routine investigations, each one with some limitations.

PLAIN RADIOGRAPHY

Plain films are essential and highly predictive. Up to 80% of patients with cord compression have abnormal spinal films, and normal films do not exclude the diagnosis. About 60% of lymphomas and 65% of pediatric tumors have normal plain films. However, abnormal films are found more often in breast cancer (94%) and lung cancer (74%). The features correlated with epidural disease were a greater than 50% vertebral collapse (85%), a pedicular lesion (31%), and a tumor limited to the vertebral body without collapse (7%). The frequency of epidural disease in a cancer patient with back pain alone with no neurologic deficit and metastases on radiography is greater than 60%. However, the same patient with normal films has a 10% chance of epidural disease. The sensitivity and specificity for prediction of epidural disease are 91% and 86%, respectively. However, abnormal radiographs do not indicate all the levels of cord compression.

BONE SCAN

A bone scan is more sensitive than plain radiography, but the specificity is only 53%, with a high false-positive rate. A negative radiograph and a negative bone scan in an asymptomatic patient reduces the risk of epidural disease to less than 1%. A bone scan is not required in the presence of neurologic signs and abnormal plain films, however, it may indicate tumor at other sites of the bone. In addition, bone scans do not indicate the level of compression.

SPINAL COMPUTED TOMOGRAPHY

Computed tomography (CT) is more sensitive and specific than plain films and bone scans in identifying benign disease. In one study of patients with abnormal bone scans, normal plain films, and a normal neurologic examination, CT revealed benign disease in 33% of them. Cortical bone discontinuity around the neural canal was highly associated with epidural compression. This is an important diagnostic test in determining which patients are at high risk for epidural tumor. However, myelography or MRI is superior to spinal CT alone in assessing cord compression.

MYELOGRAPHY

Until recently myelography had been the definitive test. Presently, magnetic resonance imaging (MRI) is used extensively for imaging the spinal cord. Myelograms are invasive in that they require a lumbar puncture, which can be associated with a 16% to 24% chance of rapid neurologic deterioration. Myelograms cannot delineate the upper extent of the lesion in cases of complete block and require a C1-C2 puncture for complete visualization. Also, when two or more areas of cord compression are present, it is almost impossible to examine the intervening area with myelography. It also can not identify a paraspinal tumor and requires spinal CT to identify and design the radiation fields. However, it provides cerebrospinal fluid for analysis and can be used when patients are unable to undergo MRI. In a prospective study of 70 patients, the sensitivity and specificity for myelography were found to be 95% and 88%, respectively, compared to 92% and 90% for MRI, for detecting extradural masses causing cord compression. Similarly for extradural masses without cord compression, the sensitivity and specificity for myelography were 49% and 88%, respectively, compared with 73% and 90% for MRI. This would indicate that both are equally sensitive for epidural disease causing cord compression, but MRI tends to be more sensitive when cord compromise has not yet developed.

MAGNETIC RESONANCE IMAGING

MRI has become the standard for diagnosis because it is noninvasive, less uncomfortable, and may be cost effective. It can identify the paraspinal extension of tumor and is sensitive enough to identify bony metastases to design the fields for radiation therapy. It can also identify other asymptomatic areas of epidural compression. MRI can differentiate extradural from leptomeningeal and intramedullary lesions by gadolinium contrast.

THERAPY

Palliation is the objective (Fig 62-2). The goals are return to ambulation, prevention of progression of neurologic injury, local tumor control, and pain relief. There are no absolute recommendations for

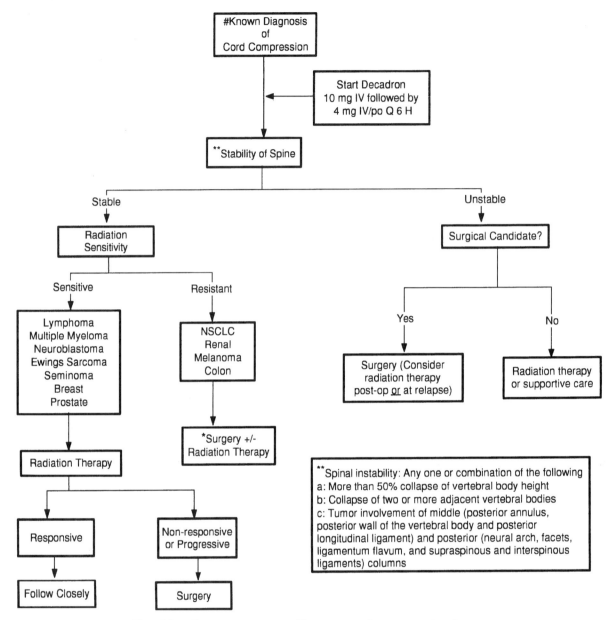

FIGURE 62-2 *Alogrithm for management of known cord compression in a cancer patient. The key reasoning principle is to determine spinal stability and tumor sensitivity to radiation therapy. The goal is palliation with maintenance or recovery of ambulatory status. Consider chemotherapy in addition to radiation therapy/surgery if the primary tumor is chemosensitive. The evidence supporting these recommendations is level III and IV. (A single asterisk indicates a need to consider surgery if the expected survival is at least 4 months and the patient is medically stable. A number sign [#] indicates that a specific cancer diagnosis has been made.)*

treatment because of the lack of good randomized prospective studies under similar conditions. Steroids should be started whenever the diagnosis is suspected, because they rapidly improve pain and function. Decadron is the drug of choice, but the dosage is controversial. One retrospective study using a 100-mg bolus of decadron followed by 96 mg per day for 3 days (followed by a tapering schedule), gave no indication that high-dose steroids resulted in better neurologic recovery. However, it had remarkable analgesic effect. In a small randomized prospective trial, an initial high-dose of 100 mg intravenously was found to be equally effective for the relief of pain as a conventional dose of 10 mg intravenously followed by 4 mg four times per day orally. Given the lack of a positive effect and the added toxicity for the high-dose decadron, we recommend 10 mg of decadron intravenously followed by 4 mg orally or intravenously every 6 hours.

Further treatment options include either radiation, surgery, or a combination of both. In general this should be a team approach involving medical oncology, radiation oncology, and neurosurgery. Review of the data before 1979 shows that radiation therapy alone may be as effective as surgery combined with radiation, with 40% to 60% of all patients ambulatory after therapy. A small prospective randomized comparison of laminectomy followed by radiation therapy to radiation therapy alone showed no difference in effectiveness. Recent radiation therapy results show that up to 80% of the patients remain ambulatory, and about 20% of paraperitic nonambulatory and 5% of paraplegic patients regained ambulation. Similarly, 75% of the patients maintain sphincter function, and a third with bladder dysfunction will regain normal function. There is a recent renewed interest in a selective surgical approach as primary therapy because anterior stabilization, or posterior decompression followed by stabilization, has a 70% to 74% chance of neurologic improvement. A recent retrospective surgical study showed 46% survival at 2 years, with an overall median survival duration of 16 months, compared with less than 30% survival at one year for most radiation series. However, the results continue to be poor with either therapy for plegic patients, with less than a 5% response. The prognostic factors include functional status at the start of therapy and radiosensitivity of the tumor. In some series the median survival for breast cancer is up to 14 months and up to 50% survival at one year in another series.

RECOMMENDATIONS

Radiation therapy only (Consider only in patients with a stable spine. The optimal dose and fractionation are not established yet. Usual dose is about 3000 cGy.)

1. Radiosensitive tumors

2. Spine involvement with no neurologic defect

3. Multiple sites of compression

4. Poor medical status in a nonsurgical candidate

5. Slowly evolving cord compression

Surgery only

1. New compression with neurologic deterioration at a previously irradiated level

2. Progressive deterioration during radiation therapy

Surgery followed by radiation

1. Pathologic fracture with instability or cord compression by a bone

2. Solitary site of relapse

3. Unknown diagnosis

4. Radiation-resistant tumor

5. Paravertebral tumor with direct extension

Chemotherapy

1. Chemosensitive tumor in association with surgery or radiation therapy

2. Relapse of a chemosensitive tumor at sites of previous surgery or radiation

SUGGESTED READINGS

Boogerd W, van der Sande JJ: Diagnosis and treatment of spinal cord compression in malignant disease. Cancer Treatment Reviews 19:129–150, 1993

Cybllski GR: Methods of surgical stabilization for metastatic disease of spine, Review article. Neurosurgery 25:240–252, 1989

Delaney TF Oldfield EH: Spinal cord compression. pp. 2118–2127. In Devita VT Jr, Hellman S, Rosenberg SA (eds): Cancer: Principles & Practice of Oncology. Lippincott-Raven, Philadelphia, 1993

Desforges JF Bryne TN: Spinal cord compression from epidural mets, N Engl J med 327:614–619, 1992

Grant R, Greenberg HS Papadopoulos SM: Metastatic epidural cord compression. Neurologic Clinics 9:825–840, 1991

Jordan JE, Donaldson SS Enzmann DR: Cost effectiveness and outcome assessment of MRI. Cancer 75:2579–2586, 1995

Maranzano E, Latini P, Checcaglini F et al: Radiation therapy in metastatic spinal cord compression. Cancer 67:1311–1317, 1991

Rodichok LD, Harper GR, Ruckdeschel JC et al: Early diagnosis of spinal epidural metastases. Am J Med 70:1181–1187, 1981

Sundaresan N, Digiacinto GV, Hughes JEO, Cafferty M, Vallejo A: Treatment of neoplastic spinal cord compression, prospective study. Neurosurgery 29:645–650, 1991

Vecht Ch J, Vries EP, Haaxma-Reiche H et al: Initial bolus of conventional vs. high-dose dexamethasone in metastatic spinal cord compression. Neurology 39:1255–1257, 1989

Young RF, King GA, Post EM: Treatment of spinal epidural metastases. Randomized comparison of laminectomy and radiotherapy. J Neurosurg 53: 741–748, 1980

63 Hypercalcemia

Rambabu Tummala

Incidence/prevalence: The overall incidence of hypercalcemia of malignancy is less than 2% and is more common in solid tumors. Higher prevalence rates are seen in non-small-cell lung cancer, breast cancer, and genitourinary cancers.

Goals of treatment: To identify patients for whom specific effective therapy for the underlying disease is available and to treat them aggressively. In refractory cases, *palliation* of symptoms is the objective. Survival is not affected if there is no specific treatment available for the primary disease.

Main modality of treatment: Pamidronate is the most commonly used drug because of its ease of administration. It is relatively less toxic and highly effective with prolonged duration of action. Hydration is an important part of any therapy.

Prognosis: Most of these patients have end stage cancer that is refractory to any form of therapy. Treatment of hypercalcemia has no effect on the underlying tumor. Survival is 4 to 6 weeks unless specific antitumor therapy is available.

Hypercalcemia is the most common metabolic disorder in malignancy that requires emergency therapy when severe or symptomatic. It has been estimated that hypercalcemia occurs in 10% to 20% of cancer patients at some time during the course of their disease. Blomqvist et al. reported an overall incidence of 1.5% (111 of 7,610 patients), whereas a retrospective analysis from M.D. Anderson Cancer Center in 1993 reported an incidence of 0.52% for severe and 0.63% for moderate hypercalcemia. The incidence is higher in renal cell carcinoma, non-small-cell lung carcinoma, and myeloma. In a retrospective report from China on 218 renal cell carcinoma patients over 20 years, an incidence of 9.2% was reported. Table 63-1 shows the prevalence of hypercalcemia in different malignancies.

Hypercalcemia occurs most commonly in solid tumors, especially squamous cell carcinoma of the lung and adenocarcinoma of breast. Most hypercalcemic patients have advanced disease, and more than 80% of these patients with solid tumors have obvious metastatic bone disease. Hypercalcemia is almost always associated with a large tumor mass in non-small-cell lung cancer. Hormonal therapy for breast carcinoma may sometimes trigger hypercalcemia, often accompanied by a "flare" reaction. Hypercalcemia is rarely seen in either small-cell lung cancer or adenocarcinoma of prostate, which frequently metastasize to bone. However, some uncommon tumors are frequently associated with hypercalcemia. These include small-cell carcinoma of the ovary and cholangiocarcinoma.

TABLE 63-1   HYPERCALCEMIA IN DIFFERENT MALIGNANCIES

Primary Site	Fisken et al. (1980) %	Blomqvist et al. (1986) %	Ralston et al. (1990) %
Lung	24	28	45
Breast	20	38	17
Genitourinary	18	6	12
Head and Neck	6	6	4
Unknown primary	4	not available	8
Multiple myeloma	6	9	6
Lymphoma	4	3	3

Hypercalcemia is less common in hematologic malignancies. Approximately 20% to 40% of patients with myeloma develop hypercalcemia at some time during the course of the disease. In Hodgkin's disease, an incidence of 1.6% to 5.4% has been reported. These patients are generally older, 75% have either stage III or IV bulky disease, which is predominantly infradiaphragmatic. At least 4.1% of all newly registered non-Hodgkin's lymphoma (NHL) patients at M.D. Anderson Cancer Center are hypercalcemic. It is very uncommon in low-grade NHL, complicating only 1% to 2% of cases. However, the incidence may be as high as 30% in inter-mediate-and high-grade lymphomas. Hypercalcemia occurs in both B- and T-cell phenotypes and is more common with bulky disease. In addition, adult T-cell lymphoma related to HTLV-1 is commonly associated with hypercalcemia.

J. Suzumiya et al. reported evidence of hyper-calcemia in 21 patients at autopsy of 47 cases of adult T-cell leukemia/lymphoma. It is not uncommon in leukemias. J.F. Seymour et al. reported an incidence of 1.8% (17/937) in acute myelogenous leukemia (AML), 5.8% (20/346) in acute lym-phoblastic leukemia (ALL), 7% (26/369) in blastic phase of chronic myelogenous leukemia (CML), and 3.8% (6/159) in chronic lymphocytic leukemia (CLL) among previously untreated patients.

CLINICAL MANIFESTATIONS

The diagnosis of hypercalcemia is often overlooked because of nonspecific or vague symptoms. It affects multiple systems, and the severity of presentation is not necessarily related to the degree of hypercalcemia. Patients with an acute elevation of serum calcium may present with more serious symptoms than patients with long-standing increases. Table 63-2 shows the common presenting signs and symptoms.

DIFFERENTIAL DIAGNOSIS

Hypercalcemia in hospitalized patients is usually malignancy associated, while among outpatients, hyperparathyroidism is the most common cause. Together, they account for 80% to 90% of the cases of hypercalcemia. Spurious hypercalcemia can be secondary to hemoconcentration and from prolonged pressure of the tourniquet for venipuncture. As serum calcium is highly bound to albumin, its level should be measured to make a correction for the serum calcium level.

$$\text{Corrected calcium (mg/dL)} =$$
$$\text{measured calcium (mg/dL)} +$$
$$0.8[4.0 - \text{S. albumin (g/dL)}]$$

TABLE 63-2   COMMON SIGNS AND SYMPTOMS OF HYPERCALCEMIA

General: dehydration, weakness, pruritus
Gastrointestinal: loss of appetite, nausea, vomiting, weight loss, constipation
Kidney: polyuria, polydipsia, azotemia
Neuromuscular: weakness, tiredness, confusion, weakened reflexes, seizures, somnolence, coma
Cardiovascular: shortened QT interval, arrhythmia, cardiac arrest

Fisken et al. reported that in only four out of 219 cases (1.8%), hypercalcemia was found before the malignancy was apparent. There is no single definitive test or symptom complex that can establish the etiology of hypercalcemia. A good history, physical examination, and laboratory data can provide valuable information. A normal or low serum immunoreactive PTH level with an elevated serum PTH-related peptide will exclude the diagnosis of primary hyperparathyroidism. Table 63-3 lists the other causes of hypercalcemia.

PATHOPHYSIOLOGY

It is useful to divide malignancy-associated hypercalcemia into three major categories. *Humoral hypercalcemia of malignancy* is the most common form, and is seen in solid tumors and is mediated by PTH-related peptide. This causes generalized osteoclastic bone resorption and increased renal resorption of calcium. The second common form is *local osteolytic hypercalcemia*, which causes localized bone resorption in the vicinity of tumor cells metastatic to bone. Various cytokines and local factors have been implicated in this type. Examples include non-small-cell lung cancer (NSCLC), breast carcinoma, and myeloma. The third most common form is *calcitriol mediated* and is seen in Hodgkin's disease and NHL. Calcitriol increases the intestinal absorption of calcium and enhances osteoclast activity. In most tumors more than one mechanism is involved.

TABLE 63-3   NONMALIGNANCY-RELATED CAUSES OF HYPERCALCEMIA

Type	Cause
Endocrine	Hyperparathyroidism
	Hyperthyroidism
	Adrenal insufficiency
Medications	Thiazide diuretics
	Lithium
	Tamoxifen in breast cancer patients
	Theophylline
	Hypervitaminosis A or D
Others	Renal disease
	Granulomatous diseases like sarcoidosis, histoplasmosis, etc.
	Immobilization

TREATMENT

Hypercalcemia can be divided into *mild* (serum calcium <12 mg/dL, but above the normal range), *moderate* (12–13.5 mg/dL) and *severe* (> 13.5 mg/dL) categories on the basis of corrected serum calcium levels. However, the symptom onset and severity may not necessarily be related to the serum calcium level, and any symptomatic patient should be treated as a severe case, irrespective of the level. It most commonly occurs in patients with advanced cancer who have failed prior therapies for the underlying disease. Correction of hypercalcemia, however, improves the symptoms and may allow the patients to return home during their terminal stage. Successful management of hypercalcemia provides time to plan for the management of the underlying disease, but has no effect on survival, unless specific antitumor therapy is available. Ralston et al. reported a median survival of 30 days, with no difference between antihypercalcemic regimens when no specific antitumor therapy was instituted. A median survival of 135 days was found when specific anticancer therapy is available. Survival was even shorter in the study by Warrell et al., with a median survival of only 29 days, mostly in patients with solid tumors. Blomqvist et al. reported a 44% survival at 3 months and 31% at one year. An improvement in survival in this group is attributed to specific chemotherapy, received by more than one third of the patients. A median survival of 38 days for squamous cell lung cancer and 30 days for breast cancer has been reported. Brada et al. reported a median survival of 8.5 months for 93 breast cancer patients. They reported that the presence of symptoms, visceral disease, and level of serum calcium are independent prognostic indicators for survival. The median survival was 3.5 years for patients with no adverse prognostic factors, 16 months with one prognostic factor, and 2.5 months with two or more adverse prognostic factors. In most situations, failure of therapy with progressive disease is the cause of death.

GENERAL MEASURES

The best treatment is one directed at the underlying disease. The goal is to correct dehydration, enhance urinary calcium excretion, and to prevent bone resorption by inhibiting osteoclasts. Early mobilization is encouraged and medications should be adjusted (Table 63-3). Nonsteroidal anti-inflammatory drugs (NSAIDs) can decrease renal blood flow and should be avoided.

SPECIFIC MEASURES

The literature on therapy contains only a few carefully controlled studies. The major defeciencies are variability in patient selection, underlying primary diagnosis, and reporting of results. The duration of normocalcemia is often difficult to assess because of intercurrent therapy.

HYDRATION

Most patients are dehydrated because of anorexia, emesis, and calciuresis. Intravenous rehydration with isotonic saline is the first step in their management. Hosking et al. first reported the beneficial effect of rehydration in severe hypercalcemia when he noted a mean decrease of 2.4 mg/dL in serum calcium levels in thirteen of sixteen patients. However, similar results were not reproduced in other studies. Two prospective, randomized studies, with one arm consisting of infusion of normal saline alone, have shown a complete response rate varying from 7% to 22% in the saline only arm. Among patients with severe hypercalcemia, the complete response was only 15%. The mean duration of complete response was 6 days, and 91% of the patients relapsed by day 7. These studies demonstrate that hydration alone rarely leads to normalization of serum calcium levels in hypercalcemic patients. The reductions usually range from 1.6 to 2.4 mg/dL.

The rate of saline administration depends upon the severity of hypercalcemia and the status of the cardiovascular system. In general, about 2.5 to 4 L of saline per day are recommended, with cautious use of diuretics.

LOOP DIURETICS

The indications for loop diuretics are to prevent volume overload and to promote calciuria. Suki et al. first reported a reduction in serum calcium levels by increasing urinary excretion with furosemide-induced diuresis in 1970. However, there are no controlled studies showing a benefit of diuretics, even though they are commonly used. These drugs can potentially aggravate the existing hypercalcemia by causing hypovolemia, if the patient is not adequately hydrated. Frequent monitoring of electrolytes is required during their use. Given the risks of these drugs and the availability of new and safer therapy for hypercalcemia, loop diuretics should be reserved for situations of fluid overload.

PHOSPHATES

An increase in serum phosphorous concentration decreases osteoclastic activity and decreases calcium resorption from bone. Intravenous phosphate is very effective and has a rapid onset of action.

TABLE 63-4   TREATMENT OF CANCER-RELATED HYPERCALCEMIA

Treatment Characteristics	Normal Saline	Oral Phosphorus	Corticosteroids	Calcitonin
Dose	200–400(+) ml/h	1–3 g/day orally, divided doses	40–100 mg/d prednisone or equivalent	2–8 U/kg SC or IM every 6–12 hours
Indications	Hypovolemia, dehydration	Mild or moderate hypercalcemia, hypophosphatemia	Hypercalcemia from myeloma, lymphoma, hormonal flare	Mild or moderate hypercalcemia: acute control
Onset of action	12–24 hours	24–48 hours	3–5 days	1–4 hours
Relative potency[a]	20%	30%	0%–40%, depending on disease	30%
Advantages	Corrects dehydration	Orally available: minimal toxicity	Orally available	Minimal toxicity
Disadvantages toxicity	Pulmonary edema, hypernatremia, fluid overload	Nausea, diarrhea, extraosseous calcification	Hyperglycemia, gastritis, osteopenia	Nausea, hypersensitivity

Abbreviations: IM, intramuscularly; IV, intravenously; SC, subcutaneously.

[a]Potency is defined as the expected proportion of patients with a serum calcium ≥ 12.0 mg/dl who will achieve normocalcemia.

(From Warrell RP: Metabolic emergencies. pp. 2128–2141. In Devita VT Jr, Hellman S, Rosenberg SA [eds]: Cancer: Principles and Practice of Oncology. Lippincott-Raven, Philadelphia, 1993, with permission.)

However, this therapy is very dangerous because of the risk of precipitation of calcium-phosphate complexes in tissues, resulting in severe toxicity. This may also cause hypotension, renal failure, and severe hypocalcemia. Its use is restricted to extreme, life-threatening hypercalcemia not responding to any other form of therapy. Oral phosphates (0.5–3.0 g/day) are effective in mild hypercalcemia, but limited by nausea and diarrhea.

CORTICOSTEROIDS

Corticosteroids inhibit osteoclast mediated bone resorption and decrease gastrointestinal absorption of calcium. They are effective agents in the therapy of calcitriol-mediated hypercalcemia, such as in Hodgkin's disease and NHL, independent of any antitumor cytotoxicity. They are also effective in myeloma and leukemia but have no role in solid tumors. The minimum effective dose is uncertain, but generally 40 to 100 mg of prednisone per day is used.

CALCITONIN

This drug acts by inhibiting bone resorption and increasing renal excretion of calcium. The major advantages are its rapid onset of action, which is evident within 1 to 2 hours of initial dosing, and that it is safe, even in patients with dehydration and renal insufficiency. Its peak effect is seen in 24 to 48 hours and is sustained for 5 to 7 days. However, its effect is modest, reducing the serum calcium by 2 mg/dl, and resistance develops rapidly. Side effects are mild and include nausea, abdominal cramps, vomiting, and flushing. Allergic reactions to salmon calcitonin, the most widely used preparation, are unusual, but an initial skin test with 1 unit is recommended before therapy. The maximum recommended dose of calcitonin is 8 IU/kg given intramuscularly or subcutaneously every 6 hours for 1 to 2 days. For chronic use, 4 IU/kg can be given subcutaneously once or twice a day. Calcitonin has been used in combination with more potent agents, like biphosphonates. Thiebaud et al. reported that the combination of a single dose of pamidronate (45 or 60 mg) and salmon calcitonin given as suppositories for 3 days normalized serum calcium levels in all patients, with a significant decrease in serum calcium evident by day 2. This combination is safe and may be more efficacious than either alone.

PLICAMYCIN (MITHRAMYCIN)

An antitumor antibiotic that acts directly by its cytotoxic effect on osteoclasts, plicamycin is given intravenously in a dose of 25 µg/kg over 4 to 6 hours. Care should be taken to avoid extravasation

Etidronate	Plicamycin	Gallium Nitrate	Pamidronate
7.5 mg/kg IV over 4 hour daily for 3–5 days	10–50 (usually 25) µg/kg IV by brief infusion	100–200 mg/m²/ day by continuous IV infusion up to 5 days	60–90 mg IV over 24 hours
Mild or moderate hypercalcemia	Moderate or severe hypercalcemia	Moderate or severe hypercalcemia	Moderate or severe hypercalcemia
48 hours	24–48 hours	24–48 hours	24–48 hours
30%–40%	80%	80%	70%–80%
Usually well tolerated; decreases bone resorption	Highly effective	Highly effective; decreases bone resorption	Highly effective; decreases bone resorption
Occasional nephrotoxicity	Nausea, nephrotoxicity, hepatoxicity, thrombocytopenia, coagulopathy	Prolonged infusion, nephrotoxicity, hypophosphatemia	Fever, venous irritation

of the drug, because it can cause local irritation and cellulitis. The dose can be repeated at intervals of 24 to 48 hours, and the effect is seen in the first 24 hours. The response rate varies between 45% and 80%, but the duration of response is unpredictable. The serious side effects include rapid rebound hypercalcemia, occurring unpredictably. Others include nausea, hepatotoxicity, renal insufficiency, and thrombocytopenia. The toxic effects are cumulative, making its long-term use limited. This agent should be considered only when hypercalcemia is resistant to other safer drugs. Its use may limit the dose of other cytotoxic agents being used to treat the underlying disease.

BIPHOSPHONATES

Biphosphonates are analogues of pyrophosphate in which P-O-P is replaced by a stable P-C-P bond. Etidrionate, clodronate, and pamidronate are the most commonly used biphosphonates. They act by inhibiting osteoclastic activity. They bind to hydroxyapatite in bone and inhibit the dissolution of crystals. Because of their high affinity for bone mineral and their resistance to degradation, they have a long half-life. The gastrointestinal absorption is poor after oral administration and is worse if taken with food. They should be given intravenously after starting hydration as they can aggravate renal insufficiency.

Etidronate (Didronel) This was the first biphosphonate licensed for use in the management of metabolic bone disease. Oral absorption is poor and unreliable. Singer et al. in a randomized, double blind, multicenter study comparing etidronate (7.5 mg/kg/day over 2 hours for 3 days in 136 patients) to saline infusion showed normalization of corrected serum calcium levels in 24% of the patients receiving etidronate. Etidronate in two randomized and double-blind studies, compared with gallium nitrate and pamidronate, has shown a complete response rate of about 40% in both studies. Etidronate is usually administered intravenously at a maximal dose of 7.5 mg/kg/day for 3 to 5 days. Even a 24-hour infusion of 30 mg/kg has been shown to be safe, effective, and may be more convenient than standard therapy. Oral maintenance therapy is not effective.

Pamidronate (Aredia) This is highly effective in returning calcium levels to normal. Early studies demonstrated that single dose therapy achieves the same effect as divided doses over a few days. Pamidronate can be administered either as a single 24-hour infusion or as a short infusion over 2 to 4 hours. Body et al. showed a dose-response relationship in their retrospective review. The success rate for corrected serum calcium levels was 80% for the 0.5 mg/kg (35 patients) and 1.0 mg/kg (52 patients) groups combined, compared with 94% for the 1.5 mg/kg (73 patients) group. Nussbaum et al. in a randomized, double-blind, multicenter study confirmed the dose-response relationship when the drug was given as a single 24-hour infusion. The corrected serum calcium normalized in 40% of patients who received 30 mg (15 patients), in 61% of patients who received 60 mg (18 patients), and in 100% of patients who received 90 mg (17 patients) of pamidronate. In the former study, the duration of normocalcemia was prolonged in the high-dose group; however, in the latter study there was no significant difference in duration of normocalcemia between the groups. The duration of normocalcemia was between 3 to 4 weeks. The response in both studies was not influenced by the presence of skeletal metastasis. Another double-blind study showed no significant difference in response rates when 60 mg of pamidronate were infused over either 4 or 24 hours. A randomized comparative study of three intravenous biphosphonates showed the superiority of pamidronate infusion. More patients in the pamidronate group became normocalcemic, and the effect was apparent sooner and lasted longer. Similarly, a double-blind, randomized study by Gucalp et al. confirmed the superiority of 60 mg of pamidronate over the standard dose of etidronate (response rate is 70% vs. 41%). Ralston et al. compared the effect of pamidronate with that of mithramycin and a combination of corticosteroids and calcitonin. They showed that pamsidronate induced a more effective fall in serum calcium than the rest, although the time to onset of effect was longer. However, interim results of a randomized, multi-institutional study of pamidronate versus gallium nitrate suggest superiority of the latter drug, pending the final outcome.

Side Effects of Biphosphonates In general, biphosphonates are well tolerated. Low-grade pyrexia is reported in 15% to 20% of patients. Rapid infusion of etidronate has been associated with worsening renal function. While hypocalcemia is common with higher doses, hyperphosphatemia is noted with etidronate. Oral therapy may be associated with intolerance.

GALLIUM NITRATE

Patients receiving gallium nitrate for lymphoma were noted to have hypocalcemia as a side effect. It appears to inhibit bone resorption by adsorbing to and reducing the solubility of hydroxyapatite crystals. It is administered as a continuous infusion at 200 mg/m^2/day for 5 days. Two randomized, double-blind studies have demonstrated the superiority of gallium nitrate compared with either etidronate or calcitonin for acute treatment of hypercalcemia. The complete response rates to gallium nitrate were 82% and 69%, respectively, in the above studies. Median duration of normocalcemia was reported as 6 days, in one study. The incidence of renal insufficiency is similar to biphosphonates, and the drug should be administered only after rehydration. Other nephrotoxic medications should be avoided. Other side effects include nausea, vomiting, and hypophosphatemia.

PRACTICAL APPROACH

The best way to control hypercalcemia is by treating the underlying malignancy. This is difficult because most of the patients has refractory and progressive disease. In the absence of effective therapy, patient's symptoms and immediate prognosis should be used as a guide for further therapy. There should be a frank discussion with the patient and the family about further options, including no therapy. It should be emphasized that antihypercalcemic therapy is only palliative, with no effect on the primary disease.

Patients can be grouped into those who require inpatient care and those who can be managed as outpatients. Patients with a serum calcium greater then 12 mg/dL, moderate to severe symptoms, evidence of dehydration or who appear sick should be hospitalized. Other patients can be managed outside the hospital.

INPATIENT MANAGEMENT

Intravenous administration of isotonic saline is the first treatment of choice. The rate of hydration depends upon the degree of volume loss and cardiac reserve. Loop diuretics should be given only in case of fluid retention or overload. Other therapeutic agents should be considered only after an adequate urinary output. Calcitonin, however, can be given immediately for a fast and short effect. The best option is to combine a faster acting agent (calcitonin) with a slower acting agent (pamidronate or gallium nitrate). We recommend calcitonin at 4 to 8 units/kg every 6 hours for one to two days in combination with pamidronate for severe hypercalcemia associated with neurologic symptoms. We prefer a 90-mg dose of pamidronate for patients with a corrected serum calcium of greater than or equal to 13.5 mg/dL, and a 60-mg dose if the level is less than 13.5 mg/dL. In lymphomas and myeloma, which are steroid responsive, prednisone is beneficial. Patients with myeloma, severe hypercalcemia, and severe renal insufficiency should be referred for immediate dialysis. Mithramycin is reserved for refractory cases, with no other therapy available.

OUTPATIENT MANAGEMENT

Patients and their families should be well educated and have clear instructions about increased oral fluid intake. Medications that can potentially aggravate hypercalcemia should be avoided. No specific guidelines are available, as most of the studies are based on inpatient management. Oral phosphates, 1 to 3 g/day, are useful if tolerated. We prefer intermittent, intravenous infusions of pamidronate, 60 mg over 4 hours, every 2 to 3 weeks because of the ease of administration and efficacy. Steroids may be of help if the disease is responsive. An algorithm exploring the full range of management options is presented in Figure 63-1.

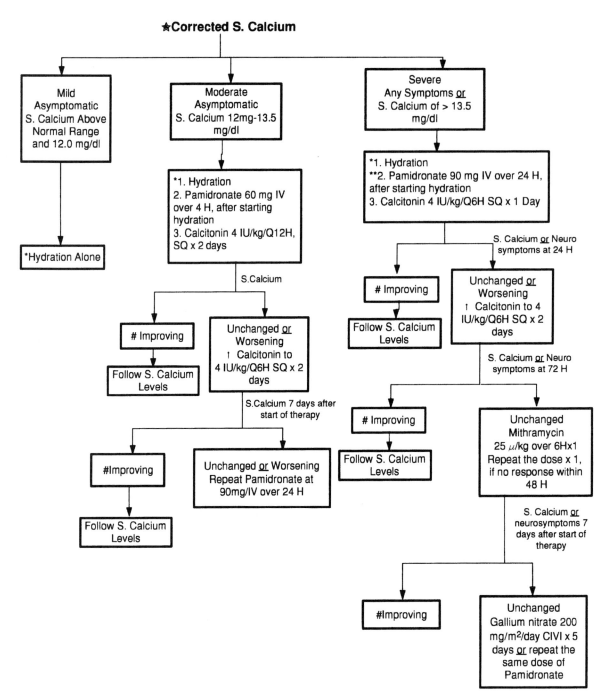

FIGURE 63-1 *Algorithm for management of hypercalcemia. The key reasoning principle is to identify patients who have specific antitumor therapy available and treat them aggressively. The goals of therapy are to give enough time for the definitive therapy of the underlying disease to work and/or for palliation of symptoms in refractory cases. Consider steroids (prednisone 40–100 mg p.o./day) in case of hematologic tumors. If neurologic symptoms do not improve after correction of hypercalcemia, consider spinal tap to rule out meningeal carcinomatosis. The evidence supporting these recommendations is level II and III. ★, corrected calcium (mg/dl) = measured calcium (mg/dL) + 0.8 (4.0-S albumin (g/dl). *NS 3–4 liters per day for the first 48 h, at least. Rate of hydration is dependent on the degree of dehydration and cardiac reserve. Once adequate hydration is noted with good urinary output, hydration can be decreased to at least 2 liters a day. Furosemide is given only in case of fluid overload or retention with dependent edema. **Pamidronate, 90 mg over 4 h, has been shown to be equally effective but is not yet approved as a 4-hour infusion. #Follow serum calcium levels for 2 to 3 days to avoid any hypocalcemia.*

SUGGESTED READINGS

Bertheault-Cvitkovic F, Tubiana-Hulin M, Chevalier B et al: Gallium nitrate vs. pamidronate for acute control of cancer-related hypercalcemia: interim results of a randomized, double-blind, multinational study (meeting abstract). Proc Annu Meet Am Soc Clin Oncol 14A:369, 1995

Bilezikian JP: Management of acute hypercalcemia. N Engl J Med 326:1196–1203, 1992

Blomqvist CP: Malignant hypercalcemia—a hospital survey. Acta Med Scand 220:455–463, 1986

Fisken RA, Heath DA, Bold AM: Hypercalcemia – a hospital survey. Quart J Med 196:405–418, 1980

Gucalp R, Ritch P, Wiernik PH, et al: Comparative study of pamidronate disodium and etidronate disodium in the treatment of cancer-related hypercalcemia. J Clin Oncol 10:134–142, 1992

Gucalp R, Theriault R, Gill I et al: Treatment of cancer-related hypercalcemia: double-blind comparison of rapid and slow intravenous infusion regimens of pamidronate disodium and saline alone. Arch Intern Med 154:1935–1944, 1994

Nussbaum SR, VandePol CJ, Younger J et al: Single-dose intravenous therapy with pamidronate for the treatment of hypercalcemia of malignancy: comparison of 30-, 60-, and 90-mg dosages. Am J Med 95:297–304, 1993

Ralston SH, Alzaid AA, Gardner MD, Boyle IT: Treatment of cancer associated hypercalcemia with combined aminohydroxypropylidene diphosphonate and calcitonin. BMJ 292:1549–1550, 1986

Ralston SH, Patel U, Fraser WD et al: Comparison of three intravenous bisphosphonates in cancer-associated hypercalcemia. Lancet 2:1180–1182, 1989

Ralston SH, Patel U, Gallacher SJ, Campbell J, Boyle IT: Cancer-associated hypercalcemia: morbidity and mortality. Ann Intern Med 112:499–504, 1990

Seymour JF, Gagel RF: Calcitriol: the major humoral mediator of hypercalcemia in Hodgkin's disease and NHL. Blood 82:1383–1394, 1993

Singer FR, Ritch PS, Lad TE, et al: Treatment of hypercalcemia of malignancy with intravenous etidronate, a controlled multicenter study. Arch Intern Med 151:471–476, 1991

Thiebaud D, Jacquet AF, Burckhardt P: Fast and effective treatment of malignant hypercalcemia: combination of suppositories of calcitonin and a single infusion of 3-amino 1-hydroxypropylidene-1-biphosphonate. Arch Intern Med 150:2125–2128, 1990

Warrell RP: Metabolic emergencies. pp. 2128–2141. In Devita VT, Jr, Hellman S, Rosenberg SA, (eds): Cancer: Principles & Practice of Oncology. Lippincott-Raven, Philadelphia, 1993

Warrell RP, Israel R, Frisone M, et al: Clin Oncol Gallium nitrate for acute treatment of cancer-related hypercalcemia: a randomized, double-blind comparison to calcitonin. Ann Intern Med 108:669–674, 1988

Warrell RP, Murphy WK, Schulman P, O'Dwyer PJ, Heller G: A randomized double-blind study of gallium nitrate compared with etidronate for acute control of cancer-related hypercalcemia. J Clin Oncol 9:1467–1475, 1991

Wisenski LA: Salmon calcitonin in the acute management of hypercalcemia. Calcif Tissue Int Suppl 46:S26–S30, 1990

64 Treatment and Prophylaxis of Graft-Versus-Host Disease

Donald R. Fleming

Graft-versus-host disease (GVHD), once known only as a dreaded phenomenon associated with allogeneic bone marrow transplant patients, is now being artificially produced in autologous transplant patients because of its potential to inhibit relapse. Nevertheless, GVHD remains a major cause of both mortality as well as morbidity in allogeneic transplant settings. Overall, between 30% and 60% of all allogeneic transplant patients experience some degree of GVHD. Without T-cell depletion of the marrow, the average incidence of GVHD is about 50%, with about one third of these patients succumbing to the disease process. While about 80% to 90% of patients with stage I-II survive the disease, only 40% to 50% of those developing stage III-IV experience long-term survival. The primary effectors involved in GVHD remain elusive. T lymphocytes, natural killer cells, as well as various cytokines released by these and additional interacting cells are felt to play a role in the histopathologic changes associated with GVHD.

Clinically, the process of GVHD can be divided into both acute and chronic phases, with the former beginning in the early engraftment period (often described as the first 100 days after transplant) and the latter occurring subsequent to this time period. Despite the definition of these two different types of GVHD, based on artificial barriers of time, definite clinical differences help in distinguishing each form.

ACUTE GVHD

Acute GVHD presents as an erythrodermatous rash associated with debilitating diarrhea and cholestatic liver dysfunction. Distinct staging and grading that are based on organ-related involvement determine the therapy of the disease (Fig. 64-1 and Table 64-1). Because of concomitant regimen-related tox-icities and infectious disease processes, the etiology of the clinical features associated with acute GVHD often remain elusive. Treatment is empiric and frequently based on potentially broad etiologies.

CHRONIC GVHD

Later in the post-transplant period a clinically distinct entity, chronic GVHD, presents itself with a spectrum of unique clinical manifestations. Chronic GVHD may occur as a continuum from acute GVHD referred to as progressive chronic GVHD; as an interrupted disease interval from acute GVHD, described as quiescent chronic GVHD, or as a *de novo* process in which the patient never had a history of acute GVHD. Once the patient has an extensive disease, the treatment is promptly initiated based on whether the patient is receiving immunosuppressive therapy and whether he or she has thrombocytopenia (see Fig. 64-2 and Table 64-2). As with acute GVHD, the most accessible areas are carefully examined for suspicious areas to biopsy to confirm the diagnosis. Skin, gut, and liver in succession of preference, are typically areas pursued diagnostically. In addition, examination of the oral mucosa for lichenoid stria, can often be helpful when searching for areas of chronic GVHD. Ocular involvement of chronic GVHD can be detected early by use of Schirmer's test as well as slit-lamp testing by an experienced ophthalmologist. Other clinical features are often a composite of sclerodermatous skin changes along with chronic gastrointestinal abnormalities. With progression, the patient's pulmonary status can deteriorate because of a progressive obstructive pulmonary disease process known as bronchiolitis obliterans. As with acute GVHD, infections remain a major factor in morbidity as well as mortality in chronic GVHD, necessitating extension of

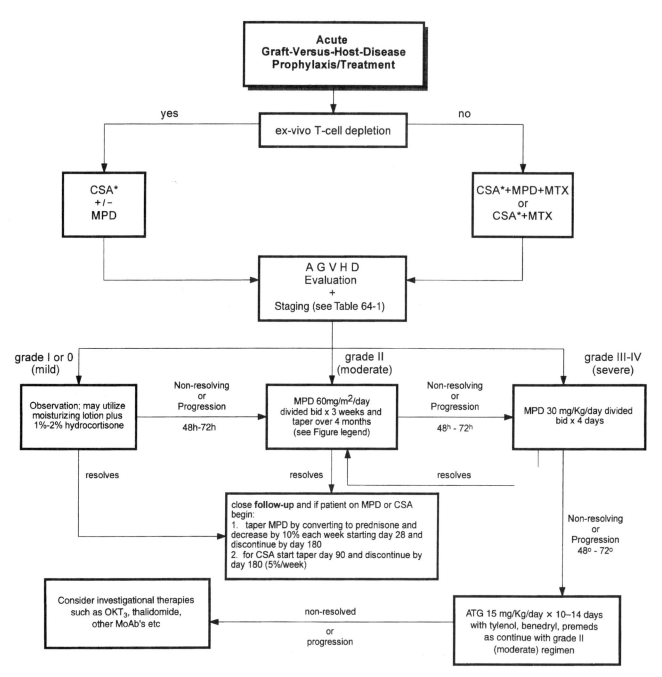

FIGURE 64-1 *Algorithm for selective prophylaxis as well as overall therapeutic approach for acute graft-versus-host disease GVHD. The ideal goal of treatment is to control the morbidity from GHVD while at the same time to allow some therapeutic effects of GVHD on malignant cells (graft versus leukemia effect). The recommended strategy, for prevention, is based on randomized controlled clinical trials and meta-analysis (level I and II evidence). The use of in vivo methods of acute GVHD prophylaxis in T-cell deplated patients is less well established and based on level III and IV data. The approach to treatment of acute GVHD is based primarily on level II and III data, which involves well-designed but nevertheless low-power randomized studies. CSA, Cyclosporin, 3 to 5 mg/kg/day (adjust levels); MPD, methylprednisolone 30mg/m²/d; convert to equal prednisone dose once taking oral medications without problems; MTX, methotrexate 15mg/m²/day intravenous day plus one, then 10 mg/m² on day of transplant +3, +6, +11 (hold day +11 for severe mucositis); ATG, antithymocyte globulin.*

TABLE 64-1   STAGING AND GRADING OF ACUTE GVHD

Stage	Skin	Liver	Intestinal (diarrhea)
1	M-P rash <25% BSA	Bilirubin, 2–3 mg/dl	<500 cc/day
2	M-P rash 25–50% BSA	Bilirubin, 3–6 mg/dl	500–1,000 cc/day
3	Generalized erythroderma	Bilirubin, 6–15 mg/dl	1,000–1,500 cc/day
4	Generalized erythroderma with bullous formation and desquamation	Bilirubin, >15 mg/dl	abdominal pain and/or ileus

Grade	
I	1–2 skin, no gut or liver; no decline in performance
II	1–3 skin, 1 gut and/or liver, mild decline in performance
III	2–3 skin, 2–3 gut, or 2–4 liver; mild decline in performance
IV	As in III with 2–4 organ involvement and extreme performance decline.

Abbreviations: M-P, maculopapular.

(From Thomas ED, Storb R, Cliff RA et al: Bone marrow transplantation. N Engl J Med 292:895–902, 1975, with permission.)

the antimicrobial prophylaxis period. Frequent, multidisciplinary interventions, including dentistry, opthamology, and physical therapy, are essential in caring for patients with extensive chronic GVHD.

Risks for GVHD are numerous; however, with some predictability, proper preventive techniques can be initiated to minimize catastrophic clinical outcomes. Characteristics attributed to both the donor as well as the recipient have been described (Table 64-3). Based on these as well as other predictive features, specific measures can be applied to present GVHD (see Fig 64-1). While the occurence of GVHD can be a major factor in poor outcome in allogeneic transplantation, its complete elimination through T-cell depletion can have just as devastating effects through the increased incidence of both pri-

mary disease relapse and graft failure. Most clinical trials have, and are continuing to arrive at, acceptable medians of GVHD and relapse. Further insight may eventually allow us to separate these two entities. The algorithms involved in this chapter focus on both prevention as well as treatment of GVHD. Data for construction of the algorithm for prevention and treatment of acute GVHD are of high quality (level I and II); initial treatment of chronic GVHD are also of high quality (level I and II). However, data for salvage treatment are of level III, IV, and V. It is evident, therefore, that modifications of current regimens will probably not result in improvement of control of GVHD. To this end, new treatment modalities are needed to improve current results of the management of GVHD.

TABLE 64-2   STAGING OF CHRONIC GVHD[2]

Limited
Localized skin involvement and/or hepatic dysfunction due to cGVHD

Extensive
Generalized skin involvement, or
Localized skin involvement and/or hepatic dysfunction caused by GVHD, plus:
    1. Liver histology consistent with aggressive hepatitis, bridging necrosis, or cirrhosis, or
    2. Involvement of eyes: Schirmer's test with less than 5 mm wetting, or
    3. Involvement of minor salivary glands of oral mucosa demonstrated by labial biopsy, or
    4. Involvement of any other target organ

Abbreviation: GVHD, graft-versus-host disease.

(From Sullivan KM, Storb R, Buckner CD et al: graft-versus-host disease as adoptive immunotherapy in patients with advanced hematologic neoplasms. N Engl J Med 320:828–834, 1989, with permission.)

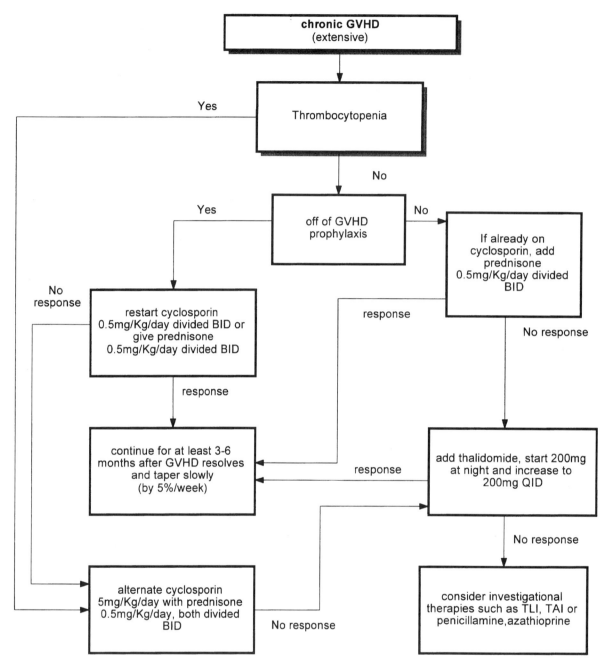

FIGURE 64-2   *Algorithm for treatment of (extensive) chronic graft-versus-host disease GVHD). It is important to continue antimicrobial prophylactic measures because of the increased immunosuppressive effects of both the treatment as well as the disease process. Decision making is based on nonrandomized, matched case-controlled trials (level I, III, and IV evidence); while, first-line salvage techniques involve matched case-controlled situations (level III and level IV evidence). Several second-line salvage regimens are based on case reports and clinical examples (level V). Note that many authors believe that because it is not life-threatening, and may decrease the relapse rate, limited chronic GVHD should not be treated unless it becomes extensive. It is important to remember that a clinical reponse may take months to detect. Thalidomide may cause significant somnolence. TLI, total lymphoid irradiation; TAI, thoracoabdominal irradiation; BID, twice a day; QID, four times a day; qhs, every night.*

TABLE 64-3   GVHD RISK ASSESSMENT (POOR RISK) BASED ON BOTH DONOR AND
RECIPIENT FEATURES

Recipient
Increased age
Increased number of transfusions
Viral shedding or active infections (CMV, HSV, VZV)
Non-T-cell depleted marrow given
Post-BMT cytokines therapy (IL-2, IFN, etc.)

Donor
Increased age
Positive viral serology (CMV, HSV, VZV)
Female
Pregnancy
Unrelated and HLA-mismatched related transplants

Abbreviation: BMT, bone marrow transplantation; CMV, cytomegalovirus; GVHD, graft-versus-host disease; HSV, herpes simplex virus; IFN, interferior; IL-2, interleukin-2; VZV, varicella zoster virus.

SUGGESTED READINGS

Barakoff SJ, Deeg HJ, Ferrara J, Atkinson K, (eds): Graft-versus-Host-Disease—Immunology, Pathophysiology and Treatment. Marcel Dekker, New York, 1990

Chao NS, Schmidt G, Niland et al: Cyclosporin, methotrexate and prednisone compared with cyclosporin and prednisone for prophylaxis of acute graft versus host disease. N Engl J Med 329:1225–1229, 1993

Nademanee A, Schmidt G, Parker P et al: The outcome of matched unrelated donor bone marrow transplantation in patient with hematologic malignancies using molecular typing for donor selection and graft-versus-host disease prophylaxis regimen of cyclosporin, methotrexate and prednisone. Blood 86:1228–1234, 1995

Santos GW, Tutschka PJ, Brookmeyer R et al: Cyclosporine plus methylprednisolone as prophylaxis for GVHD: randomized double blind study in patients undergoing bone marrow transplantation. Clin Transplant 1:21–29, 1987

Storb R, Deeg HJ, Pepe M et al; Methotrexate and cyclosporine versus cyclosporine alone for prophylaxis of graft-versus-host disease in patients given HLA identical marrow grafts for leukemia: a long term follow up of a controlled trial. Blood 73:1729–1734, 1989

Sullivan KM: Graft-versus-host disease. In: Forman SJ, Blume KG, Thomas ED (eds): Bone Marrow Transplantation. Blackwell Scientific, Boston, 1994

Sullivan KM, Storb R, Buckner CD et al: Graft-versus-host disease as adoptive immunotherapy in patients with advanced hematologic neoplasms. N Engl J Med 320:828–834, 1989

Thomas ED, Storb R, Cliff RA et al: Bone marrow transplantation. N Engl J Med 292:895–902, 1975

Vogelsang GB, Hess AD: Graft-versus-host disease: new directions for a persistent problem. Blood 84:2061–2067, 1994

Treatment Protocols

Paul Mangino
Beverly Taft
Benjamin Djulbegović

Dosages for protocols described in the following appendices are mainly based on manufacturers recommendations and references cited in the chapters describing management of a particular treatment. Note, however, that virtually no data exist comparing the methods of administration described in this section with some other methods described in the literature. Similarly, dose modifications for hematologic, renal, or liver abnormalities are based on pharmacologic understanding of the effects of various chemotherapeutics and not on outcomes favoring the recommendations described. For example, there is virtually no evidence to suggest that reducing a dose of some chemotherapeutic agents according to white cell or platelet count (see Appendix Table 2-3) produces superior clinical outcome than supporting hematopoiesis with growth factors. Therefore, recommendations provided in the next section are based on our experience and our best judgment of currently available data in the literature.

Body-Surface-Area Nomogram, Performance Scales, and Criteria for Grading Toxicity

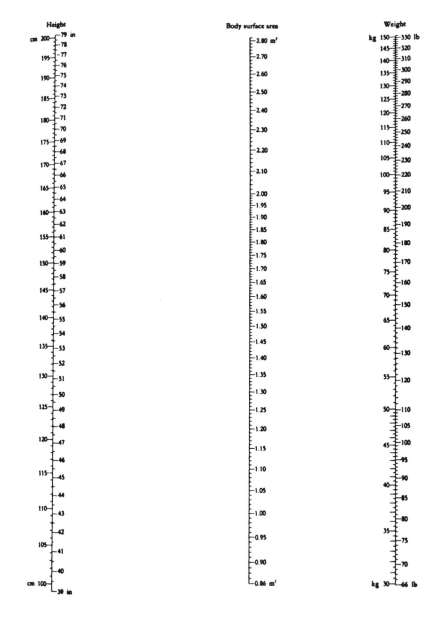

APPENDIX FIGURE 1-1 *Nomogram for the determination of body-surface area of adults from height and weight. A straight line connecting the individual's height and weight will intersect the center column at the individual's body-surface area. (From Hubbard SM, Gross J: Principles of clinical research. p. 195. In Gross J, Johnson BL: Handbook of Oncology Nursing. 2nd Ed. Jones and Bartlett, Sudbury, MA, 1994, with permission.)*

APPENDIX TABLE 1-1 KARNOFSKY AND ZUBROD (ECOG) PERFORMANCE SCALES

Karnofsky

100%	No evidence of disease
90%	Normal activity with minor signs of disease
80%	Normal activity with effort; signs of disease
70%	Cannot do normal activity but cares for self
60%	Requires occasional assistance
50%	Requires considerable assistance; frequent medical care
40%	Disabled; requires special care
30%	Severely disabled; hospitalization may be indicated
20%	Very sick; hospitalization necessary for supportive treatment
10%	Moribund

Zubrod (Eastern Cooperative Oncology Group [ECOG])

0	Asymptomatic, normal activity
1	Symptomatic but fully ambulatory
2	Symptomatic; in bed less than 50% of time
3	Symptomatic; in bed more than 50% of time; not bedridden
4	100% bedridden

Approximate relationship of Karnofsky to Zubrod scales
0 Zubrod = 100% Karnofsky
1 Zubrod = 85% Karnofsky
2 Zubrod = 65% Karnofsky
3 Zubrod = 40% Karnofsky
4 Zubrod = 15% Karnofsky

(From Yarbro JW: The Oncologist's Pocket Guide. WB Saunders, Philadelphia, 1993, with permission.)

APPENDIX TABLE 1-2 CRITERIA FOR GRADING TOXICITY

A variety of scales are currently in use by various clinical trials groups for grading the toxicity associated with chemotherapeutic agents. These scales are quite similar, but not identical. The scales included in Table 1-1, for the most part, follow the South West Oncology Group (SWOG) toxicity criteria and are identical in most places to scales used by Cancer Acute Leukemia Group B (CALGB), ECOG, World Health Organization (WHO), etc.

The toxicity grades apply only to changes thought to be induced by drugs, not by the disease itself. Symptoms of the disease are coded using the Performance Scales of Karnofsky and Zubrod, which are shown in Table 1-1.

Toxic grade 0 indicates normal or no change from the pretreatment state. Toxic grade 5 indicates death resulting from drug-induced toxicity. The maximum grade encountered during therapy is scored.

Toxicity	Grade 0	Grade 1	Grade 2	Grade 3	Grade 4
Hematologic					
WBC ($\times 10^9$/L)	4.0	3.0–3.9	2.0–2.9	1.0–1.9	<1.0
Platelets ($\times 10^9$/L)	WNL	75–normal	50–74.9	25–49.9	<25
Hemoglobin (g/dL)	WNL	10–normal	8–10	6.5–7.9	<6.5
Granulocytes ($\times 10^9$/L)	>2.0	1.5–1.9	1.0–1.4	0.5–0.9	<0.5
Lymphocytes ($\times 10^9$/L)	>2.0	1.5–1.9	1.0–1.4	0.5–0.9	<0.5
Hematologic, other (specify)		Mild	Moderate	Severe	Life threatening
Clotting					
Fibrinogen	WNL	75%–99% NL	50%–74% NL	25%–49% NL	<24% NL
Prothrombin time	WNL	101%–125% NL	126%–150% NL	151%–200% NL	>200% NL
PTT	WNL	101%–166% NL	167%–233% NL	234%–300% NL	>300% NL
Clotting, other (specify)		Mild	Moderate	Severe	Life threatening
Hemorrhage	None	No transfusion	Transfusion, 1–2 units	Transfusion, 3–4 units	Transfusion, >4 units
Infection	None	Mild	Moderate	IV antibiotics or antifungal	Life threatening (eg, septic shock)
Miscellaneous					
Alopecia		Mild	Pronounced		
Weight gain	<5%	5%–9.9%	10%–19.9%	>20%	
Weight loss	<5%	5%–9.9%	10%–19.9%	>20%	
Laryngitis		Mild, intermittent	Persistent hoarseness	Whispered speech	
Salivary		Mild dryness	Moderate to complete dryness		Salivary gland necrosis
Anorexia		Present			
Wound dehiscence		Skin or subcutaneous		Fascia	
Wound necrosis				Present	
Rectal laceration				Present	
Miscellaneous, other		Mild	Moderate	Severe	Life threatening

	Grade 0	Grade 1	Grade 2	Grade 3	Grade 4
Pain					
Specify site	No	Nonnarcotics	PO narcotics	IM/IV narcotics	Uncontrollable
Tumor flare pain	None	Redness or needs nonnarcotics	PO narcotics	IM/IV narcotics	Uncontrollable
Mucosal					
Stomatitis	None	Painless ulcers Mild soreness	Painful erythema and edema but can eat	Pain and edema prevent eating	Needs enteral or parenteral support
Pharyngitis esophagitis	None	Painless ulcers Mild dysphagia	Dysphagia but can eat without narcotics	Cannot eat solids or needs narcotics to eat	Needs enteral or parenteral support
Vaginitis or other mucositis	None	Erythema, mild pain; but no treatment is required	Serosanguinous discharge or pain requires treatment with nonnarcotic	Confluent fibrinous, or requires narcotic for pain	Necrosis
Gastrointestinal					
Nausea	None	Mild, but able to eat	Oral intake reduced significantly		No significant oral intake
Vomiting	None	1 episode/24 hours	2–5 episodes/24 hours	6–10 episodes/24 hours	>10 episodes/24 hours
Diarrhea	None	2–3 stools/day over normal	4–6 stools/day or nocturnal, or cramping	7–9 stools/day, or incontinence, or severe cramping	>10 stools/day or bloody or needs IV fluid
Constipation	None	Needs stool softener	Needs laxatives	Needs enema or manual evacuation	
Ileus	None			Yes, <96 hours	Yes, >96 hours
Gastritis/ulcer	No	Needs antacid	Needs vigorous medical management	Needs surgical management	Perforation or hemorrhage
Small bowel obstruction	No		Intermittent, but no treatment	Requires treatment	Requires surgery
Intestinal fistula	No			Yes	
Other (specify)		Mild	Moderate	Severe	Life threatening
Liver					
Bilirubin	WNL		1.5 × NL	1.5–3.0 × NL	>3.0 × NL
SGOT/SGPT	WNL	2.5 × NL	2.6–5.0 × NL	5.1–20 × NL	>20 × NL
Alkaline phosphatase or 5' nucleotidase	WNL	2.5 × NL	2.6–5.0 × NL	5.1–20 × NL	>20 × NL
Clinical status				Precoma	Hepatic coma
Other		Mild	Moderate	Severe	Life threatening

(Continued)

457

Toxicity	Grade 0	Grade 1	Grade 2	Grade 3	Grade 4
Lung					
Dyspnea	No change		Dyspnea with significant exertion	Dyspnea with normal activity	Dyspnea at rest
pO_2/pCO_2	No change or pO_2 > 85 and pCO_2 <40	pO_2 70–85 pCO_2 40–50	pO_2 60–70 pCO_2 50–60	pO_2 50–60 pCO_2 60–70	pO_2 < 50 or pCO_2 > 70
CO diffusion	>90% pre-Rx	76%–90% pre-Rx	51%–75% pre-Rx	26%–50% pre-Rx	<25% pre-Rx
Pulmonary fibrosis	None	asymptomatic, radiographic		Symptomatic	
Pulmonary edema	None	Radiographic changes only	Steroids required	Diuretics required	Intubation required
Pneumonitis (noninfectious)	None			Oxygen required	Assisted ventilation
Cough	None	Mild, OTC medications	Requires narcotic medications	Uncontrolled spasms	
Other (specify)	None	Mild	Moderate	Severe	Life threatening
Cardiac					
Dysrhythmia	None	Asymptomatic, transient; no treatment	Recurrent or persistent, no treatment	Requires treatment	Requires monitor or V-tach or V-fib or hypotension
Ejection fraction or heart failure	None	Decline of EF < 20%	Decline of EF > 20% but asymptomatic	Mild CHF that responds to treatment	Severe CHF or refractory to treatment
Ischemia	None	Nonspecific T-wave flattening	ST- and T-wave ischemic changes	Angina but no infarction	Acute myocardial infarction
Pericarditis	None	Asymptomatic	Symptoms, signs mild, moderate	Drainage required	Tamponade Life threatening
Other (specify)		Mild	Moderate	Severe	Life threatening
Circulatory					
Hypertension	No change	Asymptomatic or transient by >20 mmHg or >150/100 if NL	Recurrent or persistent by > 20 mmHg or >150/100 if NL	Requires therapy	Hypertensive crisis
Hypotension	No change	No therapy (transient orthostatic hypotension)	Requires fluids but not hospitalization	Requires hospitalization but resolves in <48 hours after stopping drug	Requires hospitalization, lasts >48 hours after stopping drug
Phlebitis/thrombosis		Superficial		Deep vein	Major event Pulmonary Embolism (PE)
Edema	None	1+ (PM only)	2+ (during day)	3+	4+
Veno-occlusive disease	None			Present	
Other (specify)		Mild	Moderate	Severe	Life threatening

Renal and bladder				
Incontinence	None	With cough/sneeze	Spontaneous	No control
Dysuria	None	Mild	Moderate, but pyridium controls	Not controlled by pyridium
Urinary retention	None	Residual < 100 cc, or occasionally needs catheter; or difficulty starting stream	Catheter always required	Surgical procedure required	Life threatening
Frequency or urgency	No change	Increased or nocturia to $2 \times NL$	More than $2 \times NL$ but < hourly	Urgency hourly or requires catheter
Hemorrhagic cystitis	None	Microscopic hematuria	Frank blood but no Rx required	Irrigation of bladder required	Life threatening
Bladder cramps	None	Present (code pain as applicable)	Moderate	Severe
Bladder, other				
Creatinine	WNL	$<1.5 \times NL$	$1.5–3.0 \times NL$	$3.1–6.0 \times NL$	$>6 \times NL$
Proteinuria	None	1 + or <3 g/L	2–3+ or 3–10 g/L	4+ or >10 g/L	Nephrotic syndrome
Hematuria	None	Microscopic only	Gross, no clots	Gross with clots	Transfusion
Renal failure					Dialysis required
Renal, other (specify)		Mild	Moderate	Severe	Life threatening
Ureteral obstruction	None	Unilateral No surgery	Bilateral, no surgery	Incomplete, stints or surgery	Complete bilateral
Genitourinary fistula				Present
Genitourinary, other (specify)		Mild	Moderate	Severe	Life threatening
Metabolic				
Hyponatremia (mEq/L)	No change	131–135	126–130	121–125	<120
Hypokalemia (mEq/L)	No change	3.1–3.5	2.6–3.0	2.1–2.5	<2.0
Hyperglycemia (mg/dL)	No change	116–160	161–250	251–500	>500 or ketoacidosis
Hypoglycemia (mg/dL)	No change	55–64	40–54	30–39	<30
Amylase	WNL	$1.5 \times NL$	$1.5–2 \times NL$	$2.1–5 \times NL$	$>5 \times NL$
Hypercalcemia (mg/dL)	No change	10.6–11.5	11.6–12.5	12.6–13.5	>13.5
Hypocalcemia (mg/dL)	No change	8.4–7.8	7.7–7.0	6.9–6.1	<6.0
Hypomagnesemia (mg/dL)	No change	1.4–1.2	1.1–0.9	0.8–0.6	<0.5
Other, metabolic		Mild	Moderate	Severe	Life threatening
Neurologic (motor)				
Weakness	None	Subjective weakness with no objective findings	Mild objective weakness without significant impairment	Objective weakness with functional impairment	Paralysis
Incoordination or ataxia	None	Slight incoordination, dysdiadokinesis	Intention tremor, dysmetria nystagmus	Locomotor ataxia

(Continued)

Toxicity	Grade 0	Grade 1	Grade 2	Grade 3	Grade 4
Speech impairment	None		Slurred speech	Expressive aphasia	Mute
Cerebellar necrosis					Present
Neurologic (sensory)					
Paresthesia	None	Mild	Moderate	Interferes with function	
Numbness/other peripheral nervous system abnormality			Nondisabling objective sensory loss	Disabling, objective sensory loss	
Reflexes		Diminished	Loss of deep tendon		
Hearing	None or no change	Asymptomatic (audiometry only)	Tinnitus	Interferes with function, correctable with hearing aid	Deafness not correctable
Vision				Symptomatic subtotal loss; blurred vision	Blindness
Taste		Slight change	Marked change		
Neurologic (central)					
Disorientation	None	Confusion or disorientation; easily reoriented	Confusion requires supervision	Requires admission to institution; or hallucinations	
Somnolence or agitation	None	Nondisabling	Requires care giver	Requires admission to institution	Coma
Personality change	None	Not disruptive	Disruptive	Harmful to self or others	Psychosis
Convulsions	None	Focal without impairment of consciousness	Focal with impairment of consciousness	Generalized, tonic–clonic, or absence attack	With loss of consciousness >10 minutes
Malaise/fatigue lethargy	None	Mild Normal activity	Change in daily activities	In bed or chair >50% waking hours	
Anxiety/depression	None	Mild Normal activity	Change in normal activities	Unable to function	
Cerebral necrosis					Present
Neurologic (other)					
Headache	None	Mild	Moderate/severe but transient	Severe and unrelenting	
Dizzyness/vertigo	None	Nondisabling		Disabling	
Insomnia	Normal	Occasional, may need sedative		Insomnia even with sedation	
Restlessness	Normal		Requires sedation		
Other, (specify)		Mild	Moderate	Severe	Life threatening
Dermatologic					
Injection site	None	Pain	Inflammation or phlebitis	Ulceration or necrosis	Plastic surgery indicated
Skin rash	None	Asymptomatic Maculopapular	With pruritis or other symptom	Generalized eruption	Exfoliative dermatitis

Category	None	Mild	Moderate	Severe	Life threatening
Blistering	None	Asymptomatic	Symptomatic, limited	Symptomatic, generalized	
Erythema		Asymptomatic	Pruritis/tenderness		
Erythema in XRT field (same as erythema)					
Desquamation		Peeling, dry	Patchy, moist	Confluent, moist	
Desquamation in XRT field (same as desquamation)					
Skin necrosis					Present
Skin ulceration					Present
Chronic skin changes	None		Telangiectasia or atrophy	Fibrosis, contractures, scars	Nonhealing ulcers
Pigmentation		Mild	Pronounced		
Photosensitivity	None	Mild sunburn / Mild photophobia	Sunburn with edema / Severe photophobia	Blistering in sun or desquamation	
Dry skin		Controlled with emollients	Uncontrolled with emollients		
Other, dermatologic		Mild	Moderate	Severe	Life threatening
Hand-foot syndrome		(also grade appropriate dermatologic phenomena)	Present		
Granuloma		Mild	Present		
Yellowing			Prominent		
Immunologic					
Allergy (also code rash)		Transient rash / Drug fever < 38°C	Urticaria / Drug fever > 38°C / Mild bronchospasm	Serum sickness / Bronchospasm requires Rx	Anaphylaxis
Other		Mild	Moderate	Severe	Life threatening
Flu-like symptoms					
Fever (in absence of infection)		37.1–38.0°C	38.1–40.0°C	> 40.0°C for less than 24 hours	> 40.0°C over 24 hours or hypotension
Chills		Mild, brief	Severe or prolonged		
Myalgia/arthralgia		Mild	Decreased movement	Disabled	
Sweats		Mild, occasional	Drenching, frequent		
Facial flushing		Present			
Other		Mild	Moderate	Severe	Life threatening
Eye					
Conjunctivitis/keratitis		Steroids or antibiotics not needed	Requires steroids or antibiotics	Corneal ulcers or opacification	
Dry eyes			Requires artificial tears		Requires enucleation
Glaucoma				Present	
Other (specify)		Mild	Moderate	Severe	Life threatening

(Continued)

Toxicity	Grade 0	Grade 1	Grade 2	Grade 3	Grade 4
Endocrine					
Libido		Decrease		Absence	
Erectile impotence		Mild	Moderate	No erections	
Sterility				Present	
Gynecomastia		Mild	Pronounced or painful		
Hot flashes		Mild or <1/day	Moderate and >1/day	Frequent and interferes with normal function	
Menses		Occasional irregularity	Very irregular	Amenorrhea for at least 6 months	
Cushingoid		Mild	Pronounced		
Other		Mild	Moderate	Severe	Life threatening

Abbreviations: CHF, congestive heart failure; EF, ejection fraction; IM, intramuscular; IV, intravenous; NC, no change (due to drug toxicity); NL, normal; OTC, over the counter; pre-Rx, pretreatment; Rx, treatment; SGOT, serum glutamic-oxaloacetic transaminase; SGPT, serum glutamic-pyruvic transaminase; V-fib, ventricular fibrillation; V-tach, ventricular tachycardia; WNL, within normal limits.

(From Yarbro JW: The Oncologist's Pocket Guide. WB Saunders, Philadelphia, 1993, with permission.)

APPENDIX 2 — Antineoplastic Drug Dose Modifications

APPENDIX TABLE 2-1   DRUGS REQUIRING DOSE MODIFICATION FOR ORGAN DYSFUNCTION

Agent	Organ Dysfunction	Suggested Dose Modification
Methotrexate[a]	Renal insufficiency	
Cisplatin	Renal insufficiency	In proportion to $C_{Cr}/100$ when $C_{Cr} < 60$ ml/min
Carboplatin	Renal insufficiency	Target AUC of 5–7 mg/ml × min; AUC = Dose/($C_{Cr} + 25$)
Cyclophosphamide and ifosfamide	Renal failure (GFR < 25% normal)	50%–75% decrease
Bleomycin	Renal failure (GFR < 25% normal)	50%–75% decrease
mAMSA	Renal failure (GFR < 25% normal)	50%–75% decrease
Streptozotocin	Renal failure (GFR < 25% normal)	50%–75% decrease
Hydroxyurea, Etoposide, Deoxycoformycin, Fludarabine, Chlorodeoxyadenosine	Renal insufficiency	In proportion to $C_{Cr}/100$ when $C_{Cr} < 60$ ml/min
Doxorubicin and daunorubicin	Hepatic dysfunction (no clear correlation of pharmacokinetics or toxicity proven)	Use caution with bilirubin ≥ 2.5; advisable to begin with reduced dose and escalate as tolerated
Paclitaxel (Taxol)	Hepatic dysfunction	25%–50% decrease for patients with hepatic metastases > 2 cm
Vincristine, Vinblastine, mAMSA, ThioTEPA, Epirubicin	Hepatic dysfunction	1. Only approximate guidelines can be offered and are probably inaccurate. 2. For bilirubin > 1.5 mg/dl, reduce initial dose by 50%. 3. For bilirubin > 3.0 mg/dl, reduce initial dose by 75%

Abbreviations: AUC, area under curve; C_{Cr}, creatinine clearance; GFR, glomerular filtration rate.

[a]See also Appendix Table 2-2.

(From Chabner BA, Longo DL: Cancer Chemotherapy and Biotherapy: Principles and Practice. Lippincott-Raven Publishers, Philadelphia, 1996, with permission.)

APPENDIX TABLE 2-2   DOSE MODIFICATION WITH ORGAN DYSFUNCTION

Hepatic Dysfunction: % of usual dose to administer if, on day of treatment

Drug	Bili <1.5 and SGOT <60	Bili 1.5–3.0 and SGOT 60–180	Bili 3.1–5.0 and SGOT > 180	Bili >5.0
5-Fluorouracil[a]	100	100	100	omit
Cyclophosphamide	100	100	75	omit
Methotrexate	100	100	75	omit
Daunorubicin	100	75	50	omit
Adriamycin	100	50	25	omit
Vinblastine Vincristine VP-16	100	50	omit	omit

Renal Dysfunction: % of usual dose to administer if GFR (ml/min) is

Drug	>50	10–50	<10
Methotrexate	100	50	0
Cisplatin	100	50	0
Nitrosoureas	100	0	0
Cyclophosphamide	100	100	50
Mithramycin	100	75	50
Bleomycin	100	75	50

[a] *See also Appendix Table 2–1.*

Abbreviations: SGOT, Serum Glutamic-Oxaloacetic Transaminase; Bili, bilirubin; GFR, glomerular filtration rate.

APPENDIX TABLE 2-3   SLIDING SCALE FOR DOSE ADJUSTMENT OF COMMONLY USED CHEMOTHERAPEUTIC AGENTS BASED ON HEMATOLOGIC TOXICITY[a]

Leukocyte count (/mm³)	Platelet Count (/mm³)	Dose Adjustment
> 4,000	> 100,000	100% all drugs
3,000–3,900	> 100,000	100% vincristine,[b] 100% bleomycin; 75% mechlorethamine, 75% procarbazine (after MOPP only; 50% after hybrid program); 50% doxorubicin
2,000–2,900	50,000–100,000	100% vincristine; 25% mechlorethamine, 25% procarbazine 50% bleomycin; 25% doxorubicin
1,000–1,900	50,000–100,000	50% vincristine, 25% mechlorethamine, 25% procarbazine, 25% bleomycin, 25% doxorubicin
< 1,000	< 50,000	No drug

[a] *Alternative practice is to administer G(M)-CSF for several days before next cycle of chemotherapy (e.g., GM-CSF was used in doses of 8 or 16 µg/kg for 5 days beginning on day 17 of the MOPP treatment for Hodgkin's disease [J Clin Oncol 1992;10:390]; G-CSF in a dose of 5 µg/kg SQ was used on days 15–19 of each subsequent chemotherapy cycle for breast cancer, starting chemotherapy 2 days after completion of G-CSF if: WBC > 3,000/mm³, ANC > 1,500/mm³, platelet count > 100,000/mm³ and hemoglobin > 8 g/dl [J Clin Oncol 1996;14:1573]). It appears that a dose-intensity of chemotherapeutic agents is increased when growth-factor support is used.*

For dose modification in case of hepatic and renal dysfunction (see Appendix Tables 2-1 and 2-2).

Note if the bone marrow contains tumor cells, full doses should be given.

[b] *If signs of peripheral neuropathy develop (inability to button clothes), dose is reduced to 50%; if patient develops ileus or has difficulty ambulating, vincristine should be held until symptoms improve and then resume at a 50% dose.*

(Modified from Djulbegović B: Reasoning and Decision Making in Hematology. Churchill Livingstone, New York, 1992, with permission.)

APPENDIX TABLE 2-4   DOSE MODIFICATIONS FOR VARIOUS ADMINISTRATION SCHEDULES OF 5-FLUO-ROURACIL [5-FU] (ACCORDING TO SOUTH WEST ONCOLOGY GROUP RECOMMENDATIONS)

BOLUS 5-FU

Dosage modification of 5-FU when given alone (not during combined radiation therapy and chemotherapy).

If multiple toxicities are seen, the dose administered should be based on the most severe toxicity experienced. Dosage reductions are based on the dose of chemotherapy given on the preceding treatment and on toxicities observed since the previous dose of chemotherapy.

Modifications based on interval toxicity (if no hematologic toxicity, stomatitis, diarrhea, or other side effects attributed to 5-FU): increase 5-FU dose by 10%. Dose reescalation is allowed.

Toxicity	5-FU Dose Reduction[a]
Hematologic Nadirs (/μl)	
WBC 1,000–2,500	–20%
WBC < 1,000	–30%
PLT 25,000–75,000	–20%
PLT < 25,000	–30%
Diarrhea	
Grade 2	–20%
Grade 3–4	–30%
Stomatitis	
Grade 2	–20%
Grade 3–4	–30%
Dermatitis	
Mild (Grade 1)	None
Moderate (Grade 2)	–20%
Severe (Grade 3–4)	–30%

If Grade 2 or greater diarrhea or stomatitis is present at the scheduled time for the next cycle, chemotherapy should be postponed until the toxicity clears.

If WBC < 3,500/μl and/or platelets < 100,000/μl at the start of a treatment cycle, stop therapy and repeat counts weekly $\times$ 2. If the blood counts are still below these levels after two weeks, adjuvant therapy should be discontinued unless platelet count is > 100,000 and the absolute granulocyte count is $\geq$ 2,000/μl.

[a] Dose reduction is based on dose of 5-FU given on the preceding chemotherapy-alone treatment cycle. Dose of chemotherapy following combined XRT-PVI 5-FU should be 450 mg/m²/day or the dose received during week 5 of treatment (plus any necessary dose modifications based on toxicity), whichever is lowest.

In the event that a central venous catheter is used for this portion of therapy it should be flushed daily with 5 cc NS containing 500 units heparin or per standard Institutional guidelines to prevent catheter occlusion.

PROTRACTED VENOUS INFUSION OF 5-FU (PVI)

Dose modification of 5-FU when given alone (not during combined radiation therapy and chemotherapy).

If any toxicities occur, treatment should be interrupted for 1 week or until resolution of the observed toxicity. Treatment will then be restarted at a 50 mg/m²/day reduction in dose (250 mg/m²/day). The dose will be reduced by an additional 50 mg/m²/day after each subsequent treatment interruption.

The following toxicities will constitute sufficient criteria to interrupt continuous infusion 5-FU alone and to reduce daily dose of 5-FU by 50 mg/m²/day at the time the 5-FU is restarted.[b]

1. Gastrointestinal grade 2 or greater toxicity. (Resume therapy when $\leq$ grade 1 toxicity occurs.)
2. Palmar-plantar erythrodysesthesia. If $\geq$ grade 1 symptoms occur, start pyridoxine 50 mg daily. $\geq$ grade 3 symptoms, despite pyridoxine, constitute sufficient criteria to interrupt treatment until toxicity resolves and to resume therapy at a 50 mg/m²/day dose reduction once toxicity has resolved. (Resume therapy when $\leq$ grade 1 toxicity occurs.)
3. Hematologic: WBC < 2,000/μL or platelet count <75,000/μL or hemoglobin < 8 g/dL. (Resume therapy when WBC $\geq$ 3,500/μL and platelet count $\geq$ 100,000/μL.)
4. Coagulation: prothrombin or partial thrombin time > twice the institutional upper limit of normal — omit heparin.
5. Stomatitis/mucositis/esophagitis — grade 2 or greater toxicity. (Resume therapy when $\leq$ grade 1 toxicity occurs.)

Chemotherapy cycles after combined XRT-PVI 5-FU should not be reinitiated until WBC is ≥ 3,500/μL (or, alternatively, absolute granulocyte count ≥ 2,000/μL), and platelet count ≥ 100,000/μL and patient has ≥ 1,500 calories/day intake and has no other medical contraindication to reinitiation of therapy. Chemotherapy following combined modality therapy should be reinitiated at the same dose the patient was receiving during week 6.

[b]When PVI 5-FU is interrupted, the central venous catheter should be flushed daily with 5 cc NS containing 500 units heparin or per standard institutional guidelines to prevent catheter occlusion.

BOLUS 5-FU + LEUCOVORIN (LV) + LEVAMISOLE

Dose modifications of 5-FU + LV + levamisole when given alone (not during combined radiation therapy and chemotherapy).

Patients should be prophylactically treated with ice chips and all patients who require hospitalization for chemotherapy-induced diarrhea should be considered for somatostatin analogue therapy.

If multiple toxicities are seen, the dose administered should be based on the most severe toxicity experienced. Dosage reductions are based on the dose of chemotherapy given on the preceding treatment and on toxicities observed since the previous dose of chemotherapy.

Only the dose of 5-FU may be altered. The doses of leucovorin and levamisole are not modified for chemotherapy toxicity.

Modifications based on interval toxicity (if no hematologic toxicity, stomatitis, diarrhea, or other side effects attributed to 5-FU, increase 5-FU dose by 10%). Dose re-escalation is allowed.

Toxicity	5-FU Dose Reduction[a]
Hematologic Nadirs (/μl)	
WBC 1,000–2,500	–20%
WBC < 1,000	–30%
Platelets 25,000–75,000	–20%
Platelets < 25,000	–30%
Diarrhea	
Mild (grade 1)	None
Moderate (grade 2)	–20%
Severe (grade 3–4)	–30%
Stomatitis	
Mild (grade 1)	None
Moderate (grade 2)	–20%
Severe (grade 3–4)	–30%
Dermatitis	
Mild (grade 1)	None
Moderate (grade 2)	–20%
Severe (grade 3–4)	–30%
Nausea, Vomiting	
Mild (grade 1)	None
Moderate (grade 2)	None
Severe and uncontrolled by antiemetics (grade 3–4)[b]	–20%

[a] *Dose reduction is based on dose of 5-FU given on the preceding chemotherapy alone-treatment cycle. Following combined XRT 5-FU chemotherapy should be reinitiated at 380 mg/m²/day 5-FU or the dose received during week 5 (days 29–33) of treatment (plus any necessary dose modifications based on toxicity), whichever is lowest.*

[b] *Chemotherapy doses should be decreased only if vomiting is considered clinically severe and is unresponsive to antiemetics.*

Modifications based on toxicity at time cycle is repeated:

If WBC < 3,500/μl or platelets < 100,000/μL at the start of the treatment cycle, stop all protocol treatment and repeat counts twice a week. If the blood counts are still below these levels after two weeks, adjuvant therapy should be discontinued unless platelet count is > 100,000 and the AGC is ≥ 2,000/μl.

If grade 2 or greater diarrhea or stomatitis is present at the scheduled time of the next cycle, chemotherapy should be postponed until toxicity clears (to ≤ grade 1).

DOSE MODIFICATIONS DURING COMBINED XRT-CONTINUOUS INFUSION 5-FU

Patients must have WBC ≥ 3,500/µl (or, alternatively, AGC ≥ 2,000/µl) and platelet count ≥ 100,000/µl and ≥ 1,500 kilocalories food intake/day prior to the initiation of combined XRT-continuous infusion 5-FU. Treatment will be interrupted and doses modified as follows:

Hematologic (/µL)

WBC < 2,000 or PLT < 50,000	Radiation and 5-FU	Hold all therapy until WBC ≥ 2,000 and PLT ≥ 50,000. Resume both at full dose when radiation is resumed.[a]

Stomatitis or Diarrhea

≥ 6 stools/day above postoperative baseline (or ≥ grade 3 diarrhea)	XRT and 5-FU	Temporarily discontinue; resume with 5-FU when diarrhea resolves to grade 1.[a]
≥ grade 2 mucositis, or stomatitis, or esophagitis or ≥ grade 2 weight loss	XRT and 5-FU	Temporarily discontinue. Resume at 50 mg/m² /day dose reduction when symptoms have subsided (to grade 1 toxicity).[a]

If toxicities have not resolved within 3 weeks of stopping treatment, the patient should be removed from protocol treatment.

[a] *In the event that PVI 5-FU is interrupted, the central venous catheter should be flushed daily with 5 cc NS containing 500 units heparin or per standard institutional guidelines to prevent catheter occlusion.*

DOSE MODIFICATIONS DURING COMBINED XRT PLUS BOLUS 5-FU PLUS LV

Patients must have WBC ≥ 3,500/µL (or, alternatively, AGC ≥ 2,000/µl) and platelet count ≥ 100,000/µl and ≥ 1,500 kilocalories food intake/day before initiation of combined XRT plus bolus 5-FU plus LV.

If multiple toxicities are seen, the dose administered should be based on the most severe toxicity experienced. If the radiation therapy is delayed, the chemotherapy should be delayed similarly so that the chemotherapy is always given during the first and fifth week of radiation therapy. Different drug alterations will be made depending on whether the toxicity is the maximal toxicity seen during the interval between the two doses of chemotherapy or the toxicity at the time of delivery of the second dose of chemotherapy (with week-5 radiation therapy).

RADIOTHERAPY INTERRUPTION

For any hematologic, GI, or other toxicity of grade 3 or greater, radiation therapy will be interrupted until toxicity with therapy has decreased to grade 1. Radiation therapy and chemotherapy will then resume as previously planned, with dose modifications as listed below.

Maximum toxicity during interval between courses of 5-FU given during radiation therapy

Toxicity	5-FU Dose Reduction
Hematologic nadirs (/µl)	
WBC 1,000–2,500	–20%
WBC < 1,000	–30%
PLT 25,000–75,000	–20%
PLT < 25,000	–30%
Diarrhea	
Grade 3	–20%
Grade 4	–30%
Stomatitis	
Grade 2	–20%
Grade 3–4	–30%

Toxicity at time of second dose of chemotherapy during radiation therapy

Stomatitis — grade 2–4	5-FU	Do not administer second course
	Leucovorin	
WBC < 3,500/μL[a]	5-FU	Do not administer second course
Platelets < 75,000/μL	Leucovorin	
Diarrhea — grade 2 (with loose, watery bowel movements) or grade 3–4	5-FU	Delay chemotherapy with the radiation therapy delay until diarrhea returns to grade 1. Reinitiate XRT and chemotherapy with appropriate 5-FU dose reduction after resolution of diarrhea.
	Leucovorin	

[a] *May give second dose of chemotherapy if AGC > 2,000/μL.*

Abbreviation: AGC, absolute granulocyte count; GI, gastrointestinal; NS, normal saline; PLT, platelets; PVI, prolonged venous infusion; WBC, whole blood count; XRT, radiation therapy.

APPENDIX TABLE 2-5   GUIDELINES FOR MONITORING THE CARDIAC TOXICITY OF ANTHRACYCLINES

Numerous chemotherapeutic agents have been described to cause cardiac toxicity. The best documented cases relate to anthracyclines and cyclophosphamide. Cyclophosphamide-associated cardiotoxicity is not cumulative. The onset of cardiac toxicity is acute. The treatment is supportive. Anthracyclines, on the other hand, cause cardiac damage in a cumulative manner. The probability of developing impaired myocardial function, based on a combined index of signs, symptoms, and decline in left ventricular ejection fraction (LVEF) is about 1% to 2% at a total cumulative dose of 300 mg/m^2, 3% to 5% at a dose of 400 mg/m^2, 5% to 8% at a dose of 450 mg/m^2, 6% to 20% at a dose of 500 mg/m^2, and nearly 50% for patients who had cumulative dose of doxorubicin of 1000 mg/m^2. Similar dose-related cardiotoxicity has been described for daunorubicin. Clinical evidence of congestive heart failure (CHF) can be seen immediately after the last dose of doxorubicin or can be delayed for up to 230 days (mean delay of 33 days). Radionuclide ventriculography (RNV) (gated blood pool imaging; multiply gated acquisition [MUGA]) has been traditionally considered a standard test for assessment and early detection of anthracyclin-induced cardiac damage. It is associated with a 5% error in assessment of LVEF. It is nearly equivalent to the "gold standard" test of invasive cardiac catheterization in determining functional status but is much less sensitive than endomyocardial biopsy in assessing early myocyte damage. Treatment is the same as for other forms of CHF. Below are guidelines for monitoring the cardiotoxicity of doxorubicin. The quality of medical evidence supporting these guidelines are of level III and IV. Other guidelines have been described in the literature, such as switching to less cardiotoxic agents with similar antitumor activity (e.g., mitoxantrone, whose cardiotoxicity does not appear to rise significantly until a dose of 160 mg/m^2 has been reached, which is equivalent to about 800 mg/m^2 of doxorubicin).

(From manufacturer recommendations and Allen A: The cardiotoxicity of chemotherapeutic drugs. pp. 582–597. In Perry MC (ed): The Chemotherapy Sourcebook. Williams & Willkins, 1992, with permission).

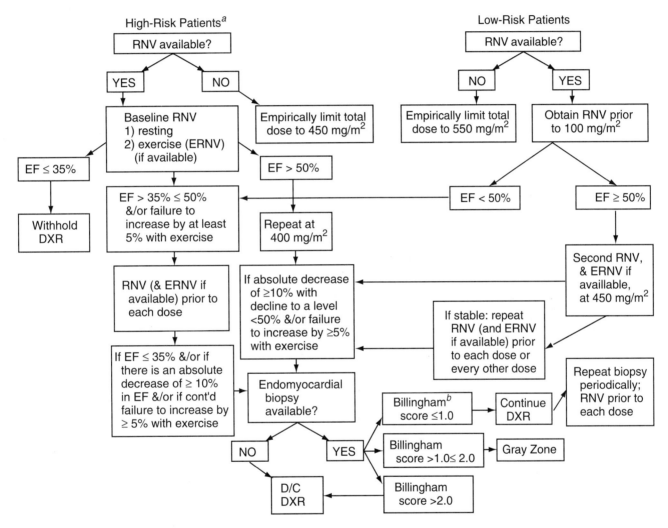

APPENDIX FIGURE 2-1. *Guideline for monitoring the cardiotoxicity of doxorubicin.*
[a]High-risk: prior mediastinal irradiation; hypertension; age > 70 years; coronary, valvular, or myocardial disease. [b]See Appendix Table 2-6. RNV, radionuclide ventriculogram; EF, ejection fraction; DXR, doxorubicin

APPENDIX TABLE 2-6 BILLINGHAM SCALE OF ANTHRACYCLINE DAMAGE

Grade	Characteristics
0	No change from normal
1	Minimal number of cells (<5% of total number of cells per block) with early changes (early myofibrillar loss and/or distended sarcoplasmic reticulum)
1.5	Small groups of cells involved (5%–15% of total number), some of which have definite changes (marked myofibrillar loss and/or cytoplasmic vacuolization)
2	Groups of cells (16%–25% of total number), some of which have definite changes (marked myofibrillar loss and/or myofibrillar loss and/or cytoplasmic vacuolization)
2.5	Groups of cells involved (26%–35%), some of which have definite changes (marked myofibrillar loss and/or cytoplasmic vacuollzation)
3	Diffuse cell damage (>35% of total number of cells) with marked changes (total loss of contractile elements, loss of organelles, mitochondrial and nuclear degeneration)

APPENDIX TABLE 2-7 CARBOPLATIN DOSE CHART BASED UPON THE CALVERT FORMULA

Creatinine Clearance (CrCl) (mL/min)	AUC = 4	AUC = 5 (mg/mL • min)	AUC = 6	AUC = 7
20	180	225	270	315
25	200	250	300	350
30	220	275	330	385
35	240	300	360	420
40	260	325	390	455
45	280	350	420	490
50	300	375	450	525
55	320	400	480	560
60	340	425	510	595
65	360	450	540	630
70	380	475	570	665
75	400	500	600	700
80	420	525	630	735
85	440	550	660	770
90	460	575	690	805
95	480	600	720	840
100	500	625	750	875
105	520	650	780	910
110	540	675	810	945
115	560	700	840	980
120	580	725	870	1015
125	600	750	900	1050
130	620	775	930	1085
135	640	800	960	1120
140	660	825	990	1155
145	680	850	1020	1190
150	700	875	1050	1225
155	720	900	1080	1260
160	740	925	1110	1295
165	760	950	1140	1330
170	780	975	1170	1365
175	800	1000	1200	1400

(From Calvert AH, Newell DR, Gumbrell LA, et al. Carboplatin dosage: prospective evaluation of a simple formula based on renal function. J Clin Oncol. 1989;7:1748–1756, with permission.)

Total Carboplatin Dose (mg) = Target AUC × (GFR + 25). Stable renal function is important for accurate determination of GFR or CrCl for AUC dosing.

Note: With the Calvert formula, the total dose of Carboplatin is calculated in mg, not mg/m².

Individualized Dosing of Carboplatin

Two dosing strategies can be employed with Carboplatin, empiric dosing or dosing based upon area under the curve (AUC). The empiric dosing approach calculates dosage according to a recommended dose received from clinical experience and determined by a patient's body surface area (BSA).[a] Subsequent dosage modification is based upon observed toxicity and therapeutic effect.

Another approach for determining the initial dose of Carboplatin is the use of mathematical formulae, which are based on a patient's preexisting renal function[1-3] or renal function and desired platelet nadir.[4] Renal excretion is the major route of elimination for Carboplatin. The use of dosing formulae, as compared with empirical dose calculation based on BSA, allows compensation for patient variations in pretreatment renal function that might otherwise result in either underdosing (in patients with above average renal function) or overdosing (in patients with impaired renal function).

A simple formula for calculating dosage, based upon a patient's glomerular filtration rate (GFR) in mL/min and Paraplatin target AUC in mg/ml • min, has been proposed by Calvert et al.[1-3] In these studies, GFR was measured by ^{51}Cr-EDTA.[5]

Calvert Formula for Carboplatin Dosing

$$\text{Total Dose (mg)} = \text{Target AUC} \times (\text{GFR} + 25)^1$$

The target AUC of 4 to 6 mg/ml • min using single-agent Paraplatin appears to provide the most appropriate dose range in previously treated patients.[2] This study also showed a trend between the AUC of single-agent Carboplatin administered to previously treated patients and the likelihood of developing toxicity.[2]

CARBOPLATIN DOSE CALCULATION CHART

The dose chart on the preceding page (Appendix Table 2-7) provides Carboplatin doses, as calculated by the formula of Calvert et al.[1] This formula provides individual dosages for patients based upon GFR or creatinine clearance (CrCl) and AUC. GFR approximates CrCl, and CrCl values can be measured by various methods or estimated by published mathematical formulae, based upon the patient's serum creatinine, age, sex, height, and body weight.

To use this chart

1. Choose the target AUC.
2. Determine the patient's CrCl value.
3. Cross-reference the CrCl value with the target AUC to arrive at the Carboplatin dose in milligrams, *not milligrams per square meter*.

REFERENCES

1. Calvert AH, Newell DR, Gumbrell LA et al: Carboplatin dosage: prospective evaluation of a simple for-

---

[a]The dosing regimen for patients with recurrent ovarian carcinoma currently listed in the Paraplatin package insert is 360 mg/m² intravenously (IV), given every 4 weeks. In general, however, single intermittent courses of Paraplatin should not be repeated until the neutrophil count is at least 2,000 and the platelet count is at least 100,000.

mula based on renal function. J Clin Oncol 7:1748–1756, 1989

2. Jodrell DI, Egorin MJ, Canetta RM et al: Relationships between carboplatin exposure and tumor response and toxicity in patients with ovarian cancer. J Clin Oncol 10:520–528, 1992

3. Sørensen BT, Strömgren A, Jakobsen P et al: Dose-toxicity relationship of carboplatin in combination with cyclophosphamide in ovarian cancer patients. Cancer Chemother Pharmacol 28:397–401, 1991

4. Egorin MJ, Van Echo DA, Olmon EA et al: Prospective validation of a pharmacologically based dosing scheme for the *cis*-diamminedichloroplatinum (II) analogue diamminecyclobutanedicarboxylatoplatinum. Cancer Res 45:6502–6506, 1985

5. Daugaard G, Rossing N, Rørth M: Effects of cisplatin on different measures of glomerular function in the human kidney with special emphasis on high-dose. Cancer Chemother Pharmacol 21:163–167, 1988

Protocols for Treatment of Acute Lymphoblastic Leukemia

Alfonso Cervera

Tumor lysis syndrome is more frequent in patients with acute lymphoblastic leukemia (ALL) than in patients with acute myelogenous leukemia. It is especially frequent in patients with B-cell ALL. An adequate amount of fluid should be provided to ensure a urine output of at least 100 mL/hr. The addition of sodium bicarbonate 50 mEq/L of solution will favor an alkaline urine, which improves solubility of uric acid. Allopurinol 300 to 600 mg/day should also be given; however, it must be remembered that it can induce severe allergic reactions. The dose of allopurinol should be reduced if concomitant use of 6 mercaptopurine is planned.

Broad spectrum antibiotics should be started immediately in the febrile neutropenic patient, after obtaining adequate cultures. Blood cultures should be obtained every 24 hours if fever persists. Ceftazidime alone or ceftazidime with vancomycin in the patient with a long-term vascular device are adequate most of the time. Fungal prophylaxis with fluconazole and an oral quinolone antibiotic should be started in the neutropenic patient. If after three days of adequate antibiotic coverage the patient continues to be febrile, amphotericin B should be started, particularly in those patients who have been neutropenic for a prolonged period (see Ch. 56).

Hemorrhage caused by thrombocytopenia is also a concern in ALL. Platelets either from random donors or from single donors should be provided if the platelet count drops below $15 \times 10^9/L$ or if it drops below $20 \times 10^9/L$ in the patient who is febrile or who has severe mucositis. If there is clinical bleeding, enough platelets should be transfused to keep them above $50 \times 10^9/L$.

For doses of antiemetics, see Chapter 53 to 60.

THE GERMAN MULTICENTER TRIALS FOR THE TREATMENT OF ACUTE LYMPHOBLASTIC LEUKEMIA OF ADULTS (GMALL): PROTOCOL FOR MATURE B-CELL ALL (SEE CH. 3).

The chemotherapy consists of 6 alternate 5-day cycles, A and B, that are given every 21 days. For central nervous system prophylaxis, 24 Gy radiation is given between cycles 2 and 3.

BLOCK A

Vincristine 2 mg IV day 1
Methotrexate 1,500 mg/m² with leucovorin (LV) rescue IV day 1*
Ifosfamide 800 mg/m² IV days 1 through 5
VM-26 100 mg/m² IV days 4 and 5
Ara C 150 mg/m² IV bid days 4 and 5
Dexamethasone 10 mg/m² po days 1 through 5
Triple intrathecal chemotherapy days 1 and 5**

BLOCK B

Triple intrathecal chemotherapy day 1**
Vincristine 2 mg IV day 1
Methotrexate 1,500 mg/m² with LV rescue IV day 1*
Cyclophosphamide 200 mg/m² IV days 1 through 5
Adriamycin 25 mg/m² IV days 4 and 5
Dexamethasone 10 mg/m² po days 1 through 5

If at diagnosis the white blood cell count is above 25,000 or if there is a large tumor mass, cyclophosphamide 200 mg/m² IV every 24 hours for 5 days and prednisone 20 mg/m² po tid for 5 days should be given before starting the protocol.

---

*Methotrexate administration: one tenth of the total dose is given over half an hour and the rest is given as a 23.5-hour infusion. The LV rescue starts 36 hours after the beginning of the methotrexate infusion with 30 mg/m² IV, followed by oral doses of 30 mg/m², 15 mg/m², and 3 doses of 5 mg/m² given at 42, 48, 54, 68, and 78 hours. In patients with a slower clearance of methotrexate and levels of more than 0.5 to 5 μmol/L at 42 hours, LV 50 mg/m² IV every 6 hours up to 60 hours should be given. If at 68 hours the serum methotrexate level is more than 0.01 μmol/L, LV 30 mg/m² IV every 6 hours should be continued for 4 to 6 more doses.
**Triple intrathecal chemotherapy: methotrexate 15 mg, cytarabine 40 mg, and dexamethasone 4 mg.

THE GERMAN MULTICENTER TRIALS FOR TREATMENT OF ACUTE LYMPHOBLASTIC LEUKEMIA IN ADULTS (GMALL): PROTOCOL FOR STANDARD RISK ALL EXCLUDING MATURE B-CELL ALL (SEE CH. 3)

Induction (weeks 1–8)

PHASE I

Prednisone 60 mg/m² po days 1–29
Asparaginase 5,000 U/m² IV days 15–29
Vincristine 2 mg IV days 1, 8, 15, 22
Daunorubicin 45 mg/m² IV days 1, 8, 15, 22

PHASE II

Cyclophosphamide 650 mg/m² IV days 29, 43, 57
Cytarabine 75 mg/m² IV days 31–34, 38–41, 45–48, 52–55
6-Mercaptopurine 60 mg/m² po days 29–57

CNS PROPHYLAXIS (ONCE REMISSION HAS BEEN ACHIEVED)[a]

Cranial irradiation (24 Gy over 4 weeks)
Methotrexate 15 mg, intrathecal once a week during phase II of induction therapy

CONSOLIDATION THERAPY[b]

Cytosine Arabinoside 75 mg/m² IV days 1–5
VM-26 60 mg/m² IV days 1–5

MAINTENANCE THERAPY

6-mercaptopurine 60 mg/m² po daily
Methotrexate 20 mg/m² IV once a week

---

[a]In the case of involvement of the CNS at diagnosis, the dose of radiation is increased to 30 Gy and the field extended to include the spinal column; weekly intrathecal methotrexate is started at diagnosis, until the cerebrospinal fluid is cleared of blasts.
[b]There is currently an ongoing study for high-risk patients (see below) in which consolidation is given as follows: Arm A (week 13): cytarabine 3 g/m² IV twice a day (as a 3-hour infusion) on days 1–4, mitoxantrone 10 mg/m² IV days 2–5. (The dose of cytarabine is reduced to 1 g/m² in patients older than 50 years.)
Compared to
Arm B (days 13, 15, and 17): Methotrexate 1,500 mg/m² IV day 1 (see previous section for high-dose methotrexate rescue). Asparaginase 10,000 U/m² IV day 2. The preliminary results suggest that those patients who receive cytarabine and mitoxantrone fare better than those who get any other consolidation.
High-dose Cytarabine and Mitoxantrone for the Treatment of Relapsed or Refractory ALL.
Cytarabine 3 g/m² every 12 hours IV on days 1–4
Mitoxantrone 10 mg/m² IV on days 2–5
Dexamethasone eye drops should be given during the 4 days of high-dose cytarabine treatment and discontinued 24 hours after the last dose (see Ch. 4 and Appendix 4 for details on administration of high-dose cytarabine).

Protocols for Management of Acute Myelogenous Leukemia (AML)

Alfonso Cervera

SUPPORTIVE CARE

Vigorous hydration (125–150 ml/m²/h) with solutions containing 50 mEq of sodium bicarbonate per 1000 ml should be done before chemotherapy. Alkalinization should be avoided in the presence of severe hyperphosphatemia (especially if the product of the serum calcium and phosphate exceeds 60), as the crystals of calcium phosphate become less soluble at a urine pH above 6. Allopurinol should be given (200–400 mg/day) if there is hyperuricemia or if the white blood cell (WBC) count is above 10,000/mm³; it should be discontinued if a rash appears.

Anemia should be corrected and the hemoglobin level should be kept above 10 g/dL. This provides some reserve in case of a major hemorrhage. However, transfusions should be done very carefully in the presence of hyperleukocytosis, especially if the WBC count is above 50,000/mm³, given the risk of inducing complications of blood hyperviscosity.

Platelets should be transfused to keep the platelet count above 15,000 in the patient who has no mucositis. When mucositis appears as a result of chemotherapy, it is probably safer to maintain the count above 20,000. If bleeding or disseminated intravascular coagulation (DIC) is present, platelets should be given when the count is below 50,000.

All blood products should be leukopoor to decrease the number of febrile episodes after transfusions and exposure to alloantigens. Transfusion-associated graft-versus-host disease is very rare in AML; however, it is safer to use irradiated products. Determine cytomegalovirus (CMV) serology in young patients who can be candidates for bone marrow transplant; those who have not been infected with it should be transfused only with CMV-negative products (some evidence suggests that when CMV negative products are not available, leukocyte-depleted units are safe).

Leukapheresis is begun when the WBC count is above 100,000/mm³ or below that if there are symptoms of leukostasis. Reducing the WBC count may also prevent the development of tumor lysis syndrome.

Prophylaxis with a quinolone antibiotic and fluconazole 400 mg/day is important if the patient is afebrile. In the presence of fever and neutropenia, wide spectrum antibiotic coverage should be instituted. Ceftazidime with vancomycin is a good choice; vancomycin is especially important if the fever was noticed after long-term vascular devices have been implanted. However, it must be mentioned that the current trend is to avoid it, when unnecessary, given the emergence of resistant strains of enterococcus and *Staphylococcus*. Blood cultures should be done before starting antibiotic therapy and every day while fever persists. If the temperature continues to be elevated after 3 days of antibiotic administration and the cultures are unrevealing, amphotericin B 0.6 to 1 mg/kg/day should be added; premedication with diphenhydramine, acetaminophen, and low-dose hydrocortisone may help if fever and chills occur during its administration. Adequate hydration is extremely important to reduce the nephrotoxicity of this drug. Consideration should also be given to using liposomal preparations of amphotericin B. (See also Chs. 53 through 60.)

AML: Standard Induction Therapy

Alfonso Cervera

1. Hydration to begin at ___ (at least 24 hours before chemotherapy). D51/2NS + KCl 10 mEq/L + NaHCO$_3$ 50 mEq/L to run at (150 mL/m²/h).

2. Cytarabine (200 mg/m²) ___ mg in NS 500 mL to run at 21 mL/h qd for 7 days (100 mg/m² can be used in elderly or debilitated patients).

3. Idarubicin (12 mg/m²) ___ mg IV slow push qd for 3 days (starting on day 1 of cytarabine). The dose should be reduced by 50% if serum bilirubin is between 2.5 and 5 mg/dL. Do not administer if serum bilirubin is above 5 mg/dL, as little experience in the presence of severe hepatic dysfunction exists. (See Appendix 2).

4. Granisetron 1 mg + dexamethasone 10 mg in D5W 50 mL over 1/2 hour before the first dose of cytarabine and then every morning through the last day of cytarabine infusion.

5. Lorazepam 1 to 2 mg IV before each dose of idarubicin.

6. Droperidol 1.25 to 2.5 mg IV every 6 hours if nausea is not controlled by lorazepam.

7. Obtain complete blood count and serum chemistry and electrolytes before chemotherapy starts and then every morning.

8. Norethindrone 10 mg po per day while the platelet count is below 50,000/mm³ (to prevent menstrual bleeding) in premenopausal females.

9. Ciprofloxacin 500 mg po q12h or 400 mg IV q12h if the absolute neutrophil count is below 1,000/mm³. Continue until recovery of neutrophil count. Discontinue if antibiotics are initiated for fever.

10. Fluconazole 400 mg po or IV qam if the absolute neutrophil count is below 1,000/mm³. Continue until neutrophil count recovery. Discontinue if amphotericin B is started.

11. Allopurinol 300 mg po qam if the serum uric acid is elevated or if the pretreatment WBC count is above 10,000/mm³.

12. Transfuse one single-donor, leukopoor, irradiated, apheresis-platelet product or eight pooled random-donor, leukopoor, irradiated-platelet units if the platelet count is below 15,000 or below 20,000 if there is severe mucositis or fever.

13. Transfuse 2 units of leukopoor, packed red blood cells if the hemoglobin level falls below 10 g/dl.

Abbreviations: IV, intravenous; NS, normal saline; D5W, 5% dextrose in water; qam, every morning.

APPENDIX 4-3

AML: Consolidation Therapy

Alfonso Cervera

Note 1: High-dose cytarabine (HDAC) can be used for induction therapy when a large tumor burden exists. The precautions and treatment of tumor lysis syndrome, such as hydration and administration of allopurinol, should be observed.

1. Cytarabine (3g/m^2) ___ g in NS 250 mL IV over 2 hours every 12 hours for 12 doses starting at ___ on ___ (patients older than 50 years should receive 1.5 g/m^2 to reduce the incidence of severe central nervous system toxicity).

2. Idarubicin (12 mg/m^2) ___ mg slow IV push every 24 hours for 3 doses after the 3rd, 5th and 7th doses of cytarabine.

3. Check electrolytes and complete blood count every 24 hours.

4. Ciprofloxacin 500 po q12h or 400 mg IV q12h if the neutrophil count is below 1,000/mm^3. Continue until recovery of neutrophil count. Discontinue if antibiotics are initiated for fever.

5. Fluconazole 400 mg po or IV qam if the absolute neutrophil count is below 1,000/mm^3. Continue until neutrophil recovery. Discontinue if amphotericin B is initiated.

6. Dexamethasone eye drops 0.1%. Instill 2 drops in each eye every 6 hours. Discontinue 6 hours after last dose of cytarabine (to reduce ocular toxicity of HDAC).

4. Granisetron 1 mg + dexamethasone 10 mg in D5W 50 cc over 1/2 hour before the first dose of cytarabine and then qam through the last dose of cytarabine.

5. Lorazepam 1 to 2 mg IV before each dose of cytarabine and idarubicin.

6. Droperidol 1.25 to 2.5 mg IV every 6 hours for nausea not controlled by lorazepam.

7. Norethindrone 10 mg po every day while the platelet count is below 50,000/mm^3 (to prevent menstrual bleeding) in premenopausal females.

Note 2: The same principles for adjusting the dose of idarubicin would apply for this regimen, but high-dose cytarabine should be used very carefully, if at all, in the presence of significant hepatic dysfunction (see Appendix 2).

Abbreviations: IV, intravenous; NS, normal saline; D5W, 5% dextrose in water; qam, every morning.

APPENDIX 4-4

AML: Treatment of Relapsed or Refractory Disease

Alfonso Cervera

1. VP-16 (4.2 g/m²) ___ mg total dose. Mix 400 mg/L NS for ___ bags (of 1,000 cc), plus one additional bag of ___ mg in ___ ml NS. Infuse IV at 175 mL/m²/h ___ ml/h. (VP-16 at a concentration of 0.4 mg/mL will be stable for 48 hours.)

2. After VP-16 finishes, start hydration with D51/2 NS + KCl 10 mEq/L and NaHCO₃ 50 mEq/L (at 150 mL/m²/hr) ___. Continue this rate until 24 hours after last dose of cyclophosphamide has been infused.

3. Cyclophosphamide (50 mg/kg) ___ gm in NS 500 mL IV over 2 hours every 24 hours for 4 doses starting at least 6 hours after the end of the VP-16 infusion. (Hydration fluids should be reduced to 100 mL/m²/h during cyclophophamide infusion.)

5. Mesna (10 mg/kg) ___ mg IV every 4 hours, starting 30 minutes before first dose of cyclophosphamide and ending 24 hours after last dose of cyclophosphamide.

6. Granisetron 1 mg + dexamethasone 10 mg in D5W 50 mL IV over 1/2 hour before each dose of cyclophosphamide.

7. Lorazepam 1 to 2 mg IV every 4 to 6 hours for breakthrough nausea and vomiting.

8. Obtain complete blood count, serum electrolytes, and serum chemistry every 24 hours.

9. Weigh patient twice every day and report if there is weight gain or loss greater than 2 kg.

10. Determine fluid balance every 4 hours. If urine output is less than 400 mL/4 hrs or if fluid input is greater than fluid output by more than 500 mL, give furosemide 20 mg IV. Report if urine output is less than 100 cc after furosemide.

11. Ciprofloxacin 500 mg po or 400 mg IV q12h if absolute neutrophil count is below 1,000/mm³. Continue until recovery of neutrophil count. Discontinue if antibiotics are initiated for fever.

12. Fluconazole 400 mg po or IV if absolute neutrophil count is below 1,000/mm³. Continue until recovery of neutrophil count. Discontinue if amphotericin B is initiated.

13. Norethindrone 10 mg po every day while the platelet count is below 50,000/mm³ (to prevent menstrual bleeding) in premenopausal females.

14. Filgrastim (G-CSF) (5 µg/kg) — µg sc every 24 hours. Start 24 hours after the last dose of cyclophosphamide and continue until the absolute neutrophil count has been above 1,500/mm³ for three consecutive days.

15. Continous bladder irrigation with NS at 250 mL/h is used at some centers during cyclophosphamide infusion.

Abbreviation: NS, normal saline; IV, intravenous; D5W, 5% dextrose in water, SC, subcutaneous.

APPENDIX
4-5

Treatment of M3 Subtype of AML

Alfonso Cervera

1. Retinoic acid (45 mg/m²/day in two divided doses (round off to the nearest 10 mg) ___ mg po with meals twice a day until remission. Discontinue if remission has not been achieved by day 90 of treatment.

2. Obtain complete blood count, prothrombin time, partial thromboplastin time, fibrinogen, D dimer, serum electrolytes, and serum chemistry qam.

3. Ciprofloxacin 500 mg po q12h or 400 mg IV q12h if the absolute neutrophil count is under 1000/mm³. Discontinue if antibiotics are started for fever.

4. Fluconazole 400 mg po or IV qam if the absolute neutrophil count drops below 1000/mm³. Discontinue if amphotericin B is initiated.

5. Transfuse one single-donor, leukopoor, irradiated, apheresis-platelet product or 8 units of pooled, leukopoor, random-donor platelets if the platelet count is below 15,000 and there is no evidence of DIC. In the presence of laboratory evidence of DIC, but without bleeding, it is preferable to keep the platelet count above 30,000. In the presence of laboratory evidence of DIC and clinical bleeding, the platelet count must be kept above 50,000/mm³.

6. Transfuse 2 units of leukopoor, irradiated, packed red blood cells if the hemoglobin is below 10 g/dL.

Note 1: Pregnancy should be ruled out before initiation of the drug in women of reproductive age. Two reliable forms of contraception should be used during treatment unless abstinence is the chosen method. A pregnancy test should be obtained monthly during treatment.

Note 2: Treatment in the patient who presents with a WBC count of more than 10,000/mm³ is still controversial, since these patients are at particular risk of retinoic acid syndrome. Most authorities would agree that retinoic acid be given in conjunction with standard chemotherapy, and that steroids be added from the beginning. However, treatment strategies in this setting have not been defined rigorously. For the patient whose WBC is below 10,000 at the time of diagnosis, we advocate the use of dexamethasone 10 mg twice a day for three days; this can be repeated later if necessary. A recently published trial reports very good results with prednisolone 75 mg every day as long as the WBC is above 10,000/mm³; however, this means longer exposure to steroids.

Note 3: The use of heparin remains controversial. It can be used in low to moderate doses.

Note 4: Fresh frozen plasma and even cryoprecipitate may be indicated in the patient with DIC and persistently low fibrinogen. The use of heparin is still controversial; however, given in intermediate dose (15,000 U/day IV) it may be beneficial if the D dimer is persistently elevated. Antifibrinolytic agents should not be given concomitantly with ATRA.

Abbreviations: ATRA, all-trans retinous acid; DIC, disseminated intravascular coagulation; IV, intravenous; WBC, white blood cell; qam, every morning.

APPENDIX 5

Treatment of Chronic Myelogenous Leukemia
(see also Fig. 5-2 and Table 5-1)

Allopurinol: 300 mg qd until WBC (white blood cell) count is less than 15,000/mm³ or uric acid is within normal range.

Hydroxyurea (HU): 5 to 2.0 g/day. Adjust according to WBC count as follows:

WBC Count	HU Dose
> 100K (100,000/mm³)	4 g/d
> 75K	3 g/d
> 50K	2 g/d
> 30K	1.5 g/d
> 15K	1.0 g/d
> 7.5K	0.5 g/d
≤ 7.5K	0

Obtain CBC weekly until WBC is less than 20K, then monthly. Try to keep WBC count between 5 and 15K. An average maintenance dose is 1 to 1.5 g/d. Obtain liver function tests (SMA-18) every month to monitor side effects of HU (other reported side effects are painful tongue, hyperkeratosis, reversible skin rash).

a-interferon (IFN): (5 million units/m² daily = ___). Before IFN is begun, reduce WBC to 10 to 20K with HU to minimize leukocytosis-associated side effects (chills, fever, musculoskeletal pain, etc.). Administer at bedtime with acetaminophen 650 mg to minimize flulike symptoms. Begin at 50% of the dose for the first week. Tachyphylaxis develops within 1 to 2 weeks. If depression, fatigue, or insomnia persist, administer small dose of antidepressant (e.g., amitriptyline 25 mg qhs).

IFN dose reductions: 1) hold therapy for any grade 3 or 4 toxicity (see Appendix 1) until recovery and then start at 50% of dose; 2) reduce dose by 25% if grade 2 toxicity does not improve with symptomatic support; 3) reduce dose by 25% if WBC count decreases below 2K or platelets below 60K.

Note that immune-mediated hypothyroidism does not require discontinuation of IFN and is managed by replacement therapy.

If the patient is a young woman, start contraception (IFN is teratogenic in animals although some case reports have been published about normal delivery while patient was on IFN; similarly HU has been used in the later stages of pregnancy without apparent untoward effects).

In patients with thrombocytosis refractory to IFN and HU, use anagrelide (1 mg q 6 h for 5–7 days) or thiotepa (75 mg/m² IV q 2–3 weeks until response occurs).

APPENDIX 6

Treatment of Chronic Lymphocytic Leukemia
(see also Fig. 6-1 and Table 6-5)

Allopurinol: 300 mg qd for 7 days with each monthly cycle (to prevent tumor lysis syndrome).

TREATMENT I

Chlorambucil*: 0.7 mg/kg orally over 4 days, every 3 to 4 weeks. Escalate dose by 0.1 mg/kg with each cycle as tolerated. Monitor CBC (complete blood count) every 1 to 2 weeks for the first 8 weeks (or after each dose escalation), then every month. Reduce dose by 50% when absolute neutrophil count (ANC) falls below 1,500/mm³ or platelet count drops below 100,000/mm³. Discontinue treatment when ANC < 1,000 or platelet < 60,000/mm³.
Prednisone: 0.5 mg/kg po in one dose or divided in two doses for 7 days of each cycle. (Note that chlorambucil + prednisone is probably not superior to chlorambucil alone).

Response to therapy is usually seen within 3 to 8 months of therapy. Continue therapy as long as the response is being noted (usually not longer than 1 year).

TREATMENT II

Fludarabine, 25 mg/m² IV over 30 minutes daily for 5 consecutive days every 28 days; provide allopurinol as above. Assess response after 3 cycles. If there is no response or if disease has progressed, stop therapy and go to the next line of treatment (Fig. 6-1). If complete response is noted, continue therapy for additional 3 months. If partial response is noted, continue therapy until a plateau in response is reached, but generally not beyond 1 year of therapy.

To prevent opportunistic infection, administer sulfamethoxazole/trimethoprim 1 DS three times a week. CD4 count usually normalizes about 1 year after cessation of therapy.

Monitor CBC as described above and obtain baseline renal function tests. If creatinine is increased, obtain creatinine clearance. If creatinine clearance is above 70 ml/min a full dose may be given. If creatinine clearance is 50 ml/min, reduce dose to 50%.

If patient requires transfusion while undergoing fludarabine treatment, the manufacturer recommends using irradiated blood products to avoid transfusion-associated graft-versus-host disease, which has been observed after transfusion of nonirradiated blood in fludarabine-treated patients.

Cladribine: 0.1 mg/kg/day as continuous infusion for 7 days or 0.14 mg/kg daily in 2- hour infusion for 5 consecutive days. Monitor CBC carefully (thrombocytopenia is cumulative and patient may require permanent platelet transfusion). Administer up to 8 cycles to responding patients or until side effects occur. Provide allopurinol and Bactrim as described above (see Appendix 7).

ORDERS FOR TREATMENT OF CHRONIC LYMPHOCYTIC LEUKEMIA

TREATMENT WITH CHLORAMBUCIL + PREDNISONE

1. Allopurinol 100 mg tid for 7 days.
2. Administer chlorambucil only if ANC is above 1,500/mm³ and platelets above 100,000/mm³. If ANC < 1,500/mm³ and platelets < 100,000/mm³, call a physician.

---

*In the United States this is sold as 2-mg tablets (Leukeran).

3. Chlorambucil (Leukeran) (0.7 mg/kg) (= total dose ___ mg). (Give this dose over 4 days as Leukeran 2-mg tablets.) Leukeran 2-mg tablets # ___. Take ___ tablets po tid for 4 days.

4. Prednisone (0.5 mg/kg) (= total dose ___ mg) (Give this dose in one or divided doses each day for 7 days as tablets of 2.5, 5, 10, 20, or 50 mg) Prednisone 5 mg tablets # ___. Take ___ tablets po bid for 7 days.

5. CBC every 1 to 2 weeks, and then before the next cycle of chemotherapy.

TREATMENT WITH FLUDARABINE

1. Allopurinol 100 mg tid for 7 days.

2. Administer fludarabine only if ANC is above 1,500/mm^3, platelets above 100,000/mm^3, and creatinine normal. If creatinine is increased, obtain creatinine clearance and call a physician. If ANC < 1,500/mm^3 and platelets < 100,000/mm^3, call a physician.

3. Fludarabine 25 mg/m^2 (= ___ mg) in 100 mL of normal saline, IV over 30 minutes daily for 5 consecutive days.

4. Trimethoprim/sulfamethoxazole 1 DS tablet three times a week for 1 year.

5. CBC every 1 to 2 weeks, and then before next cycle of chemotherapy with SMA-18.

6. If ANC > 1,500/mm^3, and creatinine clearance > 70 mL/min, treat every 4 weeks × 3, then reevaluate (see above, Treatment II).

APPENDIX 7

Treatment of Hairy Cell Leukemia

INDUCTION TREATMENT

1. *Cladribine:* 0.1 mg/kg/day (= ___ mg) in 500 ml normal saline (not Dextrose) to infuse over 24 hours. Infuse daily for a total of 7 days.

Allopurinol*: 100 mg tid on the first day of treatment and continue for 2 weeks (to prevent tumor lysis syndrome). To prevent opportunistic infection, administer sulfamethoxazole/trimethoprim* 1 DS tablet three times a week. CD4 count may take up to 40 to 45 months to normalize after cessation of therapy (Blood 1994; 83:2906).

2. Obtain complete blood count (CBC) and SMA-18 weekly. Usual time to remission is about 8 to 12 weeks. Repeat bone marrow biopsy and flow cytometry studies at 3 months.** If neutropenic patient develops fever > 38°C,*** hospitalize the patient, start empirical treatment with broad-spectrum antibiotics (see Ch. 56); transfuse red blood cell products or platelets as needed (see Ch. 58).

---

*Evidences for this practice are indirect based on deduction from treatment of chronic lymphocytic leukemia (CLL) and increased risk for infections in patients treated with purine analogues (see Ch. 6).
**Complete remission is defined as complete normalization of CBC and bone marrow with absence of all constitutional symptoms and lymphadenopathy/splenomegaly (patients with mild residual splenomegaly, > 12 but < 14 cm in craniocaudal dimension, or minimal soft tissue abnormality, ≤ 2 cm, are also considered to be in complete remission).
***Fever occurs in about 45% of patients treated with cladribine. Most patients have culture-negative fever believed to be secondary to cytokine release during destruction of hairy cells with the drug. Nevertheless, most authors believe that the benefit/risk ratio of empirical treatment of neutropenic fever with antibiotics is greater than to wait to treat until the infection is documented as a source of fever.

TREATMENT OF RELAPSE

As discussed in Chapter 7, this is not well defined. Pentostatin and alfa-interferon are known active agents in hairy cell leukemia. If interferon is selected, lower dose (0.2 MU/m² qd for 28 days, followed by tiw for 6 months) is as effective as higher dose (Blood 1991;78:3133) (for method of interferon administration, see Appendix 5).

APPENDIX 8

Treatment of Hodgkin's Disease[1]

MOPP[2] (REPEAT CYCLE EVERY 28 DAYS)

Mechlorethamine (nitrogen mustard): (6 mg/m²) = ___ mg IV on day 1 and day 8 as slow push through freely flowing IV (FFIV)
Vincristine: (1.4 mg/m²) = ___ mg IV push through FFIV day 1 and day 8
Prednisone: (40 mg/m²) ___ po days 1–14
Procarbazine[3]: (100 mg/m²) ___ po days 1–14

ABVD[1] (REPEAT CYCLE EVERY 28 DAYS)

Doxorubicin: (25 mg/m²)[4] = ___ mg IV push through FFIV on days 1 and 15
Bleomycin: (10 units/m²) = ___ units IV push through FFIV on days 1 and 15
Vinblastine: (6 mg/m²) = ___ mg IV push through FFIV on days 1 and 15
Dacarbazine: (DTIC) (375 mg/m²) = ___ mg IV in 250–500 cc of normal saline (NS); IVPB (IV piggyback) through FFIV of NS to help dilute and decrease irritation of administration

MOPP/ABV

Mechlorethamine: (nitrogen mustard) (6 mg/m²) = ___ mg IV on day 1
Vincristine: (1.4 mg/m²; not to exceed 2 mg) = ___ mg IV push through FF IV day 1
Procarbazine[3]: (100 mg/m²) ___ po days 1–7
Prednisone: (40 mg/m²) ___ po days 1–14
Doxorubicin: (35 mg/m²)[4] = ___ mg IV push through FFIV on day 8
Bleomycin: (10 units/m²) = ___ units IV push through FFIV on day 8
Vinblastine: (6 mg/m²) = ___ mg IV push through FFIV on day 8

PRIOR TO CHEMOTHERAPY

1. Check complete blood count with differential (if complete blood count not normal, adjust the dose or use growth factors [see Appendix 2.])

2. Check renal and liver function tests (if not normal adjust the dose according to Appendix 2).

3. Perform neurologic examination (if not normal adjust the dose according to Appendix 2).

4. Radionuclide ventriculogram in patients at high risk for cardiac disease (see Appendix 2.)

ANTIEMETICS

Prior to chemotherapy:
Granisetron: 2 mg po
Dexamethasone: 20 mg po
Lorazepam: 1 mg IV (if indicated for apprehension); prescribe prochlorperazine spansules 15 mg bid for 3 days (for prevention of delayed nausea and vomiting).
ranitidine 150 mg bid while taking prednisone (other H₂ blocker alternative equally acceptable)[5] (see Ch. 54 for alternative regimens).

NURSING

Extravasion precautions with vesicant drugs (e.g., nitrogen mustard and vincristine)

[1] Administer as many cycles as required to achieve full documented remission (this may include repetition of biopsies of tissues initially involved) followed by 2 additional cycles as treatment consolidation (usually 6 + 2 cycles); if a patient progresses or does not respond at all after 2 to 3 cycles, consider it a refractory disease; see Appendix 2 for sliding scale for drug dose adjustment based on hematologic toxicities.

[2] *MVPP:* vinblastine (6 mg/m²) is substituted for vincristine.

LOPP: chlorambucil (6 mg/m²) is substituted for mechlorethamine and vinblastine (6 mg/m²) for vincristine.

[3] Avoid tyramine-containing foods such as cheese, red wine, beer, etc. while taking procarbazine (to avoid MAO-inhibitor-like effect).

[4] Limit total dose to 450–550 mg/m² to reduce risk of cardiotoxicity (see Appendix 2).

[5] Note that data on prevention of steroid-induced ulcer by H_2 blockers are not convincing. In our practice we usually prescribe H_2 blockers to those patients with history of peptic ulcer disease or to those who complain of dyspeptic symptoms while taking steroids.

APPENDIX 9

Treatment of Non-Hodgkin's Lymphoma[1]

PROTOCOL FOR AGGRESSIVE NHL (SEE ALSO CH. 9)

CHOP (REPEAT CYCLE Q 21 OR 28 DAYS)

Cyclophosphamide: (750 mg/m²) = ___ mg through FF (free flowing) IV or in 100 cc normal saline IV over 30 minutes.
Doxorubicin: (50 mg/m²) = ___ mg IV through FFIV over 10–15 minutes.
Vincristine: (1.4 mg/m²) = ___ mg IV push through FFIV (maximum dose 2 mg)
Prednisone: (100 mg/day in divided doses) po on days 1–5

PRIOR TO CHEMOTHERAPY

1. Check complete blood count (CBC) with differential (if CBC not normal adjust the dose or use growth factors, see Appendix 2)

2. Check renal and liver function tests (if not normal adjust the dose according to Appendix 2)

3. Perform neurologic exam (if not normal adjust the dose according to Appendix 2)

4. Radionuclide ventriculogram in patients at high risk for cardiac disease (see Appendix 2)

ANTIEMETICS PLUS OTHER SUPPORTIVE THERAPY

(See Ch. 54 for alternative regimens)
Prior to chemotherapy:
Granisetron: 2 mg po
Dexamethasone: 20 mg po
Lorazepam: 1 mg IV (if indicated for apprehension); prescribe prochlorperazine spansules 15 mg bid for 3 days (for prevention of delayed nausea and vomiting).
Ranitidine: 150 mg bid while taking prednisone (other H_2 blocker alternative equally acceptable)[2].
Allopurinol: 300 mg/day for 7 days, to prevent tumor lysis syndrome.

---

[1] Administer as many cycles as required to achieve full documented remission (this may include repetition of biopsies of tissues initially involved), followed by two additional cycles as treatment consolidation (usually 6 + 2 cycles); if a patient progresses or does not respond at all after two to three cycles, consider it a refractory disease; see Appendix 2 for sliding scale for drug dose adjustment based upon hematologic toxicities.
[2] Note that data on prevention of steroid-induced ulcer by H_2 blockers are not convincing. In our practice we usually prescribe H_2 blockers to those patients with history of peptic ulcer disease or to those who complain of dyspeptic symptoms while taking steroids.

NURSING

Extravasation precautions with vesicant drugs (e.g., nitrogen mustard and vincristine). Also, encourage oral fluids 2,000 mL/day × 2 days; avoid barbiturates with cyclophosphamide; dose of anticoagulants and digoxin may need to be altered during treatment with cyclophosphamide.

PROTOCOL FOR HELICOBACTER PYLORI-RELATED GASTRIC MUCOSA-ASSOCIATED LYMPHOID TISSUE LYMPHOMA[3]

Amoxicillin: 500 mg tid
Metronidazole: 400 mg tid
Collodial bismuth: 120 mg qid
  or omeprazole 20 mg bid
} for 2 weeks

Reevaluate within 3–6 months of treatment; repeat biopsy of abnormal areas. If *H. pylori* still detected, administer

Omeprazole: 20 mg bid
Metronidazole: 400 mg tid
Azithromycin: 500 mg; qd for 3 consecutive days
  (every week for duration of treatment)
} for two weeks

The United States Food and Drug Administration has recently approved the combination of the following for the eradication of *H. pylori*:[4]

Clarithromycin: 500 mg tid
Omeprazole: 40 mg qd
} for two weeks

[3] From Ann Intern Med 1995;122:767. *H. pylori* was completely eradicated in 25 of 26 patients; 4 patients required second-line antibiotic treatment. Total regression of lymphoma was found in 15 of 25 patients (60%). Total regression of lymphoma was evident in 8 of 15 patients after first treatment with antibiotics.
[4] The Medical Letter 1996;38:51–52

INTENSIVE INDUCTION CHEMOTHERAPY FOR SMALL-NONCLEAVED LYMPHOMA*

FIRST COURSE

1. Start IV fluid: D5½NS with KCl 20 mEq/L and sodium bicarbonate 50 mEq/L at 150 mL/hr.

2. First day of chemotherapy is day 1

3. Allopurinol 300 mg po qd × 7 days

4. Ranitidine 150 mg orally bid

5. Sulfamethoxazole/trimethoprim (Bactrim) DS one tablet bid

6. Before each dose of cyclophosphamide premedicate with

   a. Ondansetron 12 mg in D5W 50 ml IV or granisetron 10 µg/kg IV
   b. Lorazepam 1 mg IV
   c. Dexamethasone 20 mg in D5W 50 ml IV

7. Cyclophosphamide (1500 mg/m²) = ___ mg in normal saline (NS) 500 ml IV over 2 hours qd × 2 days starting at ___ on days 1 and 2.

8. Etoposide (200 mg/m²) = ___ mg in NS 1,000 mL by continuous infusion over 12 hours every 12 hours for 6 bags (1 bag = 1 L). Start first bag immediately after first dose of cyclophosphamide.

9. Prednisone (60 mg/m²) = ___ mg orally qd for 7 days, starting on day 1 (may divide into 2 doses/day).

10. Vincristine (1.4 mg/m²) = ___ mg (maximum 2 mg) IV push on ___ and ___ (day 8 and day 22).

11. Bleomycin (10 mg/m²) = ___ mg IV bolus on ___ and ___ (day 8 and 22).

12. Methotrexate (200 mg/m²) = ___ mg IV push on ___ (day 15).

13. Leucovorin (15 mg/m²) = ___ mg orally every 6 hours for 6 doses starting 24 hours after methotrexate dose.

14. Methotrexate level 48 hours and 72 hours after methotrexate dose.

(see Appendix 3 for interpretations of methotrexate levels).

15. Acetaminophen 650 mg every 4 hours prn pain or fever.

16. Lorazepam 1–2 mg IV every 4 hours prn nausea/vomiting.

17. Prochlorperazine (Compazine) 10 mg po or IV every 6 hours prn breakthrough nausea.

18. Peridex mouthwash 10 ml swish and spit qid.

SECOND COURSE

1. Second course starts on day 29 or delay until ANC is greater than 1,000/mm³

2. Start IV fluid: D5 1/2 NS with KCl 20 mEq/L and sodium bicarbonate 50 mEq/L at 150 ml/hr

3. First day of chemotherapy is day 1

4. Allopurinol 300 mg po qd × 7 days

5. Ranitidine 150 mg orally bid

6. Sulfamethoxazole/trimethoprim (Bactrim) DS one tablet bid

7. Premedication before cyclophosphamide with

    a. Ondansetron 12 mg in D5W 50 ml IV (or granisetron 10 μg/kg IV)
    b. Lorazepam 1 mg IV
    c. Dexamethasone 20 mg in D5W 50 ml IV

8. Cyclophosphamide (1,500 mg/m²) = ___ mg in NS 500 ml over 2 hours starting at ___ on day 1.

9. Etoposide (100 mg/m²) = ___ mg in NS 500 ml IV over 2 hours qd for 3 days starting at ___ on days 1,2, and 3.

10. Doxorubicin (45 mg/m²) = ___ mg IV push qd × 2 days at ___ on days 1 and 2.

11. Prednisone (60 mg/m²) = ___ mg orally qd for 7 days, starting on day 1; may divide into 2 doses/day).

12. Vincristine (1.4 mg/m²) = ___ mg (maximum 2 mg) IV push on ___ and ___ (day 8 and day 22)

13. Bleomycin (10 mg/m²) = ___ mg IV bolus on ___ and ___ (day 8 and 22)

14. Methotrexate (200 mg/m²) = ___ mg IV push on ___ (day 15)

15. Leucovorin (15 mg/m²) = ___ mg orally every 6 hours for 6 doses starting 24 hours after methotrexate dose.

16. Methotrexate level 48 hours and 72 hours after methotrexate dose. (See also Appendix 3.)

17. Acetaminophen 650 mg every 4 hours prn pain or fever

18. Lorazepam 1–2 mg IV every 4 hours prn nausea/vomiting

19. Prochlorperazine 10 mg po or IV every 6 hours prn breakthrough nausea

20. Peridex mouthwash 10 ml swish and spit qid

21. G-CSF 5 μg/kg sq qd until ANC greater than 1500/mm³. Start 2 days after chemotherapy completed.

*Check laboratory test results and adjust dosage of drugs as described under **PRIOR TO CHEMOTHERAPY** section.

SALVAGE PROTOCOL FOR AGGRESSIVE NHL

DEXAMETHASONE/ARA-C/CISPLATIN OR CARBOPLATIN (DAP)

HT:___ WT:___ IBW:___ BSA:___

1. Allopurinol 300 mg qd. Discontinue on ___.

2. Dexamethasone eye drops 0.1%. Instill 2 drops in each eye q6 hours. Discontinue after ___.

3. Hydration: D5½ NS + KCl 10 mEq/L + NaHCO₃ 50 mEq/Lto run at (150 ml/m²/hr) = ___ ml/hr except when ARA-C is infusing. Continue this rate until ___, unless otherwise ordered.

4. Dexamethasone (15 mg/m²) = ___ mg in D5W 50 ml IV q 6 hours × 8 doses. First dose at ___ on ___.

5. Cytosine arabinoside (ARA-C) (3 g/m²) = ___ g in NS 250 ml and infused IV over exactly 2 hours q 12 hours × 4 doses starting ___ on ___.

(NOTE: Patients > 50 years should receive 1.5 g/m²)

6. Circle one:

    a. Cisplatin (50 mg/m²) = ___ mg + mannitol 50 g in normal saline (NS) 1,000 ml by continuous intravenous infusion at 100 ml/hr qd × 2 days starting at ___ on ___. (Immediately after 1st & 3rd ARA-C)
    b. Carboplatin (200 mg/m²) = ___ mg in 250 ml NS by continous intravenous infusion at 25 ml/hr qd × 2

7. Granisetron 1 mg in D5W 50 ml IV before the first dose of dexamethasone each day

8. Ranitidine 150 mg po bid

9. Sulfamethoxazole/trimethoprim (Bactrim) DS one tablet po bid

10. Two days after chemotherapy has been completed, start G-CSF 5 μg/kg subcutaneously qd × 10 days

Check prior chemotherapy laboratory test results as described under **PRIOR TO CHEMOTHERAPY** section.

APPENDIX 10 Treatment of Mycosis Fungoides and Sézary Syndrome

TOPICAL TREATMENT

Mechlorethamine: Prepare solution of 10–20 mg dissolved in 50–100 mL of tap water (vesicant activity is absent at this low concentration). Paint with a brush entire skin (not just the involved sites) after bathing each day. Continue as long as there is a response. First response is usually seen in 1 to 2 weeks, but long-term administration may be necessary for maximum effect: daily treatment for 6 months to a year, followed by treatment every other day for an additional 2 years. (Br J Dermatol 1977;97:547)

If hypersensitivity reaction occurs (in about 35–40% of patients), one may initially try to dilute concentration to 10 mg in 100 mL and use topical steroids. If this does not control symptoms, next step is to mix in petroleum base (Cancer 1983;52:2214) or polyethylene glycol, or to switch to topical use of Carmustine (J Am Acad Dermatol 1990;22:802, J Am Acad Dermatol 1983;9:363).

PUVA (psoralen + ultraviolet A light): (8-methoxypsoralen (8-MOP) will inhibit DNA synthesis only if photoactivated). Methoxypsoralen is given in 0.6 mg/kg BW 2 hours before exposure to UV light. The initial UVA dose, between 1.5 to 3.0 J/cm², can be increased by approximately 0.5 J/cm² per treatment as tolerated. UV light-blocking eye glasses should be worn for 24 hours after administration of 8-MOP. Therapy is typically given three times a week until complete clearance occurs, followed by maintenance therapy once every 2 to 4 weeks for about 1 year. If interferon-α is combined with PUVA, give 3–18 million units three times a week according to the method described in Appendix 5.

TSEB (total skin electron beam therapy): refer to a specialized center.

Photopheresis: refer to a specialized center.

SYSTEMIC TREATMENT

Oral methotrexate: (20 mg/m² = ___ mg) twice weekly. Monitor complete blood count, liver function tests, and creatinine function (SMA-18) at least once a month.

COP (cyclophosphamide, vincristine, prednisone): see Appendix 9 for details on dosage and monitoring. Administer 8 to 12 courses if response is obtained.

CHOP (cyclophosphamide, doxorubicin, vincristine, prednisone): See Appendix 9 for details on dosage and monitoring. Administer between 12 to 16 cycles if response is obtained. (Omit doxorubicin from the regimen after a cumulative dose of 450 mg/m² is reached to avoid cardiotoxicity) (see Appendix 2).

Purine analogues (fludarabine, cladribine): see Appendices 6 and 7 for dosage and a method of administration.

APPENDIX

11   Treatment of Multiple Myeloma

MP PROTOCOL

Melphalan	9 mg/m²/day po × 4 days
Prednisone	50 mg bid po × 4 days
or	
Melphalan	6 mg/m²/day po × 7 days
Prednisone	100 mg/m²/day po × 7 days

Administer MP every 28 days or modify according to complete blood count (CBC). In clinical practice, MP is often administered q 5–6 weeks. Take melphalan in fasting state because food reduces absorption (> 1/3). Encourage patient to walk and to drink at least 2–3 L of fluids daily.

> Avoid diuretics
> Analgesic on fixed schedule
> Obtain CBC q 2–3 weeks after 1 cycle to monitor melphalan bioavailability.

If some degree of leukopenia and thrombocytopenia is observed, continue with same dose. If CBC is unchanged, increase dose of melphalan 2–4 mg/day until leukopenia/thrombocytopenia is observed; withhold treatment if white blood cells < 2,500/mm³ (ANC < 1,800/mm³) or platelet < 100,000/mm³

VAD FOR MULTIPLE MYELOMA (EVERY 28 DAYS)

1. Admission laboratory tests: complete blood count (CBC) with differential, chem-18, serum protein electrophoresis, quantitative immunoglobin, beta 2 microglobulin

2. Daily laboratory tests: CBC with differential, chem-7

3. Ondansetron 0.15 mg/kg IV before chemotherapy and q8h prn N&V (or granisetron; see Ch. 54)

4. Lorazepam 0.5–1.0 mg IV before chemotherapy, then q8h prn nausea or anxiety

5. Vincristine 0.4 mg in 1000 ml D5 1/2 normal saline (NS) by continuous infusion over 24 hours daily for 4 days

6. Doxorubicin 9 mg/m² = ___ mg in 1000 ml D5 1/2 NS by continuous infusion over 24 hours daily for 4 days

7. Dexamethasone 40 mg po daily on days 1–4, 9–12, and 17–20

8. Bactrim DS one tablet po on Mon, Wed, Fri. Continue after discharge.

9. Ranitidine 150 mg po bid. Continue after discharge.

10. Omit Dexamethasone on days 9–12 and 17–20 every other course.

11. MUGA scan every third cycle (see Appendix 2)

12. Mouth care as per protocol (e.g., salt and soda mouthwash qid) (see Ch. 57)

13. Allopurinol 300 mg qd × 7 days (adjust dose for renal insufficiency)

14. Use growth factors with each subsequent cycle if ANC < 1,500/mm³ on next cycle (see Ch. 60)

APPENDIX 12

Surgical Biopsy of Nonmelanoma Skin Cancer

Zoran Potparić

Definitive diagnosis of skin cancers is by pathologic examination of a tissue specimen. Local anesthetic, 1% lidocaine with 1:100,000 epinephrine is injected intradermally and beneath the lesion to elevate the lesion above the normal skin. After satisfactory anesthesia and vasoconstriction are achieved (5–10 minutes, until normal injected skin around lesion becomes white) the suspected skin lesion may be sampled by punch biopsy with a 2- to 5-mm disposable Keys punch, wedge biopsy, or excision in toto. The lesion should be removed by incising through the full thickness of dermis into the subcutaneous fat. The resulting defects after punch or wedge biopsy are dressed with antibiotic ointment and Band-Aid. Large defects after excisional biopsy require simple closure with 5/0 or 6/0 nylon suture. Sutures may be removed after 3 to 21 days depending on the site and size of the wound.

Shave biopsy can be easily performed for most of the skin tumors less then 0.5 cm in size. After local anesthesia, a #15 blade is used to remove the tumor by cutting in a horizontal plane through the dermis and including a partial thickness of dermis with the lesion. The resulting defect is covered with antibiotic ointment and Band-Aid for 2 days and then washed with mild soap and water to remove debris and crust. The wound is then redressed with antibiotic ointment and left exposed. Tissue specimen is best preserved in a well-sealed container with 10% formaldehyde.

APPENDIX 13

Treatment of Melanoma

ADJUVANT THERAPY

Adjuvant treatment with α-interferon 2b (IFN) for high-risk melanoma (see Ch. 13). IFN 20 million units IV 5 days/week for 4 weeks, followed by 10 million units subcutaneously 3 days/week for 48 weeks

DOSE REDUCTION

(See also Appendix 5 for details on side-effects of IFN)

If absolute neutrophil count (ANC) < 500/mm³, stop IFN; resume when ANC > 500 at 50% dose. If ANC <250/mm³, discontinue IFN

If liver function tests (LFT) > 5 times normal, stop IFN; resume when LFT < 5 times normal at 50% dose. If LFT > 10 times normal, stop IFN for any grade 3/4 toxicity (e.g., fatigue, neurologic toxicity), 25% dose reduction may be necessary (see Appendix 5)

BIOCHEMOTHERAPY FOR METASTATIC MELANOMA (IL-2/IFN/DTIC/CDPP FOR METASTATIC MELANOMA) (NOT FOR CNS DISEASE)

Repeat cycles at 21 days. Evaluate disease after two to three cycles. If no response, discontinue treatment

1. Input and output every shift; call attending physician if output is less than 500 mL per 8-hour shift.

2. Daily weights before breakfast.

3. Vital signs every 4 hours (repeat blood pressure in 15 minutes for SBP < 90 and proceed with order #4B)

4. IVF: continuous infusion 1,000 mL D5½ normal saline (NS) with 20 mEq/L KCl and 1 g MgSO$_4$/L at 100 mL/hr via pump.

a. Increase rate to 125 mL/hour if SBP < 100 mmHg

b. Give 500 mL NS IV bolus × 1 if SBP < 90 mmHg and notify attending physician if SBP remains < 90 mmHg

5. Kytril (granisetron) 1 mg IV before chemo daily (days 1–4); repeat prn day 5 if necessary. Ativan (lorazepam) 1 mg IV before chemotherapy day 1; then every 8 hrs during IL-2 administration. Reglan (metoclopramide) 10 mg and Benadryl (diphenhydramine) 25 mg IV every 4 hours prn for "breakthrough" N/V

6. DTIC (800 mg/m²) = ___ mg in 250 ml D5W IV over 1 hour (day 1 only)

7. Prehydrate cisplatin daily with 1 L NS IV over 2 hours via pump.

8. Cisplatin (20 mg/m²) = ___ mg IV in 250 mL NS over 1 hour via pump on days 1–4; on day 1 administer before initiating IL-2 infusion

9. Start IL-2 immediately after chemotherapy on day 1 and continue uninterrupted (do not interrupt IL-2 for chemotherapy).

10. Start dopamine drip at 2 µg/kg/min IV with pump when IL-2 is initiated. Discontinue dopamine 6 hours after last IL-2 bag is completed.

11. IL-2 (9 million units/m²) = ___ million units in 50 mL D5W only, IV via syringe pump over 24 hours daily × 4 days.

12. Interferon alpha (5 million units/M²) = ___ million units daily (days 1–5).

13. Ativan 0.5 mg IV every 4 hours prn N/V, immediately followed with Compazine (prochlorperazine) 10 mg IV every 4 hours prn N/V.

14. Demerol (meperidine) 50 mg IV every 6 hours prn chills.

15. NO STEROIDS!

16. Naprosyn (naproxyn) 250 mg every 12 hours (start upon admission and continue until discharged).

17. Tylenol (acetaminophen) 650 mg every 4 hours prn.

18. Atarax (hydroxyzine) 50 mg po every 6 hrs prn itching.

19. Lomotil (diphenoxycate/atropine) 2 tabs at start of diarrhea; then one after each loose bowel movement, not to exceed 8/day.

20. Paregoric (opium tincture) 5 to 10 mL po every 4 hours prn diarrhea if not controlled with Lomotil

21. Eucerin lotion at bedside (please encourage use)

22. Lanolin to lips

23. Basis soap at bedside

24. Complete blood count (CBC) with differential/SMA18 before starting chemotherapy. Do not administer cisplatin if creatinine > 1.6 mg

25. CBC with differential, SMA18, and magnesium daily

26. EKG every morning

27. O_2 saturation

28. Protime, partial thromboplastin time day 2 of chemotherapy; also day 9

29. Weekly CBCs should be arranged at discharge.

APPENDIX
14 # Protocols for Treatment of Head and Neck Cancers

Srdjan Denić

NEOADJUVANT CHEMOTHERAPY

CISPLATINUM + 5-FU (5-FLUOROURACIL)

Larynx, hypopharynx, oral cavity and oropharynx
Height ___   Weight ___   BSA ___

1. *Day 1 laboratory tests:* Complete blood count (CBC) with differential, SMA 18, Mg^{++}, 12-hour creatinine clearance

2. *Daily laboratory tests:* CBC with diff, SMA 7, Mg^{++}

3. *IV fluids:* 1,000 ml D5½ normal saline (NS) with 20 mEq/L KCl and 1 g $MgSO_4$/L at 150 mL/hr continuously

4. *5 FU (1,000 mg/m²)* = —- mg in 1,000 mL NS to infuse as 24-hour continuous infusion days 1 through 5

5. Give cisplatin on day 2 if Cr Cl > 60 mL/min: 30 minutes before cisplatin premedicate with

   a. Granisetron 2 mg po (or 1 mg IV) (or, ondansetron 32 mg IV piggy back 15 to 30 min before treatment)
   b. Dexamethasone 20 mg po
   c. Mannitol 25% 50 mL IV over 10 minutes (must be filtered)
   d. Cisplatin (100 mg/m²) = —- mg in 250 mL NS IV over 1 hour
   e. Mannitol 20% 500 mL IV over 3 hours after cisplatin

6. At 6 AM the morning following chemotherapy, begin delayed-emesis antiemetics (see also Ch. 54 for alternative protocols):
   a. Prochloperazine spansules 15 mg po bid
   b. Dexamethasone 8 mg po bid × 2 days, tapered to 4 mg po bid × 2 days
   c. Lorazepam 1 to 2 mg po or IV q 6 to 8 hour for prn anxiety or nausea/vomiting

7. CBC and SMA-18 before each cycle; adjust dose according to Appendix[2] or according to the following scheme (J Clin Oncol 1994;12:385)

Delay treatment until leukocytes > 4,000/mm³ and platelets > 100,000/mm³

Nadir leukocytes/mm³,	*platelets/mm³,*	*reduce cisplatin dose by*
2,000–2,900	50,000–75,000	25%
<2,000	<50,000	50%

if creatinine 2.0–2.5 mg/dL, then reduce cisplatin dose by 50%
if mucositis grade 2 or 3, then reduce 5-fluorouracil dose by 25%
(Taylor SG et al. J Clin Oncol 1994; 12:385)

8. Repeat treatment q 4 weeks × 2–3; then reassess

If complete remission (CR) or partial remission (PR) after 2 cycles is achieved, administer 3rd cycle followed by radiation therapy; if residual tumor after radiation therapy is seen, consider resection.

CISPLATINUM, 5-FU, AND BLEOMYCIN + RADIATION THERAPY (EUR J CANCER 1992;28:1792)

Nasopharyngeal carcinoma
(Expected outcomes based on 30 treated pts: CR, 10%, PR, 73% after 2 cycles of chemotherapy)
Height ___   Weight ___   BSA ___

1. *Day 1 laboratory tests:* CBC with differential, SMA 18, Mg++, 12-hour creatinine clearance

2. *Daily laboratory tests:* CBC with differential, SMA 7, Mg++

3. *IV fluids:* 1,000 mL D$_5$ 1/2 NS with 20 mEq/L KCl and 1 g MgSO$_4$/L at 150 mL/hr continuously

4. *5-FU (650 mg/m^2)* = ___ mg in 1,000 mL NS to infuse as 24-hour continuous IV infusion days 1 through 5

5. Give cisplatin on day 1 if Cr Cl > 60 mL/min: 30 minutes before cisplatin premedicate with

    a. Granisetron 2 mg po (or 1 mg IV) (or, ondansetron 32 mg IV piggy back 15–30 min before treatment)
    b. Dexamethasone 20 mg po
    c. Mannitol 25% 50 mL IV over 10 minutes (must be filtered)
    d. Cisplatin (100 mg/m^2) = —- mg in 250 mL NS IV over 1 hour
    e. Mannitol 20% 500 mL IV over 3 hours after cisplatin

6. *Bleomycin:* 15 mg IV push through free flowing IV on day 1, followed by (16 mg/m^2/day) = —- as a continuous IV infusion days 1 through 5

7. At 6 AM the morning after chemotherapy, begin delayed-emesis antiemetics (see also Ch. 54 for alternative protocols):

    a. Prochloperazine spansules 15 mg po bid
    b. Dexamethasone 8 mg po bid × 2 days, tapered to 4 mg po bid × 2 days
    c. Lorazepam 1 to 2 mg po or IV q 6 to 8 hours prn for anxiety or nausea/vomiting

CBC and SMA-18 before each cycle (adjust the dose according to Appendix 2 or according to the scheme on the preceding page)
Administer 2 cycles of chemotherapy q 4 weeks; then give radiation therapy 200 cGy/day, five days/wk

8. Administer third cycle of chemotherapy, followed by radiation therapy 200 cGy/d, five days/wk

PALLIATIVE TREATMENT

WEEKLY METHOTREXATE FOR HEAD/NECK CANCER

HT ___   WT ___   BSA ___

1. *Day 1 laboratory tests:* CBC with differential SMA 18 — repeat every 4 weeks

2. *Weekly laboratory tests:* CBC with differential

3. *Methotrexate (40–60 mg/m^2)* = ___ mg IV push through freely flowing IV

4. Escalate dose if no toxicity by 20%

5. *For severe toxicity:* Leucovorin 10 mg po q 6 hours × 6 doses, then reevaluate

6. Pain control (as described in Chapter 55)

CISPLATIN EVERY 21 DAYS

Height ___   Weight ___   BSA ___

1. *Day 1 laboratory tests:* CBC with differential, SMA 18, 12-hour creatinine clearance and Mg++

2. *Daily laboratory tests:* CBC with differential, SMA-17, and Mg++

3. *IV fluids:* 1000 mL D$_5$ 1/2 NS with 20 mEq/L KCl, 1 g MgSO$_4$/L at 150 mL/hr continuously

4. Give cisplatin on day 2 if CrCl > 60 mL/min: 30 minutes before cisplatin premedicate with

    a. Granisetron 2 mg po (or 1 mg IV) or, ondansetron 32 mg IV piggy back 15 to 30 minutes prior to treatment
    b. Dexamethasone 20 mg po
    c. Mannitol 25% 50 mL IV over 10 minutes (must be filtered)
    d. Cisplatin (100 mg/m^2) = —- mg in 250 mL NS IV over 1 hour
    e. Mannitol 20% 500 mL IV over 3 hours after cisplatin

5. At 6 AM the morning after chemotherapy, begin delayed-emesis antiemetics (see also Ch. 54 for alternative protocols):

   a. Prochloperazine spansules 15 mg po bid

   b. Dexamethasone 8 mg po bid × 2 days, tapered to 4 mg po bid × 2 days

   c. Lorazepam 1 to 2 mg po or IV q 6 to 8 hours prn for anxiety or nausea/vomiting

6. CBC and SMA-18 before each cycle; adjust dose according to Appendix 2 or according to the following scheme (J Clin Oncol 1994;12:385)

Delay treatment until leukocytes > 4,000/mm³ and platelets > 100,000/mm³

Nadir leukocytes/mm³,	platelets/mm³,	reduce cisplatin dose by
2,000–2,900	50,000–75,000	25%
<2,000	<50,000	50%

if creatinine 2.0 to 2.5 mg/dL, then reduce cisplatin dose by 50%

7. Pain control (as described in Ch. 55)

APPENDIX
15

Protocols for Treatment of Lung Cancer

TREATMENT OF NON-SMALL CELL LUNG CANCER WITH CISPLATIN AND VP-16 [ETOPOSIDE]

Height ___   Weight ___   BSA ___

1. *Day 1:* Complete blood count (CBC) with differential, SMA-18, 12-hour urine collection for creatinine clearance

2. Obtain daily SMA-7 and Mg++ levels

3. *IV fluid:* D5½ normal saline (NS) with 20 mEq/L of KCL and 1 g $MgSO_4$/L to run at 150 mL/hr

4. *VP-16* (100 mg/m²)= ___ mg in 250 ml of NS IV over two hours qd × 3 days. Infuse at 2 mg/min (to avoid hypotension)

6. Cisplatin on day 2 (if creatinine clearance > 60 mL/min); 30 minutes before cisplatin, premedicate with
   a. Granisetron 2 mg po (or 1 mg IV) or, ondansetron 32 mg IV piggy back 15 to 30 minutes before treatment
   b. Dexamethasone 20 mg po
   c. Mannitol 25% 50 ml IV over 10 minutes (must be filtered)
   d. Cisplatin (100 mg/m²)= ―- mg in 250 mL NS IV over 1 hour
   e. Mannitol 20% 500 mL IV over 3 hours after cisplatin

7. At 6 AM the morning after chemotherapy, begin delayed-emesis antiemetics (see also Ch. 54 for alternative protocols).
   a. Prochloperazine spansules 15 mg po bid
   b. Dexamethasone 8 mg po bid × 2 days, tapered to 4 mg po bid × 2 days
   c. Lorazepam 1 to 2 mg IV or po q 6 to 8 hours prn for anxiety or nausea/vomiting

8. Repeat chemotherapy at 3 to 4 week intervals for 4 cycles

TREATMENT OF SMALL CELL LUNG CANCER WITH CYCLOPHOSPHAMIDE, DOXORUBICIN AND VINCRISTINE

Height ___   Weight ___   BSA ___

1. MUGA scan in high-risk patients (see Appendix 2)

2. Day 1: CBC with differential, SMA-18

3. CBC at nadir (first cycle): day 7 to 10 after chemotherapy

4. Fifteen to 30 minutes before chemotherapy, premedicate with
   a. Granisetron 2 mg po (or 1 mg IV) or, ondansetron 32 mg IV piggy back
   b. Dexamethasone 20 mg po

5. Cyclophosphamide 1000 mg/m² = ___ mg in 100 mL NS IV over 30 minutes

7. Adriamycin (doxorubicin) 40 mg/m² = ___ mg IV push

8. Vincristine (1.4 mg/m²; not to exceed 2 mg) = ___ mg IV push

9. Prochloperazine spansules 15 mg po bid prn for nausea/vomiting

10. Repeat treatment every 3 weeks for 6 cycles

(See Appendix 2 for dose adjustment and monitoring of cardiac toxicity.)

TREATMENT OF NON-SMALL CELL LUNG CANCER WITH CARBOPLATIN AND PACLITAXEL

Height ___   Weight ___   BSA ___

AUC (creatinine clearance +25) $\times$ 6 = ___ mg (See Appendix 2 and Table 2-6)

1. Day 1: Complete blood count (CBC) with differential, SMA-18, 12-hour urine collection for creatinine clearance

2. Carboplatin (AUC 6) = ___ mg in 250 mL NS IV over 1 hour

3. Paclitaxel (225 mg/m^2) = ___ mg in 250 mL NS IV over 3 hours
   a. Dexamethasone 20 mg IV 30 min pre-paclitaxel
   b. Diphenhydramine 50 mg IV with Ranitidine 50 mg IV in 50 mL NS pre-paclitaxel
   c. Lorazepam 1 mg pre-paclitaxel
   d. Granisetron 2 mg pre-paclitaxel (optional for nausea/vomiting)

4. CBC with differential on day 7 or 8

5. G-CSF may be required if patient develops clinically significant neutropenia

6. Repeat treatment every 3 weeks for 6 cycles

(See Vafai D et al. Phase I/II trial of combination carboplatin and taxol in NSCLC. Presented at 31st Annual Meeting of ASCO, May 20–23, 1995, Los Angeles, CA.)

NOTE:
Optimal regimens for the management of NSCLC are not yet identified. Protocols in this appendix are most commonly used in our practice.

LOW-DOSE CISPLATINUM WITH RADIATION THERAPY FOR NONSMALL-CELL LUNG CANCER

1. *Cisplatin:* 1 to 2 hours before radiation therapy (XRT) at 5 mg/m^2 = ___ mg IV qd as a bolus for 5 days per week concurrently with XRT (total XRT dose usually delivered over 6.5 weeks)

2. Encourage patient to drink at least 2 L of fluids per day

3. CBC, SMA-18 q week

4. Withhold cisplatinum or XRT for grade 4 hematologic toxicity (see Appendix 1) and for increase in serum creatinine

5. Resume treatment when hematologic toxicity $\leq$2 and when creatinine returns to baseline

6. Evaluate disease 3 to 4 weeks after treatment completion. If patient has complete or partial response or stable disease administer consolidation treatment with

Cisplatin 50 mg/m^2 = ___ mg IV on days 1 and 8 (as shown below) every 28 days
Give chemotherapy if white blood cell count >3,500/mm^3, platelet count > 100,000/mm^3 and creatine clearance > 50 mL/min; 30 minutes before cisplatin premedicate with
   a. Granisetron 2 mg po (or 1 mg IV) or ondansetron 32 mg IV piggy back 15 to 30 minutes before treatment
   b. Dexamethasone 20 mg po
   c. Mannitol 25% 50 mL IV over 10 minutes (must be filtered)
   d. *cisplatin* (50 mg/m^2)= —- mg in 250 mL NS IV over 1 hour
   e. Mannitol 20% 500 mL IV over 3 hours after cisplatin

7. At 6 AM the morning after chemotherapy begins, delayed-emesis antiemetics (see also ch. 54 for alternative protocol):
   a. Prochloperazine spansules 15 mg po bid
   b. Dexamethasone 8 mg po bid $\times$ 2 days, tapered to 4 mg po bid $\times$ 2 days
   c. Lorazepam 1 to 2 mg IV q 6 to 8 hours prn for anxiety or nausea/vomiting

8. Follow-up: q 2 months for the first year, q 3 months for the second and third year, and at 6-month intervals thereafter

(From J Clin Oncol 1994;12:1814, with permission.)

Protocol for Treatment of Esophageal Cancer

Rambabu Tummala

Height___   Weight___   BSA___

For chemotherapy + radiation therapy as primary therapy: We suggest a regimen similar to RTOG study (Herskovic A et al; see Ch. 23) with 4 courses of combined 5-FU (5-fluorouracil): continuous infusion for the first four days of weeks 1, 5, 8, and 11 and cisplatin (on the first day of each course) plus 50 Gy of XRT (daily fractionation of 2 Gy given five days a week, beginning with day 1 of first cycle of chemotherapy).

1. *Before cisplatin:* Decadron (dexamethasone) 20 mg po or IV over 30 minutes; Kytril (granisetron) 2 mg po or 1 mg IV or Zofran (ondansetron) 32 mg IV; Normal saline (NS) 1 L IV over 3 to 4 hours; Mannitol 25% 50 mL IV over 10 minutes (must be filtered)

2. *After cisplatin:* Mannitol 20% 500 mL IV over 3 hours, starting immediately after completion of cisplatin

3. *Chemotherapy:* Cisplatin (75 mg/m²) = ___ mg in 500 mL NS IV over 2 hours × 1 on day 1; 5-FU (1,000 mg/m²/day)=___ mg in 1 L of D_5W (5% dextrose) continuous infusion over 24 hours × 4 days starting on day 1

4. *PRN orders:* At 6 AM the morning after chemotherapy begins, delayed-emesis antiemetics (see also Ch. 54 for an alternative protocol):
   a. Prochloperazine spansules 15 mg po bid
   b. Dexamethasone 8 mg po bid for 2 days, tapered to 4 mg po bid for 2 days
   c. Lorazepam 1 to 2 mg IV q 6 to 8 hours prn for anxiety or nausea/vomiting

Complete blood count, SMA-18 before each course of chemotherapy and prn (see Appendix 2 for dose adjustment)

APPENDIX 17

Protocols for Treatment of Metastatic Gastric Cancer

5-FU-LEUCOVORIN[1]

Height___   Weight___   BSA___

1. Laboratory tests day 1: complete blood count, SMA 18, CEA every other cycle

2. 5-FU (5-fluorouracil) (400 mg/m²/d) = ___ mg IV push through free flowing (FF), normal saline IV days 1 through 5

3. Leucovorin (200 mg/m²/d) = ___ mg IV push through FFIV days 1 through 5

4. Antiemetics prn (not routinely needed; e.g., prochloperazine 10 mg po qid prn for nausea/vomiting)

5. Repeat q 21 days if gastrointestinal toxicity, central nervous system, and hematologic status within acceptable limits (see Appendix 2 for dose adjustment) until progression of a disease

---

(Adapted from J Clin Oncol 4:685–696, 1986, with permission.)

Alternatively, one may administer 5-FU (500 mg/m²) = ___ mg IV push IV for 5 consecutive days and repeat q 5 weeks until progression of disease

[1] Note that despite higher response rates seen with combined therapy, none of the protocols based on combined chemotherapy has demonstrated survival superiority over 5-FU alone (see Ch. 24). However, in one randomized study, FAMTX protocol showed survival advantage over FAM (J Clin Oncol 1991;9:827), leading some authors to recommend FAMTX as a standard protocol. However, FAMTX was not associated with a survival advantage when compared with EAP (etoposide-Adriamycin-cisplatin) but had a better toxicity profile than EAP (see next protocol for details on administration).

FAMTX

Height___   Weight___   BSA___

1. *Laboratory tests day 1:* CBC, SMA18; CEA every other cycle

2. *Day 15 Laboratory tests:* CBC, SMA-7

3. A physician may choose to order methotrexate (MTX) levels q AM until MTX level < 0.1 μmol/L

4. MTX (1.5 g/m²) = ___ mg IV on day 1

(Dilute 1,000 mg vial with 19.4 mL to provide a concentration of 50 mg/mL, then dilute further with 50 mL D5W or NS)

(i.e., 3,000 mg in at least 100 mL)

5. 5-FU (1.5 g/m²) = ___ mg IV push (given 1 hour after MTX infusion)

6. Leucovorin (15 mg/m²)= ___ mg po q 6 hrs × 48 hours starting 24 hours after MTX

7. *Antiemetics:* 30 minutes before chemotherapy premedicate with

   a. Granisetron 2 mg po (or 1 mg IV) or, ondansetron 32 mg IV piggy back 15 to 30 minutes prior to treatment

   b. Dexamethasone 20 mg po
      Antiemetics on prn basis:

   c. Prochloperazine spansules 15 mg po bid

   d. Lorazepam 1 to 2 mg po or IV q 6 to 8 hours prn for anxiety or nausea/vomiting

8. *On day 15:* Adriamycin (30 mg/m²) = ___ mg IV push through FF IV

9. Repeat q 28 days × 2 cycles. If partial response is noted, continue until progression of tumor or unacceptable toxicity. For patients achieving complete remission, continue 12 to 14 months of therapy and then observe (see Ch. 24)

Adjust doses of drugs according to Appendix 2

Outcomes reported with FAMTX: response rates: 33% (16%-50%); CR 10%; median survival, 7.3 months; 1-year survival, 17%

(Adapted from J Clin Oncol 10:541–548, 1992, with permission.)

<table>
<tr><td>APPENDIX
18</td><td># Protocols for Treatment of Pancreatic Cancer</td></tr>
</table>

Height___   Weight___   BSA___

RESECTABLE DISEASE

WHIPPLE PROCEDURE PLUS ADJUVANT RADIATION THERAPY WITH 5-FU (5-FLUOROURACIL)/LEUCOVORIN

1. Leucovorin (500 mg/m^2) = ___mg in normal saline (NS) 100 mL. Infuse IV over 2 hours.

2. One hour after leucovorin started, give 5-fluorouracil (500 mg/m^2) = ___ mg IV over 3 to 5 minutes.

3. Repeat above treatment weekly × 6 weeks during radiation therapy, then rest 2 weeks, then repeat another 6-week cycle with 2-week rest for at least 6 months

4. Complete blood count (CBC) with differential, chem-18 weekly during chemotherapy

5. Monitor diarrhea and mucositis weekly

6. For modification of doses for hematologic, gastrointestinal, neurologic, or dermatologic toxicity see below or refer to Appendix 2

7. Antiemetics usually provided on prn (as needed) basis (e.g., prochlorperazine 15 mg spansules po bid, or metoclopramide 30 mg po qid with or without diphenhydramine 50 mg po q 4 hours prn for restlessness; lorazepam 1 to 2 mg po or IV q 6 to 8 hours) (see Chapter 54)

DOSAGE MODIFICATIONS FOR 5-FU AND LEUCOVORIN

1. White blood cell (WBC) count 3,499/mm^3 to 2,500/mm^3 or platelet count 75,000/mm^3 to 99,000/mm^3: delay chemotherapy and repeat counts weekly.

When WBC > 3,500 and platelet count > 100,000, resume 5-FU at dosage 400 mg/m^2 with 100% of leucovorin for remaining weeks of treatment.

2. WBC count < 2,499/mm^3 or platelets < 74,999/mm^3: delay therapy for at least three weeks and until WBC count > 3,500 and platelets > 100,000. Begin next cycle at 400 mg/m^2 of 5FU.

DOSAGE MODIFICATION FOR GASTROINTESTINAL TOXICITY

Stomatitis with mild to moderate ulcers and/or diarrhea, with two watery stools per day if symptoms are present at the time of treatment: hold treatment.

If symptoms occur between treatments and there are no symptoms at the time of treatment, no adjustments should be made. Intravenous supportive care when indicated. Resume treatment at 400 mg/m^2 5-FU and 100% of leucovorin for remaining weeks of treatment cycle.

For severe stomatitis and diarrhea (three to six stools per day) with no evidence of occult blood: hold therapy at least three weeks and until full recovery; then begin the next cycle at 400 mg/m^2 of 5FU and 100% of leucovorin. Hospitalization with aggressive IV supportive care may be indicated.

Gastrointestinal bleeding and > 7 stools per day, discontinue further therapy. Hospitalization with aggressive IV support.

DOSAGE MODIFICATION FOR SKIN TOXICITY: SEE APPENDIX 2

LOCALIZED UNRESECTABLE DISEASE AND ADVANCED DISEASE[a]

1. *Gemcitabine* (Gemzar) (1000 mg/m²) = ___ mg in 100 mL of NS to run IV over 30 minutes once weekly for up to 7 weeks, followed by a week of rest.

2. Repeat above treatment once a week for 3 weeks of every 4 weeks. (The first series of weekly doses up to 7 weeks plus the initial rest week defines cycle 1. Subsequently, each cycle consists of 3 weekly doses given over a period of 4 weeks with the fourth week as a week of rest.)

3. Continue treatment as long as there is a response. (See Ch. 25, Table 25-2 for assessment of response) or until progression of disease or unacceptable treatment side effects.

4. CBC with differential, Chem-18 weekly during chemotherapy.

---

[a] Preliminary data suggest slight superiority over 5-FU (median survival:5.65 vs 4.41 months; the quality of life improved (23.8% vs 4.8%); further studies are needed to establish gemcitabine as a standard of the treatment over 5-FU (see Ch. 25).

DOSE ADJUSTMENTS OF GEMCITABINE IN A CYCLE*

Dose adjustments within a cycle are made following the guidelines shown below based on platelet, leukocyte, and absolute granulocyte counts (AGC) monitored every week before each dose of gemcitabine.

* According to the manfacturer's preliminary recommendations.

APPENDIX TABLE 18-1 HEMATOLOGIC TOXICITIES

AGC (× 10⁶/L)		Platelets (× 10⁶/L)	Percent of Full Dose
> 1000	and	> 100,000	100
500	or	50,000–100,000	75
< 500	or	< 50,000	Hold

APPENDIX TABLE 18-2 NONHEMATOLOGIC TOXICITIES

WHO Grade (See Appendix)	Percent of Full Dose
0–2 (and Grade 3 nausea/vomiting and alopecia)	100
3 (except nausea/vomiting and alopecia)	50 or hold[a]
4	Hold[a]

[a] *This decision will depend upon the type of nonhematologic toxicity seen and which course is medically most sound in the judgment of the physician.*

DOSE ADJUSTMENTS OF GEMCITABINE FOR SUBSEQUENT CYCLES

The following guidelines should be followed:

Hematologic toxicity: Patients who sustained either febrile neutropenia, WHO grade 4 thrombocytopenia, or bleeding associated with thrombocytopenia should be dosed at 50% of the commencing dose of the previous cycle. Subsequent dose escalation may be allowed provided the patient tolerates the doses given at the 50% level.

Nonhematologic toxicity: The table below provides guidelines for subsequent dosing following the worst WHO grade of toxicity demonstrated in the previous cycle.

APPENDIX TABLE 18-3   NONHEMATOLOGIC TOXICITIES

WHO Grade	Percent of Full Dose
0–2 (and grade 3 nausea/vomiting and alopecia)	100
3 (except nausea/vomiting and alopecia)	75
4	50 or hold[a]

[a] *This decision will depend upon the type of nonhematologic toxicity seen and which course is medically most sound in the judgment of the physician. Doses held because of toxicity or missed are not given at a later time. If the dose held or missed was to be given on day 1 of the next cycle, that next cycle will not be considered to start until the day the first dose is actually administered to the patient (i.e., 1-2-3-R, X-1-2-3-R, etc.). If the second (day 9) dose is held or missed, the cycle would continue per protocol with one dose not given (i.e., 1-2-3-R, 1-X-3-R, 1-2-3-R, etc.). If the third (day 15) dose is held or missed, this would be considered the week of rest. The following week a dose would be administered (if toxicity permits) and considered the beginning (day 1) of a new cycle. This set of circumstances would result in a 21-day cycle (i.e., 1-2-3-R, 1-2-X, 1-2-3-R, etc.).*

Protocol for Treatment of Colon Cancer

ADJUVANT TREATMENT OF COLON CANCER

5-FU + LEVAMISOLE

Height___   Weight___   BSA___

1. 5-fluorouracil (450 mg/m^2) = ___ mg IV over 3 to 5 minutes daily for 5 days, followed four weeks later by the same dose weekly for 48 weeks

2. Levamisole 50 mg po tid for 3 days every other week

3. Complete blood count (CBC) with differential, chem-18 weekly during chemotherapy

4. Monitor diarrhea and mucositis weekly

5. For modification of doses for hematologic, gastrointestinal, neurologic, or dermatologic toxicity refer to Appendix 2

6. Antiemetics routinely not required (provide on prn basis); (e.g., prochlorperazine 15 mg spansules po bid or metoclopramide 30 mg po qid with or without diphenhydramine 50 mg po q 4 hours prn for restlessness) (see Ch. 54)

TREATMENT OF METASTATIC COLON CANCER[a]

PROTOCOL WITH 5-FU (5-FLUOROURACIL)/LEUCOVORIN[b]

Height___   Weight___   BSA___

1. Leucovorin (500 mg/m^2) = ___ mg in normal saline (NS) 100 mL. Infuse over 2 hours.

2. One hour after leucovorin started, give 5-fluorouracil (600 mg/m^2) = ___ mg IV over 3 to 5 minutes.

3. Repeat above treatment weekly × 6 weeks, rest 2 weeks, then repeat another 6-week cycle with 2-week rest for one year.

4. CBC with differential, chem-18 weekly during chemotherapy.

5. Monitor diarrhea and mucositis weekly.

6. For modification of doses for hematologic, gastrointestinal, neurologic, or dermatologic toxicity refer to Appendix 2.

7. Antiemetics routinely not required (provide on prn basis); (e.g., prochlorperazine 15 mg spansules po bid or metoclopramide 30 mg po qid with or without diphenhydramine 50 mg po q 4 hours prn for restlessness) (See Ch. 54).

---

[a] Note that the FDA (Food and Drug Administration) has recently approved CPT-11 (irinotecan) as a second line treatment for metastic colorectal cancer.

[b] A recent randomized trial (level II evidence) showed that high-dose leucovorin (LV) (500 mg/m^2) is not superior to low-dose leucovorin (20 mg/m^2) and could be even more toxic. Median survival was 55.1 weeks in high-dose LV group and 54.1 weeks in low-dose LV group. Twenty-seven percent of patients in high-dose LV group experienced grade III|IV diarrhea as opposed to 16% treated with low-dose LV. (J Clin Oncol 1996;14:2274.)

APPENDIX 20

Protocol for Treatment of Rectal Cancer

ADJUVANT TREATMENT WITH 5-FU AND CONCOMITANT RADIATION THERAPY[a]

See Ch. 29 (SWOG 9304 protocol)

Height___   Weight___   BSA___m^2

1. Day 1 (and before each chemotherapy): Complete blood count with differential, SMA 18

2. Premedication: Antiemetics given on as needed basis (e.g.,) prochloperazine 10 mg po qid prn nausea/vomiting

3. 5-FU (425 mg/m^2) = ___ mg IV push through FF (free flowing) normal saline (NS) IV days 1 through 5; repeat days 29 through 33

Note: restart 5-FU after completion of XRT (28 days after completion of XRT)

Repeat 5-FU (400 mg/m^2) = ___ mg IV push through FFIV days 1 through 5 (Start day 57 through 61; continue q28d for 1 year)

Leucovorin (20 mg/m^2/day) = ___ mg IV push before 5-FU daily on days 1 through 5 (days 57 through 61; continue q28d for 1 year)

4. See Appendix 2 for dose adjustment

---

[a]Radiation therapy starts day 1 of the treatment cycle and continues for 6–8 weeks.

PROTOCOL FOR TREATMENT OF METASTATIC DISEASE

See Appendix 19.

APPENDIX

21

Protocol for Treatment of Anal Cancer

COMBINED TREATMENT WITH 5-FU, MITOMYCIN C AND CONCOMITANT XRT[a]

Height____   Weight____   BSA____m^2

1. Day 1 (and before each chemotherapy): Complete blood count with differential, SMA 18

2. *Premedication:* Antiemetics given on as needed basis (e.g., prochloperazine 10 mg po qid prn nausea/vomiting; dexamethasone 20 mg po if mitomycin is given as well).

3. *5-FU (1000 mg/m^2)* = ____ mg IV in 1000 ml normal saline as a continuous infusion days 1 through 4 (maximum dose 1500 mg/day)

4. *Mitomycin C* (10 mg/m^2) =____ mg IV push on day 1 (some clinicians omit it)

5. *Radiation therapy:* may be delivered in a single course of 250 cGy/d for 5 days × 4 weeks or in split course with 2500 cGy in 2 weeks

6. Repeat treatment (radiation + chemotherapy) on day 43 (See Appendix 2 for toxicity and dose adjustment) (Adopted from Int J Rad Oncol Biol Phys 1991;21:1115, with permission.)

---

[a]There is level II evidence to support inclusion of MMC (mitomycin C) in the protocol for the treatment of anal cancer. In the recent randomized trial evaluating 5-FU + MMC + XRT vs. 5-FU + XRT, the treatment that included MMC lead to increases in disease-free survival (73% vs. 51%) and colostomy-free survival (71% vs. 59%), with lower colostomy rates (9% vs. 22%); however, no signficant difference in overall survival was noted (J Clin Oncol 1996;14:2527).

APPENDIX 22	# Iodine[131] in the Management of Thyroid Carcinoma

Nolan Sakow

Surgical resection alone of thyroid cancer is rarely definitive. Optimal results are usually achieved with surgery and iodine[131] treatment. When a subtotal or near total thyroidectomy is combined with ^{131}I treatment, the probability of thyroid cancer recurrence decreases to 1.3%, which compares favorably with thyroidectomy without [131]I (3%), and partial thyroidectomy alone (11%). Most authors believe that these benefits outweigh the risks associated with a total thyroidectomy (such as iatrogenic hypoparathyroidism, recurrent laryngeal nerve paralysis; see Ch. 31). Other specific indications for ^{131}I therapy in thyroid cancer patients include postoperative residual tumor in the neck that cannot be removed surgically, distant metastases, invasion of the thyroid capsule, cervical or mediastinal lymph node metastasis, and recurrent thyroid carcinoma. (If the surgical oncologist performs a pure lobectomy, the role of nuclear medicine and radioiodine has been significantly diminished as adjunct therapy. This is because the normal remaining thyroid lobe will be avid for the radioiodine and, as such, there will be no ability to diagnose and treat the metastasis.)

Protocol for use of radioiodine as a treatment for thyroid carcinoma is described below. These recommendations are primarily based on level III and IV evidence, since there are virtually no prospective trials addressing the role of ^{131}I in the management of thyroid cancer. However, indirect evidence (see Ch. 1) on the role of iodine in the physiology of thyroid hormone synthesis are so strong that current recommendations for the use of ^{131}I may be considered quite solid.

First, the patient must have a near total thyroidectomy. The patient should not be placed on thyroid supplements postoperatively. This is to increase the thyroid stimulating hormone (TSH) level to approximately 40 to 50mTu/l (the higher the better) to enhance the avidity of the radioiodine into possible residual tumor bed or to ablate remaining normal thyroid remnants. Therefore, approximately 6 weeks after surgery the patient should be scheduled for a diagnostic whole body ^{131}I scan. TSH levels should be drawn several days before the small diagnostic tracer dose of [131]I. If the patient's symptomatology associated with hypothyroidism is extreme (i.e., lethargy, weight gain, and edema), Cytomel (T3) can be given for 2 to 3 weeks postoperatively and then stopped several weeks before the radioiodine imaging. Exogenous dosing with bovine TSH is expensive and does not appear to enhance radioiodine uptake. Similarly, the results with TSH are inconclusive.

The patient should not receive any iodinated contrast from radiographic procedures as this will cause competitive inhibition of the ^{131}I into the thyroid remnants and the thyroid metastases. Also, the patient should be placed on a low-iodine diet. Some have advocated the use of diuretics to increase the amount of iodine in the urine to decrease the total iodine body pool.

If the patient is of childbearing age, a pregnancy test should be done before the radioiodine dosing. Radioiodine does cross the placenta and can ablate the fetal thyroid and could potentially cause other abnormalities.

The patient will then be given a 2- to 5-millicurie dose of ^{131}I; imaging follows approximately 48 to 72 hours later. Frequently, there is a small remnant of normal thyroid tissue or possibly regional or distant metastasis. If there is significant tumor burden, the patient will need to be admitted to the hospital by Nuclear Regulatory Commission regulations for high dose ^{131}I therapy. High dose, by definition, is greater than 30 mCi [131]I. If there is only a small remnant of normal thyroid, some have advocated an outpatient approach of less than 30 millicuries in an attempt to eradicate the small remnant of tissue and to decrease hospital costs. This may be a good approach, but additional doses may be necessary to ablate these small remnants. If a tumor burden is large, the patient will need much larger doses as an inpatient. Hospitalization in a private room will usually be 2 to 3 days, and the patient is encouraged to be well hydrated and to urinate frequently. When the patient is ready to be discharged, a repeat whole body ^{131}I scan is performed to see if the biodistribution has changed from that of the initial evaluation. The patient can be discharged when radiation exposure is less than 5 mrem/hour at 1 m distance.

The patient should remain off thyroid supplements for an additional 3 to 5 days after hospitalization, continue to drink abundant fluids, and urinate frequently as the patient will be significantly radioactive for at least a week after ablation. The patient can then be placed on thyroid supplements.

An additional advantage to this approach is that serum thyroglobulin levels can be measured after a patient has received a subtotal-total thyroidectomy, and with appropriate ablation therapy, the patient is athyroid. If the thyroglobulin levels rise, this indicates disease recurrence. Some authors suggest using ^{131}I therapy with thyroglobulin greater than 8 ng/ml even if the ^{131}I whole-body scan is negative. This monitoring can only be accomplished in the patient who has received complete ablation as patients who have a lobectomy without radioiodine will have normal circulating thyroglobulin levels.

The risks associated with high dose radioiodine are minimal but cumulative. There is some suggestion that ^{131}I in the 100 to 200 mCi range may induce a second malignancy in the form of leukemia or bladder cancer or, less likely, breast carcinoma. As the ablative doses increase, this risk of second malignancy increases. The total bone marrow exposure with a 100 millicurie dosing is less than 50 rems, although this dose may occasionally produce transitory pancytopenia and, as such, a complete blood count is probably indicated several weeks after ablation. Upper limits of safe dose of ^{131}I administration are empirically derived to be exposure to less than 200 rem with whole-body retention of less than 120 mCi at 48 hours; lung retention of less than 80 mCi at 48 hours is the upper safe limit for development of pulmonary fibrosis. However, there was one report of a death associated with ablation in a patient who had extensive pulmonary metastasis, received a high dose of radioiodine, and developed pneumonitis and respiratory failure.

The total dose received in patients who have bone and brain metastasis in association with follicular carcinoma is minimal, and in these cases the external beam radiation should be used.

It is recommended that the patient have a repeat whole body ^{131}I scan 6 to 12 months after ablation. The patient must again be taken off thyroid supplements, and the TSH level ideally should be greater than 50; no contrast should be given to the patient 4 to 6 weeks before imaging. If the whole body ^{131}I scan is completely unremarkable, with no thyroid remnants or metastasis, the patient can be followed up yearly. Once several scans are negative, scanning can be done every 3 to 5 years or serum thyroglobulin levels can be followed.

If there is a question about skeletal metastasis, the whole body ^{131}I scan can be positive for skeletal metastasis, but it assumes that the tumor burden within the skeleton will be large enough to accumulate enough radioiodine to be visualized with the scan. Frequently, this is not the case and since metastasis associated with primary thyroid malignancies are, for the most part, lytic, a bone scan is of limited value. Therefore, in both the diagnosis and treatment of skeletal metastasis from a well-differentiated thyroid carcinoma, treatment with ^{131}I has a limited role. In these cases palliative external beam radiation is usually performed.

SUGGESTED READING

Ain KB: Strategies for managing differentiated thyroid cancer. IM January:45–58, 1996

| APPENDIX 23 | # Palliative Systemic Treatment of Disseminated Adrenocortical Carcinoma |

Renato V. La Rocca

o,p-DDD (Mitotane): start at 2 to 6 g/day and titrate up to 6 to 12 g/day, in divided doses; provide replacement doses of hydrocortisone

Possible role for achieving serum mitotane levels >14 µg/mL; levels > 20 µg/mL are associated with increased neurotoxicity

Dose reduction for clinical toxicity may be necessary over the long term.

Adverse reactions:

Gastrointestinal (80%): anorexia, nausea, diarrhea

Neuromuscular (50%): headache, depression, tremors, confusion

Skin rash (15%): Abnormalities in platelet function (see Ch. 32.)

Protocols for Treatment of Endocrine Cancers (Carcinoid Tumors and Metastatic Gastrinoma)

APPENDIX 24

Ivana Pavlić-Renar

SOMATOSTATIN ANALOGUES

A.

1. Octreotide: start at a dose of 150 to 500 μg subcutaneously (SC) tid (half life: 2 to 3 hours after SC administration)
   Evaluate in 3 months; escalate dose according to treatment response

2. Follow-up and evaluation of a response: measure biochemical marker(s) present at diagnosis q 3 months (e.g., 5-HIAA or serotonin for carcinoid tumor) + routine laboratory tests (complete blood count, SMA-18; check glucose levels periodically)

Gall blader ultrasound q 6 months (biliary stones reported as a side effect)
Thyroid function test as clinically needed (hypothyroidism reported as a side effect)
Electrocardiogram as clinically indicated (bradycardia reported as a side effect)
Definitions of a response:
   a. *Biochemical*
      Normalization: complete response
      Reduction of 50% or more: partial response
      Increase of 25% or more: progression
   b. *Radiologic:*
      Tumor size estimated as the calculated product of two perpendicular diameters of the two largest metastases
      Disappearance of tumor: complete response
      Reduction of 50% or more in tumor size: partial response
      Increase of 25% or more in tumor size: progression
   c. *Symptom relief:* analogue visual scales for flushing and diarrhea severity
   d. No need for additional treatment routinely. Pancreatic enzymes in persistent steatorrhea, loperamide for diarrhea, hypoglycemic agents for hyperglycemia if present on follow-up.
B. *Somatuline* (less experience than with octreotide) Starting dose: 2250 μg tid; escalation possible to 9,000 μg tid

STREPTOZOCIN

Height___   Weight___   BSA___m^2

1. Complete blood count (CBC), SMA-18 before chemotherapy

2. *Antiemetics:*
   a. Granisetron 2 mg po (or 1 mg IV) or ondansetron 32 mg IV piggy back 15 to 30 minutes before treatment
   b. Dexamethasone 20 mg po

3. Streptozocin (500 mg/m^2) = ___ mg in 100 mL normal saline IV over 15 minutes for 5 days

4. Prescribe antiemetics on as needed basis for nausea/vomiting:

   a. Prochloperazine spansules 15 mg po bid or capsules 10 mg po qid
   b. Lorazepam 1 to 2 mg IV or po q 6 to 8 hours prn for anxiety or nausea/vomiting

5. May reduce a dose by 50 to 75% in patients with renal failure (creatinine clearance < 25 ml/min); repeat a cycle q 6 weeks until maximal benefit or dose-limiting toxicity

APPENDIX 25

Protocols for Treatment of Breast Cancer

Steven C. Goldstein
Karen K. Fields
Daniel M. Sullivan

Height___   Weight___   BSA___

ADJUVANT OR INITIAL TREATMENT OF METASTATIC DISEASE

AC (ADRIAMYCIN + CYCLOPHOSPHAMIDE) (Q 21 DAYS X 4 CYCLES)

Chemotherapy:
Doxorubicin (Adriamycin) (60 mg/m^2) = ___mg IV push through free flowing (FF) IV on day 1
Cyclophosphamide (600 mg/m^2) = ___mg IV push through FFIV or as 100 mL normal saline (NS) infusion over 15 minutes on day 1.

Antiemetics prior to chemotherapy:
1. Granisetron 2 mg po (or 1 mg IV) or, ondansetron 32 mg IV piggy back 15 to 30 minutes before treatment
2. Dexamethasone 20 mg po

Antiemetics prn:
1. Prochloperazine spansules 15 mg po bid
2. Lorazepam 1 to 2 mg po or IV q 6 to 8 hours prn for anxiety or nausea/vomiting

Laboratory:
Complete blood count (CBC) and SMA-18 before each cycle (adjust the dose as necessary; see Appendix 2)
Other measures:
Assess carefully cardiac status before each treatment (see Appendix 2)
Encourage increased oral fluid intake (~ 3 L/day) for 48 hours after chemotherapy

CMF (Q 21 DAYS X 6 TO 8 CYCLES)

Chemotherapy:
Cyclophosphamide (600 mg/m^2) = ___ mg IV push through FFIV or as 100 mL NS infusion over 15 minutes day 1
or Cyclophosphamide (100 mg/m^2) tablets = ___mg po on days 1 through 14
Methotrexate (40 mg/m^2) = ___mg IV through FFIV day 1
5-FU (fluorouracil) (600 mg/m^2) = ___mg IV through FFIV day 1

Antiemetics prior to chemotherapy:
1. Granisetron 2 mg po (or 1 mg IV) or, ondansetron 32 mg IV piggy back 15 to 30 minutes before treatment
2. Dexamethasone 20 mg po

Antiemetics prn:
1. Prochloperazine spansules 15 mg po bid
2. Lorazepam 1 to 2 mg po or IV q 6 to 8 hours prn for anxiety or nausea/vomiting

Laboratory:
CBC and SMA-18 before each cycle (adjust the dose as necessary; see Appendix 2)
Other measures:
Prevention of alopecia: Kold Kap application 15 minutes before cyclophosphamide; leave on throughout chemotherapy and 30 minutes after chemotherapy
Encourage increased oral fluid intake (~ 3 L/day) for 48 hours after chemotherapy

SEQUENTIAL ADRIA/CMF

Chemotherapy
Adriamycin (75 mg/m²) = ___ mg IV push through FF IV q 21 days for 4 cycles
then CMF q 21 days for 8 cycles given as:
Cyclophosphamide (600 mg/m²) = ___ mg IV push through FFIV or as 100 mL NS infusion over 15 minutes day 1
Methotrexate (40 mg/m²) = ___ mg IV push through FFIV day 1
5-FU (fluorouracil) (600 mg/m²) = ___ mg IV thru FFIV day 1

Antiemetics prior to chemotherapy:
1. Granisetron 2 mg po (or 1 mg IV) or, ondansetron 32 mg IV piggy back 15 to 30 minutes before treatment
2. Dexamethasone 20 mg po

Antiemetics prn:
1. Prochloperazine spansules 15 mg po bid
2. Lorazepam 1 to 2 mg po or IV q 6 to 8 hours prn for anxiety or nausea/vomiting

Laboratory:
CBC and SMA-18 before each cycle (adjust the dose as necessary; see Appendix 2)
Other measures:
Assess carefully cardiac status before each treatment (see Appendix 2)
Encourage increased oral fluid intake (~ 3 L/day) for 48 hours after chemotherapy

CAF (Q 21 DAYS X 4 TO 6 CYCLES)

Chemotherapy:
Doxorubicin (Adriamycin) (60 mg/m²) = ___ mg IV push through FFIV on day 1
Cyclophosphamide (600 mg/m²) = ___ mg IV push through FFIV or as 100 mL NS infusion over 15 minutes on day 1
5-FU (fluorouracil) (600 mg/m²) = ___ mg IV through FFIV day 1

Antiemetics prior to chemotherapy:
1. Granisetron 2 mg po (or 1 mg iv) or, ondansetron 32 mg IV piggy back 15 to 30 minutes before treatment
2. Dexamethasone 20 mg po

Antiemetics prn:
1. Prochloperazine spansules 15 mg po bid
2. Lorazepam 1 to 2 mg po or IV q 6 to 8 hours prn for anxiety or nausea/vomiting

Laboratory:
CBC and SMA-18 before each cycle (adjust the dose as necessary; see Appendix 2)
Other measures:
Assess carefully cardiac status before each treatment (see Appendix 2)
Encourage increased oral fluid intake (~ 3 L/day) for 48 hours after chemotherapy

SALVAGE TREATMENT

a. *Taxol (Paclitaxel) (q 3 weeks)*
Premedicate with:
Dexamethasone 20 mg po 12 hrs and 6 hrs before Taxol
Benadryl (diphenhydramine) 50 mg IV 30 min before Taxol
Zantac (ranitidine) 50 mg IV 30 minutes before Taxol or Tagamet (cimetidine) 300 mg IV 30 minutes before Taxol
Taxol (150–250 mg/m²; usually 175 mg/m²) = ___mg in 500 mL NS IV over 3 hours via pump

b. *Navelbine (30 mg/m²)* = ___ mg in 100 mL NS through FF IV to run over 10 minutes
Antiemetics: prochloperazine 10 mg po q 6 hours prn
Repeat q week for 4 cycles, then 1 week break (reevaluate)
CBC before each chemotherapy

c. *NFL*
Chemotherapy
Novantrone (mitoxantrone) (12 mg/m²) = ___ mg in 50 mL NS to run IV over 10 minutes day 1
Leucovorin (300 mg/m²) = ___ mg in 100 ml of NS to run IV over 2 hours on days 1–3
5-FU (350 mg/m²) = ___ mg one hour into leucovorin infusion, over 3–5 min

Antiemetics (before chemotherapy)
Prochlorperazine 15 mg po bid
Dexamethasone 20 mg po
Laboratory:
CBC and SMA-18 before each cycle (adjust the dose as necessary; see Appendix 2)

Other measures:
Assess carefully cardiac status before each treatment (see Appendix 2)
Assess for signs and symptoms of stomatitis/diarrhea
Encourage increased oral fluid intake (~ 3 L/day) for 48 hours after chemotherapy

APPENDIX TABLE 25-1   COMMONLY USED ANTIHORMONAL AGENTS

Drug	Dose
Tamoxifen (Nolvadex)	10 mg po BID (20 mg po qD)
Anastrozole (Arimidex)	1 mg po qD
Megestrol acetate (Megace)	40 mg po QID
Aminoglutethimide (Cytadren)	250 mg po QID with hydrocortisone 40 mg qD
Diethylstilbestrol (DES)	15 mg po qD
LH-RH analogues (Zoladex, Lupron)	SQ or SQ depot monthly
Fluoxymesterone (Halotestin)	10–20 mg po qD

Legend: Frequently employed antihormonal drugs and usual doses are listed. Tamoxifen is the most commonly used antihormonal drug in the adjuvant setting but is also useful in patients with estrogen receptor-positive tumors in the metastatic setting. Other drugs listed are also active and, since each drug represents a different class of antihormonal agents, can be useful in succession especially in treating patients with estrogen receptor-positive tumors with primarily bone, soft tissue, and lung metastases. A treatment strategy in appropriate patients with metastatic breast cancer responding to an initial course of antihormonal therapy such as tamoxifen is to change to an alternative antihormonal agent at the time of progression. Response rates to such salvage therapies are similar among the various agents. Response rates up to 50% have been reported, although, in general, the chances of response diminish with each subsequent drug. Decisions concerning the number of trials of different agents should be based on the patient's performance status and extent of disease. Generally after failing 2 to 3 agents, further responses are unlikely. Common side effects are related to the antiestrogen effects of these drugs. Flareup of bone pain can also be seen at the initiation of therapy in occasional patients with extensive bony involvement including the development of transient hypercalcemia in some patients, especially following therapy with tamoxifen or DES. Additionally, prolonged administration of tamoxifen has been associated with an increased risk of developing endometrial cancer and therefore its use should be limited to 5 years or less. The goals of antihormonal therapy are curative in the adjuvant setting but palliative in the metastatic setting. The key reasoning principle is that patients with estrogen receptor-positive tumors are likely to benefit in both the adjuvant and metastatic settings from antihormonal therapy and, given that these agents are relatively free of side effects, the potential benefits justify the use of these agents. The evidence to support the use of these agents is generally level I and II.

SUGGESTED READING

Henderson IC: *Endocrine Therapy of Metastatic Breast Cancer*. In: Harris JR, Hellman S, Henderson IC and Kinne DW (eds). Breast Diseases. Second Edition. JB Lippincott Company. Philadelphia. pp 559–603 (1991).

SUMMARY

This appendix summarizes the dosing schemes for some of the most commonly used chemotherapy regimens in the treatment of breast cancer. See text for indications and risk/benefit analysis. A comparative study to assess the relative efficacy of different high-dose regimens has not been performed.

In light of the potential for cardiotoxicity of anthracycline-containing regimens, one should consider obtaining a baseline MUGA evaluations in patients who ultimately may be considered eligible for high-dose therapy, patients who have received greater than 300 mg/m² Adriamycin, or patients with a clinical history suggesting cardiac disease (see Appendix 2).

Further clinical studies are required to define optimally the use of cardioprotective agents such as Dexrazoxane (Zinecard, Pharmacia) in the management of patients with breast cancer receiving anthracycline therapy beyond 300 mg/m².

APPENDIX 26

Protocols for Treatment of Ovarian Cancer

TAXOL (PACLITAXEL) -CISPLATIN

Height____   Weight____   BSA =____m²

1. *Day 1 laboratory tests:* Complete blood count (CBC), SMA 18, 12-hour creatinine clearance

2. 12 hours before Taxol: dexamethasone 20 mg po or IV 6 hours before Taxol

3. 1,000 ml D5½ normal saline (NS) with 20 mEq/L KCl + 1 g MgSO₄/L @ 150 mL/hr; start immediately upon admission (decrease rate to 100 mL/hour during Taxol administration)

4. *Premedication:* 30 minutes before Taxol: Benadryl (diphenhydramine) 50 mg +Zantac (ranitidine) 50 mg; mix in 50 mL NS and infuse over 10 minutes (Tagamet [cimetidine] 300 mg IV may be given instead of Zantac)

5. *Taxol* (135–210 mg/m²) = ____mg IV in 500 ml NS over 3 hours via pump

6. 30 minutes before cisplatin, premedicate with

   a. Granisetron 2 mg po (or 1 mg IV) or, ondansetron 32 mg IV piggy back 15 to 30 minutes before treatment
   b. Dexamethasone 20 mg po
   c. Mannitol 25% 50 mL IV over 10 minutes (must be filtered)
   d. Cisplatin (100 mg/m²) = ____mg in 250 mL NS IV over 1 hour
   e. Mannitol 20% 500 mL over 3 hours after cisplatin

At 6 AM the morning after chemotherapy, begin delayed-emesis antiemetics (see also Ch. 54 for an alternative protocol):

   a. Prochloperazine spansules 15 mg po bid
   b. Lorazepam 1 to 2 mg IV or po q 6 to 8 hours prn for anxiety or nausea/vomiting

7. SMA-7 and Mg²⁺ day 2

8. Continue hydration fluids until able to take oral fluids (if chemotherapy given as outpatient, IVF is administered @ 150 to 250 mL/hour [1000 mL D5½ NS with 20 mEq/L KCl & 1 g MgSO₄/L])

9. Repeat q 3 weeks for 6 cycles (see Ch. 37) (adjust dose according to CBC and creatinine clearance; see Appendix 2.)

TAXOL-CARBOPLATINUM

Height____   Weight____   BSA = ____m²

1. Day 1: CBC, SMA-18

2. Calculate AUC using Calvert formula (see Appendix 2, Table 2-6)

3. 12 hours & 6 hours before Taxol: Dexamethasone 20 mg po or IV

4. Premedication: 30 minutes before Taxol: Benadryl (diphenhydramine) 50 mg + Zantac (ranitidine) 50 mg; mix in 50 ml NS and infuse over 10 minutes

5. Taxol (135 to 175 mg/m²) = ____mg IV in 500 mL NS over 3 hours via pump

6. Carboplatin (AUC 5–7.5) = ____mg IV in 250 mL NS over 1 hour

7. Repeat every 3 to 4 weeks for 6 cycles (see Ch. 37) (adjust dose according to CBC and creatinine clearance; see Appendix 2.)

APPENDIX TABLE 26-1   OTHER COMMONLY USED CHEMOTHERAPY REGIMENS

Epithelial Ovarian Cancers

PC	Cisplatin (75–100 mg/m²) Cytoxan (650–1000 mg/m²)	Q 3 weeks
CC	Carboplatin (AUC = 5–7) Cytoxan (600 mg/m²)	Q 4 weeks
PT	Cisplatin (75–100 mg/m²) Taxol (135–210 mg/m²)	Q 3 weeks
CT	Carboplatin (AUC 5–7.5) Taxol (135–175 mg/m²)	Q 3–4 weeks

Germ Cell and Sex Cord-Stromal Tumors

VAC	Vincristine	1–1.5 mg/m² on day 1 every 4 weeks
	Actinomycin-D	0.5 mg/day for 5 days every 4 weeks
	Cytoxan	150 mg/m²/day for 5 days every 4 weeks

APPENDIX 27

Combination Chemotherapy for High-Risk and Advanced Malignant Trophoblastic Disease

Height___   Weight___   BSA___m²

1. *Day 1 Laboratory tests:* Complete blood count (CBC) with differential, SMA 18

2. *Antiemetics:*

   a. Granisetron 2 mg po (or 1 mg IV) or, ondansetron 32 mg IV piggy back 15–30 min prior to treatment; dactinomycin most emetogenic)

   b. Dexamethasone 20 mg po

   c. Prochloperazine 10 mg po qid prn for nausea/vomiting

   d. Lorazepam 1 to 2 mg po or IV q 6 to 8 hours prn for anxiety or nausea/vomiting

3. VP16 (Etoposide) (100 mg/m²) = ___mg IV in 250 ml normal soline (NS) @ 2 mg/min to avoid rate-dependent hypotension, days 1 and 2

4. Methotrexate (100 mg/m²) = ___mg IV bolus, day 1 then

   Methotrexate (200 mg/m²) = ___mg IV in 500 mL NS as 12-hour infusion day 1

5. Dactinomycin (300 mg/m²) = ___mg IV bolus on days 1 and 2

6. Folinic acid 15 mg po or intramusculorly (IM) q 12 hours × 4 doses starting 24 hours after methotrexate bolus infusion

7. On day 7 of cycle: CBC with differential, SMA 18

8. Cyclophosphamide (Cytoxan) (600 mg/m²) = ___mg IV in 100 mL of NS over 15 minutes on day 7

9. Vincristine (1 mg/m²) = ___mg IV push day 7

10. If no toxicity by laboratory tests and clinical examination, begin next cycle on day 15

11. Continue treatment until 3 consecutive normal hCG titers are achieved. Administer 2 courses of therapy after attainment of normal hCG levels.

SINGLE-AGENT CHEMOTHERAPY REGIMENS FOR NONMETASTATIC AND GOOD-PROGNOSIS METASTATIC TROPHOBLASTIC DISEASE

Methotrexate-folinic acid (for orders see below):

        Methotrexate 1.0 mg/kg IM days 1, 3, 5, and 7

        Folinic acid 0.1 mg/kg IM days 2, 4, 6, and 8

5-day regimens:

        Actinomycin D 0.4–0.8 mg/m² IV daily for 5 days

        CBC, platelet count, liver function tests (SGOT, SGPT) daily

        OR

        Methotrexate 16 mg/m² daily for 5 days

        CBC, platelet daily

        OR

        Etoposide 100 mg/m² po daily for 5 days

        Repeat cycles every 2 weeks if toxicity resolved

        Treat for 1 to 3 cycles past normal hCG titer

Pulse Regimens:

        Actinomycin D 1.25 mg/m² IV every 2 weeks

        OR

        Methotrexate 40 mg/m² IM weekly

        Repeat cycles every 2 weeks if toxicity resolved

        Treat for 1 to 3 cycles past normal hCG titer

Protocol with methotrexate (MTX) – folinic acid

1. *Laboratory tests*: day 1: CBC with differential, SMA 18; CBC before day 7 dose

2. *Methotrexate (1 mg/kg)* = ___mg IM days 1, 3, 5, and 7

3. *Folinic acid (0.1 mg/kg)* = ___mg IM days 2, 4, 6, and 8 (exactly 24 hours after each methotrepxaote dose)

4. *Premedication:*

Antiemetics given prn (e.g., prochloperazine 10 mg po qid prn nausea/vomiting)

5. hCG levels in 2 weeks

6. Repeat cycle:___ (A second course is given if hCG titer does not fall by one log within 18 days, if the HCG level plateaus for more than 2 weeks, or becomes reelevated, or if new sites of disease develop)

    CBC with differential, SMA-18 before chemotherapy (adjust the dose according to Appendix 2)

APPENDIX
28

Protocols for Treatment of Metastatic Renal Cancer

IMMUNOTHERAPY WITH INTERLEUKIN-2 (IL-2)

Admit to TCU (transitional care unit) or other intensive-monitoring unit

1. Strict input and output measurement; call physician if urine output < 500 mL/8 hrs

2. Daily 6 AM weight

3. *Vital signs:* q 4 hours, if temp > 38.5°, respiration rate (RR) > 30 min; blood pressure (BP) <100 mmHg systolic, BP >100 diastolic mmHg, call physician

4. Electrocardiogram q AM

5. *Day 1 laboratory tests*: Complete blood count (CBC) with differential, SMA 18

6. *Daily laboratory tests:* CBC with differential, SMA 18 and magnesium levels

7. PT/PTT day 2 and day 9 of cycle

8. 1000 ml of D5W 1/2 normal saline (NS) with 20 mEq/L KCl and 500 mg MgSO4/L @ 150 mL/hr for 6 hrs before first dose of IL-2; when IL-2 initiated, decrease IV to 40 mL/hr

9. Dopamine drip for renal perfusion @ 2 µg/kg/min when IL-2 initiated; discontinue drip 6 hours after IL-2 is completed

10. IL-2 720,000 I U/kg = ___IU q 8 hours over 15 minutes for 15 doses (mix in 100 ml D5W with 0.4 mL of albumin; no filter)

11. Acetaminophen 650 mg po q 4 hrs A T C (around the clock)

12. Indomethacin 50 mg po q 8 hours A T C

13. Ranitidine (Zantac) 150 mg po q 12 hrs

14. No steroids!

15. Granisetron 2 mg po or 1 mg IV before IL-2

16. Prochlorperazine (Compazine) 10 mg po or IV q 4 to 6 hours prn "breakthrough" nausea/vomiting

17. Lorazepam (Ativan) 1mg IV q 8 hrs during IL-2, start before IL-2, then give 0.5 mg IV q 4 to 6 hrs prn anxiety or nausea/vomiting

18. Eucerin lotion at bedside, encourage use, at least bid, to take supply home

19. Basis soap @ bedside

20. Lanolin to lips prn

21. Lomotil 2 tabs po q 6 hrs prn diarrhea

22. Demerol (meperidine) 25 mg IV q 4 to 6 hrs prn chills

23. Atarax (hydroxyzine) 50 mg po q 6 hrs prn itching

24. O_2 sats during first 24 hours; then prn

25. Rest 10 days & repeat once

26. Repeat cycle every 10 weeks if stable or responding disease

CHEMO-IMMUNO-BIO-THERAPY WITH INTERFERON, INTERLEUKIN-2, AND 5-FU*

1. Admit to intensive care unit

2. Course #:___ Height___ Weight___   BSA___

3. Diagnosis: metastatic renal cell carcinoma

4. Strict input and output and daily weights

5. Vital signs q 4 hours

6. Regular diet

7. Inform physician when temperature >38.5°C; respiration rate >30/min

   BP <100 mmHg systolic or > 100 mmHg diastolic

8. CBC, Chem 18, Mg levels daily

9. IV: D5½ NS with 20 mEq/L KCl and 500 mg $MgSO_4$/L at rate of 150 mL/hour

10. IL-2 (6 million IU/m^2) = ___ IU (mix in 100 ml D5W with 0.4 ml of albumin, no filter) IV over 24 hours daily, days 1 to 5

11. 5-FU (600 mg/m^2) = ___ mg IV over 24 hours, days 1 to 5

    Administer 5 FU and IL-2 through double lumen central catheter

12. Interferon (4×10^6 units/m^2) = ___ units sq days 1 to 5

13. Renal dose dopamine 2 μg/kg/min when IL-2 is initiated.

    Discontinue dopamine 6 hours after last IL-2 is finished

14. Acetaminophen 650 mg po when starting IL-2 and q 4 hours during infusion × 5 days, to include one dose following completion of IL-2

15. Naprosyn (naproxen) 250 mg po q 12 hours

16. Zantac (ranitidine) 150 mg po q 12 hours

17. Mylanta 30 ml po q 4 hours prn

18. Kytril (granisetron) 1 mg IV qd before therapy

19. Reglan (metoclopramide) 10 mg po/IV + Benadryl (diphenhydramine) 50 mg IV before therapy, then prn q-6 h

20. Ativan (lorazepam) 1 to 2 mg po or IV q 6 to 8 hours during IL-2 prn anxiety or nausea /vomiting

21. Compazine (prochlorperazine) 10 mg IV or po q 4 to 6 hours prn nausea/vomiting

22. Atarax (hydroxizine) 25 to 50 mg po q 6 hours prn itching

23. Eucerin lotion at bedside, encourage its use; at least bid; to take supply home

24. Lomotil 2 tabs po q 6 h prn diarrhea

25. Demerol (meperidine) 25 mg IVPB Q 4 to 6 hours prn chills

26. No steroids!

27. Repeat q 4 weeks until progression of a disease or intolerable toxicity

Preliminary results as reported by MD Anderson group (ASCO 1994): Overall response rate 47% (95% C.I 24–71%); CR-3 pts (16%) pts, PR-6 pts (31%). Responses by sites: lung-6 (42%, CR-1 PR-5), soft tissue-3/4 (75%, CR-1, PR-2), bone-1/3 (33%, CR-1), lymph nodes-2/6 (33%, CR-1, PR-1), liver 0/3. Grade III-IV toxicity included stomatitis (26%), neutropenia (16%), skin (11%). CNS toxicity composed of confusion (5%) and hallucinations (26%). Gram + bacteremia occurred in 11/77 (14.2%) courses. One patient had a sudden cardiac death.

———————————

*There is no convincing data to suggest that combined treatment is superior over single-agent IL-2 or interferon. The protocol for combined treatment is included because it appears to show higher responses to single agent therapies, that usually do not produce tumor regression in more than 15–20% cases (level IV evidence).

APPENDIX 29

Protocol for Treatment of Bladder Cancer

MVAC

Height___   Weight___   BSA___

Hydration: 1,000 mL D5½ NS with 20 mEq/L KCl + 1 g of MgSO$_4$/L to run at 150 mL/hr continuously

Labs: CBC/SMA 18, 12 hr creatinine clearance — start immediately on admission. Repeat CBC and SMA-18 on days 14, 21 and prior to each new cycle of chemotherapy.

Antiemetics: Prior to cisplatinum:

1. granisetron 2 mg po (or 1 mg IV) (or, ondansetron 32 mg IV piggy back 15–30 min prior to treatment)

2. dexamethasone 20 mg po.

Followed by protocol for prevention of delayed emesis

3. prochlorperazine spansules 15 mg po bid

4. lorazepam 1–2 mg IV q 6–8 h prn anxiety or nausea/vomiting

5. dexamethasone 8 mg po bid for 2 days, tapered to 4 mg po bid for 2 days

Chemotherapy (for dose modification see Appendix 2):

Methotrexate (30 mg/m^2) = ___ mg IV push on days 1, 15 & 22 (day 15 & 22 will be arranged outpatient)
Vinblastine (3 mg/m^2) = ___ mg IV push on days day 2, 15 & 22 (day 15 & 22 will be arranged outpatient)
Adriamycin (30 mg/m^2) = ___ mg IV push on day 2
Cisplatinum* (70 mg/m^2) = ___ mg IV in 100 mL NS administer over 30 min on day 2
Mannitol 25% 50 ml IV pre-cisplatinum
Mannitol 20% 500 ml IV over 3 hr post cisplatinum
Repeat every 28 days (see Ch. 44)

*If (on day 2) Carboplatin is used instead of cisplatinum, administer at a dose of 200 mg/m^2 IV in 250 ml of NS over 1 hour or use AUC (area under curve) of 6 according to nomogram shown in Appendix 2.

<table>
<tr><td>

APPENDIX

30

</td><td>

Protocols for Treatment of Prostate Cancer

</td></tr>
</table>

Renato V. La Rocca

Chemohormonal Regimens in Hormone Refractory Prostate Cancer

1. Estramustine 280–420 mg po in 2–3 divided doses

Avoid milk products when taking estramustine so as not to impair its absorption
Prochlorperazine 10 mg bid prn nausea/vomiting

2. Estramustine 10 mg/kg po in 3 divided doses for 6 weeks, then off for 2 weeks

Vinblastine 4 mg/m^2 IV q week for 6 weeks, then off for 2 weeks
Avoid milk products when taking estramustine so as not to impair its absorption; hold vinblastine for ANC < 2000/uL or a platelet count < 75,000/uL

3. Oral estramustine 15 mg/kg/d in four divided doses on days 1 to 21

Oral VP-16 50 mg/M^2/d in two divided doses on days 1 to 21
Avoid milk products when taking estramustine so as not to impair its absorption; hold both meds for ANC <1,000/uL or platelet count <50,000/uL

4. Ketoconazole 400 mg po tid
Adriamycin 20 mg/m^2 IV (most often via 24 hr continuous infusion) q week (often for 6 weeks in a row then off for 2 weeks)
Add hydrocortisone 30 mg po at 8 am, 20 mg po at 8 pm.
Avoid H$_2$-antagonists while taking ketoconazole; ascorbic acid (250 mg) po can be administered simultaneously with ketoconazole to enhance its absorption.
Limit cumulative dose of adriamycin to 400 mg/m^2
Hold adriamycin for ANC < 1,500/uL or platelet count < 100,000/uL.
— Prochlorperazine 10 mg po prior to Adriamycin and prn nausea/vomiting
— Metoclopramide 30 mg po qid prior to Adriamycin and prn nausea/vomiting

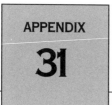

APPENDIX 31

Protocols for Treatment of Metastatic Penile/Urethral Cancer

HT___ WT___ BSA___-m²

1. *Day 1:* CBC/SMA 18/ 12 hr. creatinine clearance

2. *Daily Labs:* SMA-7 and Mg levels

3. Methotrexate (200 mg/m²) = ___mg IV in 50 ml of NS over 30 min *on days 1, 15 & 22*

4. Bleomycin (20 units/m²) = ___ units IV in 1,000 ml of NS as 24-hr continuous infusion *days 2–6*

5. Mannitol 12.5 grams (50 ml of 25% solution) IV before each Cisplatin dose

6. *Antiemetics:* Prior to cisplatinum:

   a. granisetron 2 mg po (or 1 mg iv) (or, ondansetron 32 mg IV piggy back 15–30 min prior to treatment)
   b. dexamethasone 20 mg po

Followed by protocol for prevention of delayed emesis:

   c. Prochlorperazine spansules 15 mg po bid
   d. Lorazepam 1–2 mg po or IV q 6–8 h prn anxiety or nausea/vomiting
   e. Dexamethasone 8 mg po bid × 2 days, tapered to 4 mg po bid × 2 days

7. Cisplatin (20 mg/m²) = ___mg IV in 100 ml NS over 1 hour on *days 2–6*

8. Leucovorin 25 mg po every 6 hrs × 72 hours (if unable to take orally — administer IV)

9. Repeat every—days until progression of tumor or unacceptable toxicity (adjust dose according to Appendix 2)

APPENDIX 32

Protocols for Treatment of Testicular Cancer

INITIAL TREATMENT PROTOCOL

PE±B (EINHORN PROTOCOLs)

HT___   WT___   BSA___ = m²

1. Day 1 Labs: CBC with diff/ SMA-18/ 12 hr. creat. clearance/αFP/βhCG

2. Days 2–5 Labs: SMA-7 & Mg levels (while in hospital)

3. 1,000 mL D5½ NS with 20 mEq/L KCl and 1 gm MgSO₄/L @ 150 mL/hr continuously (start upon admission)

4. *Premeds*: dexamethasone 20 mg po prior to ifosfamide daily 1–5; granisetron 2 mg po prior to ifosfamide daily 1–5 (or, ondansetron 32 mg IV piggy back 15–30 min prior to treatment); prochlorperazine 10 mg po or iv q 4–6 hr prn "breakthrough" nausea/vomiting

5. Mannitol 25% 50 mL IV daily prior to cisplatinum

6. If creatinine clearance > 60 mL/min: *Platinol* (Cisplatinum)(20 mg/m²/day) = ___mg IV in 100 mL NS over 30 min days 1–5

7. *VP-16* (Etoposide) (100 mg/m²) = ___mg IV in 250 mL NS at rate of ≤ 2 mg/min (to avoid rate-dependent hypotension) Days 1–5

8. *(Blenoxane)* Bleomycin 30 units IV bolus on days 2, 9 & 16 (Total life time dose allowed: 400 units)

9. Administer aceteminophen (Tylenol) 500–1,000 mg po prior to Bleomycin then q 4 h for 2 doses following Bleomycin

10. Repeat every 3 weeks for 4 cycles if CBC, SMA-18 within acceptable limits (If prior XRT or granulocytopenia & fever after earlier dose of VP-16, then reduce the dose by 20%; see Appendix 2 for further details on dose adjustment)

11. Obtain αFP/βhCG prior to each cycle

(Adapted from N Eng J Med 316: 1435–1440, 1987.)

SALVAGE REGIMEN VIP (VP-16, IFOSFAMIDE, CISPLATINUM)— REPEAT Q 21 DAYS FOR 4 CYCLES

HT___   WT___   BSA___ = m²

1. Day 1 Labs: CBC (complete blood count) with differential, SMA 18; 12 hr creatinine clearance

2. Daily Labs (while in hospital): SMA-7 with magnesium levels

3. 1,000 mL of D5½ NS with 20 mEq/L KCl and 1 gm MgSO₄/L to run at 150 mL/hr continuously

4. VP-16 (Etoposide) (75 mg/m²/day) = ___mg IV in 250 mL NS to be administered at rate not to exceed 2 mg/min (to avoid rate-dependent hypotension) days 1–5

5. Mesna 400 mg IV bolus on day 1 in 50 mL of NS over 15 minutes prior to start of ifosfamide on day 1; then 1200 mg/day as continuous infusion on days 1–5

6. Dexamethasone 20 mg po prior to ifosfamide daily 1–5; granisetron 2 mg po prior to ifosfamide daily 1–5 (or, ondansetron 32 mg IV piggy back 15–30 min prior to treatment); prochlorperazine 10 mg po or IV q 4–6 hr prn "breakthrough" nausea/vomiting

7. Ifosfamide (1200 mg/m²/day) = ___mg IV in 500–1000 mL NS as continuous infusion on days 1–5

8. Mannitol 25% 50mL IV prior to cisplatinum daily

9. Cisplatinum (20 mg/m²/day) = ___mg IV in 100 mL NS over 30 minutes days 1–5

10. Administer cisplatinum if creatinine clearance > 60 ml/min, SMA-18 and CBC within acceptable range (see Appendix 2 for dose adjustment)

APPENDIX 33

Protocols for Treatment of Brain Tumors

RTOG 90-05 PROTOCOL FOR TREATMENT OF GLIOMA:BCNU + XRT*

HT___   WT___   BSA___m²

1. Day 1 Labs: CBC/SMA 18

2. Thirty minutes prior to chemotherapy premedicate with

   a. granisetron 2 mg po (or 1 mg IV) (or, ondansetron 32 mg IV piggy back 15–30 min prior to treatment)
   b. dexamethasone 20 mg po At 6 am the morning following chemotherapy, begin delayed-emesis antiemetics (see also chapter 54 for an alternative protocol):
   c. prochlorperazine spansules 15 mg po bid
   d. dexamethasone 8 mg po bid for 2 days, tapered to 4 mg po bid for 2 days
   e. lorazepam 1–2 mg IV q 6–8 h prn anxiety or nausea/vomiting

3. BCNU (Carmustine) (80 mg/m²) = ___mg IV in 500 mL NS over 2 hours running through FF (free flowing) fluid of NS (to avoid burning at IV site) daily for 3 days
   Calculate BCNU on actual weight (wt); If wt > 125% ideal body wt (IBW), then maximum BCNU dose is IBW *plus* 25% (Maximum cummulative dose of BCNU is 1,440 mg/m²)

4. XRT per radiation oncology protocol (starting on same day as chemotherapy)

5. Repeat BCNU every 8 weeks X 6 cycles if CBC within acceptable limits and no pulmonary toxicity is noted
   Hematological Dose Modification:

ANC (× 10⁶/L)		Platelets (× 10⁶/L)	Dose (%)
>750	and	>75,000	100%
250–750	or	25–75,000	50%–75%
<250	or	<25,000	10%

6. Chest X-ray every 4 months

7. Neuro examination weekly during treatment; then monthly

PCV PLUS WHOLE BRAIN XRT (WITH HYDREA) FOR GLIOMA*

HT___   WT___   BSA___m²

1. Day 1: CBC/SMA 18

2. Hydrea (Hydroxyurea) = 400 mg/m² po = ___mg every other day of XRT (available as 500 mg capsules)

3. Within 14 days of completion of XRT – give the following:

   A. Lomustine (CCNU) (110 mg/m²) = ___mg po Day 1 (available as 10, 40 and 100 mg capsules)
   B. Procarbazine (Matulane) (60 mg/m²) = ___mg po days 8 to 21 (available as 50 mg capsules) (See Appendix 8 for list of food/drugs to avoid with procarbazine)

---

*Note that PCV regimen was superior to BCNU in a randomized trial following surgery and radiotherapy to patients with anaplastic gliomas leading to longer time to progression and longer survival (Int J Radiol Oncol Biol Phys 18:321, 1990)

    C. Vincristine (Oncovin) (1.4 mg/m²) = ___mg IV on Days 8 and 29 (maximum 2 mg IV per dose)

4. Administer antiemetics on as needed basis for nausea/vomiting (see Chapter 54):

    a. prochlorperazine spansules 15 mg po bid or 10 mg capsules po qid

    b. lorazepam 1–2 mg po q 6–8 h prn anxiety

5. Repeat PCV q 6–8 weeks X 1 year or until tumor progression if CBC, SMA-18 and neurological exam within accpetable limits (See Appendix 2 for details on a dose adjustment)

(Adapted from Int J Rad Onc Biol Phys 18:321–324, 1990, with permission.)

APPENDIX

34

Protocol for Treatment of Osteosarcoma

NEOADJUVANT HIGH DOSE METHOTREXATE (HDMTX) WITH OR WITHOUT VINCRISTINE (VCR)*†

HT___ WT___ BSA___m²

Induction

Weeks 0,1, 2 & 3 HdMTX with Rescue ± Vincristine

1. CBC & SMA-18 Weekly

2. *Hydration* IVF'S: 1,000 mL D5½ NS at 200 mL/hr

3. *Antiemetics*:

   a. Granisetron 2 mg PO (or 1 mg IV) (or, ondansetron 32 mg IV piggy back 15–30 min prior to treatment)
   b. Dexamethasone 20 mg PO
   c. Lorazepam 1–2 mg IV or PO q 6–8 h prn anxiety or nausea/vomiting

4. Sodium bicarbonate (1 mEq/kg) = ___ mEq IV in 100 mL NS over 15 min before HdMTX

5. High dose methotrexate (8–12 g/m²) = ___ g IV in 1000 mL D5W with 1 mEq/kg sodium bicarbonate = ___ mEq over 4 hrs.

6. If randomized to receive Vincristine (1.5 mg/m²) = ___mg IV push 24 hrs post HdMTX (call for antiemetic if needed — none indicated for VCR alone)

7. Oral calcium leucovorin 10 mg po q 6 hrs for 10 doses — starting 20 hours following HdMTX infusion

8. Oral sodium bicarbonate 2–3 mEq/kg/24 hrs in 4 divided doses for 3 days post HdMTX

9. Force fluids to have urine output 1600 mL/m² day 1 and 2,000 mL/m² days 2 & 3

10. Check urine pH post each voiding — If urine pH <7.0 instruct to take additional dose of oral sodium bicarbonate

11. *Lab*: Serum creatinine and methotrexate level daily

12. If the 72 hour MTX level >2.0×10^{-7} M-instruct to take additional oral calcium leukovorin @ same dose for 24 hrs, until MTX level is < 2.0×10^{-7} M

13. If serum creatinine is elevated and MTX level abnormally high on day 1 or 2 following HdMTX admit for IV fluids — also give higher doses of calcium leucovorin, which is calculated by multiplying the usual calcium leukovorin dose by the serum MTX level divided by normal MTX level

    This dose is continued until MTX level is <1.0×10^{-7} M

14. If weekly labs within acceptable limits – repeat above chemoRx at weeks 0, 1, 2 & 3

Week 6 "BCD" (bleomycin, cyclophosphamide, dactinomycin)

1. CBC/SMA 18 prior to chemotherapy

---

*Optimal treatment protocol not identified; physicians are strongly encourage to refer patients to clinical trials/centers with strong interest in the treatment of sarcomas. We present here one protocol which we have used in our practice.

†See Overall Schema of Protocol

2. *Antiemetics*:

    a. Granisetron 2 mg PO (or 1 mg IV) (or, ondansetron 32 mg IV piggy back 15–30 min prior to treatment)

    b. Dexamethasone 20 mg PO

    c. Lorazepam 1–2 mg IV or q 6–8 h prn anxiety or nausea/vomiting

3. Bleomycin (15 units/m²/day) = ___units IV push through freely flowing (FF) IV

Cyclophosphamide (Cytoxan) (600 mg/m²/day) = ___mg IV in 100 mL NS over 30 minutes (if dose > 1000 mg increase dilution to 250 mL NS)

Dactinomycin (600 mg/m²/day) = ___mg IV through FFIV

Weeks 9 & 10

HdMTX (same as Week 0)

Echo or MUGA scan prior to week 11 (starting Adriamycin (see Appendix 2)

Week 11:

Antiemetics:

    a. Granisetron 2 mg PO (or 1 mg IV) (or, ondansetron 32 mg IV piggy back 15–30 min prior to treatment)

    b. Dexamethasone 20 mg PO

Adriamycin (30 mg/m²/day) = ___mg IV thru FFJV daily for 3 days

Check CBC prior to day 1 chemotherapy

Week 14 & 15:

HdMTX (Same as Week 0)

*Break for surgery — recovery

Maintenance Treatment

Start maintenance course A group vs. B group pending grade of sarcoma.

OSTEOSARCOMA (GRADE I/II) MAINTENANCE REGIMEN A

Week 0	Adria/Platinol	
Week 3	Adria/Platinol	} Repeat total 3 cycles
Week 6	BCD	

Week 0: Echocardiogram Prior to Starting Maintenance

1. CBC/SMA18/12 hr. creatinine clearance

2. *Antiemetics*:

    a. Granisetron 2 mg po (or 1 mg iv) (or, ondansetron 32 mg IV piggy back 15–30 min prior to treatment)

    b. Dexamethasone 20 mg po

    c. Lorazepam 1–2 mg IV or q 6–8 h prn anxiety or nausea/vomiting

3. Adriamycin (30 mg/m²/day) = ___mg IV thru FFIV day 1, prior to Platinol

4. Instructed to have oral intake in excess of 3,000 mL between 6PM and 6AM the morning of treatment

5. Upon arrival to outpatient area — start IV fluids: 1,000 mL D5 1/2 NS with 30 mEq/L KCl, 250 mg calcium gluconate/L, 500 mg MgSO₄/L @ 200 mL/m²/hr for 2 hours

6. Mannitol bolus 8 g/m² = ___g IV

7. Platinol (120 mg/m²) = ___mg IV over 20 min in 100 mL NS

8. Mannitol 20% @ rate of 35 mL/m² IV for 6 hours

9. Continue above IV fluids for additional 2 hours post completion of 6 hr of Mannitol infusion

10. At 3 PM obtain SMA-7, Ca, Mg levels STAT; if within normal limits — the patient can go home and return next day for repeat electrolytes and continued hydration with fluids if necessary.

11. When cumulative Adriamycin dose > 300 mg/m² — repeat echocardiogram/MUGA scan (see Appendix 2)

Week 6 BCD

1. CBC/SMA 18 prior to chemotherapy

2. *Antiemetics*:

    a. Granisetron 2 mg PO (or 1 mg IV) (or, ondansetron 32 mg IV piggy back 15–30 min prior to treatment)

    b. Dexamethasone 20 mg PO

    c. Lorazepam 1–2 mg IV or q 6–8 h prn anxiety or nausea/vomiting

3. Bleomycin (15 units/m²/day) = ___ units IV push through FFIV. Cytoxan (cyclophosphamide) (600 mg/m²/day) = ___ mg IV in 100 mL NS over 30 minutes (if dose > 1,000 mg — dilute in 250 mL NS) Dactinomycin (600 mg/m²/day) = ___ mg IV through FFIV

4. 2–3 week rest period post BCD, then recycle week 0 – week 6 (total 3 cycles)

OSTEOSARCOMA (GRADE III/IV) MAINTENANCE THERAPY: REGIMEN B

Week 0	BCD ± VCR
Week 3 & 4	HdMTX
Week 5	Adriamycin
Week 8 & 9	HdMTX —* Delete HdMTX after 1 vs 2 Cycles
	Repeat above total 3 cycles

1. CBC/SMA 18 prior to Chemotherapy

2. *Antiemetics*:

    a. Granisetron 2 mg po (or 1 mg IV) (or, ondansetron 32 mg IV piggy back 15–30 min prior to treatment)

    b. Dexamethasone 20 mg po

    c. Lorazepam 1–2 mg IV q 6–8 h prn anxiety or nausea/vomiting

3. Bleomycin (15 units/m²/day) =—-units IV thru FFIV

Cytoxan (600 mg/m²/day) = ___mg IV in 100 mL NS over 30 minutes (if dose > 1000 mg dilute in 250 mL NS)

Dactinomycin (600 mg/m²/day) = ___mg IV thru FFIV

Week 3—HdMTX (Same as HdMTX ± vincristine at Week 0)

Week 4—Same as Week 3

Week 5—CBC prior to chemotherapy day 1

    a. Granisetron 2 mg po (or 1 mg IV) (or, ondansetron 32 mg IV piggy back 15–30 min prior to treatment)

    b. Dexamethasone 20 mg po

    c. Adriamycin (30 mg/m²/day) = ___ mg IV push thru FFIV days 1–3

        Week 8 & 9—same as week 0 - HdMTX ± VCR

*Delete HdMTX after cycle 1 vs 2 cycles

Regimen B — repeated for total of 3 cycles

Examples of Nutritional Interventions in Oncology

Ellen Gesser

PATIENT WITH NUTRITIONAL DEFICIT

Patient A: Diagnosis: Lung Cancer
Treatment: Radiation (XRT)
WT=70 kg, HT=70, Age=65, Sex=Male, UBW=74 kg, IBW= 149–183 lbs (68–83Kg) (See Table 53-1)
24 hour food intake recall:

Breakfast	*Lunch*	*Evening Meal*
Banana (1)	Homemade veg soup (1 c)	Roast (3 oz)
Wheaties (¾ c)	Peanut butter/jelly sandwich	Potatoes (½ c)
Skim milk (1 c)	Water (2–8 oz)	Carrots (½ c)
Sugar (1 tsp)		Muffin (1)
	Snack	
	Ice cream (½ c)	
	Crackers (6)	

Actual calories/protein intake (see Tables 53-2 and 53-3) = 1,621 cals/64 g
Energy requirement: BEE*=1,478 Kcals + 20%AF+30%IF=2,306 kcal
Protein requirement: 70 g (1 g/kg)
Fluid requirement: 2,100–2,450cc (1 cc/kcal or 30–35 cc/kg)
Deficit: minimal (estimated p.o. intake = 70% of calculated needs) (1,621/2,306 = 2,306 =70%)
Intervention: Diet manipulation, increased calories, increase protein, frequent smaller feedings and Nutrashake 4 oz BID (see Table 53-4)

Patient B: Diagnosis: Squamous Cell Cancer of Nasopharynx
Treatment: Concomitant XRT and chemotherapy
WT=70kg, Ht=70', Age=65, Sex=Male, UBW=75kg IBW=68–83kg
24 hour food intake recall:

Breakfast	*Lunch*	*Evening Meal*
Scrambled egg (2)	Lemonade (1 c)	Clam Chowder (1c)
Whole Milk (1c)		Whole Milk (1c)

---

*Calculated by Harris Benedict equations (see Fig. 53-1). Male-BEE = 66 + (13.7×wt) + (5×ht) – (6.8×age);
Female-BEE = 655 + (9.6×wt) + (1.8×ht) – (4.7×age) (wt in kg; ht in cm; age in years)
AF = activity factor: restricted = 10%, sedentary = 20%, aerobic 3for/wk = 30%, aerobic
5×wk = 50%, aerobic 7×week=60%, true athlete = 70%
Kg = lbs÷2.2

1 inch = 2.5 cm	c = Cup	PO = per os (by mouth)
UBW = Usual Body Weight	tsp = teaspoon	
IBW = Ideal Body Weight	oz = 29.57 ml	

Snack
Nutrashake (4 oz)
Pudding (½c)
Nutrashake (2 oz)

Actual calorie/protein intake = 1165 cals/46g

Energy requirement: BEE=1478 kcals + 10% AF + 30% IF=2,114 kcal

Protein requirement: 84 g (1.2g/kg)

Fluid requirement: =2,100–2,450 cc (1cc/kcal or 30–35cc/kg)

Deficit: Moderate (estimated p.o. intake = 55% of calculated needs (1,165/2,114 = 55%)

Additional considerations:

6% nonvolitional weight loss

Predictable need for nutrition support because of type of cancer and XRT and chemotherapy; likely to be greater over next several weeks because of dysphagia

Intervention: Increase calories, increase protein content as soft solids and liquids as tolerated in frequent small feedings. PEG feeding of Nutren 1.5 6×250 mL/24 hr (+ additional water to fulfill calculated requirements of 2,100–2,450 cc water: 1,164 cc free water from Nutren 1.5 and remainder p.o. or as water flush through PEG).

Patient C: Diagnosis: Colon cancer s/p colon resection

Wt = 54.5 kg, Ht = 68', Age = 38, Sex = Female, UBW = 59kg, IBW = 57–70kg

24 hour food intake recall:

Breakfast	*Lunch*	*Evening Meal*
Banana (1)	(Nothing)	Cornbread (1)
Juice (1/2c)		Buttermilk (1c)
Toast w/jelly (1)		Beans (1/2 c)
Scrambled egg (1)		
2% milk (1c)		

Actual calorie/protein intake = 810 cal/32 g

Energy requirement: BEE = 1318 + 20% AF+ 30% IF = 2057 kcal

Protein requirement: 81g (1.5g/kg)

Fluid requirement: 1636–2057cc (1 cc/kcal or 30–35 cc/kg)

Deficit: Severe (estimated p.o. intake 39% of calculated needs) (810/2,057 = 39%)

Additional considerations:

7% nonvolitional weight loss

Diarrhea

Duke's C colon cancer

Intervention: Decrease fiber diet as tolerated; TPN (see Table 53-5)

(Planned to meet estimated nutritional requirement without consideration to p.o. intake)*

916 cc 50% dextrose = 458 g dextrose × 3.4 kcal/kg = 1,557 kcal

953 cc 8.5% amino acids = 81 g protein

250 cc 20 oz lipids @ 2 kcal/cc = 500 kcal

2,119 cc total volume in 24 hours. Total NPC = 2057 kcal

(Administered @ 88 cc/hr)

Carbohydrate kcals provided @ 5.8 mg/kg/min (within maximum oxidative capacity of 5–7 mg/kg/min.) Balance of kcals are supplied by lipids providing 24% of total kcals (within 4–60% recommended range).

*May alternately plan TPN to fulfill calculated requirement with consideration to current p.o. contribution and adjust as appropriate.

Index

Page numbers followed by f *indicate figures; those followed by* t *indicate tables.*